Toxicology: Clinical Principles

Toxicology: Clinical Principles

Editor: Bradley Delk

FOSTER ACADEMICS
www.fosteracademics.com

www.fosteracademics.com

FOSTER
ACADEMICS

Cataloging-in-Publication Data

Toxicology : clinical principles / edited by Bradley Delk.
p. cm.
Includes bibliographical references and index.
ISBN 978-1-63242-838-7
1. Drugs--Toxicology. 2. Toxicology. 3. Clinical toxicology. 4. Pharmacology. I. Delk, Bradley.
RA1238 .T69 2019
615.704 072 4--dc23

Foster Academics,
118-35 Queens Blvd., Suite 400,
Forest Hills, NY 11375, USA

ISBN 978-1-63242-838-7 (Hardback)

Printed and bound in China.

Contents

Preface

Toxicology is a discipline that is concerned with the study of the adverse effects of chemical substances on an organism. The practice of diagnosing and treating exposures to toxins and toxicants is also under the scope of its study. The correlation of the dose and its effect on the exposed organism is a crucial study in this domain. Medical toxicologists deal with adverse drug reactions, acute or chronic poisoning, substance abuse, drug overdoses, and chemical exposures. Practitioners of medical toxicology are physicians specialized primarily in occupational medicine, emergency medicine or pediatrics. This book elucidates new techniques and applications of toxicology in a multidisciplinary manner. It strives to provide a fair idea about toxicology and help develop a better understanding of the latest advances in this field. It is a vital tool for all researching or studying toxicology as it gives incredible insights into emerging trends and concepts.

Various studies have approached the subject by analyzing it with a single perspective, but the present book provides diverse methodologies and techniques to address this field. This book contains theories and applications needed for understanding the subject from different perspectives. The aim is to keep the readers informed about the progresses in the field; therefore, the contributions were carefully examined to compile novel researches by specialists from across the globe.

Indeed, the job of the editor is the most crucial and challenging in compiling all chapters into a single book. In the end, I would extend my sincere thanks to the chapter authors for their profound work. I am also thankful for the support provided by my family and colleagues during the compilation of this book.

Editor

Dihydroisotanshinone I combined with radiation inhibits the migration ability of prostate cancer cells through DNA damage and CCL2 pathway

I-Yun Lee[1†], Yin-Yin Lin[1†], Yao-Hsu Yang[1], Yu-Shin Lin[3], Chun-Liang Lin[4,5], Wei-Yu Lin[6,7], Yu-Ching Cheng[1], Li-Hsin Shu[1] and Ching-Yuan Wu[1,2*]

Abstract

Background: Radiotherapy plays an important role in the treatment of prostate cancer. Despite that sophisticated techniques of radiotherapy and radiation combined with chemotherapy were applied to the patients, some tumors may recur. Therefore, the study investigated the effect of dihydroisotanshinone I (DT) and the combination treatment of 5 μM DT and 5Gy irradiation (IR) against the migration ability of prostate cancer cells.

Methods: DT and the combination treatment were studied for its biological activity against migration ability of prostate cancer cells with transwell migration assay. Subsequently, we tried to explore the underlying mechanism with ELISA, flow cytometry and Western's blotting assay.

Results: The results showed that DT and the combination treatment substantially inhibited the migration ability of prostate cancer cells. DT and the combined treatment can decrease the ability of macrophages to recruit prostate cancer cells. Mechanistically, DT and the combination treatment reduced the secretion of chemokine (C-C Motif) Ligand 2 (CCL2) from prostate cancer cells. We also found that DT treatment induced the cell cycle of prostate cancer cells entering S phase and increased the protein expression of DNA damage response proteins (*r*H2AX and phosphorylated ataxia telangiectasia-mutated [ATM]) in DU145 cells and PC-3 cells.

Conclusions: DT displays radiosensitization and antimigration effects in prostate cancer cells by inducing DNA damage and inhibiting CCL2 secretion. We suggest that DT can be used as a novel antimetastatic cancer drug or radiosensitizer in the armamentarium of prostate cancer management.

Keywords: Dihydroisotanshinone I, Radiosensitive, Prostate cancer, DNA damage, CCL2

Background

Radiotherapy is an effective form of local cancer treatment because it induces the DNA damage response (DDR) [1]. However, a fraction of tumors recur after such treatment, usually in more aggressive and metastatic forms [2]. Sensors inside cells can recognize DNA damage and start the DDR process, which induces cell cycle arrest to allow the damaged DNA to be repaired. Among the different types of DNA damage events, DNA double-strand breaks (DDBs) are the most lethal. During DDBs, ATM (previously known as ataxia–telangiectasia mutated) is phosphorylated and activated, serving as a pivotal regulator for the execution of DDR in the maintenance of genomic stability. Another protein, H2AX, acts as an important platform for recruiting DDR proteins. Activated ATM then phosphorylates histone H2AX at S139 (known as *r*H2AX), which recruits a mediator of DNA damage, checking protein 1 (MDC1), to the sites of DNA breaks, which in turn recruits downstream repair proteins to DNA damage foci for repair [3–5]. During DDBs, the S

* Correspondence: smbepigwu77@gmail.com
†Equal contributors
[1]Department of Chinese Medicine, Chiayi Chang Gung Memorial Hospital, No.6, W. Sec., Jiapu Rd., Puzi City, Chiayi County 613, Taiwan, Republic of China
[2]School of Chinese medicine, College of Medicine, Chang Gung University, Tao-Yuan, Taiwan
Full list of author information is available at the end of the article

phase can be delayed. Notably, these DDR proteins can be crucial in cancer treatment with chemotherapy agents and radiotherapy. Despite the sophisticated radiation techniques that have been developed, as well as the combination of radiation with chemotherapy, some tumors do recur. Thus, a method that improves the local control of primary or metastasized tumors with a combination of radiotherapy and radiosensitizer may be beneficial for patients with cancer.

Tumor-associated macrophages are derived from peripheral blood monocytes that are recruited into the tumor and potentiate the seeding and establishment of metastatic cells [6]. C-C motif chemokine ligand 2 (CCL2), also known as monocyte chemoattractant protein-1, was first identified by its ability to attract monocytes in vitro [7, 8]. CCL2 recruits prostate cancer epithelial cells to the bone microenvironment and regulates their rate of proliferation [9, 10]. Dihydroisotanshinone I (DT) (Fig. 1a), a substance extracted from the dried root of Salvia miltiorrhiza Bunge, contains abietane-type diterpene quinone. In a previous study [11], tanshinone IIA inhibited the metastasis of hepatocellular carcinoma and was identified as a potential means of increasing survival rates. In our previous study, we noted that DT substantially inhibited the migratory ability of prostate cancer cells in both a macrophage-conditioned medium and a macrophage/prostate cancer coculture medium [12]. However, the effect of DT combined with radiotherapy on prostate cancer cells and the underlying mechanism remain unclear. In this study, we investigated the effect of DT in combination with ionizing radiation (IR) on the migration of prostate cancer cells in a macrophage medium. We also observed the exact mechanism for combining DT with radiation therapy.

Methods

Cell culture and treatment

The human prostate cancer cell lines (DU145 cells and PC-3 cells), human acute monocytic leukaemia cell line (THP-1 cells), IMR-9 cells (human normal lung fibroblast) were obtained from the American Type Culture Collection. The DU145 cells and PC-3 cells were cultured in Dulbecco's Modified Eagle's medium (DMEM) (Invitrogen Corp., Carlsbad, CA), supplemented with 10% FBS at 37 °C and 5% CO_2. The THP1 cells were cultured in RPMI-1640 medium (RPMI) (Invitrogen Corp., Carlsbad, CA), supplemented with 10% fetal bovine serum (FBS) at 37 °C and 5% CO_2. IMR-90 cells were cultured in Minimum essential medium Eagle (Invitrogen Corp., Carlsbad, CA), supplemented with 10% fetal bovine serum (FBS) at 37 °C and 5% CO2. Recombinant Human CCL2 was obtained from Peprotech. Dihydroisotanshinone I (DT) was obtained from ChemFaces Natural Products Co., Ltd., China (Catalog number: CFN-90162, the purity of dihydroisotanshinone is 98% and its solubility in DMSO is > 5 mg/mL). Human prostate cancer cells and macrophages were cultured to 60–70% confluence prior to treatment. Medium was then replaced with fresh medium containing dihydroisotanshinone in DMSO (dimethyl sulfoxide) at the indicated concentrations. Cells treated with DMSO alone were used as untreated controls.

Cell migration assay

Cell migration assays were performed as described previously [13]. For the migration of human prostate cancer cells in monoculture, the indicated cell lines (DU145 cells, PC-3 cells, or IMR-90 cells) (1×10^5 cells/well) were plated in the upper chambers of Transwell plates with 8-μm pore polycarbonate membrane inserts in a medium without fetal bovine serum (FBS). A medium with FBS was plated in the lower chambers. After treatment or no treatment with dimethyl sulfoxide (DMSO) and with the indicated treatment for 16–24 h, the cells that had migrated to the bottom were fixed and stained using 1% toluidine blue. The numbers of cells were averaged after six randomly selected fields were counted. For the prostate cancer recruitment assay, THP-1 cells (1×10^5 cells/well) were cultured for 24 h. The THP-1 cell medium was then collected and plated in the lower chambers. After treatment or no treatment with DMSO and with the indicated treatment for 24 h, the human prostate cancer cells (DU145 cells or PC-3 cells) (1×10^5 cells/well) were plated in the upper chambers in the medium without FBS. After incubation for 16–24 h, the cells that had migrated into the bottom were fixed and stained using 1% toluidine blue, and the numbers were averaged after six randomly selected fields were counted. Each sample was assayed in triplicate, and each experiment was repeated at least twice.

Enzyme-linked immunosorbent assay

Enzyme-linked immunosorbent assays (ELISAs) were performed as described previously [14]. The medium was collected from a monoculture of prostate cancer cells with or without DMSO treatment, the indicated concentration of DT, or the indicated dose of IR for 24 h. Human CCL2 or human interleukin 8 (IL-8) in medium were detected with human CCL2 ELISA kits (eBioscience, catalog number: 88–7399) or human IL-8 ELISA kits (eBioscience, catalog number: 88–8086) according to the manufacturer's instructions.

Western blot analysis

Western blot analyses were performed as described previously [15]. Cellular extracts of the human prostate cancer cell line (DU145 cells and PC-3 cells) that had been treated with DMSO or 10 μM of DT for 0 or 6 h were prepared according to the manufacturer's instructions. Equal amounts of protein were fractionated via 6% or 12% SDS-PAGE and transferred to polyvinylidene difluoride (PVDF) membranes. The membranes were then blocked with 5% nonfat dried milk for 30 min and incubated in primary antibody for 3 h at room

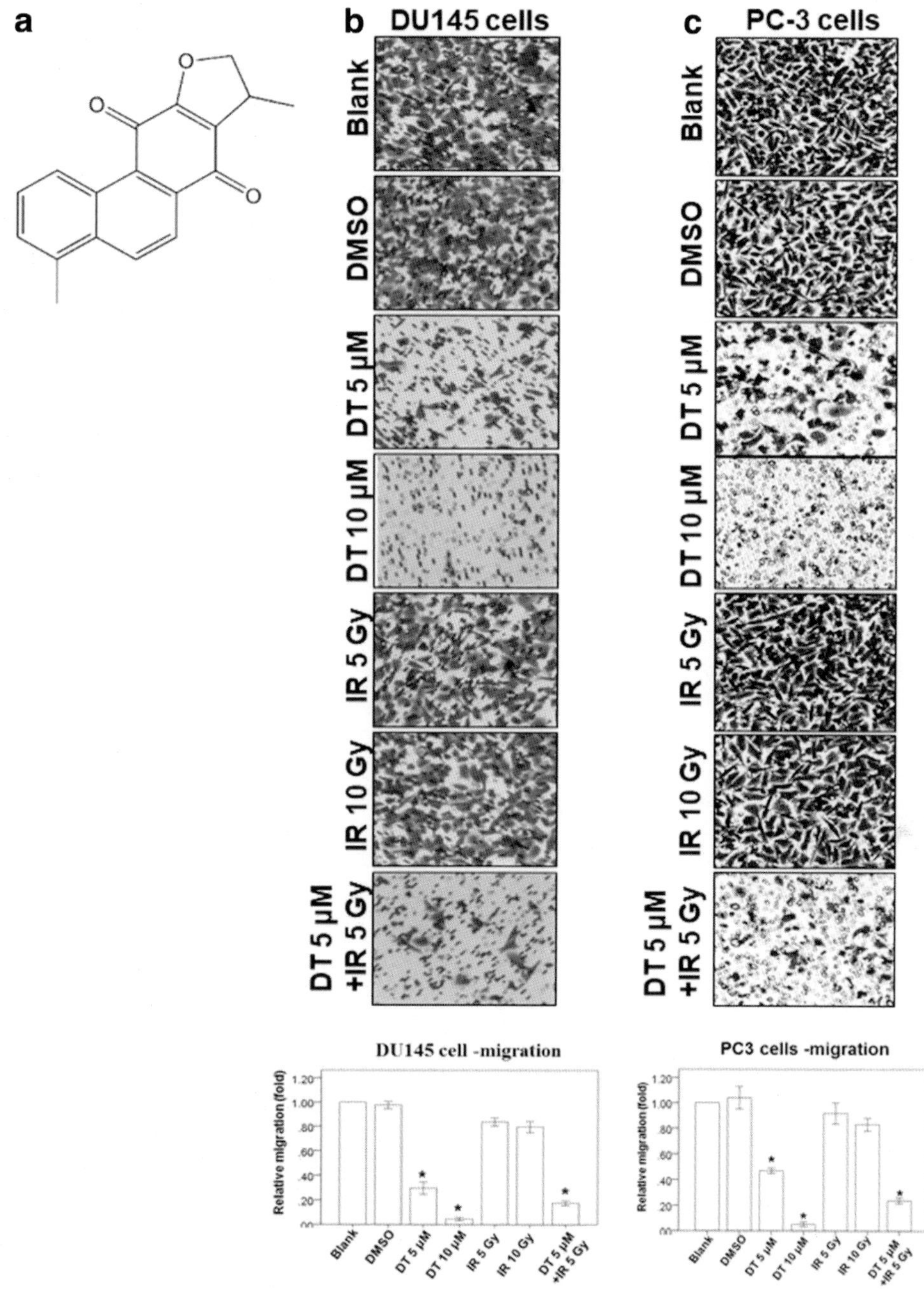

Fig. 1 DT blocks different human prostate cancer cells migration on in vitro Transwell migration assay. **a** The structure of dihydroisotanshinone I (DT). **b**, **c**, The migration ability of DU145 cells (**b**) and PC-3 cells (**c**) were measured with the transwell migration assay. After treated with indicated drugs for 24 h, the photographs (× 100) were taken and the migratory cells were measured using AlphaEase®FC StandAlone Software. Numbers of the migratory DU145 cells and PC-3 cells in each group were normalized to the control. The results were from three independent experiments. (Error bar = mean ± S.E.M. Asterisks (*) mark samples significantly different from blank group with $p < 0.05$)

temperature. The primary antibodies used were anti-H2AX antibody (Cell Signaling, ratio: 1:1000), antiphosphorylated (S139)-H2AX antibody (Cell Signaling, ratio: 1:1000), anti-ATM antibody (Cell Signaling, ratio: 1:1000), antiphosphorylated (S1981)-ATM antibody (Rockland, ratio:1:2000), and anti-α-tubulin antibody (Santa Cruz, IB: 1:10,000). The primary and secondary antibodies were diluted with 1% nonfat dried milk in 0.1% tris-buffered saline with Tween 20 (TBST). Blots were washed with 0.1% TBST and incubated in horseradish peroxidase-conjugated secondary antimouse or antirabbit antibodies (Santa Cruz, ratio: 1:5000) for 1 h at room temperature. After washing with 1X TBST again, protein signals were detected by chemiluminescence with the SuperSignal Substrate (Pierce, Number: 34,087).

Cell cycle assay

DU145 cells or PC-3 cells (1×10^6 cells) were seeded in a 100-mm plate and cultured overnight before treatment. The cells were then treated with 10 μM of DT for 0–6 h. After incubation, the cells were analyzed using flow cytometry with propidium iodide (PI) staining to determine the distribution of the G0/G1, G2/M, and S phases of the cell cycle. Briefly, the medium was removed and harvested after washing with phosphate-buffered saline (PBS). The supernatant was removed by centrifugation. Cell pellets were washed with PBS and fixed in 75% ethanol overnight at − 20 °C. The next day, the treated cells were washed with cold PBS and stained with PI solution (50 μg/mL PI [Sigma-Aldrich] and 0.5 μg/mL ribonuclease [Sigma-Aldrich] in PBS) in a 37 °C water bath for 15 min. The cell cycle stages were measured by flow cytometry.

Statistical analyses

All values were the means ± standard error of mean (SEM) of the replicate samples ($n = 3$ to 6, depending on the experiment) and experiments were repeated by a minimum of three times. Differences between two groups were assessed using the unpaired two-tailed Student's t-test or by ANOVA if more than two groups were analyzed. The Tukey test was used as a post-hoc test in ANOVA for testing the significance of pairwise group comparisons. P-values < 0.05 were considered statistically significant in all comparisons. SPSS version 13.0 for windows (LEAD technologies, Inc.) was used for all calculations.

Results

DT and the combination treatment can block cell motility in different human prostate cancer cells

To study the effect of DT on the migration ability of prostate cancer cells, we used two prostate cancer cell lines (PC-3 and DU145) to study the function of DT, IR, and the combined therapy with 5 μM DT and 5 Gy IR in the migration assay (Fig. 1b, c). The results showed that 5–10 μM DT considerably inhibited the migration ability of prostate cancer cells in a dose-dependent manner. We also used 5–10 Gy IR to compare the effects of DT on migration. Our results showed that neither 5 nor 10 Gy IR were able to inhibit the migration ability of prostate cancer cells, whereas 10 μM DT was able to do so. Combination treatment with 5 μM DT and 5 Gy IR substantially inhibited the migration ability of prostate cancer cell as 10 μM DT did. These data suggest that DT and the combined therapy can inhibit the migration of prostate cancer cells in an effective manner.

Effects of DT and the combined therapy on prostate cancer cell migration in the THP-1 cell medium

Previous studies have shown that macrophages promote tumor invasion and metastasis and that the motility of human prostate cancer cells is inhibited by DT. Therefore, we investigated the effect of DT and the combined therapy on the ability of macrophages to promote tumor migration. Because THP-1 cells are extensively used to study monocyte/macrophage functions, mechanisms, signaling pathways, and drug activities [16, 17], we used THP-1 cells as our model (Fig. 2a). In the control group, DU145 cells and PC-3 cells were recruited by the conditioned medium. This demonstrated that THP-1 cell medium can promote the migration ability of prostate cancer cells. However, 5–10 μM DT markedly inhibited the migration of prostate cancer cells in a dose-dependent manner in the THP-1 cell medium (Fig. 2b, c). Moreover, 5 and 10 Gy IR alone did not inhibit the migration ability of DU145 cells and PC-3 cells. However, combined treatment (5 μM DT plus 5 Gy IR) was able to inhibit the migration ability of prostate cancer cells. These data suggested that DT or combined treatment may diminish the ability of macrophages to recruit prostate cancer cells.

DT and combined therapy inhibit the secretion of CCL2 by prostate cancer cells

Our results indicated that DT inhibits the motility of prostate cancer cells, even in the THP-1 cell medium. In previous studies, increased CCL2 expression in prostate cancer cells encouraged metastasis through macrophage recruitment [18–20]. In another study, IL-8 was demonstrated to be an important molecule for androgen-independent prostate cancer growth and progression [21]. We subsequently used ELISA to examine the effects of different treatments on the secretion of IL-8 or CCL2 by prostate cancer cells. After conducting the indicated treatment for 24 h, we found that IL-8 secretion was not inhibited (Fig. 3a, c). However, DT and combined treatment with IR (5 μM DT plus 5 Gy IR) considerably inhibited the secretion of CCL2 by prostate cancer cells (Fig. 3b, d). To validate the critical role of CCL2 in controlling the migration ability of DT-treated prostate cancer cells, we investigated the effects of DT or combined treatment with IR (5 μM DT plus 5 Gy IR) and with or without CCL2 on the migration ability of prostate cancer cells. After adding 5 pg/mL of CCL2 to the conditioned medium, we observed that CCL2 partially rescued the migration ability of DT- or combination-treated PC-3 cells (relative migration: from 30 to 40% to 60%) (Fig. 3f). Our results suggest that CCL2 is among the cytokines that control the migration ability of DT- or combination-treated prostate cancer cells, and that DT and combined treatment inhibit the migration of prostate cancer cells through their effects on CCL2. In our previous study, we found that the proliferation of IMR-90 cells (normal human lung fibroblasts) was mildly inhibited by 5 μM DT treatment for 24 h [22]. In addition, we discovered that 5 μM DT inhibits the migration ability of IMR-90 cells (Fig. 3e). The migration ability of IMR-90 cells was mildly inhibited by 5 Gy IR. In the present study,

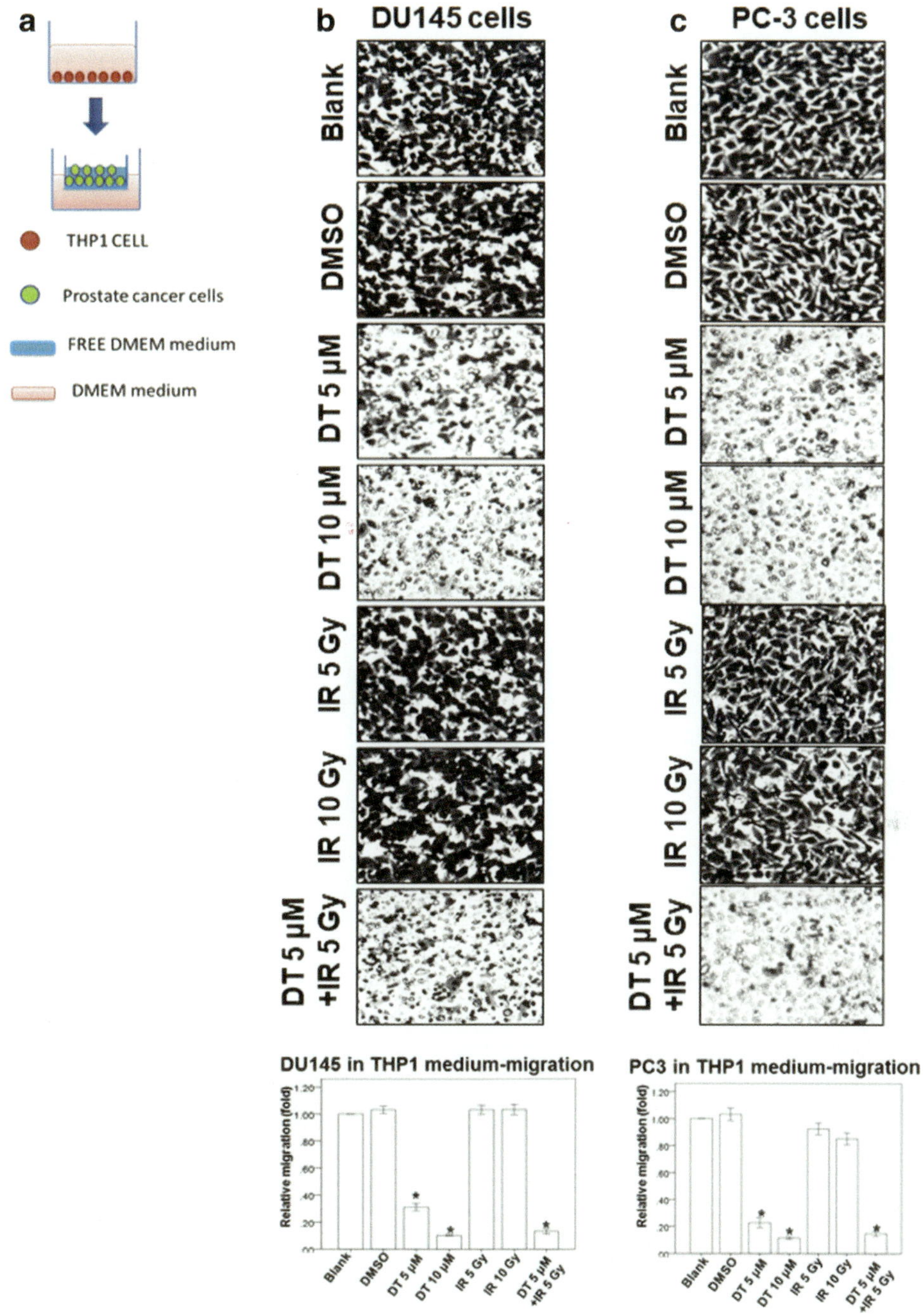

Fig. 2 The effect of DT on prostate cancer cell migration in the THP1 cell medium. The migration ability of human prostate cancers in the THP1 cells medium were measured with the transwell migration assay. **a** THP1 cells were cultured for 24 h. Then the condition medium were collected and placed in the lower chamber. **b**, **c** The DU145 cells (**b**) and PC-3 cells (**c**) were then placed on the upper chamber for the migration assay. After incubation for 24 h, the photographs (× 100) were taken and the migratory cells were measured using AlphaEase®FC StandAlone Software. Numbers of the migratory DU145 cells and PC-3 cells in each group were normalized to the control. The results were from three independent experiments. (Error bars = mean ± S.E.M. Asterisks (*) mark samples significantly different from blank group with $p < 0.05$)

combination treatment with 5 μM DT and 5 Gy IR was also able to inhibit the migration ability of prostate cancer cells. These data suggest that DT and the combined therapy can inhibit the migration ability of both prostate cancer cells and normal human lung fibroblasts.

Effects of DT on cell cycle progression of prostate cancer cells in vitro

Because DT demonstrated potential antimigration effects on prostate cancer cells, we further investigated the mechanism of DT on prostate cancer cells. First, we determined

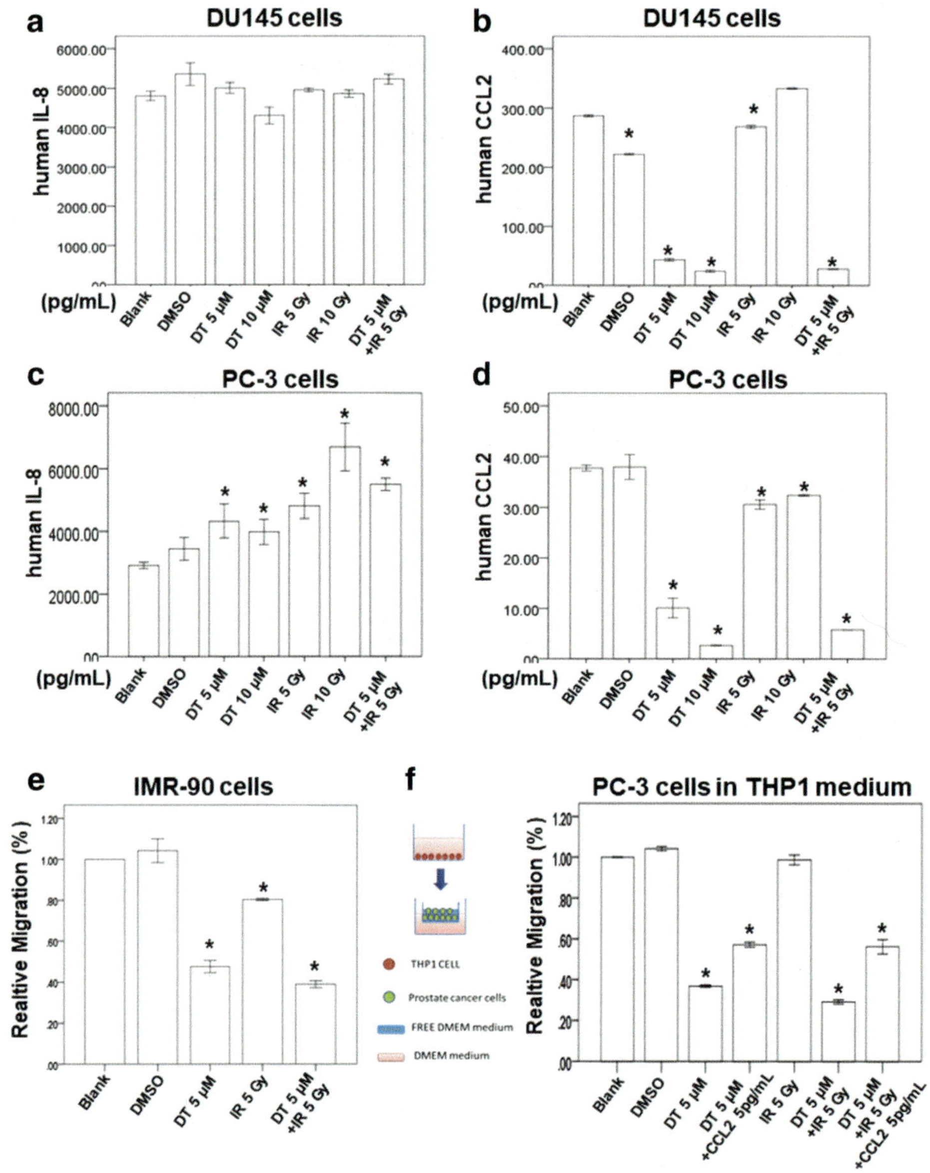

Fig. 3 Effects of DT on the protein secretion of IL8 or CCL2 from prostate cancer cells and on human normal fibroblasts migration in the THP1 cell medium. The condition medium of coculture with DU145 cell or PC-3 cells were collected from untreated cells, cells treated with DMSO or indicated treatment for 24 h. The secretion of human IL8 was measured with ELISA kits (**a**, **c**). The secretion of human CCL2 was measured with ELISA kits (**b**, **d**). **e** The migration ability of IMR-90 cells were measured with the transwell migration assay. After treated with indicated drugs for 24 h, the photographs (× 100) were taken and the migratory cells were measured using AlphaEase®FC StandAlone Software. Numbers of the migratory IMR-90 cells in each group were normalized to the control. **f** The migration ability of human prostate cancers in the macrophages medium were measured by the transwell migration assay. THP1 cells were treated with DMSO or DT for 24 h. Then the conditioned medium was collected and placed in the lower chamber. In the group of DT+ 5 pg/mL CCL2, 5 pg/mL CCL2 was added into the condition medium of this group. Then, PC-3 cells were then placed on the upper chamber for the migration assay. After incubation for 24 h, the photographs (× 100) were taken and the migratory cells were measured using AlphaEase®FC StandAlone Software. The quantification of the indicated migratory cells numbers in each group were normalized to the control. All the results are representative of at least three independent experiments. (Error bars = mean ± S.E.M. Asterisks (*) mark samples significantly different from blank group with $p < 0.05$)

the effect of DT on the cell cycle progression of prostate cancer cells. Compared with the control cells, the S-phase proportion of cells treated with 10 μM DT increased from 30% to 40–50% in 6 h (Fig. 4). The results showed that DT treatments were able to prolong or arrest the S phase of the prostate cancer cell cycle.

DT regulates DDR proteins in prostate cancer cells

During DDBs, ATM is autophosphorylated at serine 1981 and phosphorylates H2AX at serine 139, which then recruits downstream repair proteins to DNA damage foci for repair. In this stage, the S phase can be delayed. Several cellular factors that are directly phosphorylated by ATM

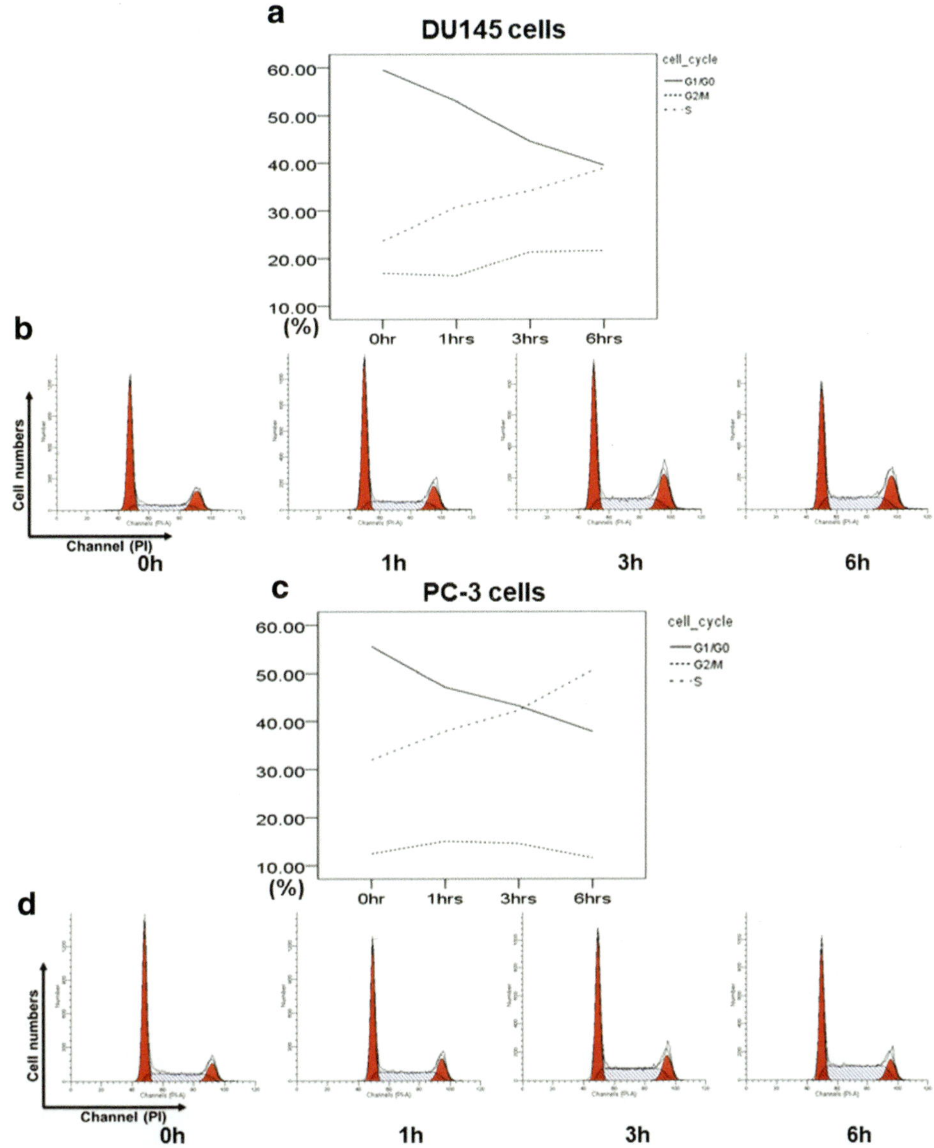

Fig. 4 Effects of DT on human prostate cancer cell cycle. DU145 cells or PC-3 cells were treated with 10 μM of DT for 0, 1, 3, 6 h and then subjected to flow cytometry with PI staining. The cell cycle phase distribution of DU145 cells (**a**) or PC-3 cells (**c**) after treatment with DT were measured in the indicated hours. The representative histograms between PI intensity and cell numbers of DU145 cells (**b**) or PC-3 cells (**d**) were measured by flow cytometry

contribute to the S-phase checkpoint. Considering how the previous data showed that DT may prolong the S phase of the cell cycle in prostate cancer cells after 6 h, we used a western blot assay to investigate its effect on these DNA damage proteins, phosphorylated (S1981)-ATM (p-ATM) and H2AX, in DU145 cells and PC-3 cells. We found that 10 μM DT induced the protein expression of H2AX and p-ATM in DU145 cells (Fig. 5a) or PC-3 cells (Fig. 5b) within 6 h. These data suggested DT has the potential to induce DDR in prostate cancer cells.

Discussion

In previous studies, various members of the tanshinone family were demonstrated to be capable of inhibiting the growth of several types of cancer cells, including prostate cancer cells [23–25]. Moreover, tanshinone IIA can suppress the migration ability of osteosarcoma MG-63 cells and gastric cancer AGS cells [26, 27]. Another recent study showed that 15,16-dihydrotanshinone I has a structure similar to that of DT and induces endoplasmic reticulum stress in prostate carcinoma cells (DU145 cells) [28].

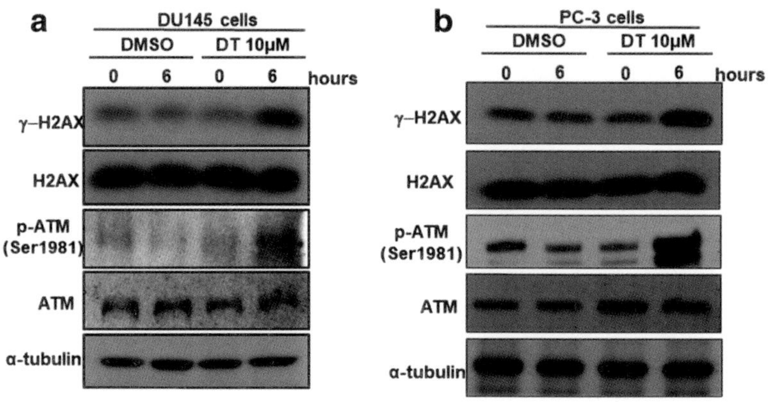

Fig. 5 DT inhibits the protein expression of DNA damage response proteins in prostate cancer cells. Total cell extracts of DU145 cells (**a**) or PC-3 cell (**b**) were harvested from untreated cells and cells treated with DMSO or DT for 0, 6 h. The protein was immunoblotted with polyclonal antibodies specific for DNA damage response proteins (γ-H2AX and phosphorylated-ATM). α-tubulin was used as an internal loading control

Tanshinone IIA and DT possess an ortho-quinone and an intact ring D, respectively, suggesting that the structure of tanshinones may influence the ways in which they inhibit migration ability in tumors. In our previous study, we also found that DT substantially inhibited the migratory ability of prostate cancer cells in both a macrophage-conditioned medium and macrophage/prostate cancer coculture medium [12]. In this study, we discovered that the combination treatment with 5 μM DT and 5 Gy IR more strongly inhibited the migration ability of prostate cancer cells compared with 5 μM DT (Figs. 1 and 2). These results suggest that DT cooperates with radiation therapy and demonstrate the effectiveness of the combined therapy in inhibiting the migration of prostate cancer cells.

CCL2 regulates macrophage differentiation, growth, and chemotaxis [29]. Furthermore, CCL2 was previously shown to inhibit the generation of tumor-reactive T cells [30]. Tanshinone IIA was found to have considerable growth-inhibiting effects on U-937 cells through the induction of apoptosis by downregulation of CCL2 expression [25]. In our previous studies, DT reduced the secretion of CCL2 by both lung cancer cells and prostate cancer cells [12, 22], yet the effect of the combined therapy on CCL2 secretion by prostate cancer cells is unclear. In the present study, we discovered that IR 5 Gy mildly decreased CCL2 secretion by both PC-3 and DU145 cells. Moreover, the combination treatment inhibited CCL2 secretion by prostate cancer cells more strongly than 5 μM DT did (Fig. 3 b and d). These results suggest that DT cooperates with radiation therapy to affect CCL2 secretion. The previous report showed that tanshinone IIA inhibited cyclic strain-induced IL-8 expression by the induction of heme oxygenase (HO-1) in endothelial cells [31]. Tanshinone I also reduced the transcriptional activity of IL-8 [32]. In our results, DT did not decrease the secretion of IL-8 by either PC-3 or DU145 cells. In a previous study, fluorouracil, which interrupts the action of this enzyme and blocks synthesis of the pyrimidine thymidine, increased the levels of IL-8 secreted from PC-3 cells [33]. Notably, increased IL-8 expression was also observed after treatment with DT only, IR only, or combined therapy in PC-3 cells (Fig. 3c). These results suggest that the mechanism of DT on PC-3 cells may occur at the DNA level. By contrast, a previous study showed that the structural difference between several tanshinones at the C-15 position of the furan ring resulted in differential inhibition of CYP3A (cytochrome P450 3A) activity [34]. The positioning of the furan ring in DT and tanshinone IIA might have caused this difference. The underlying mechanism will be investigated in our future research.

Among the various types of DNA damage, the most deleterious is DNA DDBs. Double-strand breaks can be generated using exogenous sources, including IR or chemotherapeutic agents. During DDBs, ATM is phosphorylated and then phosphorylates histone H2AX at S139 (known as γH2AX). If they remain unrepaired, DDBs may induce cell death and apoptosis [35]. Numerous chemotherapeutic agents and types of radiotherapy exert cytotoxic effects by inducing DNA DDBs. According to previous studies, tanshinone IIA can bind to the DNA minor groove [36] and significantly sensitize oral squamous cell carcinoma to radiation through the autophagy pathway [37]. In one report, 5–20 μM tanshinone IIA combined with IR 6Gy was able to induce γH2AX expression. However, the effect of tanshinone monotherapy on the DNA damage pathway is still unclear. This is the first study to demonstrate that 10 μM DT increased the S phase proportion of the cell cycle and phosphorylated ATM and γH2AX expression in prostate cancer cells. The results suggest that DT can induce DNA DSBs and increase the effect of IR.

In one meta-analysis of patients with locally advanced prostate cancer, optimal oncological outcomes were obtained through radical prostatectomy with adjuvant radiotherapy or radiotherapy with adjuvant hormonal therapy [38]. These results suggest that radiotherapy is a vital treatment for locally advanced prostate cancer. However, radiotherapy can increase the risk of urinary incontinence, bladder neck contracture, and urethral stricture [39, 40], and can cause capillary destruction with reduced vascularity and tissue fibrosis [39]. To improve outcomes, in several countries radiotherapy is often combined with complementary and alternative medicine [41–43]. Notably, tanshinone IIA not only sensitizes oral squamous cell carcinoma to radiation through the autophagy pathway [37], but also has a protective effect against radiation-induced ototoxicity in HEI-OC1 cells, a mouse auditory cell line [44]. Sodium tanshinone IIA sulfonate has also been shown to prevent radiation-induced toxicity in cardiomyocytes [45]. These reports suggest that tanshinones have different effects on radiation therapy in different cell lines. However, the effects and mechanisms of these combined therapies on the immune system are still unclear. Our results first demonstrated that combined treatment (5 μM DT with 5 Gy IR) was able to diminish migration of prostate cancer cells in a more effective manner than did the larger dose of IR (10 Gy). The combination treatment reduced CCL2 in prostate cancer cells. In addition, the combined treatment decreased the ability of macrophages to recruit prostate cancer cells. In our previous study, we also discovered that DT inhibited the secretion of CCL2 by the cultured medium of macrophages, including THP-1 cells and RAW 264.7 cells [12]. These results suggest that macrophages and cytokines, like CCL2, may regulate the effect of combined treatment on prostate cancer.

Conclusions

In conclusion, DT displays radiosensitization and anti-migration effects in prostate cancer cells by inducing DNA damage and inhibiting CCL2 secretion. We suggest that DT can be used as a novel antimetastatic cancer drug or radiosensitizer in the armamentarium of prostate cancer management.

Abbreviations

ATM: Ataxia telangiectasia-mutated; CCL2: Chemokine C-C Motif Ligand 2; DDBs: DNA double-strand breaks; DDR: DNA damage response; DMEM: Dulbecco's Modified Eagle's medium; DMSO: Dimethyl sulfoxide; DT: Dihydroisotanshinone I; ELISA: Enzyme-linked immunosorbent assay; FBS: Fetal bovine serum; MDC1: Mediator of DNA damage checking protein 1; PVDF: Polyvinylidene difluoride; SDS-PAGE: Sodium dodecyl sulfate polyacrylamide gel electrophoresis; SEM: Standard error of mean; TBST: Tris-Buffered Saline Tween-20

Acknowledgements

Not applicable.

Funding

This work was supported by grant CMRPG6C0262, CMRPG6D0343, CMRPG6F0011, CMRPG6F0661, CMRPG6E0091, CMRPG6F0551 and CMRPG6F0171 from Chang Gung Memorial Hospital, and MOST 105–2320-B-182-006-MY3, NSC 101–2320-B-182A-005 and NSC 102–2320-B-182A-007 from the Ministry of Science and Technology, Taiwan.

Authors' contributions

IYL contributed to the conception and design of the entire study. IYL and YYL carried out most of the experiments, contributed to the data interpretation and wrote the initial draft of the manuscript. YHY contributed to the experimental design. YSL and WYL contributed to data interpretation and the final editing of the manuscript. YCC, MCL and LHS contributed to Western's blotting assay, migration assay and cell cycle assay. KDL participated in the project design and to the data interpretation. CYW provided grant support, funding and the final editing of the manuscript. All authors read and approved the final manuscript.

Competing interests

The authors declare that they have no competing interests.

Author details

[1]Department of Chinese Medicine, Chiayi Chang Gung Memorial Hospital, No.6, W. Sec., Jiapu Rd., Puzi City, Chiayi County 613, Taiwan, Republic of China. [2]School of Chinese medicine, College of Medicine, Chang Gung University, Tao-Yuan, Taiwan. [3]Department of Pharmacy, Chiayi Chang Gung Memorial Hospital, Chiayi, Taiwan. [4]Departments of Nephrology, Chiayi Chang Gung Memorial Hospital, Chiayi, Taiwan. [5]Kidney and Diabetic Complications Research Team (KDCRT), Chiayi Chang Gung Memorial Hospital, Chiayi, Taiwan. [6]Department of Urology, Chang Gung Memorial Hospital at Chiayi, Puzi City, Taiwan. [7]Chang Gung University of Science and Technology, Chia-Yi, Taiwan.

References

1. Bernier J, Hall EJ, Giaccia A. Radiation oncology: a century of achievements. Nat Rev Cancer. 2004;4:737–47.
2. Suit HD. Local control and patient survival. Int J Radiat Oncol Biol Phys. 1992;23:653–60.
3. Huen MS, Sy SM, Chen J. BRCA1 and its toolbox for the maintenance of genome integrity. Nat Rev Mol Cell Biol. 2010;11:138–48.
4. Panier S, Durocher D. Regulatory ubiquitylation in response to DNA double-strand breaks. DNA Repair (Amst). 2009;8:436–43.
5. Roos WP, Kaina B. DNA damage-induced cell death: from specific DNA lesions to the DNA damage response and apoptosis. Cancer Lett. 2013;332:237–48.
6. Guo R, Wang T, Shen H, Ge HM, Sun J, Huang ZH, Shu YQ. Involvement of mTOR and survivin inhibition in tamoxifen-induced apoptosis in human hepatoblastoma cell line HepG2, Biomedicine & pharmacotherapy = Biomedecine & pharmacotherapie. 2010;64:249–53.
7. Valente AJ, Graves DT, Vialle-Valentin CE, Delgado R, Schwartz CJ. Purification of a monocyte chemotactic factor secreted by nonhuman primate vascular cells in culture. Biochemistry. 1988;27:4162–8.
8. Yoshimura T, Robinson EA, Tanaka S, Appella E, Kuratsu J, Leonard EJ. Purification and amino acid analysis of two human glioma-derived monocyte chemoattractants. J Exp Med. 1989;169:1449–59.
9. Lin SJ, Yang DR, Li G, Chang C. TR4 nuclear receptor different roles in prostate cancer progression. Front Endocrinol (Lausanne). 2015;6:78.
10. Zhang J, Lu Y, Pienta KJ. Multiple roles of chemokine (C-C motif) ligand 2 in promoting prostate cancer growth. J Natl Cancer Inst. 2010;102:522–8.
11. Wang WQ, Liu L, Sun HC, Fu YL, Xu HX, Chai ZT, Zhang QB, Kong LQ, Zhu XD, Lu L, et al. Tanshinone IIA inhibits metastasis after palliative resection of hepatocellular carcinoma and prolongs survival in part via vascular normalization. J Hematol Oncol. 2012;5:69.
12. Wu CY, Yang YH, Lin YY, Kuan FC, Lin YS, Lin WY, Tsai MY, Yang JJ, Cheng YC, Shu LH, et al. Anti-cancer effect of danshen and dihydroisotanshinone I on prostate cancer: targeting the crosstalk between macrophages and cancer cells via inhibition of the STAT3/CCL2 signaling pathway. Oncotarget. 2017;8:40246–63.
13. Lin TH, Izumi K, Lee SO, Lin WJ, Yeh S, Chang C. Anti-androgen receptor ASC-J9 versus anti-androgens MDV3100 (enzalutamide) or Casodex (Bicalutamide) leads to opposite effects on prostate cancer metastasis via differential modulation of macrophage infiltration and STAT3-CCL2 signaling. Cell Death Dis. 2013;4:e764.
14. Izumi K, Fang LY, Mizokami A, Namiki M, Li L, Lin WJ, Chang C. Targeting the androgen receptor with siRNA promotes prostate cancer metastasis

through enhanced macrophage recruitment via CCL2/CCR2-induced STAT3 activation. EMBO Mol Med. 2013;5:1383–401.

15. Tsao CK, Cutting E, Martin J, Oh WK. The role of cabazitaxel in the treatment of metastatic castration-resistant prostate cancer. Ther Adv Urol. 2014;6:97–104.
16. Ide H, Hatake K, Terado Y, Tsukino H, Okegawa T, Nutahara K, Higashihara E, Horie S. Serum level of macrophage colony-stimulating factor is increased in prostate cancer patients with bone metastasis. Hum Cell. 2008;21:1–6.
17. Mizutani K, Sud S, McGregor NA, Martinovski G, Rice BT, Craig MJ, Varsos ZS, Roca H, Pienta KJ. The chemokine CCL2 increases prostate tumor growth and bone metastasis through macrophage and osteoclast recruitment. Neoplasia. 2009;11:1235–42.
18. Loberg RD, Ying C, Craig M, Yan L, Snyder LA, Pienta KJ. CCL2 as an important mediator of prostate cancer growth in vivo through the regulation of macrophage infiltration. Neoplasia. 2007;9:556–62.
19. Lindholm PF, Sivapurapu N, Jovanovic B, Kajdacsy-Balla A. Monocyte-induced prostate cancer cell invasion is mediated by chemokine ligand 2 and nuclear factor-kappaB activity. J Clin Cell Immunol. 2015;6
20. Ito Y, Ishiguro H, Kobayashi N, Hasumi H, Watanabe M, Yao M, Uemura H. Adipocyte-derived monocyte chemotactic protein-1 (MCP-1) promotes prostate cancer progression through the induction of MMP-2 activity. Prostate. 2015;75:1009–19.
21. Araki S, Omori Y, Lyn D, Singh RK, Meinbach DM, Sandman Y, Lokeshwar VB, Lokeshwar BL. Interleukin-8 is a molecular determinant of androgen independence and progression in prostate cancer. Cancer Res. 2007;67:6854–62.
22. Wu CY, Cherng JY, Yang YH, Lin CL, Kuan FC, Lin YY, Lin YS, Shu LH, Cheng YC, Liu HT, et al. Danshen improves survival of patients with advanced lung cancer and targeting the relationship between macrophages and lung cancer cells. Oncotarget. 2017;
23. Gong Y, Li Y, Lu Y, Li L, Abdolmaleky H, Blackburn GL, Zhou JR. Bioactive tanshinones in salvia miltiorrhiza inhibit the growth of prostate cancer cells in vitro and in mice. Int J Cancer J Int du cancer. 2011;129:1042–52.
24. Shin DS, Kim HN, Shin KD, Yoon YJ, Kim SJ, Han DC, Kwon BM. Cryptotanshinone inhibits constitutive signal transducer and activator of transcription 3 function through blocking the dimerization in DU145 prostate cancer cells. Cancer Res. 2009;69:193–202.
25. Liu C, Li J, Wang L, Wu F, Huang L, Xu Y, Ye J, Xiao B, Meng F, Chen S, Yang M. Analysis of tanshinone IIA induced cellular apoptosis in leukemia cells by genome-wide expression profiling. BMC Complement Altern Med. 2012;12:5.
26. Zhang Y, Wei RX, Zhu XB, Cai L, Jin W, Hu H. Tanshinone IIA induces apoptosis and inhibits the proliferation, migration, and invasion of the osteosarcoma MG-63 cell line in vitro. Anti-Cancer Drugs. 2012;23:212–9.
27. Su CC. Tanshinone IIA decreases the migratory ability of AGS cells by decreasing the protein expression of matrix metalloproteinases, nuclear factor kappaB-p65 and cyclooxygenase-2. Mol Med Rep. 2016;13:1263–8.
28. Chuang MT, Ho FM, Wu CC, Zhuang SY, Lin SY, Suk FM, Liang YC. 15,16-Dihydrotanshinone I, a compound of salvia miltiorrhiza Bunge, Induces Apoptosis through Inducing Endoplasmic Reticular Stress in Human Prostate Carcinoma Cells. eCAM. 2011;2011:865435.
29. Pollard JW. Trophic macrophages in development and disease. Nat Rev Immunol. 2009;9:259–70.
30. Peng L, Shu S, Krauss JC. Monocyte chemoattractant protein inhibits the generation of tumor-reactive T cells. Cancer Res. 1997;57:4849–54.
31. Zhuang S, Cheng TH, Shih NL, Liu JC, Chen JJ, Hong HJ, Chan P. Tanshinone IIA induces Heme oxygenase 1 expression and inhibits cyclic strain-induced interleukin 8 expression in vascular endothelial cells. Am J Chin Med. 2016;44:377–88.
32. Lee CY, Sher HF, Chen HW, Liu CC, Chen CH, Lin CS, Yang PC, Tsay HS, Chen JJ. Anticancer effects of tanshinone I in human non-small cell lung cancer. Mol Cancer Ther. 2008;7:3527–38.
33. Wilson C, Maxwell PJ, Longley DB, Wilson RH, Johnston PG, Waugh DJ. Constitutive and treatment-induced CXCL8-signalling selectively modulates the efficacy of anti-metabolite therapeutics in metastatic prostate cancer. PLoS One. 2012;7:e36545.
34. Wang X, Yeung JH. Inhibitory effect of tanshinones on rat CYP3A2 and CYP2C11 activity and its structure-activity relationship. Fitoterapia. 2011;82:539–45.
35. Zabkiewicz J, Clarke AR. DNA damage-induced apoptosis: insights from the mouse. Biochim Biophys Acta. 2004;1705:17–25.
36. Zhang Z, Zhang J, Jin L, Song T, Wu G, Gao J. Tanshinone IIA interacts with DNA by minor groove-binding. Biol Pharm Bull. 2008;31:2342–5.
37. Ding L, Wang S, Qu X, Wang J. Tanshinone IIA sensitizes oral squamous cell carcinoma to radiation due to an enhanced autophagy. Environ Toxicol Pharmacol. 2016;46:264–9.
38. Fahmy O, Khairul-Asri MG, Hadi S, Gakis G, Stenzl A. The role of radical prostatectomy and radiotherapy in treatment of locally advanced prostate cancer: a systematic review and meta-analysis. Urol Int. 2017;
39. Gabka CJ, Benhaim P, Mathes SJ, Scheuenstuhl H, Chan A, Fu KK, Hunt TK. An experimental model to determine the effect of irradiated tissue on neutrophil function. Plast Reconstr Surg. 1995;96:1676–88.
40. Sowerby RJ, Gani J, Yim H, Radomski SB, Catton C. Long-term complications in men who have early or late radiotherapy after radical prostatectomy. Can Urol Assoc J. 2014;8:253–8.
41. Yarney J, Donkor A, Opoku SY, Yarney L, Agyeman-Duah I, Abakah AC, Asampong E. Characteristics of users and implications for the use of complementary and alternative medicine in Ghanaian cancer patients undergoing radiotherapy and chemotherapy: a cross- sectional study. BMC Complement Altern Med. 2013;13:16.
42. Nissen N, Lunde A, Pedersen CG, Johannessen H. The use of complementary and alternative medicine after the completion of hospital treatment for colorectal cancer: findings from a questionnaire study in Denmark. BMC Complement Altern Med. 2014;14:388.
43. Dhanoa A, Yong TL, Yeap SJ, Lee IS, Singh VA. Complementary and alternative medicine use amongst Malaysian orthopaedic oncology patients. BMC Complement Altern Med. 2014;14:404.
44. Du S, Yao Q, Tan P, Xie G, Ren C, Sun Q, Zhang X, Zheng R, Yang K, Yuan Y, Yuan Q. Protective effect of tanshinone IIA against radiation-induced ototoxicity in HEI-OC1 cells. Oncol Lett. 2013;6:901–6.
45. Zhang W, Li Y, Li R, Wang Y, Zhu M, Wang B, Li Y, Li D, Xie P, Liu B. Sodium Tanshinone IIA sulfonate prevents radiation-induced toxicity in H9c2 cardiomyocytes. eCAM. 2017;2017:4537974.

2

Antiproliferative and proapoptotic effects of DODAC/synthetic phosphoethanolamine on hepatocellular carcinoma cells

Arthur Cássio de Lima Luna[1,2*], Greice Kelle Viegas Saraiva[3], Gilberto Orivaldo Chierice[4], Henrique Hesse[1] and Durvanei Augusto Maria[1,2*]

Abstract

Background: Current studies have demonstrated that DODAC/PHO-S (Dioctadecyldimethylammonium Chloride/Synthetic phosphoethanolamine) liposomes induces cytotoxicity in Hepa1c1c7 and B16F10 murine tumor cells, with a higher proportion than PHO-S. Therefore, our aim was to evaluate the potential of DODAC/PHO-S to elucidate the mechanism of cell death whereby the liposomes induces cytotoxicity in hepatocellular carcinoma Hepa1c1c7, compared to the PHO-S alone.

Methods: Liposomes (DODAC/PHO-S) were prepared by ultrasonication. The cell cycle phases, protein expression and types of cell's death on Hepa1c1c7 were analyzed by flow cytometry. The internalisation of liposomes, mitochondrial electrical potential and lysosomal stability were also evaluated by confocal laser scanning microscopy.

Results: After treatment with liposomes (DODAC/PHO-S), we observed a significant increase in the population of Hepa1c1c7 cells experiencing cell cycle arrest in the S and G_2/M phases, and this treatment was significantly more effective to promote cell death by apoptosis. There also was a decrease in the mitochondrial electrical potential; changes in the lysosomes; nuclear fragmentation and catastrophic changes in Hepa1c1c7 cells. The liposomes additionally promoted increases in the expression of DR4 receptor, caspases 3 and 8, cytochrome c, p53, p21, p27 and Bax. There was also a decrease in the expression of Bcl-2, cyclin D1, CD90 and CD44 proteins.

Conclusion: The overall results showed that DODAC/PHO-S liposomes were more effective than PHO-S alone, in promoting cytotoxicity Hepa1c1c7 tumor cells, activating the intrinsic and extrinsic pathways of programmed cell death.

Keywords: Liposomes, Nanomedicine, Hepatocellular carcinoma, Antitumoral alkylphospholipids

Background

Despite great advances in the research and the development of new therapeutic strategies, cancer remains one of the leading causes of death worldwide. In 2014, there were an estimated 1,665,540 new cancer cases diagnosed and 585,720 deaths were expected in the United States of America in 2014, and it is expected to increase to over 24 million by 2035 [1, 2].

With regards to the limiting factors of the therapies currently available for the treatment of cancer, new treatments that are more effective and less harmful are necessary. Therefore, antineoplastic phospholipids (AFTs) and lipid precursors have emerged as a promising new classes of antitumor agents that do not target the DNA, however they change the plasma membrane turnover, inducing cell death, with a high selectivity for cancer cell [3, 4]. Edelfosine, miltefosine, perifosine, erucylphosphocholine and erufosine, represent this new class of AFTs, structurally related antitumor agents [5–7].

Synthetic phosphoethanolamine (PHO-S), an lipid precursor, amino-ethyl phosphoric ester, has been previously synthesized by our group [8–13]. We demonstrated that

* Correspondence: arthurluna@usp.br; durvaneiaugusto@yahoo.com.br; durvanei@usp.br
[1]Department of Biochemistry and Biophysics, Butantan Institute, 1500, Vital Brasil Avenue, Sao Paulo 05503-900, Brazil
Full list of author information is available at the end of the article

the treatment of B16F10 cells with PHO-S was able to inhibit cell proliferation and induce G_{2}/M cell cycle arrest [13]. In another study, PHO-S caused anti-proliferative effects on HUVEC, by reducing cyclin D1 mRNA, VEGFR1 gene transcription and VEGFR1 receptor expression [10, 12].

In vitro studies demonstrated that PHO-S induced cytotoxicity and apoptosis via mitochondrial pathways, in leukemia cells. The results showed that PHO-S was able to provide antiproliferative effects on acute promyelocytic leukemia (APL) cell lines. PHO-S demonstrated its antiproliferative effect on APL cell lines, decreasing CD177+ and Gr-17+ in immature myeloid cells in bone marrow, spleen and liver [11]. Additionally, the PHO-S has exerted anti-tumor activities in several tumor cell lines, such B16F10 cells; Skmel-28 and Mewo cells (human melanoma); MCF-7 cells (human breast cancer) and ehrlich ascites tumor [8–10, 12, 13].

Recently, PHO-S was encapsulated in DODAC (Dioctadecyldimethylammonium Chloride) liposomes by our group and the liposomes were physico-chemically characterised [14, 15]. In vitro studies demonstrated the efficacy of DODAC/PHO-S liposomes in inducing cytotoxicity in B16F10 murine melanoma and Hepa1c1c7 murine hepatocellular carcinoma cells, with $IC_{50\%}$ values significantly lower than PHO-S treatment. It was observed that Hepa1c1c7 cells display greater sensitivity to the DODAC/PHO-S formulation when compared with B16F10 and HUVEC cells. However, the molecular mechanism responsible for the anti-tumor properties of DODAC/PHO-S has not been demonstrated [14, 15]. Consequently, our aim was to clarify the mechanism of cell death where DODAC/PHO-S liposomal formulation induces cytotoxicity in hepatocellular carcinoma Hepa1c1c17.

Methods

Liposomal formulation DODAC/PHO-S

Liposomal formulation DODAC/PHO-S were formulated (1:1) in water, in accordance with procedures previously published [8–10, 12, 13]. After sonication, the liposomes were sterilized by filtration.

Cell culture

Hepa1c1c7 murine hepatocellular carcinoma (ATCC® CRL 2026) was cultured in αMEM medium (LGC Biotecnologia, Cotia, SP, Brazil) and supplemented with 10% fetal bovine serum in a humidified incubator at 37 °C and 5% CO_2. The cell viability was verified using Trypan Blue exclusion test. Hepa1c1c7 was chosen for the study because of its easy reproduction in vivo studies.

Cell cycle phases distribution

The Hepa1c1c7 cells at a cell density of 1×10^5 cells/well (80 to 90% confluence) were treated with PHO-S (0.3–2.0 mM), DODAC/PHO-S 1:1 (0.3–2.0 mM), and empty DODAC (0.3–2.0 mM), for 12 h. After treatment, the cells were washed with PBS (phosphate buffered saline) and fixed by the addition of 3 ml of ice cold 70% ethanol. The cells cycle was evaluated after cell incubation with 1.8 μg/ml propidium iodide (PI) solution (Sigma-Aldrich, St. Louis, MO, EUA), for 30 min. in the dark. The analysis was performed using Biosciences FACSCalibur flow cytometer (Becton Dickinson, San Jose, CA, EUA) and 10,000 events were collected. Subsequently, the data was analysed by ModFit LT 3.2 software (Becton Dickinson, San Jose, CA, EUA).

Determination of apoptotic and necrotic cells percentage by flow cytometric (Annexin-V/PI)

The Hepa1c1c7 cells were plated at 1 mL 1×10^5 cells/well in 6 well plates. After 24 h, the cells were treated with PHO-S and DODAC/PHO-S, for 12 h. Then, the cells were washed three times with PBS at 4 °C and resuspended in 100 μL of PBS, following this, were incubated with 4 μg/mL of AnnexinV (Sigma Aldrich, EUA) and 1.8 μg/μL of PI (Sigma Aldrich, EUA), for 1 h at 37 °C.

Following incubation, the cells were centrifuged at 2000 rpm for 10 min at 4 °C and resuspended in 400 μL of binding buffer 1×, provided by the manufacturer. The analysis were performed using Biosciences FACSCalibur flow cytometer (Becton Dickinson, San Jose, CA, EUA) and 10,000 events were collected. Following this, the data was analysed using ModFit LT 3.2 software (Becton Dickinson, San Jose, CA, EUA).

Expression markers analysis by flow cytometry

The analysis of protein expression were performed as previously published [15, 16]. In brief, the Hepa1c1c7 cells (1×10^5 cells/well, the cell density reached 80 to 90% confluence), were treated with PHO-S (0.3–2.0 mM), DODAC/PHO-S 1:1 (0.3–2.0 mM), and empty DODAC (0.3–2.0 mM), for 12 h, were washed with PBS and resuspended in FACS buffer with 2.5% paraformaldehyde for 1 h. After washing, cells were again resuspended in a primary antibody specific for the proteins anti-CD44, anti-CD90, anti-p53, anti-p21, anti-p27, anti-Bax, anti-Bcl-2, anti-caspase-3, anti-caspase-8 (Abcam, Cambridge, MA, United States); anti- cytochrome c, anti-DR4 (Santa (Cruz Biotechnology Inc., Santa Cruz, EUA) and anti-cyclin D1 (Cell Signaling Technology, Danvers, MA), at a concentration of 1 μg/ml at 4 °C, for 1 min. The corresponding isotope antibody was used as a negative control and as a secondary antibody was used Goat anti Mouse IgG (H/L): FITC (AbD Serotec, Raleigh, NC, United States). The cells were pelleted, washed twice with PBS, then, fluorescence-activated cell sorting (FACS) analysis was performed on BD Biosciences FACs Calibur flow cytometer (Becton Dickinson, San Jose, CA, United States) using Cell Quest and Win MDI 2.9 softwares.

Analysis of the internalisation of DODAC/PHO-S fluorescent liposomes by confocal laser scanning microscopy

DODAC/PHO-S liposomes 1:1 were prepared according to the protocol as described previously, adding 0.25 mol%, in relation to DODAC, of the fluorescent probe (Dil): 1,1′-dioctadecyl-3,3,3′,3′- tetramethylindocarbocyanine perchlorate (Life Technologies, CA, United States).

Aliquots of Hepa1c1c7 cells (1×10^5 cells/well, the cell density reached 80 to 90% confluence), were plated on sterile glass slides. After adhesion, cells were treated with DODAC/PHO-S fluorescent liposomes (1:1) 0.3 and 2.0 mM. Then, cells were fixed by adding ProLong® and incubated at − 20 °C, in the dark. The analysis was realised by confocal laser scanning microscopy (Carl Zeiss LSM 700; Leica, Mannheim, Germany).

Analysis of changes in mitochondrial electrical potential ($\Delta\Psi m$) by confocal laser scanning microscopy

The analysis of the $\Delta\Psi m$ was realised by confocal laser. The Hepa1c1c7 cells were plated on sterile glass slides in 24-well plates, at concentration of 10^5. After 24 h, the cells were treated with PHO-S and DODAC/PHO-S (1:1) at 0.3 and 2.0 mM, for 6 h. Then, the incubation with rhodamine-123 and analyses were perfomed as previously published [15, 16].

Evaluation of lysosomal stability using acridine orange (AO)

The Hepa1c1c7 were plated on sterile glass slides in 24-well plates, at concentration of 1×10^5 cells/well. After 24 h, the cells were treated with PHO-S and DODAC/PHO-S, for 6 h. The cells were then incubated with OA and analysed as previously published [15, 16].

Statistical analysis

Statistical analyses were perfomed as previously detailed [15, 16]. In brief, the differences among measurements of the groups studied were analysed using One-way ANOVA (and non-parametric) and Kruskal Wallis test. *p*-values $^{*} < 0.05$, $^{**} < 0.01$, and $^{***} < 0.001$ are statistically significant.

Results

DODAC/PHO-S liposomal formulation induces cell cycle arrest in G_2/M

The compounds were evaluated for their ability to induce changes in the cell cycle. The Hepa1c1c7 cells were treated with PHO-S, DODAC/PHO-S (1:1) at a concentration of 0.3 and 2.0 mM, for 12 h. The exposure time was determined by taking into account the results of the cytotoxicity, as previously published, and performed simultaneously with this study [13, 14].

The distribution of Hepa1c1c7 cells, that were treated, suffered alterations in their percentage, compared to the control group (Fig. 1a and b). However, it is not possible to observe significant changes in the percentage of cells in the sub-G_1 phase, among the treatments and control group (Fig. 1a and b). The number of cells in the G_0/G_1 phase decreased significantly with DODAC/PHO-S treatment, in relation to the control group (74.7 ± 1.1%), presenting a percentage of 53.2 ± 1.2% (0.3 mM) and 48.9 ± 3.5% (2.0 mM) (Fig. 1b).

The treatment with DODAC/PHO-S induced significant increases in the number of cells in S-phase, when compared to previous treatments, with values of 7.1 ± 1.9% (0.3 mM) and 9.1 ± 0.8% (2.0 mM) (Fig. 1b). The percentage of cells in the G_2/M phase showed a significant increase when treated with DODAC/PHO-S liposomes, with values of 14.3 ± 1.7% (0.3 mM) and 14.3 ± 2.1% (2.0 mM) (Fig. 1b).

DODAC/PHO-S induces an increase in the number of apoptotic cells

The Hepa1c1c7 cells were treated with PHO-S, DODAC/PHO-S (1:1) and DODAC (0.3–2.0 mM), for 12 h. Subsequently, cells in apoptosis, late apoptosis and necrosis were quantified by flow cytometry using FITC Annexin V/PI apoptosis detection Kit. The treatment with PHO-S (0.3 and 2.0 mM) significantly increased the number of apoptotic and necrotic cells, with values of 13.9 ± 3.4% (0.3 mM) and 7.5 ± 0.3% (0.3 mM), respectively. In the highest concentration (PHO-S 2.0 mM), the percentage of apoptotic cells was 21.2 ± 5.4% and 7.5 ± 0.3% of necrotic cells. Only in the highest concentration (2.0 mM) was it possible to observe an increase in the number of cells in late apoptosis, presenting a percentage value of 9.7 ± 4.6% (Fig. 2b).

The treatment with DODAC/PHO-S (0.3 and 2.0 mM) significantly increased the number of necrotic cells, with values of 9.6 ± 0.14% (0.3 mM) and 12.3 ± 0.3% (2.0 mM). There was also an increase in late apoptosis, with a percentage of 30.4 ± 0.4% (0.3 mM) and 31.0 ± 1.3% (2.0 mM). The treatment with DODAC (0.3 mM) increased the number of necrotic cells to a lesser extent when compared to the other treatments, with a percentage of 6.7 ± 0.9% (Fig. 2b).

Internalisation of liposomes DODAC/PHO-S by Hep1c1c7 cells

The internalisation of DODAC/PHO-S liposomes with fluorescent probe (Dil), was evaluated by confocal laser scanning microscopy. The Hepa1c1c7 cells were treated with DODAC/PHO-S liposomes (0.3 and 2.0 mM). The fluorescently labeled liposomes were observed and easily

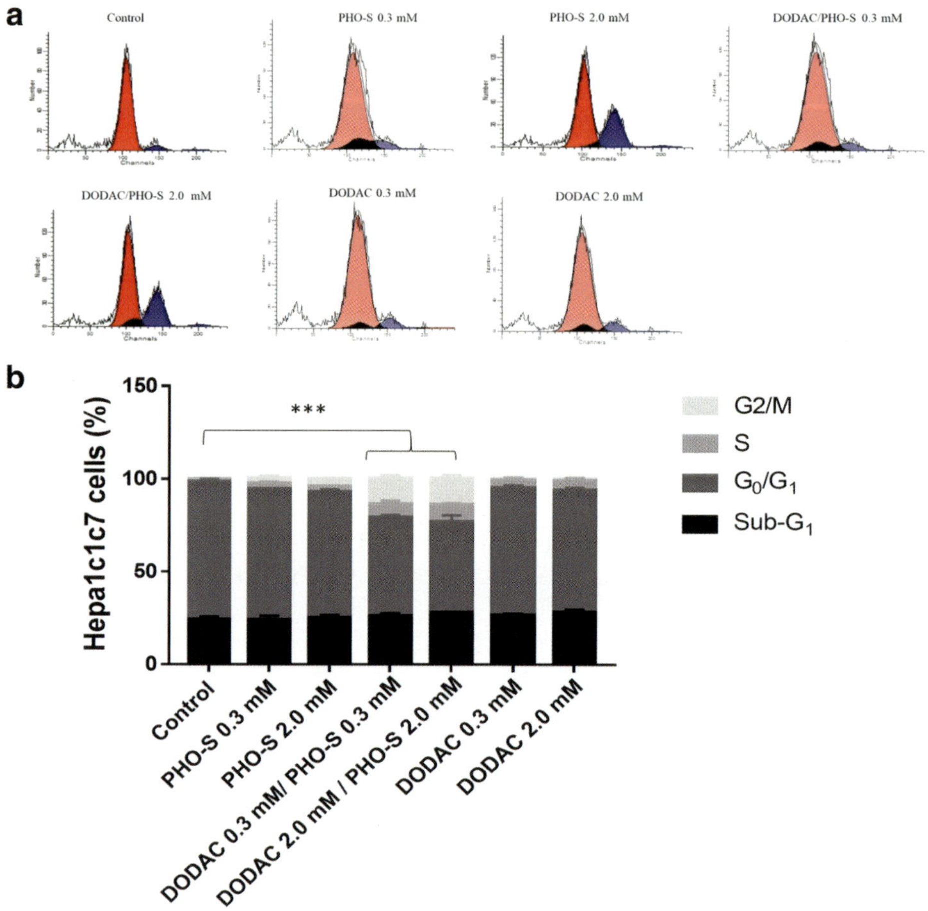

Fig. 1 Analysis of cell cycle phases of Hepa1c1c7 cells treated with PHO-S, DODAC and DODAC/PHO-S. The cells were treated with different concentrations of the formulations for a period of 12 h. The graph shows the correlation of the effect expressed as a mean ± SD of three independent experiments. **a** Representative histograms of cell cycle analysis. Y-axis represent number of cells; X-axis represents DNA content (PI intensity). **b** Population of cells in sub-G1, G_0/G_1, S and G_2/M phase. Level of statistical significance * $P < 0.05$, ** $p < 0.01$ and *** $p < 0.001$

distinguishable by their green colour. After treatment, the presence of the DODAC/PHO-S fluorescently labeled liposomes (0.3 and 2.0 mM) were observed in the cytoplasm of the Hepalclc7 cells, confirming that internalisation of the liposomes occurred, in a short period of time (Fig. 3).

DODAC/PHO-S liposomes decreases the ΔΨm

The Hepalclc7 cells were treated with PHO-S, DODAC/PHO-S (1:1) and DODAC (0.3 and 2.0 mM), for a period of 6 h. The cells treated with PHO-S and DODAC/PHO-S, demonstrated a significant decrease in ΔΨm, when compared to the control group. The cells were treated with DODAC (0.3 and 2.0 mM) and presented an attenuation of fluorescent intensity, compared to the control group. However, the positive staining demonstrated that cells had functional mitochondria (Fig. 4).

DODAC/PHO-S induces cellular morphological change

The Hepalclc7 cells were treated with PHO-S, DODAC and DODAC/PHO-S liposomes (2.0 mM), for a period of 6 h. The effects of these compounds in lysosomes were then evaluated with AO (acridine orange) assay, by confocal laser scanning microscopy. The nuclear DNA was labeled with DAPI (blue emission). For this assay, only the highest concentration (2.0 mM) was used, because it showed the greatest effectiveness in inducing cytotoxicity.

The control group cells demonstrated intense labeling of some lysosomes with a granular appearance, evenly distributed into cytoplasm (Fig. 5a). The same distribution pattern was observed in the cells treated with PHO-S. However, in this case the treatment induced an increase in the number of lysosomes (Fig. 5b and c). In the cells treated with DODAC/PHO-S liposomes, there decrease in the number of lysosomes and morphological alterations due to the apoptotic process were observed,

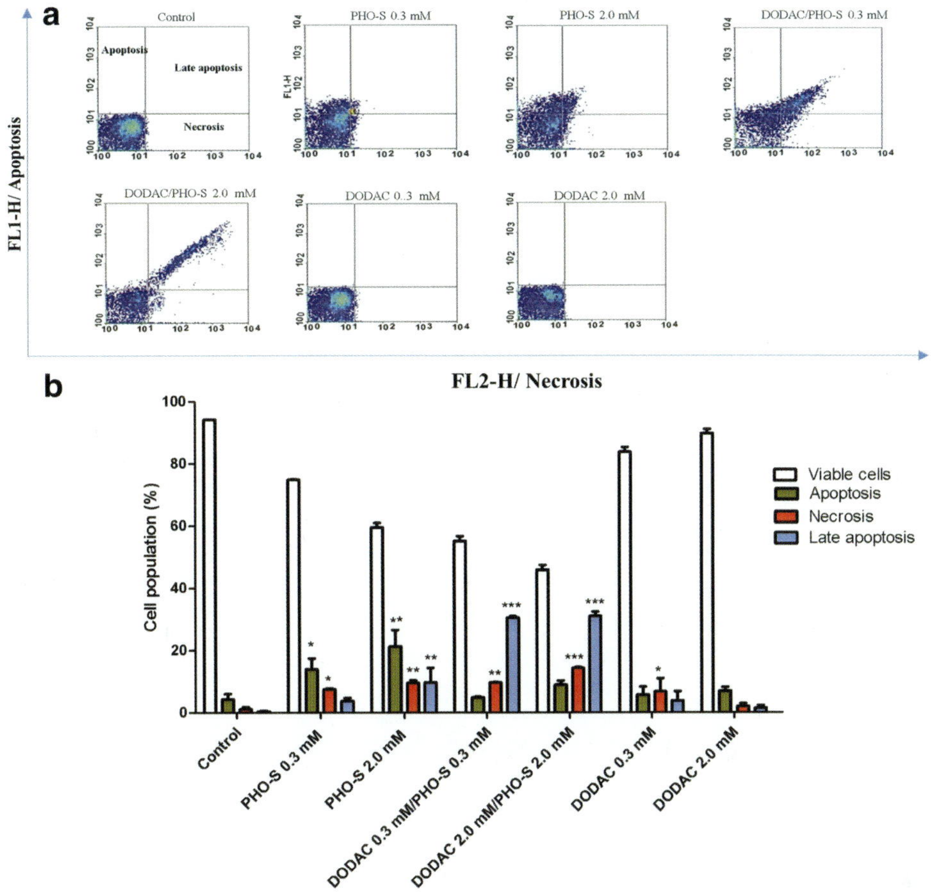

Fig. 2 Evaluation of cell death mechanism by quantifying the percentage of Hepa1c1c7 cells undergoing apoptosis, late apoptosis and necrosis, by flow cytometry using Annexin V / PI kit. The Hepa1c1c7 cells were treated with different concentrations of PHO-S, DODAC/PHO-S and DODAC, for a period of 12 h. **a** representative dot plots of fluorescence levels obtained by staining the cells for Annexin V/PI kit. **b** The bar chart shows the correlation of the effect expressed as a mean ± SD of three independent experiments. Level of statistical significance * $P < 0.05$, ** $p < 0.01$ and *** $p < 0.001$

as membrane bubbles and nuclear fragmentation (Fig. 5d and e). The cells treated with only DODAC presented a distribution pattern and labeling of lysosomes similar the cells of the control group (Fig. 5f).

Protein expression involved in programmed cell death

Hepalclc7 tumor cells were treated with PHO-S (2.0 mM), DODAC and DODAC/PHO-S (0.3 and 2.0 mM), for 24 h. The expression of proteins involved in checkpoint, cell adhesion, regulation of the cell cycle and apoptotic pathway were quantified after the treatment. These proteins are as follows: TRAIL receptors 1 (DR4), active caspases-3 and -8, free cytochrome c, p53, p21, p27, CD44, CD90, Bax, Bcl-2 and cyclin D1.

The Hepalclc7 cells treated with 2.0 mM DODAC/PHO-S, showed a significant increase in the expression of DR4 receptor, active caspases-3 and 8 and cytochrome c, with percentage values of 11.4 ± 0.1% (Fig. 6a), 13.5 ± 0.5% (Fig. 6b), 17.0 ± 0,7% (Fig. 6c) and 11.0 ± 0.7% (Fig. 6d), respectively. The treatment with empty DODAC (2.0 mM) also induced a significant growth in the expression of free cytochrome c, with value of 2.8 ± 0.1% (Fig. 6d).

Bax protein had an expression increase after treatment with 2.0 mM PHO-S (9.1 ± 1.2%), DODAC/PHO-S (11.9 ± 0.1%) and DODAC (6.5 ± 0.2%) (Fig. 6e). In contrast, antiapoptotic Bcl-2 protein had a decrease in the expression with 2.0 mM PHO-S (1.1 ± 0.9%), DODAC/PHO-S (0.3 mM - 0.1 ± 0.1%; 2.0 mM - 0.6 ± 0.1%) and 2.0 mM DODAC (1.7 ± 0.1%) (Fig. 6f).

The expression of p21 protein increased with 2.0 mM PHO-S (1.9 ± 0.1%); DODAC/PHO-S (0.3 mM - 4.3 ± 0.3% and 2.0 mM - 25.5 ± 0.7%) and empty DODAC (0.3 mM - 1.6 ± 0.3% and 2.0 mM - 18.8 ± 0.5%) (Fig. 7a). P27 protein had an increase in expression with 2.0 mM PHO-S (8.2 ± 1.6%); DODAC/PHO-S (0.3 mM - 16 ± 1.2% and 2.0 mM - 34.6 ± 0.9%) (Fig. 7b).

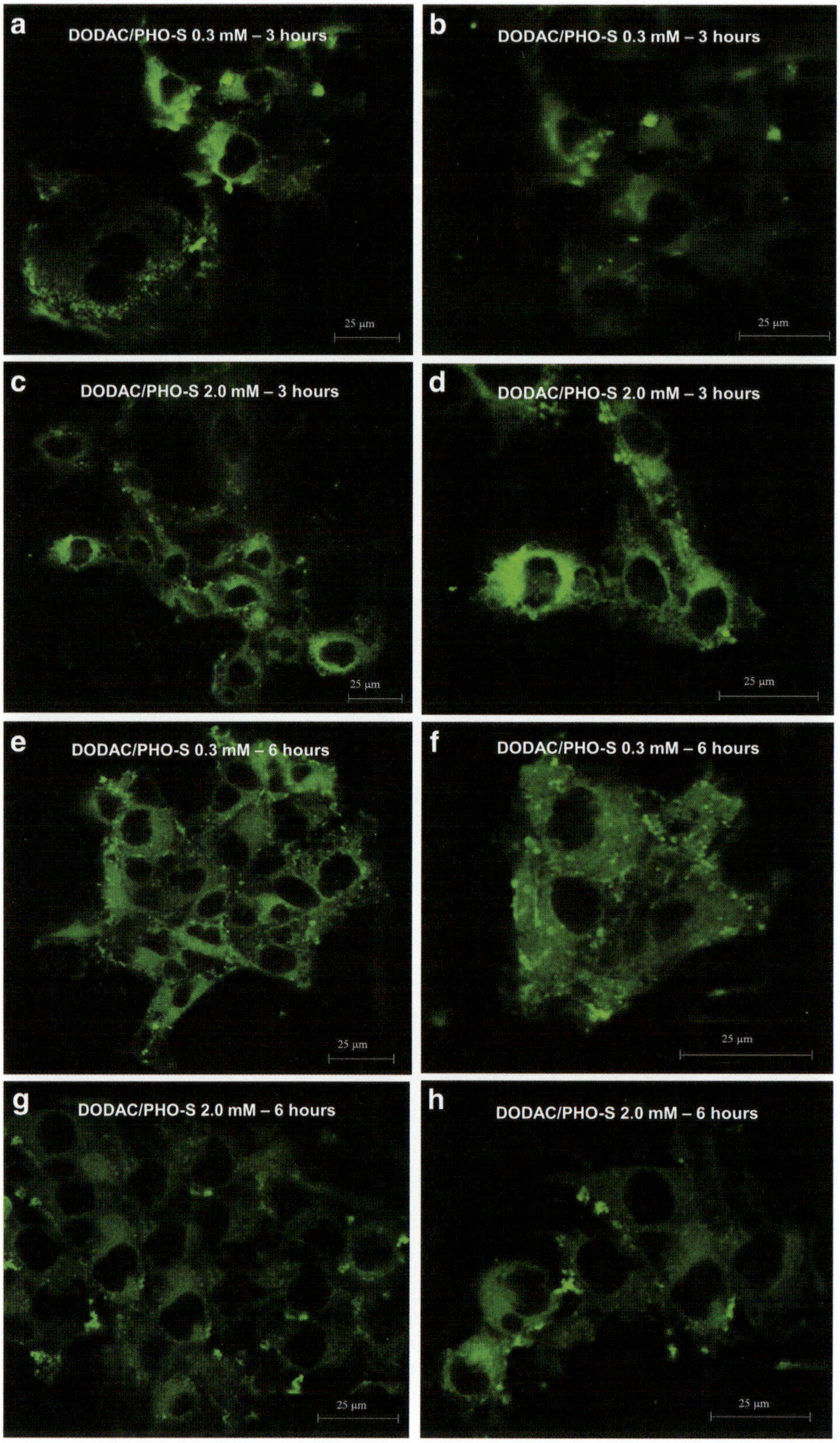

Fig. 3 Photomicrographs of liposomes DODAC/PHO-S/DiI in Hepa1c1c7 cells analyzed by confocal laser microscopy. Cells were treated with the liposomal formulation (0.3 and 2.0 mM) with a fluorescent marker for a period of 3 to 6 h. Labeled liposomes can be observed and distinguished by the colour green in the cytoplasm of the cells. Cells treated with **a** and **b** DODAC/PHO-S 0.3 mM; **c** and **d** DODAC/PHO-S 2.0 mM, for a period of 3 h. Cells treated with **e** and **f** DODAC/PHO-S 0.3 mM; **g**, **e**, **h** DODAC/PHO-S 2.0 mM, for a period of 6 h

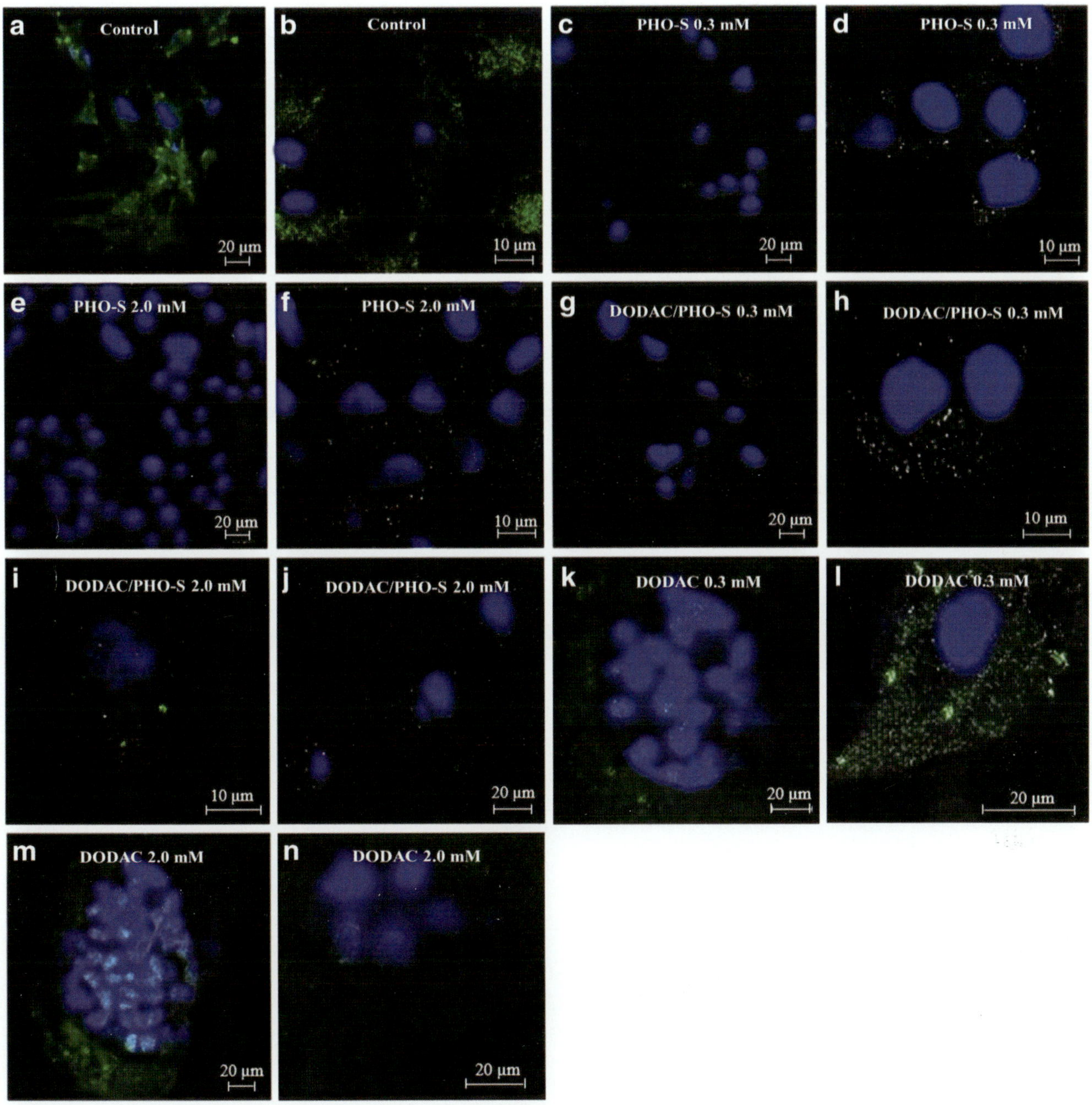

Fig. 4 Photomicrographs of the Hepa1c1c7 cells mitochondria labeled with rhodamine 123 (green) and nucleus with DAPI (blue) and analyzed by confocal laser microscopy. Cells were treated with PHO-S, DODAC and DODAC/PHO-S 1: 1, for a period of 6 h and mitochondria were labeled with rhodamine 123. **a** and **b** control; **c** and **d** PHO-S -0.3 mM; **e** and **f** PHO-S 2.0 mM; **g** and **h** DODAC/PHO-S 0.3 mM; **i** and **j** DODAC/PHO-S 2.0 mM; **k** and **l** DODAC 0.3 mM; **m** and **n** DODAC 2.0 mM. Scale bar = 10 and 20 µm

It was noticed that p53 protein increased with 2.0 mM DODAC/PHO-S (38 ± 1.7%) and 2.0 mM empty DODAC (22.9 ± 1.3%) (Fig. 7c). In contrast, the expression of cyclin D1 decreased with 2.0 mM PHO-S (16.7 ± 1.5%); 2.0 mM DODAC/PHO-S (14.8 ± 1.5%) and 2.0 mM empty DODAC (21.4 ± 0.1%) (Fig. 7d). Some markers as CD90 and CD44 were quantified after the treatment. It was possible to observe that CD90 decreased after treatment with 2.0 mM PHO-S (1.5 ± 0.9%) and DODAC/PHO-S (0.3 mM - 1.3 ± 0.1%; 2.0 mM - 1.7 ± 0.9%) (Fig. 7e). The expression of CD44 decreased significantly with

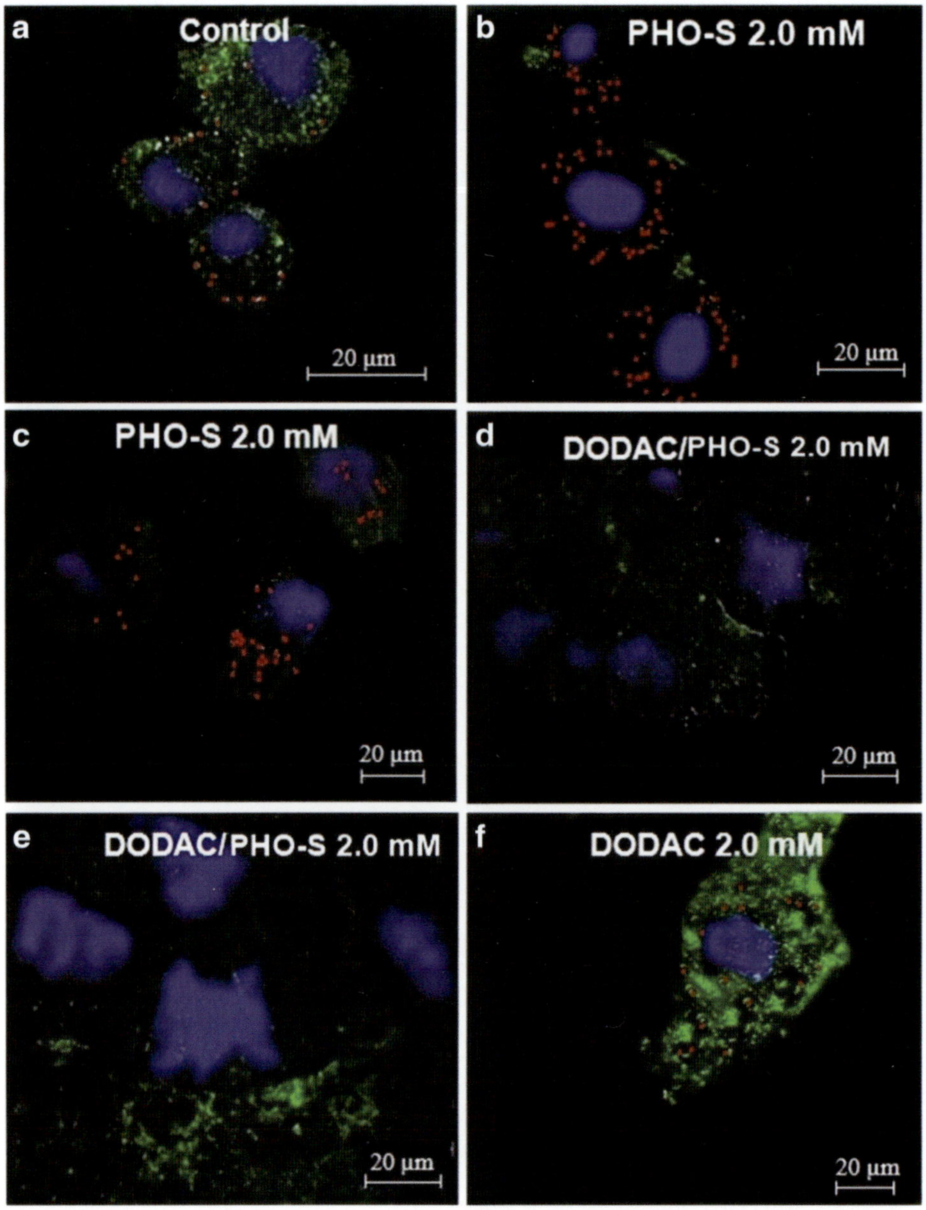

Fig. 5 Photomicrographs of the cells of murine Hepa1c1c7 hepatocarcinoma lysosomes labeled with acridine orange (green) and nucleus with DAPI (blue) and analyzed by confocal laser microscopy. Cells were treated with PHO-S, DODAC and DODAC/PHO-S 1: 1, for a period of 6 h and lysosomes and nucleus were labeled. **a** control; **b** and **c** PHO-S 2.0 mM; **d** and **e** DODAC/PHO-S 2.0 mM; **f** DODAC 2.0 mM. Scale bar = 20 µm

all treatments (Fig. 7f). There were no significant differences among the treatments.

Discussion

Several liposomal formulations containing antitumor agents are already clinically available or are under advanced stages of development, for example, Doxil® (Pegylated liposomal doxorubicin), Lipoplatin® (cisplatin) DepoCyte® (cytarabine), DaunoXome® (daunorubicin), MBP-426 (oxaliplatin), BIND (docetaxel) and MM30 (doxorubicin) [17–20]. Cationic liposomes or cationic polymers are often used in gene transfection due to their relatively easy complex formation with negatively charged genetic material [21, 22]. The complex polymer-DNA general mechanism is based on electrostatic interaction of the complex with DNA. This interaction allows internalisation of the DNA into the cells. The main advantages of these synthetic carriers are related to their versatility of their physicochemical properties, coupled with their easy handling and lower production cost [21–23].

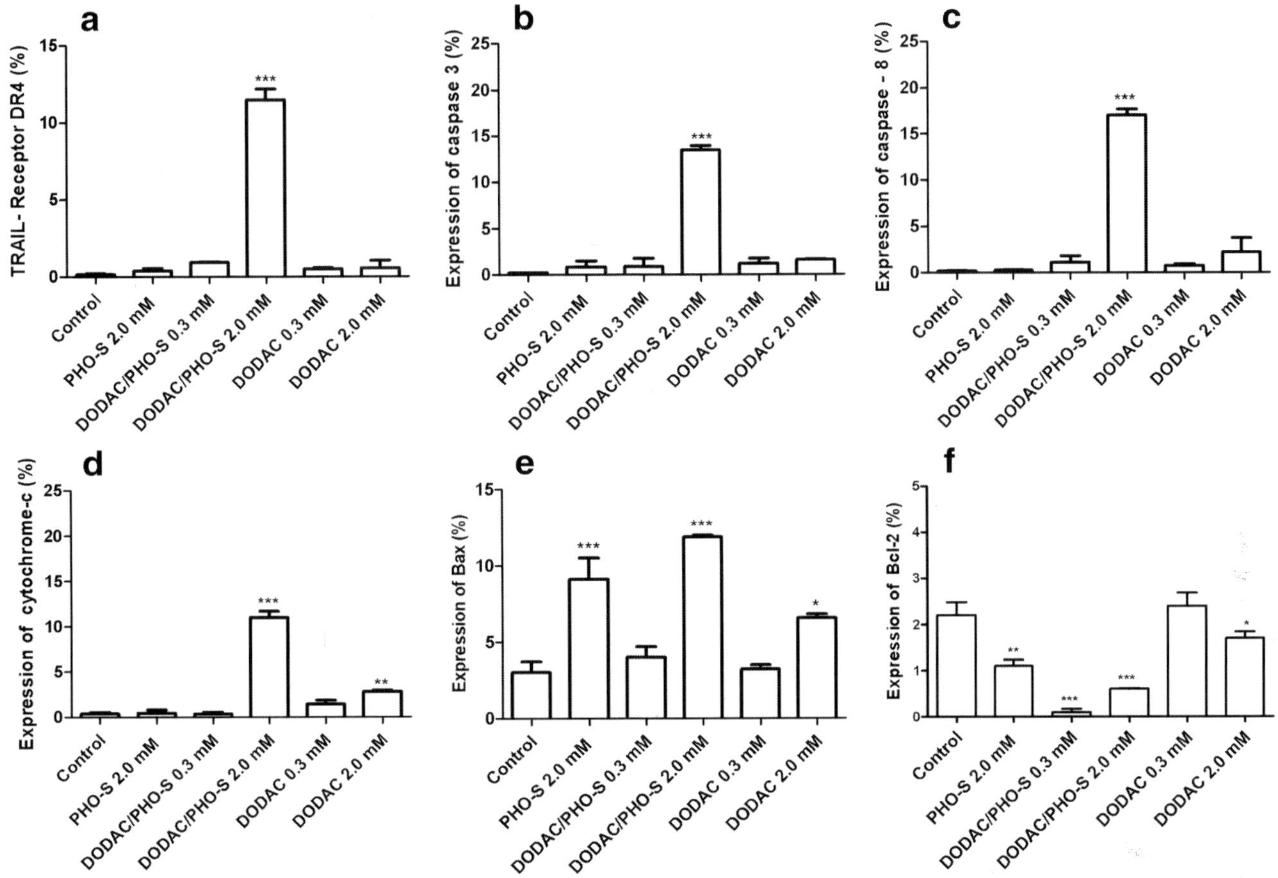

Fig. 6 Analysis of protein expression in Hepa1c1c7 cells. The expression of proteins was quantified by flow cytometry after 24 h of treatment with PHO-S, DODAC and DODAC/PHO-S. The bar graphs show the level of expression of TRAIL - DR4 receptor (**a**); protein caspase 3 (**b**); caspase-8 protein (**c**); Free cytochrome c (**d**); protein Bax (**e**); protein Bcl-2 (**f**). Values are expressed as a mean ± SD standard deviation of three independent experiments. Level of significance * $P < 0.05$, ** $p < 0.01$ and *** $p < 0.001$

In a recently published study, PHO-S was encapsulated in DODAC liposomes by our group [14, 15]. The physical, chemical stability and data relating to the characterisation of these liposomes have been mentioned before [14, 15]. This study demonstrated that PHO-S encapsulation was stable and showed an average of ~50% of PHO-S [14, 15]. In vitro studies demonstrated that DODAC/PHO-S induced cytotoxicity and inhibited cell proliferation in B16F10 and Hepa1c1c7 cells. However this was not the case with normal cells with $IC_{50\%}$ values significantly lower than PHO-S treatment. It was also observed that the liposomes were able to induce their highest level of cytotoxicity in Hepa1c1c7 tumor cells [12, 13]. This could be due to the interaction of DODAC with lipid receptors of the tumor cells.

Recent studies have demonstrated that PHO-S inhibits cell proliferation and migration, leading to the accumulation of B16F10 and MCF-7 cells in the G_2/M phase [12, 13]. As demonstrated in this study, the ability of DODAC/PHO-S liposomes to alter cell cycle phases in Hepa1c1c7 cells when compared to the control group. In the cells treated with these liposomes, there were significant increases in the population of Hepa1c1c7 cells experiencing cell cycle arrest at the S and G_2/M phases. The treatment at the lowest and highest concentrations provided the same effect on the cell population, in these phases in the cycle. Therefore, demonstrating once again the sensitivity of Hepa1c1c7 cells to the treatment with DODAC/PHO-S liposomes, in relation to the effects observed in another study with B16F10 cells, performed simultaneously [14, 15]. The treatment with this liposomes, was able to maximize the cytotoxic effect of the treatment with PHO-S by mediating alterations in cell cycle. It was possible to distinguish cells that were arrested in these phases of the cell cycle by the increase in the proportion of cells in this period. However, as determined in the analysis of the ΔΨm there was a greater number of unviable cells in the treated group, compared to the control group. This demonstrates that the cells are possibly activating the mechanism of programmed cell death.

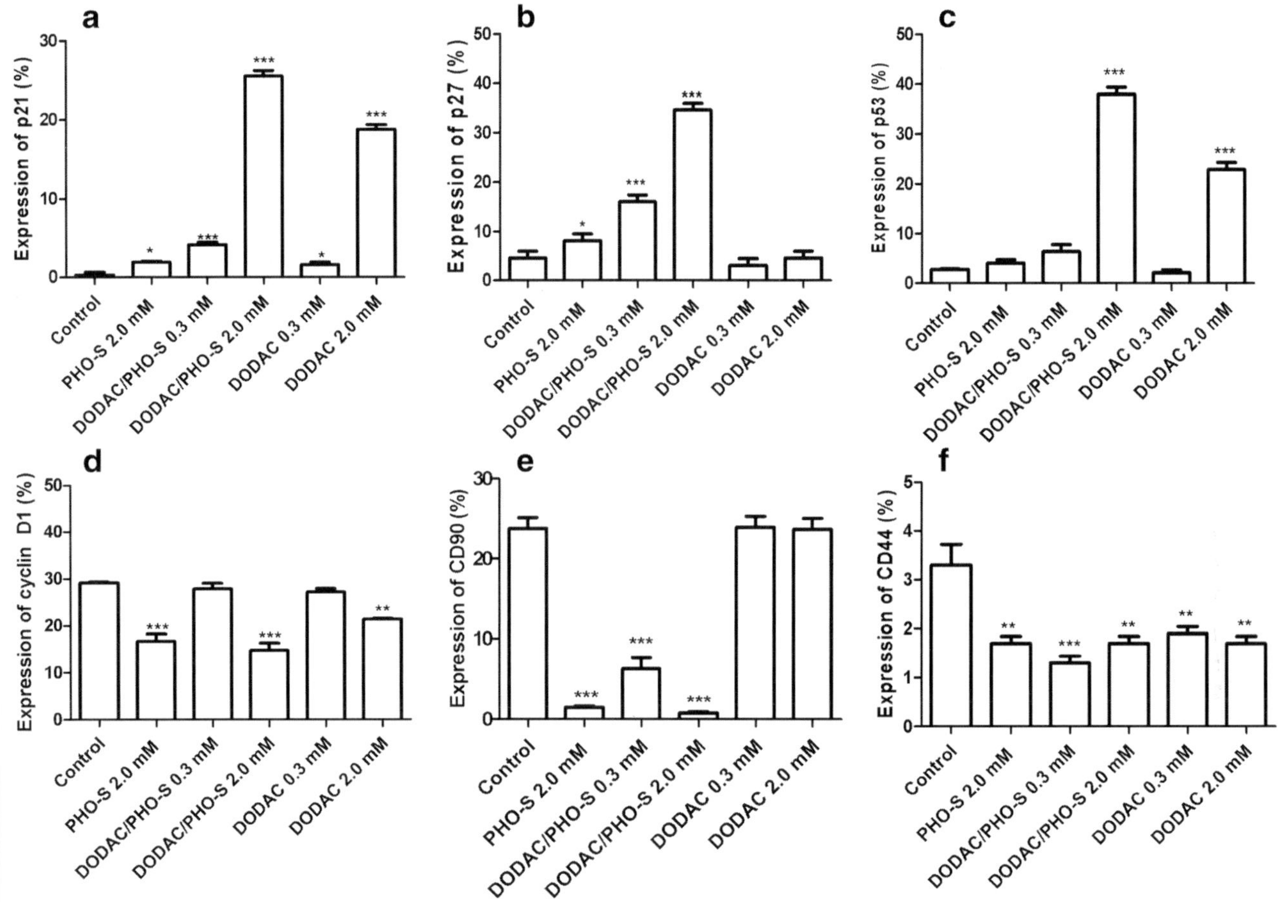

Fig. 7 Analysis of expression of proteins involved in the proliferation and metastatic process in Hepa1c1c7 cells. The expression of the proteins was quantified by flow cytometry after 24 h of treatment with PHO-S, DODAC and DODAC/PHO-S. The bar graphs show the expression level of the protein p21 protein (**a**); p27 protein (**b**); p53 protein (**c**); cyclin D1 protein (**d**); CD90 marker (**e**) and CD44 marker (**f**). Values are expressed as a mean ± SD standard deviation of three independent experiments. Level of significance ** $p < 0.01$ and *** $p < 0.001$

The treatments performed only with empty DODAC liposomes resulted in a lesser increase in the number of Hepa1c1c7 cells in the S phase, however it did not increase the number of cells stopped in the G_2/M phase, which is a specific targeted antitumor effect mediated by PHO-S [13]. This demonstrates the nonspecific effect of DODAC in promoting cytotoxicity, which is perhaps correlated with the ability of this compound to interact with electro-negatively charged molecules, including DNA [21, 22].

The induction of cell cycle arrest after DODAC/PHO-S treatment is very important, as one of the aims of the development of novel anticancer drugs is to formulate compounds that can act on cell cycle checkpoints, which are responsible for controlling cell cycle progression. The checkpoints occur at the entrance into the S phase (G_1/S checkpoint), at the entrance into mitosis (G_2/M checkpoint), as well as during replication (intra-S-phase checkpoint) [24]. A large proportion of conventional chemotherapy agents cause damage to DNA. In most cases, agents that cause DNA damage do not kill cancer cells directly, these agents act initially by activating the checkpoint and blocking cell cycle progression. This not only allows the cell to repair its DNA, but also to impede DNA synthesis or cell division in the presence of chromosome damage by initiating programmed cell death, via the intrinsic pathway [25]. To evaluate the mechanism of cell death mediated by liposomal formulation compared to PHO-S, the assay Annexin-V/PI was used. The evaluation of the integrity of the cellular membrane provides an indication whether the mechanism of cell death involves apoptosis or necrosis [26, 27]. Recent studies have shown the capacity of PHO-S in inducing death by apoptosis in different tumor cells [8–15, 28, 29]. The tests involving Annexin/PI verified these results and demonstrated that PHO-S is capable of stimulating apoptosis in greater proportion than necrosis. Substantiating the previous findings, the liposomal formulation of DODAC/PHO-S (0.3 and 2.0 mM) was significantly more effective when compared to

PHO-S, in promoting cell death by apoptosis in Hepa1c1c7 cells and in increasing the proportion cells in late apoptosis. These results demonstrates the ability of the liposomal formulation to generate cytotoxicity more efficiently than the treatment with PHO-S.

The treatments with empty DODAC liposomes did not trigger cell death by apoptosis, with only a small increase in the number of cells killed by necrosis (with treatment at lower concentrations).

In Hepa1c1c7 cells, the liposomal formulation promoted cell death by inducing the activation of the intrinsic death pathway modulated by p53 activity. This protein is likely to have induced the activity of Bax and p21 proteins, and consequently the decreased expression of cyclin D1 protein, as shown in our results. Moreover, an increase of the pro-apoptotic p27 protein and decrease of the anti-apoptotic Blc-2 protein were observed. These results demonstrate the path or route that the DODAC/PHO-S liposomes possibly uses in order to induce cellular arrest in the G_2/M phase. The expression of proteins involved in checkpoint, apoptosis and cell cycle regulation was greater in cells treated with the 2.0 mM DODAC/PHO-S than in the cells treated with PHO-S only. Thus indicating that treatment with the formulation is more effective than treatment with PHO-S.

There was no significant increase in p53 protein in the Hepa1c1c7 cells treated with PHO-S 2.0 mM. This effect was not observed probably by the exposure time of the cells to PHO-S because the expression of the proteins, which are regulated by transcriptional activation of p53, such as p21 and Bax, was changed. However, in the cells treated with the DODAC/PHO-S, the regulatory effect on p53 was sustained. This demonstrates the effectiveness of DODAC/PHO-S mediating mechanisms that cause cell cycle arrest and consequently die.

It is known that the mechanism through which p53 protein regulates the transition between the S and G_2/M phase involves the regulation of Cdc2 kinase, which is essential for cells to enter mitosis [30]. Cdc2 is inhibited simultaneously by three transcriptional targets of p53: being Gadd45, p21, and 14–3-3. p53 is a key protein that has been shown to coordinate numerous cellular signaling pathways, as cell cycle and apoptosis. p53 induces the transcription of genes that negatively regulate the progression of cell cycle, as cyclin A, polo-like kinase 1 (PLK1), cyclin B1, cyclin B2, cyclin-dependent kinase 1 (CDK1), CDC20, cell cycle phosphatases CDC25A and CDC25C, DNA replication licensing factor MCM5, CKS116 and antiapoptotic survivin (BIRC5) [30–32]. Similarly, recent studies established that PHO-S not only promoted cell cycle arrest mediated by the action of p53, but also facilitated the decrease of the anti-apoptotic protein Bcl-2 in MCF-7 cells [12].

The significant increase in the expression of protein p27 in the treatment with the DODAC/PHO-S (2.0 mM) shows an important action mechanism of this formulation, because this protein acts as an inhibitor of kinases that are dependent on cyclins and thereby negatively regulates the progress of the cell cycle from G_1 to S. In many neoplasms, the nuclear levels of p27 are reduced [33]. The downregulation of p27 occurs during the process of tumorigenesis, affecting proliferation and represents a negative response to the treatment. In normal cells, p27 blocks the progression of the cell cycle by inhibiting the activity of cyclin 2-CDK2 and cyclin A-CDK2 [33]. The induction of the expression of p27 is an important biomarker in response to chemotherapy, in this case for the liposomal formulation DODAC/PHO-S.

Considering the importance of cyclin D1 reduction in antitumor treatment, 2.0 mM liposomal formulation proved effective for this purpose because caused a decrease in cyclin expression in Hepa1c1c7 cells. Recent studies demonstrated the ability of PHO-S in reducing mRNA of cyclin D1 in MCF-7 cells and in reducing the expression of CDK4/6 in the model H460/Bcl-2 cells [12, 28]. The overexpression of cyclin D1 is associated with the development of resistance by the endocrine system in breast cancer cells. Therapeutic agents have been observed to induce the degradation of cyclin D1 in vitro, providing a useful approach for therapeutic intervention [34].

The checkpoint mechanism mediated by p53 protein may promote the repair of damaged DNA or lead to the activation of the mechanism of programed cell death. This is mediated by pro-apoptotic proteins such as Bax, PUMA and Noxa and decreased expression of anti-apoptotic proteins, including Blc-2. It was observed that treatment with DODAC/PHO-S liposomes promoted the activation of programed cell death mechanism, since there was an increase in the expression of Bax and decrease in the Bcl-2 proteins.

The treatments with empty DODAC liposomes promoted an increase in the expression of p53, p21 and Bax, and a decrease in Blc-2 proteins, though to a lower percentage that the treatment with the DODAC/PHO-S liposomes. DODAC can interact with the DNA and other negatively charged molecules, it is probably by inducing p53 protein activity and therefore the activity of p21, Bax and Blc-2. However, the use of this carrier was not cytotoxic to normal HUVEC endothelial cells, under the same proportions as compared to the B16F10 and Hepa1c1c7 tumor cell lines [15]. So, probably, indicates that it could likely, serve as an adjunct to anti-tumor effects exerted by PHO-S.

The induction of cell death by the intrinsic pathway in Hepa1c1c7 cells exerted by the DODAC/PHO-S (0.3 mM and 2.0 mM), was confirmed by the evaluation of ΔΨm. The cells treated with the liposomal formulation decreased the ΔΨm. Cells treated with only empty DODAC liposomes showed functional mitochondria. Recent study demonstrated that MCF-7 cells treated with PHO-S displayed disorders in their ΔΨm [12].

After the treatment with liposomes DODAC/PHO-S the protein expression of extrinsic pathway was also evaluated, since PHO-S has been stated as a compound capable of forming a complex with DR4 and DR5 receptors. This represents a mechanism by which the AFTs are internalized into the cytoplasm by forming coaggregation with the TNF family receptors, in particular FasL [28, 35]. In non-small cell lung adenocarcinoma cells (H460WT), PHO-S probably uses the TRAIL pathway to induce apoptosis by activating the extrinsic pathway initiated by the activation of caspase 8. This mechanism is triggered when the signal for apoptosis is irreversible or insufficient. Thus, the mitochondrial pathway is recruited by the activation of caspase-3 mediated by the cleavage of Bid, a protein with a type BH3 domain [8, 9, 13]. The results obtained from this study showed that the DODAC/PHO-S increased the expression of the DR4 receptor and activated caspases 8 and 3, resulting in the release of cytochrome c, when compared to treatment with PHO-S. TRAIL family receptors (TNF-related apoptosis-inducing ligand), are often associated with death by apoptosis through the participation of DR4 and DR5 receptors [36].

The increased expression of pro-apoptotic proteins, as caspase 3 and 8, in the cells treated with DODAC/PHO-S, demonstrated that the encapsulation of PHO-S was able to potentialise its antitumor activity. Caspases are a family of cysteine proteases that serve as primary effectors during apoptosis, and have been categorised into two groups: initiator caspases (caspases 2, 8, 9 and 10) and effector caspases (caspases 3, 6 and 7). The cleavage of different substrates by caspases is mechanically responsible for the morphological and biochemical characteristics of apoptotic cell death [27, 37]. In this context, several studies have demonstrated that PHO-S increased the expression of caspase 3 and 8 and pro-apoptotic proteins [8–10, 12, 13]. Thus, in this work we demonstrated that liposome-encapsulated PHO-S was more efficient in promoting an increase in the pro-apoptotic proteins expression, as caspase 3 and cytochrome c and, consequently, trigger apoptosis.

Recent studies have shown that apoptosis triggered by TRAIL in hepatocellular carcinoma cells (Huh-7, Hep3B) was associated with the lysosomal permeabilization and consequently the increase of cathepsin B in the cytosol. The internalisation of TRAIL and its receptors can enable factors that induce permeabilization of the lysosomal membrane and culminate in the release of cathepsin B to the cytosol [38–40]. In this context, the obtained results suggest that the lysosomal pathway may be involved in the activation of cell death mediated by DODAC/PHO-S in Hepa1c1c7 cells, given that these liposomes promoted an increase in the expression of the DR4 receptor. During the validation of these results, it was observed in photomicrographs that Hepa1c1c7 cells treated with liposomes did not show any marks of intact lysosomes after 6 h of treatment, and there was also nuclear fragmentation and major changes in the cell cycle, as noted by the AO assay. Cells treated with PHO-S showed only an increase in the number of lysosomes, which demonstrates the effectiveness of the DODAC/PHO-S in inducing cytotoxicity. Cells treated only with empty liposomes DODAC also showed lysosomes with intact membranes. However, new studies should be conducted in order to confirm the participation of the lysosomal pathway as a mechanism of action of the liposomes DODAC/PHO-S.

The internalisation of the liposomes DODAC/PHO-S (0.3 and 2.0 mM), with only 3 h of treatment, was confirmed by confocal laser microscopy. It was observed that the liposomes are rapidly internalised, which makes it a great tool for antitumor therapy. After 6 h, it was still possible to observe liposomes in the cytosol of the cells. However, within this treatment time some cells already presented morphological changes corresponding to the apoptotic process.

The potential of liposomes DODAC/PHO-S in inducing cell death in Hepa1c1c7 cells, was confirmed by significant reduction in the expression of CD90 and CD44 markers. It demonstrated the ability of this formulation in the promotion of cytotoxicity in these cells. The cells treated with empty DODAC liposomes (0.3 and 2.0 mM) did not significantly reduce the expression of the marker CD90, therefore, these cells still display tumorigenic potential. Studies of patients with liver and in 91.6% of the blood samples taken CD45 and $CD90^+$ were present. The $CD44^+/CD90^+$ cells showed a more aggressive phenotype than the $CD90^+/CD44^-$ cells and formed metastatic lesions in the lungs of immunodeficient mice. The blockade of CD44 expression avoided the local and metastatic formation of tumor nodules by $CD90^+$ cells [41].

Conclusion

The set of results demonstrate that electrostatic interaction between DODAC/PHO-S and cell membrane maximises the antitumor effects mediated by PHO-S. Thus, the overall results show that the liposomal formulation DODAC/PHO-S was effective in promoting cytotoxicity in Hepa1c1c7 cells, activating the intrinsic and extrinsic pathways of programmed cell death.

Abbreviations

AFTs: Antineoplastic phospholipids; ANOVA: Analysis of variance; AO: Acridine Orange; APL: Acute promyelocytic leukemia; BH3: Bcl-2 homology 3; CD: Cluster of differentiation; Cyclin: Cell cycle protein; DiI: 1,1'-dioctadecyl-3,3,3',3'-

tetramethylindocarbocyanine perchlorate; DODAC: Dioctadecyldimethylammonium Chloride; FACS: Fluorescence-Activated Cell Sorting ; h: hours; IgG: Immunoglobulin; Min: Minutes; PBS: Phosphate buffered saline; PHO-S: Synthetic phosphoethanolamine; PI: Propidium iodide; SD: mean ± standard deviation; TNF-α: Tumor necrosis factor alpha; αMEM: Minimum Essential Medium Eagle Alpha Modification; ΔΨm: mitochondrial electrical potential

Funding

This study was funded by Sao Paulo Research Foundation, process number: 2015/02950-1.

Authors' contributions

ACLL carried out the research and wrote the first draft of the manuscript. GKVS assisted in the research work and revised the manuscript. GOC assisted in the research work and revised the manuscript. HH revised the manuscript. DAM designed the protocol and revised the manuscript. All authors read and approved the final manuscript.

Competing interest

The authors declare that they have no competing interests.

Author details

[1]Department of Biochemistry and Biophysics, Butantan Institute, 1500, Vital Brasil Avenue, Sao Paulo 05503-900, Brazil. [2]Department of Medical Sciences, Medical School, University of Sao Paulo, Sao Paulo, Brazil. [3]Department of Biochemistry, Institute of Chemistry, University of Sao Paulo, Sao Paulo, Brazil. [4]Department of Chemistry and Molecular Physics, University of Sao Paulo, Sao Carlos, Brazil.

References

1. Vanneman M, Dranoff G. Combining immunotherapy and targeted therapies in cancer treatment. Nat Rev Cancer. 2012;12:237–51.
2. Siegel R, Ma J, Zou Z, Jemal A. Cancer statistics, 2014. CA Cancer J Clin. 2014;64:9–29.
3. Ríos-Marco P, Marco C, Gálvez X, Jiménez-López JM, Carrasco MP. Alkylphospholipids: an update on molecular mechanisms and clinical relevance. Biochim Biophys Acta. 2017;1859:1657–67.
4. Ríos-Marco P, Ríos A, Jiménez-López JM, Carrasco MP, Marco C. Cholesterol homeostasis and autophagic flux in perifosine-treated human hepatoblastoma HepG2 and glioblastoma U-87 MG cell lines. Biochem Pharmacol. 2015;96:10–9.
5. van Blitterswijk WJ, Verheij M. Anticancer alkylphospholipids. Mechanisms of action, cellular sensitivity and resistance, and clinical prospects. Curr Pharm Des. 2008;14:2061–74.
6. van Blitterswijk WJ, Verheij M. Anticancer mechanisms and clinical application of alkylphospholipids. Biochim Biophys Acta 2013; 1831:663–674.
7. Marco C, Ríos-Marco P, Jiménez-López JM, Segovia JL, Carrasco MP. Antitumoral alkylphospholipids alter cell lipid metabolism. Anti Cancer Agents Med Chem. 2014;14:545–58.
8. Ferreira AK, Meneguelo R, Neto SC, Chierice GO, Maria DA. Synthetic Phosphoethanolamine induces apoptosis through Caspase-3 pathway by decreasing expression of Bax/bad protein and changes cell cycle in melanoma. J Cancer Sci Ther. 2011;3:053–9.
9. Ferreira AK, Meneguelo R, Pereira A, Mendonça Filho O, Chierice GO, Maria DA. Anticancer effects of synthetic phosphoethanolamine on Ehrlich ascites tumor: an experimental study. Anticancer Res. 2012;32: 95–104.
10. Ferreira AK, Freitas VM, Levy D, Ruiz JL, Bydlowski SP, Rici RE, Filho OM, Chierice GO, Maria DA. Anti-angiogenic and anti-metastatic activity of synthetic phosphoethanolamine. PLoS One. 2013;8:e57937.
11. Ferreira AK, Santana-Lemos BA, Rego EM, Filho OM, Chierice GO, Maria DA. Synthetic phosphoethanolamine has in vitro and in vivo anti-leukemia effects. Br J Cancer. 2013;109:2819–28.
12. Ferreira AK, Meneguelo R, Pereira A, Filho OM, Chierice GO, Maria DA. Synthetic phosphoethanolamine induces cell cycle arrest and apoptosis in human breast cancer MCF-7 cells through the mitochondrial pathway. Biomed Pharmacother. 2013;67:481–7.
13. Ferreira AK, Meneguelo R, Marques FL, Radin A, Filho OM, Neto SC, Chierice GO, Maria DA. Synthetic phosphoethanolamine a precursor of membrane phospholipids reduce tumor growth in mice bearing melanoma B16-F10 and in vitro induce apoptosis and arrest in G2/M phase. Biomed Pharmacother. 2012;66:541–8.
14. Luna ACL, D'Agostino LG, Saraiva GKV, Claro Neto S, Cuccovia IM, Maria DA. Potential antitumoral of the novel DODAC/PHO-S liposome. In: Méndez-Vilas ADJ, editor. Microscopy: advances in scientific research and education. Badajoz: Formatex press; 2014. p. 557–63.
15. Luna AC, Saraiva GK, Filho OM, Chierice GO, Neto SC, Cuccovia IM, Maria DA. Potential antitumor activity of novel DODAC/PHO-S liposomes. Int J Nanomedicine. 2016;11:1577–91.
16. Luna ACL, Santos Filho JRA, Hesse H, Neto SC, Chierice GO, Maria DA. Modulation of pro-apoptotic effects and mitochondrial potential on B16F10 cells by DODAC/PHO-S liposomes. BMC Res Notes. 2018;11:126.
17. Tacar O, Sriamornsak P, Dass CR. Doxorubicin. An update on anticancer molecular action, toxicity and novel drug delivery systems. J Pharm Pharmacol. 2013;65:157–70.
18. Stathopoulos GP, Boulikas T. Lipoplatin formulation review article. J Drug Deliv. 2012;2012:581363.
19. Rueda Domínguez A, Olmos Hidalgo D, Viciana Garrido R, Torres Sánchez E. Liposomal cytarabine (DepoCyte) for the treatment of neoplastic meningitis. Clin Transl Oncol. 2005;7:232–8.
20. Rosenthal E, Poizot-Martin I, Saint-Marc T, Spano JP, Cacoub P, Group DS. Phase IV study of liposomal daunorubicin (DaunoXome) in AIDS-related Kaposi sarcoma. Am J Clin Oncol. 2002;25:57–9.
21. Ulrich AS. Biophysical aspects of using liposomes as delivery vehicles. Biosci Rep. 2002;22:129–50.
22. Oliveira AC, Martens TF, Raemdonck K, Adati RD, Feitosa E, Botelho C, Gomes AC, Braeckmans K, Real Oliveira ME. Dioctadecyldimethylammonium:monoolein nanocarriers for efficient in vitro gene silencing. ACS Appl Mater Interfaces. 2014; 6:6977–89.
23. Carmona-Ribeiro AM. Bilayer-forming synthetic lipids: drugs or carriers? Curr Med Chem. 2003;10:2425–46.
24. Löbrich M, Jeggo PA. The impact of a negligent G2/M checkpoint on genomic instability and cancer induction. Nat Rev Cancer. 2007;7:861–9.
25. Dijkstra KK, Cristophe B, Boonstra J. Evasion of G1 checkpoints in Cancer. In: Checkpoint controls and targets in Cancer therapy. New York: human press; 2009. p. 3–26.
26. Poon IK, Hulett MD, Parish CR. Molecular mechanisms of late apoptotic/ necrotic cell clearance. Cell Death Differ. 2010;17:381–97.
27. Elmore S. Apoptosis: a review of programmed cell death. Toxicol Pathol. 2007;35:495–516.
28. Ferreira AK: Alquil fosfatado sintético precursor dos fosfolipídios de membrana celular com potencial efeito antitumoral e apoptótico em modelos de tumores experimentais. Universidade de São Paulo, São Paulo; 2013. Programa de Fisiopatologia Experimental; 2013 http://www.teses.usp.br/teses/disponiveis/5/5160/tde-20052013-145336/pt-br.php. Accessed 5 June 2017.
29. Ferreira DS, Lopes SC, Franco MS, Oliveira MC. pH-sensitive liposomes for drug delivery in cancer treatment. Ther Deliv. 2013;4:1099–123.
30. Taylor WR, Stark GR. Regulation of the G2/M transition by p53. Oncogene. 2001;20:1803–15.
31. Kuang JWR. Mechanisms of G2 phase arrest in DNA damage-induced checkpoint response. In: zH S, editor. Checkpoint controls and targets in cancer therapy. New York: Humana Press; 2010. p. 37–52.
32. Engeland K. Cell cycle arrest through indirect transcriptional repression by p53: I have a DREAM. Cell Death Differ. 2018;25:114–32.
33. Xiao-Feng Le RCB. p27Kip1 as a Biomarker and Target for Treatment of Cancer. In: zH S, editor. Checkpoint controls and targets in cancer therapy. New York: Humana Press; 2010. p. 215–33.
34. Alao JP. The regulation of cyclin D1 degradation: roles in cancer development and the potential for therapeutic invention. Mol Cancer. 2007;6:24.
35. Lee BS, Kang SU, Hwang HS, Kim YS, Sung ES, Shin YS, Lim YC, Kim CH. An agonistic antibody to human death receptor 4 induces apoptotic cell death in head and neck cancer cells through mitochondrial ROS generation. Cancer Lett. 2012;322:45–57.
36. Nagane M, Shimizu S, Mori E, Kataoka S, Shiokawa Y. Predominant antitumor effects by fully human anti-TRAIL-receptor 2 (DR5) monoclonal antibodies in

human glioma cells in vitro and in vivo. Neuro-Oncology. 2010;12:687–700.
37. Yuan J, Najafov A, Py BF. Roles of caspases in necrotic cell death. Cell. 2016; 167:1693–704.
38. Werneburg NW, Guicciardi ME, Bronk SF, Kaufmann SH, Gores GJ. Tumor necrosis factor-related apoptosis-inducing ligand activates a lysosomal pathway of apoptosis that is regulated by Bcl-2 proteins. J Biol Chem. 2007; 282:28960–70.
39. Guicciardi ME, Bronk SF, Werneburg NW, Gores GJ. cFLIPL prevents TRAIL-induced apoptosis of hepatocellular carcinoma cells by inhibiting the lysosomal pathway of apoptosis. Am J Physiol Gastrointest Liver Physiol. 2007;292:1337–46.
40. Guicciardi ME, Werneburg NW, Bronk SF, Franke A, Yagita H, Thomas G, Gores GJ. Cellular inhibitor of apoptosis (cIAP)-mediated ubiquitination of phosphofurin acidic cluster sorting protein 2 (PACS-2) negatively regulates tumor necrosis factor-related apoptosis-inducing ligand (TRAIL) cytotoxicity. PLoS One 2014; 9:e92124.
41. Yang ZF, Ho DW, Ng MN, Lau CK, Yu WC, Ngai P, Chu PW, Lam CT, Poon RT, Fan ST. Significance of CD90+ cancer stem cells in human liver cancer. Cancer Cell. 2008;13:153–66.

3

Classification and prediction of toxicity of chemicals using an automated phenotypic profiling of *Caenorhabditis elegans*

Shan Gao[1,5†], Weiyang Chen[3†], Yingxin Zeng[1], Haiming Jing[1], Nan Zhang[1], Matthew Flavel[4], Markandeya Jois[4], Jing-Dong J. Han[2], Bo Xian[2*] and Guojun Li[1,5*]

Abstract

Background: Traditional toxicological studies have relied heavily on various animal models to understand the effect of various compounds in a biological context. Considering the great cost, complexity and time involved in experiments using higher order organisms. Researchers have been exploring alternative models that avoid these disadvantages. One example of such a model is the nematode *Caenorhabditis elegans*. There are some advantages of *C. elegans*, such as small size, short life cycle, well defined genome, ease of maintenance and efficient reproduction.

Methods: As these benefits allow large scale studies to be initiated with relative ease, the problem of how to efficiently capture, organize and analyze the resulting large volumes of data must be addressed. We have developed a new method for quantitative screening of chemicals using *C. elegans*. 33 features were identified for each chemical treatment.

Results: The compounds with different toxicities were shown to alter the phenotypes of *C. elegans* in distinct and detectable patterns. We found that phenotypic profiling revealed conserved functions to classify and predict the toxicity of different chemicals.

Conclusions: Our results demonstrate the power of phenotypic profiling in *C. elegans* under different chemical environments.

Keywords: *C. elegans*, Chemicals, Toxicity, Image analysis, Phenotype

Background

With the global development of science and technology, new chemicals are continuously synthesized and used in industrial production and human life. The need to assess the toxic effects of these chemicals on the environment, in addition to understanding the potential health impacts of these chemicals is an urgent and ongoing issue. The scientific community must take responsibility for this task and continue to re-evaluate the best methods for measuring toxicity. Assessment of the potential toxicity of chemicals is crucial for the determination of safe levels of exposure to humans. Routine methods to evaluate potential toxicity of a vast array of chemicals on humans have employed rodent animal models. Whilst very useful, this strategy is time consuming and very expensive, in addition to the ethical concerns it raises. The importance of these studies which have incorporated mammalian model animals cannot be denied as they have been integral in establishing the Globally Harmonized System (GHS) of Classification and Labeling of Chemicals [1], in addition to countless breakthrough studies. However, if the field of

* Correspondence: xianbo@picb.ac.cn; ligj@bjcdc.org
[†]Equal contributors
[2]Key Laboratory of Computational Biology, CAS Center for Excellence in Molecular Cell Science, Collaborative Innovation Center for Genetics and Developmental Biology, Chinese Academy of Sciences-Max Planck Partner Institute for Computational Biology, Shanghai Institutes for Biological Sciences, Chinese Academy of Sciences, 320 Yue Yang Road, Shanghai 200031, China
[1]Beijing Key Laboratory of Diagnostic and Traceability Technologies for Food Poisoning, Beijing Center for Disease Prevention and Control/Beijing Center of Preventive Medicine Research, Beijing 100013, China
Full list of author information is available at the end of the article

toxicology is to progress, it will first need to develop more progressive models of testing for toxicity.

Toxicity tests often utilize large numbers of rodents, and is extremely expensive and time consuming, which has resulted in a backlog of over 10,000 novel compounds that are urgently awaiting further testing [2]. Current in vivo rodent models of toxicity can no longer meet the increasing requirements of stringent toxicological evaluation. Clearly, there is a critical need to develop more rapid and efficient techniques of toxicity screening. In vivo studies in non-rodent model organisms provide a novel platform for screening a large number of chemicals for toxicity [3–10].

In recent years, the nematode *Caenorhabditis elegans* has been utilized in toxicity testing as an alternative in vivo animal model. *C. elegans* is a free-living nematode that lives mainly in the liquid phase of soils. Since it was first developed for use as a model animal in 1965 [11], it has been widely employed in various fields such as developmental biology, aging, neurobiology, etc. [12, 13]. Its widespread application is mainly due to a range of advantageous traits. Some key examples include a relatively short life and reproduction cycle, plus an extremely small body size which contribute to making it very easy and cheap to maintain large populations in the laboratory. A trait particularly useful for toxicological studies is the ease with which a vast array of *C. elegans* phenotypes are able to be quantified before and after the administration of a treatment. This includes the ability to define changes to both internal and external phenotypes due to the transparent nature of the body. In addition, *C. elegans* is the first multicellular organism whose genome has been fully sequenced. Within this genome of 20,000 genes, about 40% of *C. elegans* genes are homologous with mammals [14]. Of this homology, many integral metabolic pathways share distinct similarity between worm and mammal. From a toxicological perspective this makes *C. elegans* a very interesting prospect as it allows the metabolic effects of compounds to be incorporated into studies. This was demonstrated by our previous study [15] that showed the correlation of *C. elegans* LC50s (24 h) to rat LD50s is similar to the relationship between mouse and rat LD50s ($r = 0.879$), and was stronger than the correlation of NHK cell median inhibition concentrations (IC50)s vs. rat LD50s ($r = 0.844$). These results indicate that *C. elegans* may be a valuable model for predicting chemicals' acute toxicity in rodents.

In recent years, several studies have tried to incorporate worms into toxicological screening studies [2, 4, 6]. These studies demonstrated that *C. elegans* is able to be utilized as a model to test the effects of chemicals toxicities in vivo. However, these studies relied on the COPAS system, which is a very expensive piece of equipment that is difficult for researchers to access. In addition, COPAS system only provides a limited range of data on features such as worm length, width and fluorescence intensity. This method of processing does not meet the throughput demands of the modern chemical research community.

The need to develop and improve automated strategies to gather phenotypic data is essential to furthering our understanding of biological functions in relation to chemical compounds. Recently, there are some interesting methods emerging that can be used to quantify phenotypes observed in *C. elegans* [16, 17]. These are predominantly designed for analyzing the images from nematode growth medium (NGM) agar plate experiments and determining the expressed phenotypes. However, they mainly focus on the quantification of only four phenotypes and the images are required to be extremely uniform in nature for the image processing to be completed accurately. This requirement for strict uniformity becomes an issue when the range of conditions that *C. elegans* are housed in is considered. For example, in a situation such as a 384 well plate experiment, and the well boundary and some uneven illumination problems would impact the results of current automated methods.

A cheap, fast and quantitative method for toxicity screening in *C. elegans* would benefit the field immensely. Here we report a method that combines a liquid toxic culturing system utilizing a 384-well plate with an automated microscope stage for image acquisition. We have utilized this method to classify automatically the toxicity of 19 compounds, under multiple concentrations according to specifically identified features of worms' phenotypes. By analyzing our defined phenotypes of worms exposed to chemicals at different concentrations, we found that phenotype profiling revealed stable functions to classify and predict the toxicity of different chemicals.

Results

Phenotypes profiling

From the large amount of image data processed, 33 distinct phenotypes were quantified (methods) across the 19 chemical compounds and at each of the 3 time points (0, 12 and 24 h), respectively. All compounds tested were shown to influence phenotype at certain time points and concentrations. In the interest of keeping this article succinct, of the 19 compounds tested, only the phenotype profile observed during treatment with lactic acid has been presented graphically to demonstrate the accuracy and depth of data collection that is possible using our methodology (Fig. 1). Extra examples of phenotypic profile data have been included in the Additional file 1: Figures S1 and S2. These

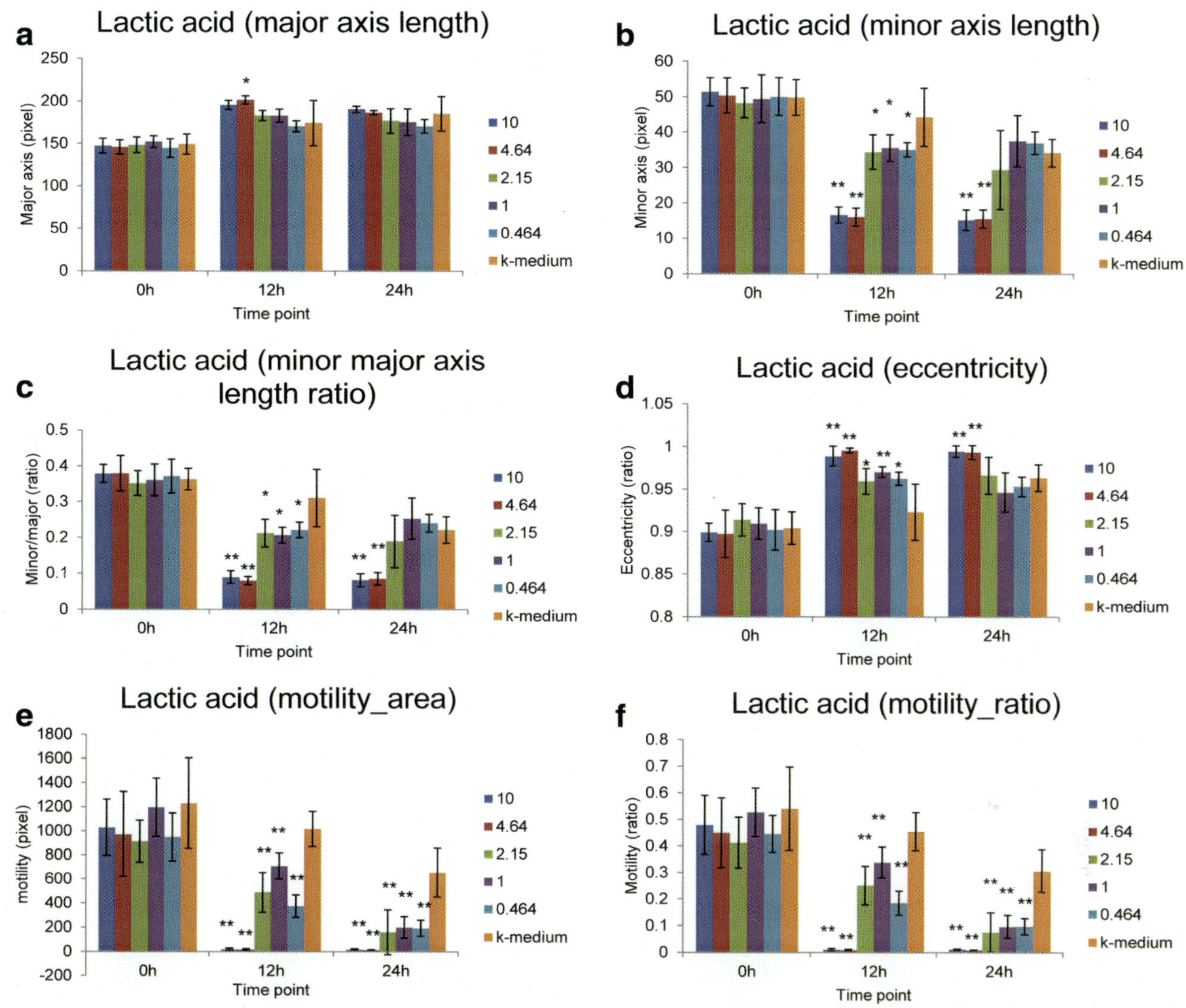

Fig. 1 Phenotypes of lactic acid under different concentrations. (**a**) Major axis length. (**b**) Minor axis length. (**c**) Minor major axis length ratio. (**d**) Eccentricity. (**e**) Motility (the moved area). (**f**) Motility (the moved area/worm size). * and ** denote unpaired two-sided Student's *t*-Test *p*-value < 0.05 and 0.01, respectively. Bar plots shows the average quantification for each phenotype on single worms. Error bars denote +/− standard deviation (SD). Concentration unit: mg/ml

supplementary figures show similar patterns to lactic acid, description of results will be limited to those observed in lactic acid.

The worms died quickly and became straighter and less curved as the chemical concentration increased. There were no significant differences between treatments and control (k-medium) for all phenotypes at the initial time point of the experiment (0 h). After 12 h of exposure to a given chemical dosage, the worms showed a range of phenotypic variations among different concentrations and control groups. For example, the major axis length (see phenotypes description) increased in all experiments. This was demonstrated by a gradient trend from higher to lower chemical concentrations (Fig. 1a). The trend is more significant in minor axis length. At 12 h, the Student's *t*-Test shows that all experiments with 5 different concentrations are significantly different from control (Fig. 1b, *p*-value = 0.02121, 0.02889, 0.01905, 1.919e-05 and 2.501e-05 for 5 concentrations from lower to higher concentrations). Our findings for the 24 h 50% lethal concentration (LC50 as determined by previous studies [15]) there is already a clear distinction between higher and lower concentrations at the time point of 12 h. Two concentrations (10 mg/ml and 4.64 mg/ml) which are both higher than the LC50, show lower level of minor axis length compared with the other three concentrations (Fig. 1b).

The ratio between single worms' minor and major axis length shows similar patterns as minor axis length (Fig. 1c), the higher values indicate the worms would be observed as more bent. The eccentricity shows the opposite pattern, because lower eccentricity values indicate the worm would appear more bent (Fig. 1d).

In terms of quantified worm motility, both the worm moved area and the moved ratio (moved area/worm size) show similar patterns (Fig. 1e, f). At the 0 h time point, there were no significant differences among worms across all experiments. As time passed, the motility of worms in control k-medium conditions showed a stable decrease. At 12 h, all the treatments showed very significant differences compared with control at that time point. We found there are drastic differences in motility for the concentrations higher or lower than the LC50 (2.79 mg/ml for Lactic Acid, see Additional file 1: Table S1.) at 24 h. Two concentrations (10 mg/ml and 4. 64 mg/ml) which are both higher than the LC50 for Lactic Acid show lower levels of motility compared with the other three concentrations. This suggests that worms died quickly and became less motile as the chemical concentration increased.

These results indicate that the phenotypes we quantified are valid potential markers for chemical toxicity identification in *C. elegans*.

Phenotypes classification

To visualize the various phenotypes and treatments' relationships among each other, all features were z-score normalized within each feature. This allowed clustering across different phenotypes and experiments using the BIC-SK algorithm [18], which is an adaptive cluster method. This method can automatically determine the optimal number of samples and feature clusters based on the Bayesian Information Criterion. With this approach, we were able to detect and visualize the various phenotypes at the same time. We find that all 33 quantified phenotypes were able to be classified accurately into distinct groupings. This grouping was also possible at each of the time points measured (0 h, 12 h and 24 h) (Fig. 2).

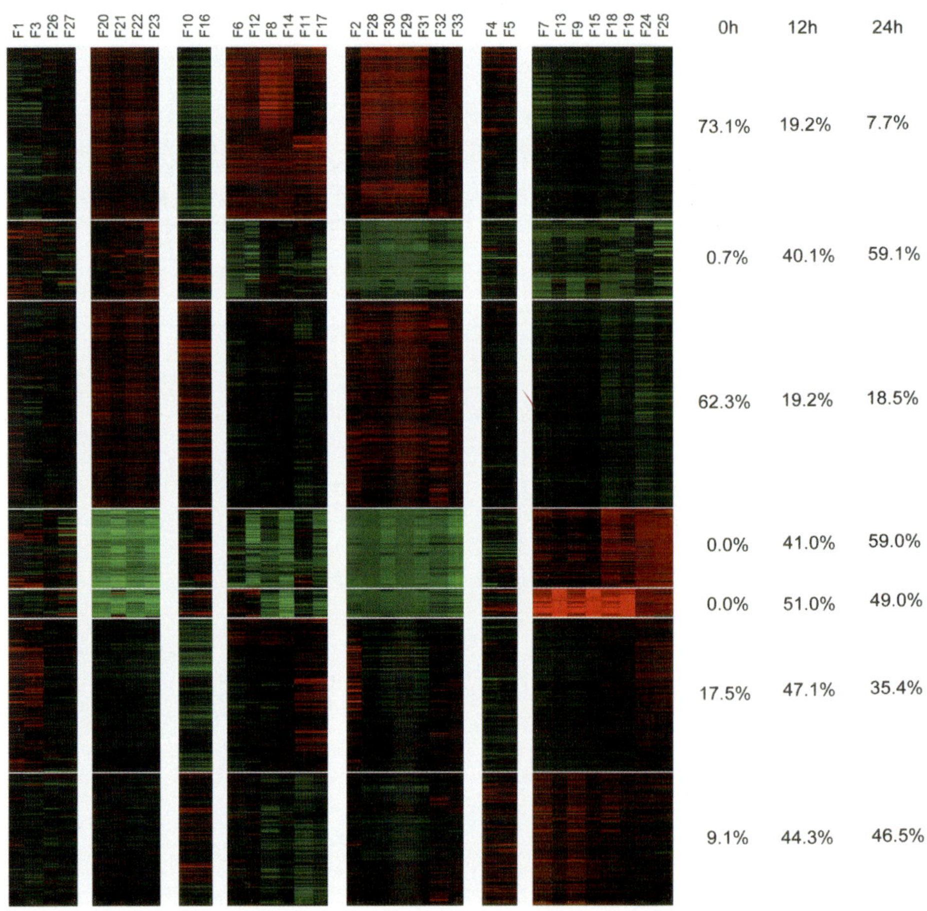

Fig. 2 Cluster on all phenotypes of all experiments (3 time points). Each column is one feature (See Methods for a detailed name and description of each feature), each row is an experiment. The proportions of each time point's experiments (in each sub-cluster) are listed in the right of heat map

We found that at 0 h experiments have different patterns compared with later time points. The features which are based on all single worms or only live single worms respectively, show similar patterns compared with other features. It indicates that it is more similar within the same measurement than different measurements.

Among these features worm length, perimeter, major axis length and eccentricity have similar patterns. Survival rate and worm motility are clustered together. Most of the 0 h data shows higher survival rate and motility compared to later time points. This is in addition to later time points showing greater length and perimeter measurements compared to 0 h observations.

In the cluster of one time point (12 h, Fig. 3a), we can see that higher concentration experiments (and therefore a higher degree of toxicity) have lower survival rate and motility than lower concentration experiments (lower toxicity). In the higher concentration experiments lower levels of minor axis length, minor/major axis length, higher levels of major axis length and eccentricity are all observed. In contrast, the lower concentration experiments show higher levels of minor axis length and minor/major axis length, lower levels of major axis length and eccentricity.

The 24-h results (Fig. 3b) are comparable to the 12-h results. It was observed that higher concentration experiments (high toxicity) have lower survival

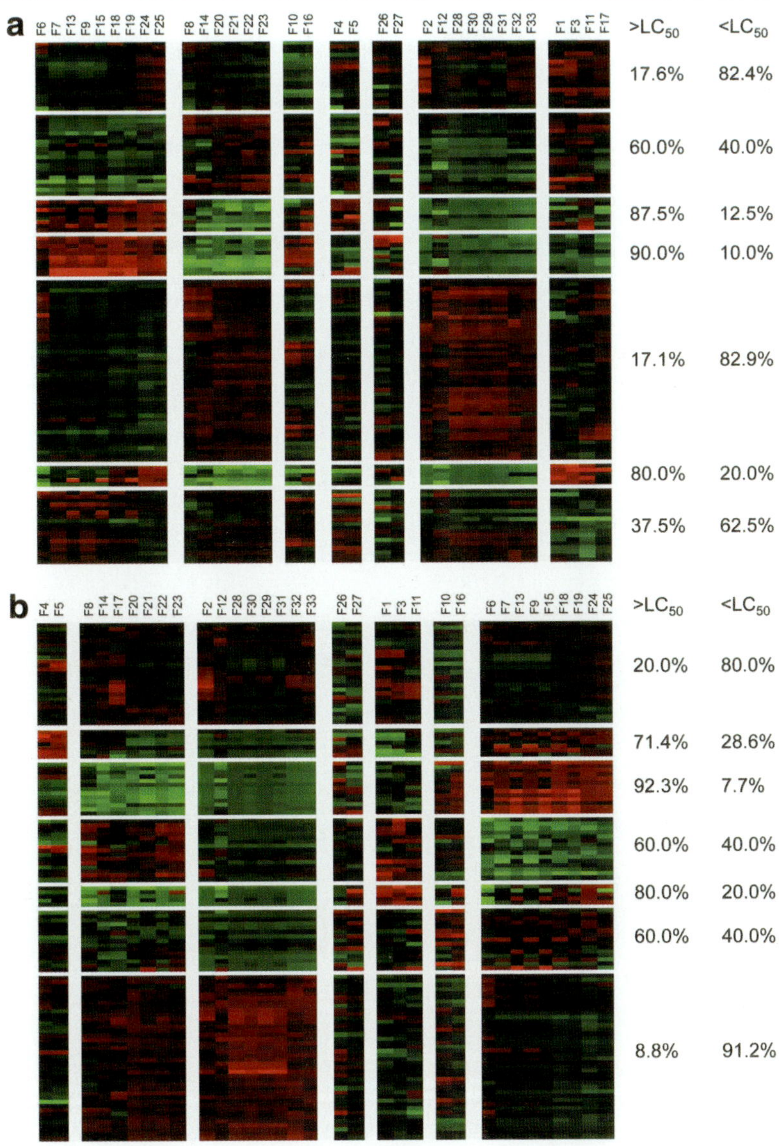

Fig. 3 **a** Cluster on the mean profile of 8 repeats, one time point (12 h). **b** Cluster on the mean profile of 8 repeats, one time point (24 h). Each column is one feature (we show the detailed name of each feature in Methods). The proportions of different concentrations' experiments (in each sub-cluster) are listed in the right of heat map. LC_{50} is 50% lethal concentration

rate and motility than lower concentration experiments (lower toxicity).

From the clustering results it appears worms died quicker, were less motile, straightened and therefore showed less body curvature as the concentration increased.

The main trends under these phenotypes

To detect whether time, concentration and toxicity associated principle components underlie these quantified phenotypes; we performed Principle Component Analysis (PCA). The advantage of using PCA is that it can summarize all phenotypes to several main components.

Firstly, PCA results on the mean profile of 8 repeats (3 time points, Fig. 4a) show some main components to distinguish different time points. Three different colors represent the experiments under different time points. We found that the first component can distinguish 0 h time point from the other two time points. The increase of the third component shows that there is one change trend from 12-h to 24-h.

The PCA on the phenotypes observed at the 12-h time point and the concentration of each experiment was ranked according to relative order for each chemical compound (Fig. 4b). We found the experiments with

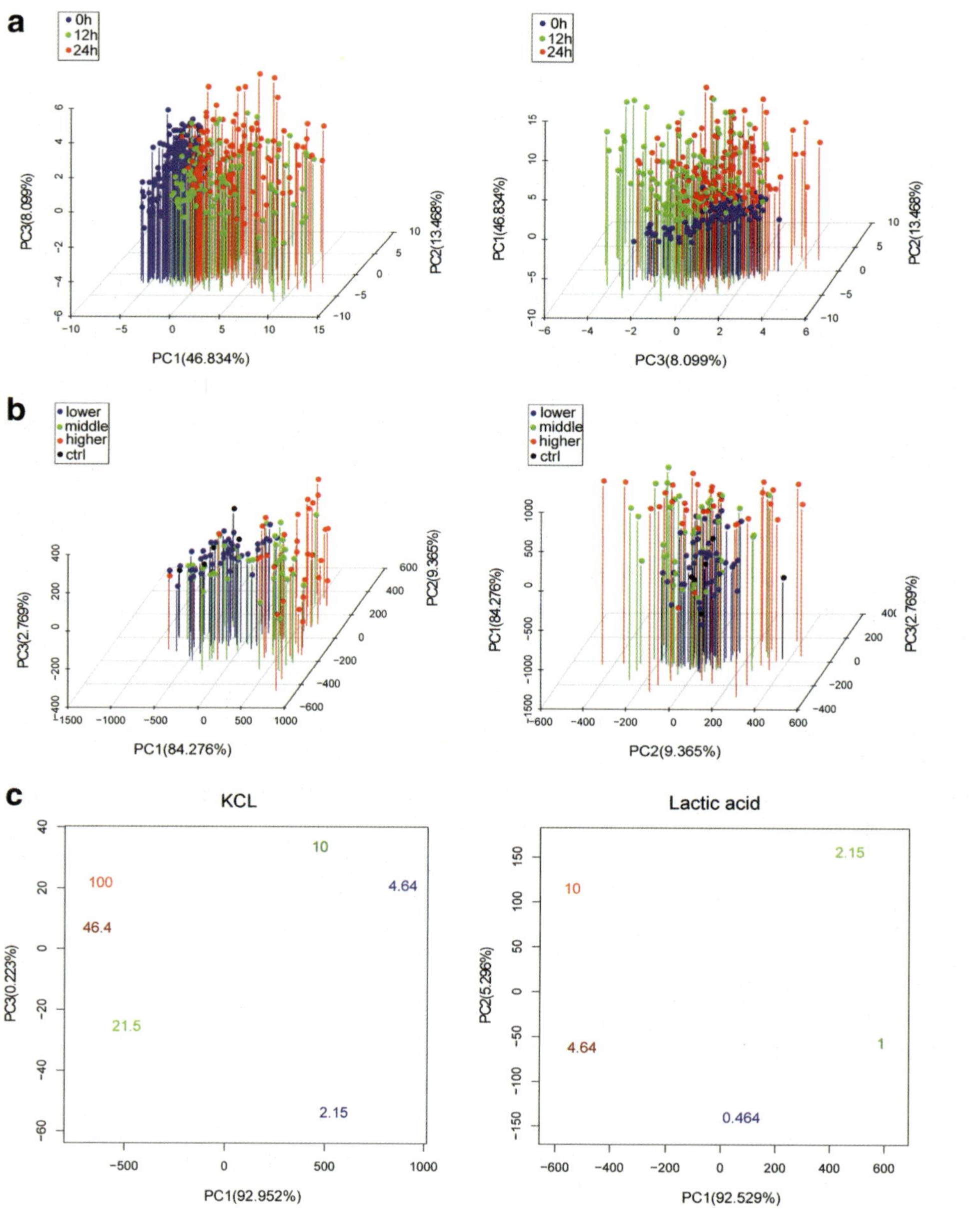

Fig. 4 a PCA on the mean profile of 8 repeats (3 time points). **b** PCA on the mean profile of 8 repeats (12 h). **c** PCA on the mean profile of single chemical compound (KCL and Lactic acid of 12 h), the value with different color is the concentration of different experiment

lower concentrations were similar to the control, whilst being drastically different from the middle and higher concentration experiments for the first main component. In the second main component, most of higher concentration experiments show marked differences from lower and middle concentrations.

From the single chemicals PCA result (Fig. 4c), we found the first main component shows considerable differences between higher and lower concentrations. Concentrations can be separated into two parts from left to right. Each part also has some difference from upper to lower shown by the third main component.

Toxicity prediction

In general, 50% lethal dosage (LD50) and 50% lethal time (LT50) are used to describe the chemicals' toxicity in rodents (rat/mouse) model in vivo. The correlation of *C. elegans* LC50s (24 h) vs. rat LD50s is equal to the correlation of mouse vs. rat LD50s ($r = 0.879$), and is stronger than the correlation of NHK cell median inhibition concentrations (IC50)s vs. rat LD50s ($r = 0.844$), which indicate that *C. elegans* may be a valuable model for predicting chemicals' acute toxicity in rodents [15].

The 24-h 50% lethal concentration is derived from previous independent experiment results [15]. Using the methods already described we found that the quantified phenotypes correlate closely with chemical concentration. Then we used these quantified phenotypes to predict if the concentration is under/above the 24 h 50% lethal concentration (LC50). For each chemical, we classified different concentration experiments to 2 classes by the concentration higher or lower than 24 h at 50% lethal concentration (LC50).

Then for each chemical we applied support vector machine (SVM) to do the 5-fold cross validation prediction tests only by the phenotypes quantified for 12 h experiments.

Results show that we can distinguish if the experiment's concentration is higher or lower than the 24 h LC50 with a high degree of accuracy only by the quantified features from the time point of 12 h (Table 1). The classifier has an average accuracy of 91.2% by 5-fold cross-validation among all chemical experiments. These results indicate that we can assess the acute toxicity only based on the phenotypes quantified for 12-h experiments. This is a useful tool which will shorten the experimental observation time in the future.

Discussion

Large numbers of novel chemicals are produced annually and current models of toxicological studies are unable to meet the demands of modern scientific research and industry.

Studies utilizing lower order in vivo model organisms (such as *C. elegans*) have the opportunity to make a large contribution to the efficient risk assessment of chemicals toxicity. The development of better computational tools outlined in this article provides an opportunity for the creation of faster toxicity screening. Testing with the nematode *C. elegans* offers a unique approach that possesses advantages over cell-based in vitro assays, which are rapid but may not be physiologically relevant in the context of a whole organism. Mammalian studies, which may better represent human responses to toxic chemicals are slow and expensive and therefore the model we present could act as a useful complementary tool to mammalian trials [4].

Our model allows the growth of nematodes exposed to water soluble compounds of known toxicity to be assessed by a screening system in combination with automated phenotype profiling methods. Modeling results were used to rank order the test compounds according to their toxicity as determined by the nematode assay. This method proved useful in identifying very toxic compounds from compounds with moderate and low toxicity.

It is clear from our results that this new method of quantitative screening on 384 well plates for chemicals can detect the degree that toxicities alter the phenotypes of *C. elegans*. We found that phenotype profiling

Table 1 The cross validation prediction performance

Compound name	Cross-validation accuracy (%)	Compound name	Cross-validation accuracy (%)
Potassium chloride	93.3	Diquat dibromide	77.4
Cadmium chloride	78.6	Glycerol	96.3
Atropine sulfate	88.9	Sodium dichromate	90
Lactic acid	100	Manganese chloride	90.6
Anhydrous two propanol	98	Sodium chloride	82.5
Ethanol	90.6	Trichloroacetic acid	100
Ethylene glycol	94.6	Citric Acid	81.8
Sodium Fluoride	100	Orthoboric acid	98.2
Sodium Hypochlorite	89.6		

revealed conserved functions to classify and predict the toxicity of different chemicals using the nematode *C. elegans* as an in vivo model organism.

In this study, 19 standard chemicals acute toxicity tests based on the 384-well plate were conducted and the movie for each well was acquired automatically by digital camera (methods). About 100GB image data was processed by our program written in MATLAB to quantify 33 phenotypic features. From these 33 phenotypic features we performed Principle Component Analysis (PCA) to get several main components and classify them to several patterns according to 3 treatment times and several treatment concentrations, respectively. Results showed that the chemical toxicity could be predicted by the treatment concentration higher or lower than the 50% lethal concentration (LC50) at 24 h.

Our previous study [15] showed that the correlation of *C. elegans* LC50s (24 h) to rat LD50s is similar to the relationship between mouse and rat LD50s ($r = 0.879$), and was stronger than the correlation of NHK cell median inhibition concentrations (IC50)s vs. rat LD50s ($r = 0.844$). Here, the automatically quantified phenotypes show significant difference among different concentrations, it is similar to the previously study [15]. We also show that the automatically quantified phenotypes can be used to distinguish the chemical concentration is under/above the 24 h 50% lethal concentration (LC50 is determined by previous studies [15]).

In summary, the methodology presented using the rapid toxicity screening and evaluation system of non-rodents correlates with the traditional animal acute toxic effects and could be used to assess new chemicals or complex mixed chemicals. The scientific principle of replacement, reduction and refinement in regards to animal ethics is the central motivator of this research as it is hoped that these findings reduce the pressure currently on higher order animals to be relied upon for toxicology research. This study is significant improvement to current system methods which use *C. elegans* to pre-screen the toxicity of new chemicals. Our method can quantify a number of phenotypes that are difficult to calculate manually, such as the worm motility, worm size, width and gray intensity. When compared with traditional methods, our method delivers a more efficient and automated collection of data. This is possible mainly due to the advancements we have made in terms of automation, level of throughput and quality of data.

Conclusions

This new method provides a powerful tool to researchers to understand the effects of chemical compounds. By combining a 384-well liquid toxic culturing plate with an automated image acquisition microscope system, we demonstrated quantitative screening of 19 chemical compounds using *C. elegans*. 33 worms' features were identified for each chemical treatment. The results demonstrate the compounds with different toxicities were shown to alter the phenotypes of *C. elegans* in distinct and detectable patterns. Moreover, the power of phenotypic profiling in *C. elegans* revealed conserved functions to classify and predict the toxicity of different chemicals. The development of better computational tools outlined in this article provides an opportunity for the creation of faster toxicity screening in *C. elegans*; therefore, the model we present could act as a useful complementary tool to mammalian trials.

Methods

Chemicals and concentrations

The 19 standard chemicals used (at the third to sixth levels of the GHS) and their respective concentrations are listed in Additional file 1: Table S1. The four to eight gradient concentration levels were designed according to Horn method. All chemicals were obtained from Sigma-Aldrich Company, and diluted by K-medium (32 mM KCL and 52 mM NaCL in 1 L ultrapure water). We used K-medium as control to compare the alterations caused by the toxicants.

Strains

All nematodes used were wild-type N2, originally obtained from the Caenorhabditis Genetics Center (CGC). Synchronized L1 worms were obtained by bleaching and then put on the nematode growth medium (NGM) plates seeded with *Escherichia coli* OP50 and kept at 20 °C. Worms at L4 stage were washed off the plate by K-medium and added into 384-well plates, each well containing ~ 20 worms. These synchronized, L4 stage worms were then ready for chemical treatment. Within 24 h of the chemical treatment experiment, we did not add bacteria to 384-well plates.

Chemical treatment

Nineteen standard chemicals were administered at concentrations a third to sixth levels of the GHS for 384-well plate acute toxicity experiment tests. According to the *C. elegans* LC50 of chemicals, worms were exposed to chemicals at a single dosage of either; 10 mg/ml, 4.64 mg/ml, 2.15 mg/ml. 1 mg/ml, 0.464 mg/ml, 0.215 mg/ml, 0.1 mg/ml or 0.0464 mg/ml. Eight parallel tests were then carried out for the specific points of the concentration gradients for each chemical. Worms were then observed with each specific chemical condition in K-medium for 0, 12 h, or 24 h.

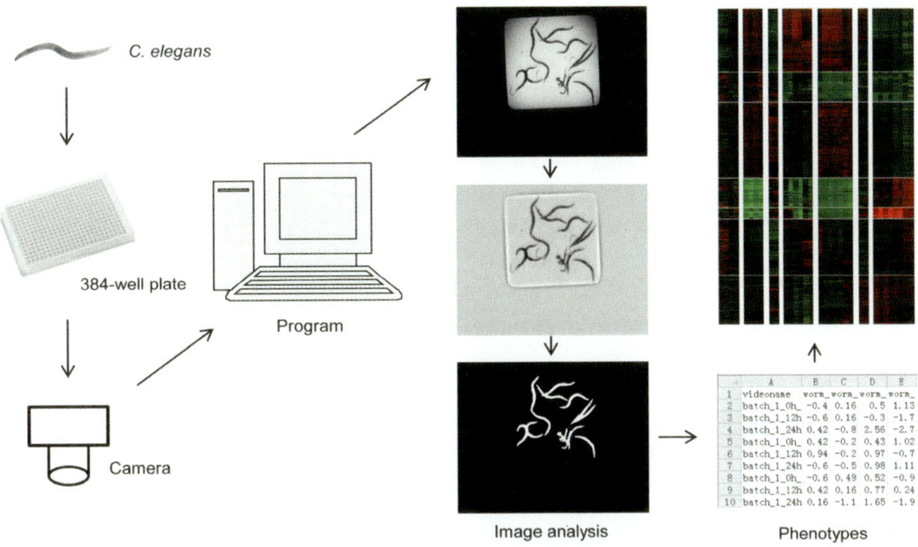

Fig. 5 Method design. Mainly there are three steps in our method: (1) culture worms in 384-well plates with different chemicals and take video for each well; (2) process these videos, get each frame, reduce the uneven illumination, segment the image, and then quantify phenotypes for worms under each chemical treatment; (3) characterize different chemicals and their toxicities based on these quantified phenotypes

Video capture

Images and video was captured at three distinct time points; 0, 12 and 24 h after noxious compounds were added. All images and videos were collected using a digital camera attached to a Nikon SMZ1000 automatic microscope.

Image processing

A program for image processing and analysis, automated worm recognition followed by automated features quantification was written using MATLAB software. The major procedures are described and shown in Fig. 5. After solving the uneven illumination problem [19], we were able to distinguish worms from the background of the well and quantify their features.

Experimental setting

Following chemical treatments, we programmed the automated acquisition of video (7 frames per second for 2 s) for each well at three time points (0 h, 12 h and 24 h) by digital camera (methods). This resulted in a tremendous amount of image data (~100GB) automatically collected through all of the tests (3 plates of 384-well plate treatments). Next, we used the image processing method we developed using MATLAB to quantify valuable phenotypic features to ultimately analyze and to classify the toxicity effect on worms.

Phenotypes definition and computation

Defined features include survival number related features, gray intensity related features, worm size, curvature, and motility related features:

F1. The single worm number in this experiment;
F2. The alive single worm number;
F3. The worms' disperse situation, which is computed by the ratio between single worm number and total worm number;
F4. The average distance of all worms' centroid;
F5. The standard deviation of distance among all worms' centroid;
F6. The single worms' average size;
F7. The single worms' average length;
F8. The single worms' average width;
F9. The single worms' average perimeter;
F10. The single worms' average gray intensity;
F11. The single worms' standard deviation of gray intensity;
F12. The alive single worms' average size;
F13. The alive single worms' average length;
F14. The alive single worms' average width;
F15. The alive single worms' average perimeter;
F16. The alive single worms' average gray intensity;
F17. The alive single worms' standard deviation of gray intensity;
F18. The single worms' major axis length, which is computed by the major axis of the ellipse that has the same normalized second central moments as the worm body region;
F19. The alive single worms' major axis length;
F20. The single worms' minor axis length, which is computed by the minor axis of the ellipse that has the same normalized second central moments as the worm body region;
F21. The alive single worms' minor axis length;

F22. The ratio between single worms' minor and major axis length, more close to 1 more close to one circle;
F23. The ratio between alive single worms' minor and major axis length;
F24. The single worms' eccentricity, which is the ratio of the distance between the foci of the ellipse and its major axis length, the value is between 0 and 1, an ellipse whose eccentricity is 0 is actually a circle, while an ellipse whose eccentricity is 1 is a line segment. It is computed from the outer ellipse of the worm's body region. We used it to show the worm body bent degree, because lower eccentricity values indicate the worm would appear more bent;
F25. The alive single worms' eccentricity;
F26. The single worms' orientation, which is the angle between the x-axis and the major axis of the ellipse;
F27. The alive single worms' orientation;
F28. The single worms' motility, which is the moved area;
F29. The single worms' motility, which is computed by the moved area/worm size;
F30. The alive single worms' motility, which is the moved area;
F31. The alive single worms' motility, which is computed by the moved area/worm size;
F32. The smoothed live worm number;
F33. Survival rate.

Statistical analysis

Results are presented as means ± SD. For the comparisons of phenotypes between each concentration treatment and control (k-medium) at each time point, we analyzed the data using unpaired two-sided Student's *t*-Test in R. P values < 0.05 were considered statistically significant. The R packages were used for PCA [20] and SVM [21] analysis.

Funding
This work was supported by "National Natural Science Foundation of China" Grant (# 31401025, 81273108, 81641184), "The capital health research and development of special" Project in Beijing (# 2011-1013-03), Opening fund of "Beijing Key Laboratory of Enviromental Toxicology" (# 2015HJDL03), grants from the Chinese Academy of Sciences (CAS; YZ201243 to J.-D.J.H), and Natural Science Foundation of Shandong Province, China (ZR2017BF041).

Authors' contributions
GL conceived the project. GL, BX, JDJH, SG and YZ designed the experiments. BX and WC designed computational analyses. BX, SG, YZ, HJ and NZ implemented the experiments. BX and WC implemented computational analyses. SG, GL, BX, WC, MF, MJ and JDJH wrote the paper. All authors read and approved the final manuscript.

Competing interests
The authors declare that they have no competing interests.

Author details
[1]Beijing Key Laboratory of Diagnostic and Traceability Technologies for Food Poisoning, Beijing Center for Disease Prevention and Control/Beijing Center of Preventive Medicine Research, Beijing 100013, China. [2]Key Laboratory of Computational Biology, CAS Center for Excellence in Molecular Cell Science, Collaborative Innovation Center for Genetics and Developmental Biology, Chinese Academy of Sciences-Max Planck Partner Institute for Computational Biology, Shanghai Institutes for Biological Sciences, Chinese Academy of Sciences, 320 Yue Yang Road, Shanghai 200031, China. [3]College of Information, Qilu University of Technology (Shandong Academy of Sciences), Jinan 250353, China. [4]School of Life Sciences, La Trobe University, Bundoora, Vic 3083, Australia. [5]Beijing Key Laboratory of Environmental Toxicology, School of Public Health, Capital Medical University, Beijing 100069, China.

References

1. Becker RA, Borgert CJ, Webb S, Ansell J, Amundson S, Portier CJ, Goldberg A, Bruner LH, Rowan A, Curren RD, et al. Report of an ISRTP workshop: progress and barriers to incorporating alternative toxicological methods in the U.S. Regul Toxicol Pharmacol. 2006;46(1):18–22.
2. Boyd WA, McBride SJ, Freedman JH. Effects of genetic mutations and chemical exposures on Caenorhabditis elegans feeding: evaluation of a novel, high-throughput screening assay. PLoS One. 2007;2(12):e1259.
3. Anderson GL, Cole RD, Williams PL. Assessing behavioral toxicity with Caenorhabditis elegans. Environ Toxicol Chem. 2004;23(5):1235–40.
4. Boyd WA, McBride SJ, Rice JR, Snyder DW, Freedman JH. A high-throughput method for assessing chemical toxicity using a Caenorhabditis elegans reproduction assay. Toxicol Appl Pharmacol. 2010;245(2):153–9.
5. Yang R, Rui Q, Kong L, Zhang N, Li Y, Wang X, Tao J, Tian P, Ma Y, Wei J, et al. Metallothioneins act downstream of insulin signaling to regulate toxicity of outdoor fine particulate matter (PM2.5) during spring festival in Beijing in nematode Caenorhabditis elegans. Toxicol Res. 2016;5(4):1097–105.
6. Boyd WA, Williams PL. Comparison of the sensitivity of three nematode species to copper and their utility in aquatic and soil toxicity tests. Environ Toxicol Chem. 2003;22(11):2768–74.
7. Dengg M, van Meel JC. Caenorhabditis elegans as model system for rapid toxicity assessment of pharmaceutical compounds. J Pharmacol Toxicol Methods. 2004;50(3):209–14.
8. Schouest K, Zitova A, Spillane C, Papkovsky D. Toxicological assessment of chemicals using Caenorhabditis elegans and optical oxygen respirometry. Environ Toxicol Chem. 2009;28(4):791–9.
9. Sprando RL, Olejnik N, Cinar HN, Ferguson M. A method to rank order water soluble compounds according to their toxicity using Caenorhabditis elegans, a complex object parametric analyzer and sorter, and axenic liquid media. Food Chem Toxicol. 2009;47(4):722–8.
10. Wang D, Xing X. Assessment of locomotion behavioral defects induced by acute toxicity from heavy metal exposure in nematode Caenorhabditis elegans. J Environ Sci (China). 2008;20(9):1132–7.
11. Brenner S. The genetics of Caenorhabditis elegans. Genetics. 1974;77(1):71–94.
12. Xian B, Shen J, Chen W, Sun N, Qiao N, Jiang D, Yu T, Men Y, Han Z, Pang Y, et al. WormFarm: a quantitative control and measurement device toward automated *Caenorhabditis elegans* aging analysis. Aging sCell. 2013;12(3): 398–409.
13. Jin C, Li J, Green CD, Yu X, Tang X, Han D, Xian B, Wang D, Huang X, Cao X, et al. Histone demethylase UTX-1 regulates *C. elegans* life span by targeting the insulin/IGF-1 signaling pathway. Cell Metab. 2011;14(2):161–72.
14. Sternberg PW. Working in the post-genomic C. elegans world. Cell. 2001; 105(2):173–6.
15. Li Y, Gao S, Jing H, Qi L, Ning J, Tan Z, Yang K, Zhao C, Ma L, Li G. Correlation of chemical acute toxicity between the nematode and the rodent. Toxicol Res. 2013;2(6):403–12.
16. Jung SK, Aleman-Meza B, Riepe C, Zhong W. QuantWorm: a comprehensive software package for Caenorhabditis elegans phenotypic assays. PLoS One. 2014;9(1):e84830.
17. Mathew MD, Mathew ND, Ebert PR. WormScan: a technique for high-throughput phenotypic analysis of Caenorhabditis elegans. PLoS One. 2012; 7(3):e33483.
18. Zhang W, Liu Y, Sun N, Wang D, Boyd-Kirkup J, Dou X, Han JD. Integrating genomic, epigenomic, and transcriptomic features reveals modular signatures underlying poor prognosis in ovarian cancer. Cell Rep. 2013;4(3): 542–53.

4

Absolute oral bioavailability and disposition kinetics of puerarin in female rats

Tosapol Anukunwithaya[1], Pilaslak Poo[1], Natthaphon Hunsakunachai[1], Ratchanee Rodsiri[1], Suchinda Malaivijitnond[2,3] and Phisit Khemawoot[1,3*]

Abstract

Background: *Pueraria candollei var. mirifica* is a medicinal plant that is promoted as a "Champion Product" by the Government of Thailand. This plant has been reported to relieve postmenopausal symptoms, prevent and reverse bone loss, inhibit the growth of breast cancer, and alleviate cardiovascular diseases in preclinical and clinical studies. However, there is little information on the oral bioavailability and tissue distribution of puerarin with respect to its pharmacodynamic activities. Therefore, the aim of this study was to determine the pharmacokinetics of puerarin, including absorption, distribution, metabolism, and elimination, in rats. Moreover, this is the first study to examine the tissue distribution of puerarin in the hippocampus, femur, tibia, and mammary gland.

Methods: Adult female rats were administered puerarin at 1 mg/kg intravenously or 5 and 10 mg/kg orally. Blood, tissue, urine, and feces were collected and analyzed by liquid chromatography–tandem mass spectrometry.

Results: Puerarin reached a maximum concentration in the blood of 140–230 μg/L within 1 h of oral dosing, and had an absolute oral bioavailability of approximately 7%. Following intravenous administration, puerarin was widely distributed in several tissues, including the hippocampus, heart, lung, stomach, liver, mammary gland, kidney, spleen, femur, and tibia. Approximately 50% of the intravenous dose was excreted as glucuronide metabolites via the urinary route.

Conclusions: The absolute oral bioavailability of puerarin was approximately 7% at doses of 5 and 10 mg/kg. Puerarin was widely distributed to several organs related to the diseases of aging, including the hippocampus, femur, tibia, and mammary gland. Glucuronides were the major metabolites of puerarin and were mainly excreted in the urine. These results are useful for the development of puerarin and *Pueraria candollei var. mirifica* as phytopharmaceutical products.

Keywords: Pharmacokinetics, Puerarin, Rats

Background

Puerarin (7,4′-dihydroxy-8-C-glucosylisoflavone, Fig. 1a) is one of the major active phytoestrogens in *Pueraria candollei var. mirifica*, an endemic Thai plant of the family Leguminosae. This plant has been reported to relieve postmenopausal symptoms [1, 2], prevent and reverse bone loss [3–5], inhibit the growth of breast cancer [6], and alleviate cardiovascular diseases [7–9] in preclinical and clinical studies. There is also increasing evidence of a beneficial role of puerarin and *Pueraria candollei var. mirifica* in the prevention of and therapy for diseases of aging such as osteoporosis, neurodegeneration, diabetes, and cardiovascular disease [5, 8, 10, 11]. However, there is little information on the oral bioavailability and tissue distribution of puerarin, with respect to its pharmacodynamic activities.

Puerarin has an aqueous solubility of 0.46 mg/mL [12] and a partition coefficient of 1.95. In pharmacokinetics studies using oral dosing in animal models, puerarin reaches a maximum plasma concentration (C_{max}) in 0.45–5.00 h and has an absorption half-life of 0.80–1.00 h after dosing [13–17]. Distribution of puerarin to the liver, spleen, kidney, lung, heart, and brain occurs within

* Correspondence: phisit.k@chula.ac.th
[1]Department of Pharmacology and Physiology, Faculty of Pharmaceutical Sciences, Chulalongkorn University, Bangkok 10330, Thailand
[3]Preclinical Pharmacokinetics and Interspecies Scaling for Drug Development Research Unit, Chulalongkorn University, Bangkok 10330, Thailand
Full list of author information is available at the end of the article

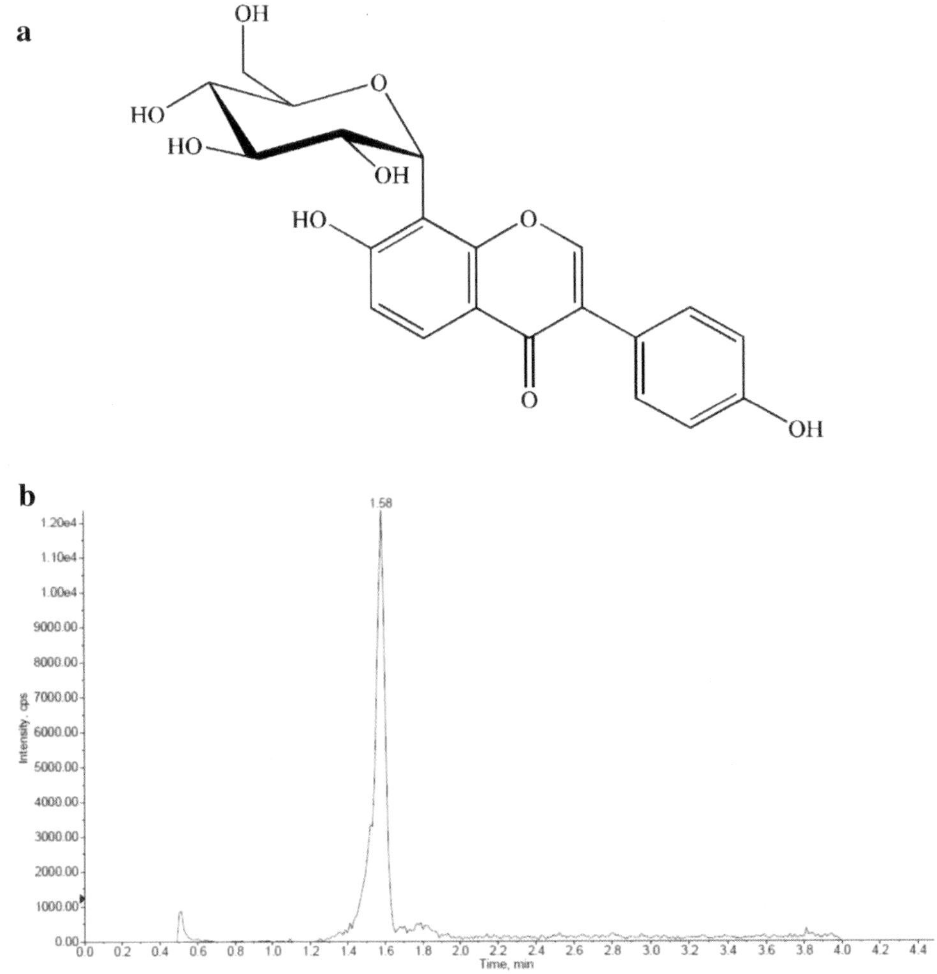

Fig. 1 **a** Structure of puerarin. **b** LC-MS/MS chromatogram of 10 ng/mL puerarin spiked in rat plasma

approximately 1 h following a single oral administration at 20 mg/kg. In the tested organs, C_{max} was reached at 2.5 h post-treatment [18]. Prasain et al. (2004) suggested that puerarin undergoes hepatic phase I metabolism via a cytochrome P450 enzyme and proposed that the metabolite was dihydroxylated puerarin [19]. However, Luo et al. reported that the major metabolic pathway of puerarin following intravenous administration is phase II glucuronidation to give puerarin-7-O-glucuronide and puerarin-4′-O-glucuronide, through glucuronidation at 7-OH and 4′-OH [20]. Excretion of puerarin has been proposed to occur mainly via the urinary system, with negligible amounts of puerarin and its glucuronide metabolites excreted via the hepatobiliary route [21].

The aim of this study was to determine the pharmacokinetics and absorption, distribution, metabolism, and elimination (ADME) properties of puerarin in the rat. The tissue distribution of puerarin in the hippocampus, femur and tibia, and mammary gland was investigated, based on the pharmacodynamic effects reported for neurodegenerative disease, osteoporosis, and breast cancer, respectively. The puerarin doses used in this study were based on estrogenic effects in the reproductive organs [22] and bone [23] in female rats. A liquid chromatography-tandem mass spectrometry (LC-MS/MS) method was developed to determine the puerarin level in biological samples following the administration of puerarin at 1 mg/kg intravenously (IV) and 5 and 10 mg/kg orally (PO) in healthy female rats.

Methods

Chemicals

Puerarin powder for the pharmacokinetic study was supplied by Dr. Suchinda Malaivijitnond, Department of Biology, Faculty of Science, Chulalongkorn University, Thailand. Glycyrrhetinic acid was purchased from Wako Pure Chemical Industries, Japan. β-Glucuronidase from *Escherichia coli* (Type VII-A) was purchased from Sigma-Aldrich (St. Louis, MO, USA). Isoflurane was purchased from Minrad International, Inc. (Orchard Park, NY, USA).

Puerarin (analytical grade) was purchased from Pure Chemistry Scientific, Inc. (Burlington, MA, USA). Dimethyl sulfoxide (DMSO) was purchased from Sigma-Aldrich.

Animals

Twenty-eight female Sprague-Dawley rats aged 12 weeks old were obtained from the National Laboratory Animal Centre, Mahidol University, Thailand. The animals were housed for 4 weeks at 25 ± 2 °C under a 12-h light/dark cycle with free access to food and water. The rats were moved to a metabolic cage one day before the experiment and kept in this cage for 72 h after the experiment. Rats weighing 300–400 g were used in pharmacokinetic studies. The sample size was four animals per experiment, based on OECD Guidelines for the Testing of Chemicals [24] and USFDA Guidance for Bioavailability and Bioequivalence Studies [25]. Experiments complied with the animal protocol guidelines of the Faculty of Pharmaceutical Sciences, Chulalongkorn University (approval number: 15–33-001, approval date: April 22, 2015).

Pharmacokinetic studies

Twelve rats were divided into three groups of four animals each for the administration of puerarin at the doses of 1 mg/kg IV, and 5 and 10 mg/kg PO. The puerarin solution for administration to animals was prepared in 20% DMSO in normal saline. Rats were anaesthetized with isoflurane by the chamber induction method before IV administration and blood collection to reduce pain and injury. Blood samples (300 μL) taken from the lateral tail vein at 0, 0.083 (5 min), 0.25, 0.50, 1, 2, 4, 8, 12, and 24 h after administration were collected in heparinized tubes, centrifuged at 1500×*g* for 10 min, and kept at − 20 °C for further analysis. Urine and feces were collected in three periods, 0–24, 24–48, and 48–72 h, following IV and PO administration and stored at − 20 °C.

To examine the tissue distribution of puerarin, another 16 rats received IV administration of 1 mg/kg puerarin and were subsequently sacrificed by cervical dislocation at 5 min and 1, 2, and 4 h after administration. Major organs including the brain (particularly hippocampus), liver, kidney, spleen, stomach, heart, lung, small intestine, mammary gland, femur, and tibia were collected, rinsed with ice-cold saline, and stored at − 20 °C until analysis.

Determination of plasma creatinine, aspartate transminase (AST), and alanine transaminase (ALT) levels at 0 and 24 h after dosing were made by the Professional Laboratory Management Corp Co., Ltd. (accredited ISO 15189) with the automated analyzer Cobas® 6000 (F. Hoffmann-La Roche, Ltd., Basel, Switzerland) using an enzymatic method (chemiluminescence) for creatinine quantitation and a kinetic method (according to the International Federation of Clinical Chemistry and Laboratory Medicine recommendations) for AST and ALT quantification to evaluate pre- and post-dose kidney and liver function.

Sample preparation

All biological samples were extracted by the protein precipitation method as previously described [26], with minor modifications. Briefly, 50 μL of plasma and urine samples were mixed directly with 200 μL of methanol containing 10 ng of glycyrrhetinic acid as the internal standard, whereas 50 mg of tissue and feces samples were chopped into small pieces, homogenized, and mixed in 200 μL methanol containing the internal standard. Then, samples were centrifuged for 10 min at 5000×*g* to precipitate proteins. A volume of 150 μL of the supernatant was transferred into a sample vial and 10 μL of the supernatant was injected into the LC-MS/MS system. For the femur and tibia, decalcified bones were prepared by soaking in 10% EDTA solution for 2 weeks, and the bones were chopped and processed in a similar manner to the other tissues [27].

For the determination of glucuronide conjugates of puerarin, 50 μL of plasma or urine was added to 50 μL of 0.1 M potassium phosphate buffer (pH 6.8) containing 1500 units of β-glucuronidase. The mixture was incubated at 37 °C for 15 min, and the reaction was stopped by adding 400 μL of methanol containing 20 ng of glycyrrhetinic acid as the internal standard. The mixture was centrifuged at 5000×*g* for 10 min, the supernatant was collected, and 10 μL of the supernatant was injected into the LC-MS/MS system. For solid samples, 50 mg of tissue and feces were chopped into small pieces, homogenized, and mixed in 50 μL of 0.1 M potassium phosphate buffer (pH 6.8) containing 1500 units of β-glucuronidase. These mixtures were then processed in a similar manner to the plasma and urine mixtures.

LC-MS/MS analysis

The analytical method was performed according to Li et al. [13] and Prasain et al. [19], with minor modifications to allow for the analysis of puerarin with good linearity, precision, and high accuracy. An Ultra LC 100 (Eksigent, Canada) system was equipped with a Synergi Fusion-RP C18 column as the stationary phase (Phenomenex, Torrance, CA, USA). The LC system used 100% methanol and 0.2% formic acid in water (pH 2.5) with a flow rate of 0.5 mL/min. The mobile phase was rinsed with 10% methanol for 0.5 min, increased to 90% methanol from 1.5 to 3.5 min, and then decreased to 10% methanol from 4 to 4.5 min. The retention time of puerarin was 1.58 min, and that of the internal standard was 2.09 min. Detection was conducted in negative ionization mode by monitoring precursor ion to product ion transitions with mass to charge ratios of 415/295 (puerarin) and 469/409 (glycyrrhetinic acid). The chromatograms were essentially free from endogenous interference (Fig. 1b). The limit of detection was estimated to be 0.16 μg/L, with a signal-to-noise ratio of 5. Calibration curves were constructed by the analysis of puerarin at 200, 100, 50, 25, 12.5, 6.25, 3.12, and 1.56 μg/L, with good correlation coefficients ($R^2 > 0.99$) for all matrices.

Data analysis

Pharmacokinetic parameters were calculated by non-compartmental analysis using PK Solutions 2.0 software (Summit Research Services, Montrose, CO, USA). The acquired results are reported as the mean ± standard deviation with a significance level of 0.05. Statistical analysis was performed by non-parametric tests using SPSS ver. 16 (SPSS, Chicago, IL, USA). The following pharmacokinetic parameters are reported: maximum plasma concentration (C_{max}), time to maximum plasma concentration (T_{max}), area under the plasma concentration-time curve from zero to the last observed time (AUC_{0-t}) or infinity ($AUC_{0-\infty}$), volume of distribution (Vd), total clearance (CL), mean residence time (MRT), and elimination half-life ($T_{1/2}$). The absolute oral bioavailability of puerarin was calculated as ($AUC_{po}/dose_{po}$) divided by ($AUC_{iv}/dose_{iv}$). The tissue-to-plasma ratio of puerarin was calculated from the tissue concentration divided by the plasma concentration in each rat at the same time point. The percentage recovery of puerarin was calculated by dividing the puerarin level found in urine or feces by the administered dose.

Results

Animal tolerability

Female rats that received puerarin at 1 mg/kg IV or 5 or 10 mg/kg PO had a normal physiological and morphological appearance pre-dose and 24 h post-dose (Table 1). Liver biochemical profiles showed no significant changes in AST and ALT levels pre-dose and 24 h post-dose in all rats, although slight decreases in AST and ALT were observed at 24 h. In the kidney biochemical profiles, blood creatinine showed no significant changes from pre-dose to post-dose following IV or PO administration of puerarin.

Plasma concentration-time profile and oral bioavailability

Mean plasma concentration-time profiles of puerarin following IV and PO administration in rats are shown in Fig. 2. Pharmacokinetic parameters of puerarin from non-compartmental analysis are summarized in Table 2. Following IV administration, the concentration declined rapidly and puerarin was cleared from the systemic circulation within 4 h, with C_{max}, 621.96 ± 170.72 μg/L; $AUC_{0-\infty}$, 292.23 ± 108.93 μg.h/L; Vd, 1.16 ± 0.56 L/kg; CL, 5.43 ± 2.66 L/h/kg; MRT, 0.24 ± 0.06 h; and $T_{1/2}$, 0.21 ± 0.06 h. Following PO administration of 5 and 10 mg/kg, the maximum concentration was reached within 1 h, and puerarin decreased to below the detection limit at 4–8 h post-dosing. C_{max} ranged from 140 to 230 μg/L and $AUC_{0-\infty}$ was 110–210 μg.h/L. The $T_{1/2}$ of puerarin ranged from 0.86–0.88 h, with no significant difference between doses. The absolute oral bioavailability of puerarin was approximately 7% at doses of 5 and 10 mg/kg.

Tissue distribution

Tissue-to-plasma ratios of puerarin in rats at 5 min and 1, 2, and 4 h after administration of puerarin at 1 mg/kg IV are shown in Fig. 3. At 5 min, the highest levels of puerarin were found in the kidney, followed by the lung, stomach, liver, mammary gland, and small intestine, all of which are highly perfused organs. The ratios in these organs were 10–100 at 5 min after IV dosing, and decreased to 1–10 at 1 h after dosing. At 2 h, puerarin was detected in most organs, including the hippocampus, heart, lung, stomach, liver, mammary gland, kidney, spleen, and tibia, but not in the femur. The ratios in most organs continued to decrease up to 4 h, but there was an increase in poorly perfused tissue such as bone. Interestingly, the tissue-to-plasma ratio of puerarin in the hippocampus and brain increased significantly and continuously from 5 min to 1, 2, and 4 h after dosing.

Metabolism

Mean plasma concentration-time profiles for puerarin glucuronide after administration of puerarin in rats are shown in Fig. 4. The $AUC_{puerarin\ glucuronide}/AUC_{puerarin}$ ratio was approximately 7 after IV dosing. The

Table 1 Physical appearance and plasma biochemical profiles before (0 h) and 24 h after administration of puerarin at 1 mg/kg IV and 5 and 10 mg/kg PO

Parameters	Administration of Puerarin					
	1 mg/kg IV		5 mg/kg PO		10 mg/kg PO	
	0 h	24 h	0 h	24 h	0 h	24 h
Physical appearance	Normal	Normal	Normal	Normal	Normal	Normal
AST (U/L)	61.67 ± 9.36	55.83 ± 2.90	57.67 ± 5.10	56.00 ± 6.84	55.60 ± 7.96	57.40 ± 5.12
ALT (U/L)	27.00 ± 26.18	11.20 ± 16.22	26.33 ± 18.78	13.17 ± 17.40	25.00 ± 13.92	12.17 ± 9.76
Creatinine (mg/dL)	0.20 ± 0.00	0.20 ± 0.00	0.21 ± 0.02	0.21 ± 0.02	0.21 ± 0.10	0.21 ± 0.08

Data are presented as mean ± S.D. ($n = 4$). $^{*}p < 0.05$, 0 h vs. 24 h

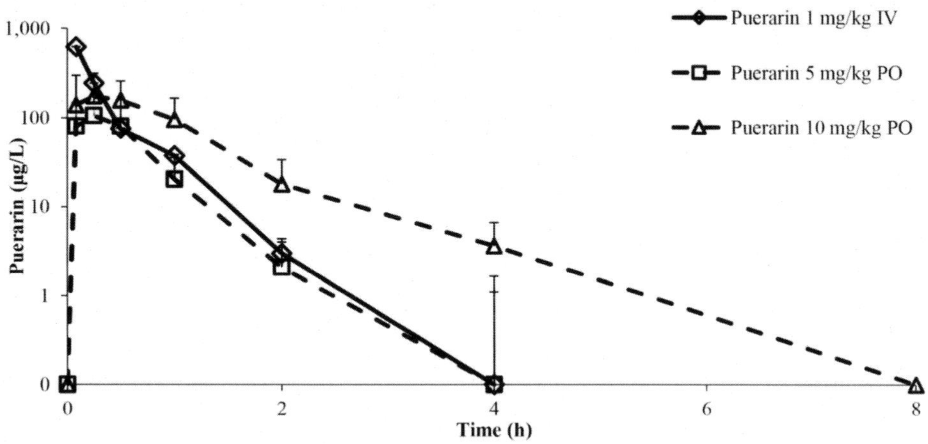

Fig. 2 Plasma concentration-time profiles of puerarin after administration of puerarin at 1 mg/kg IV (◊), 5 mg/kg PO (□) and 10 mg/kg PO (Δ). Data are shown as mean ± S.D. ($n = 4$)

concentration of puerarin glucuronide was higher than unchanged puerarin by about 30 times following PO administration of 10 mg/kg puerarin. Regarding the tissue distribution, a high ratio of glucuronide metabolites was found in most tissues at 5 min after IV dosing. The tissue-to-plasma ratio of glucuronide metabolites decreased over time in most tissues, except for the brain and bone. However, the ratios of unchanged puerarin and puerarin glucuronide in the mammary gland remained at comparable levels for 4 h after dosing.

Excretion

The percentage recovery of unchanged puerarin and puerarin glucuronide in rat urine or feces after administration are shown in Table 3. Unchanged puerarin was present in urine and feces at less than 1% following PO and IV dosing. In the IV group, puerarin glucuronide was mainly excreted in urine in the first 24 h; this accounted for almost 50% of the administered dose. Approximately 15% of puerarin glucuronide was excreted in the feces within 72 h after IV dosing. At 10 mg/kg PO, approximately 10% of puerarin glucuronide was found in the urine in the

Table 2 Pharmacokinetic parameters of puerarin and puerarin glucuronide after administration of puerarin at 1 mg/kg IV and 5 and 10 mg/kg PO

Parameters	Administration of Puerarin		
	1 mg/kg IV	5 mg/kg PO	10 mg/kg PO
Puerarin			
C_{max} (μg/L)	621.96 ± 170.72	145.47 ± 84.11	228.00 ± 164.84
T_{max} (h)	N/A	0.19 ± 0.09	0.33 ± 0.21
$AUC_{0\text{-}t}$ (μg.h/L)	291.47 ± 108.05	109.45 ± 60.61	204.57 ± 157.47
$AUC_{0\text{-}\infty}$ (μg.h/L)	292.23 ± 108.93	109.58 ± 60.55	212.20 ± 157.50
Vd (L/kg)	1.16 ± 0.56	101.59 ± 119.57	90.17 ± 18.28
MRT (h)	0.24 ± 0.06	0.67 ± 0.21	0.88 ± 0.20
$T_{1/2}$ (h)	0.21 ± 0.06	0.88 ± 0.49	0.86 ± 56.31
CL (L/h/kg)	5.43 ± 2.66	65.06 ± 52.75	74.79 ± 0.17
Absolute bioavailability (%)	100	7.50	7.29
Puerarin glucuronide			
$AUC_{0\text{-}t}$ (μg.h/L)	2133.20	73.30	7207.40
$AUC_{puerarin\ glucuronide}$ / $AUC_{puerarin}$	7.35	0.67	34.65

C_{max}, maximum concentration, T_{max}, time to reach maximum concentration, $AUC_{0\text{-}t}$, area under concentration-time curve from time 0 to last observed time, $AUC_{0\text{-}\infty}$, area under concentration-time curve from time 0 to infinity, Vd, apparent volume of distribution, MRT, mean resident time, $T_{1/2}$, half-life, CL, apparent clearance, N/A, not available

Data are presented as mean ± S.D. ($n = 4$). *$p < 0.05$ between oral doses

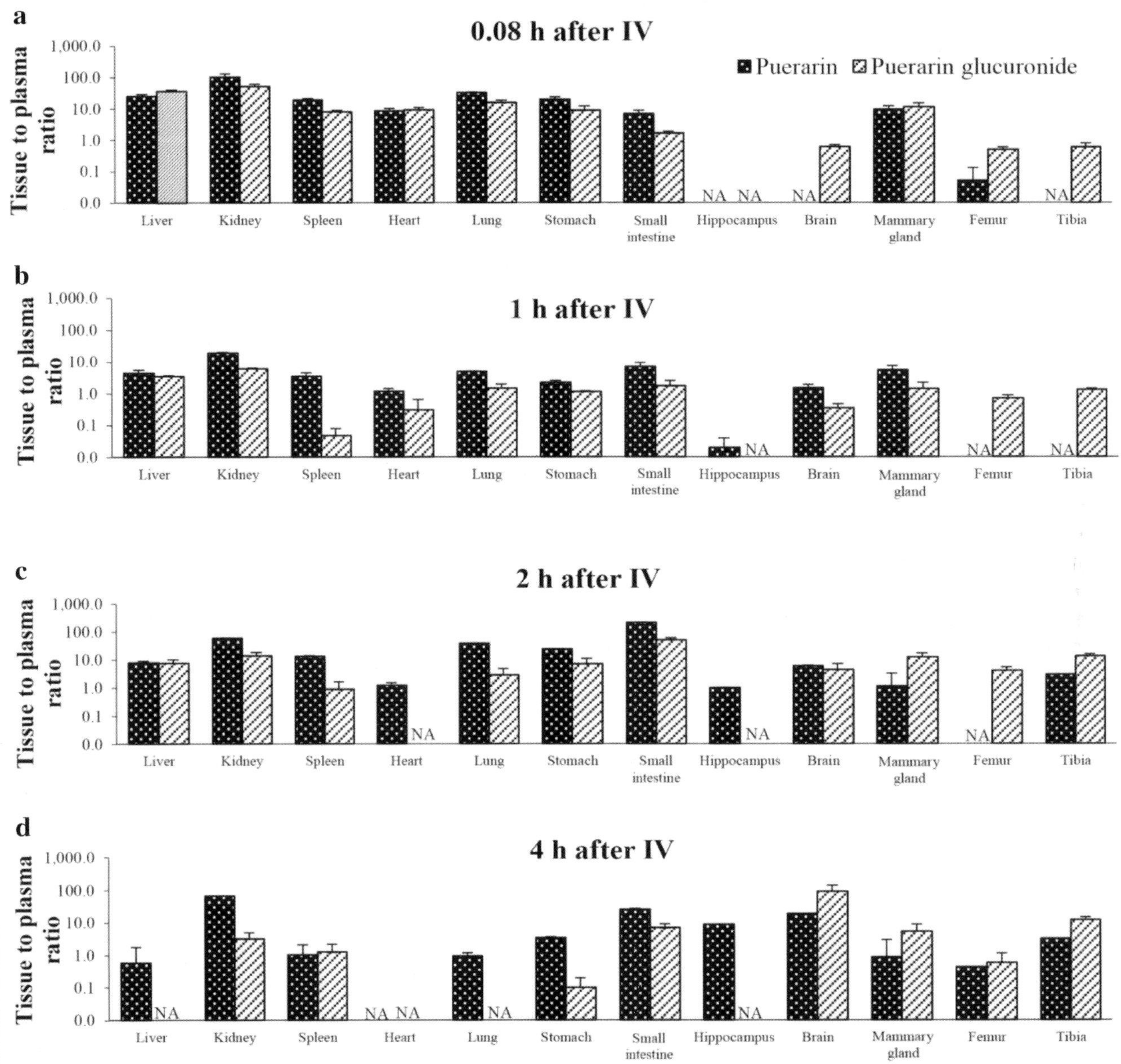

Fig. 3 Tissue-to-plasma ratios of puerarin (black bars) and puerarin glucuronide (grey bars) in internal organs at (**a**) 5 min, (**b**) 1.0 h, (**c**) 2.0 h and (**d**) 4.0 h after administration of puerarin at 1 mg/kg IV. Data are shown as mean ± S.D. ($n = 4$), NA = below limit of detection

0–24 h period. A negligible amount of puerarin glucuronide was found in feces 0–72 h after PO dosing.

Discussion

Puerarin has therapeutic effects on the cardiovascular and cerebrovascular systems and on bone [8]. Further understanding of these pharmacological activities requires information on the oral bioavailability and tissue distribution of puerarin. Therefore, this study was conducted to evaluate the ADME properties of puerarin at pharmacologically active sites in female rats. The rats could tolerate puerarin at 1 mg/kg IV and 5 and 10 mg/kg PO, which are pharmacologically active doses. All rats had a normal appearance without signs of toxicity after dosing. In addition, there were no significant changes in liver and kidney biomarkers within 24 h after dosing (Table 1). This suggests that puerarin is safe in rats in the pharmacologically active dose range, consistent with the findings of Chung et al. [28], in which male and female rats fed with puerarin for 28 days showed no toxicity at a dose up to 250 mg/kg per day.

The C_{max} of puerarin was reached within 5 min after PO dosing, and systemic clearance occurred until 8–12 h (Fig. 2). Previous studies of PO administration of a

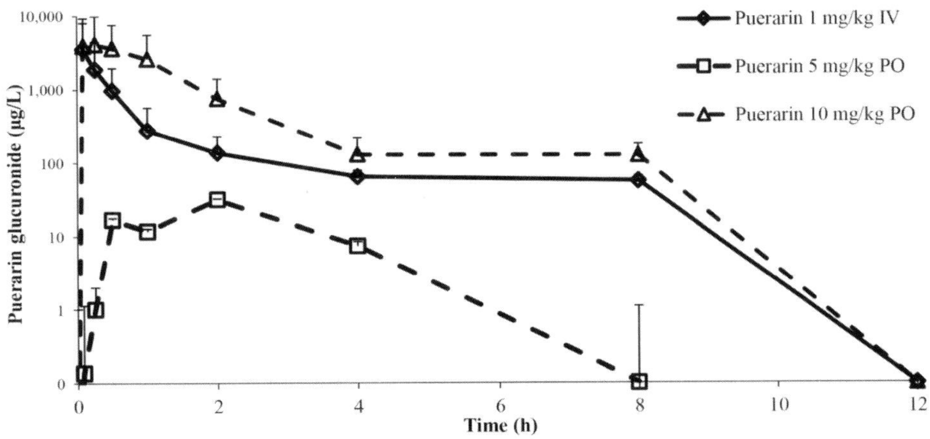

Fig. 4 Plasma concentration-time profiles of puerarin glucuronide after administration of puerarin at 1 mg/kg IV (◊), 5 mg/kg PO (□) and 10 mg/kg PO (Δ). Data are shown as mean ± S.D. ($n = 4$)

puerarin suspension resulted in C_{max} at 0.45–5.00 h [12–16]. The wider range of T_{max} in these studies might be due to the use of a puerarin suspension formulation. The puerarin used in our study was prepared as a clear solution that was readily absorbed, resulting in a shorter T_{max} compared to that for the suspension. Thus, we conclude that puerarin is absorbed rapidly from the gastrointestinal (GI) tract. Biotransformation of puerarin via the formation of glucuronide conjugates was also clearly observed within the first 5 min, indicating that the metabolism of puerarin through the glucuronidation pathway also occurs rapidly. The primary difference between puerarin glucuronides of the two oral doses could be due to the activity of distinct metabolic pathways at different doses of puerarin. At a low dose, puerarin could be metabolized via multiple metabolic pathways, e. g., sulfation and/or glucuronidation. Therefore, the level of puerarin glucuronide appeared to be low at a low dose. However, a high dose of puerarin could saturate minor metabolic pathways such as sulfation. At this point, most of the puerarin molecules might be biotransformed via a major metabolic pathway or glucuronidation, and thus the level of puerarin glucuronide was higher with a higher dose.

Table 3 Percent recovery of unchanged puerarin and puerarin glucuronide after administration of puerarin at 1 mg/kg IV and 5 and 10 mg/kg PO

Recovery (%)	Administration of Puerarin		
	1 mg/kg IV	5 mg/kg PO	10 mg/kg PO
Puerarin			
$Urine_{0\text{-}24h}$	< 1.00	< 1.00	< 1.00
$Urine_{24\text{-}48h}$	< 1.00	< 1.00	< 1.00
$Urine_{48\text{-}72h}$	< 1.00	< 1.00	< 1.00
$Faeces_{0\text{-}24h}$	< 1.00	< 1.00	< 1.00
$Faeces_{24\text{-}48h}$	< 1.00	< 1.00	< 1.00
$Faeces_{48\text{-}72h}$	< 1.00	< 1.00	< 1.00
Puerarin glucuronide			
$Urine_{0\text{-}24h}$	47.53 ± 51.37	< 1.00	12.13 ± 13.01
$Urine_{24\text{-}48h}$	2.38 ± 0.97*	< 1.00	< 1.00
$Urine_{48\text{-}72h}$	1.89 ± 0.45*	< 1.00	< 1.00
$Faeces_{0\text{-}24h}$	7.66 ± 2.51*	< 1.00	1.94 ± 2.16
$Faeces_{24\text{-}48h}$	3.55 ± 0.55*	< 1.00	< 1.00
$Faeces_{48\text{-}72h}$	3.45 ± 0.80*	< 1.00	< 1.00

Data are presented as mean ± S.D. ($n = 4$). *$p < 0.05$ among doses

The amounts of plasma puerarin and glucuronide metabolites were investigated as a function of the oral dose to examine dose proportionality. The plasma concentration of puerarin increased linearly from 5 to 10 mg/kg PO, but at a higher dose of 20–100 mg/kg, the oral bioavailability of puerarin was less than 1% (data not shown). This may be because at the higher dose, puerarin is incompletely dissolved due to precipitation in vivo. To maintain a consistent dose volume of 1 mL/kg, we varied the concentration of puerarin from 5 to 100 mg/mL in 20% DMSO in normal saline. Puerarin is in class IV of the Biopharmaceutical Classification System, indicating low solubility and low permeability, and is a weak acid that is ionized at higher pH. Thus, it will have lower solubility in the acid medium in the stomach of rats, which may cause precipitation [29]. Therefore, the lower bioavailability of puerarin at a higher oral dose may be strongly affected by the dissolution state of puerarin in GI fluid. Neither puerarin nor puerarin glucuronide were found in plasma or urine following oral dosing at 20–100 mg/kg. The low oral bioavailability of lead compounds from natural resources is a common phenomenon in herbal pharmacokinetics. Low percentage in oral bioavailability might be improved when administered in the form of crude extract or when combined with other active ingredients.

To the best of our knowledge, this is the first study on the tissue distribution of puerarin and puerarin glucuronide in the hippocampus, femur, tibia, and mammary gland (Fig. 3). Puerarin was widely distributed in several organs, and especially those with high porosity, consistent with its pharmacodynamic activities in these organs [19]. In addition, the volume of distribution of puerarin after IV dosing was approximately 1.16 L/kg, which implies a good tissue distribution. This correlates well with the physiochemical properties of puerarin including high lipophilicity (XlogP 1.95) and low water solubility (0. 46 mg/mL). The tissue distribution in the current study showed that puerarin at 1 mg/kg IV reaches appropriate levels for pharmacodynamic activities in the hippocampus, femur, tibia, and mammary gland, which are related to the prevention of and therapy for neurodegenerative diseases and osteoporosis [5, 8, 10, 11]. This tissue distribution in rats correlates well with the use of puerarin in traditional medicine. The test compound could be distributed into several organs including the hippocampus, bone, and mammary gland. However, there are some discrepancies in rat and human physiology, e.g., tissue barriers, tissue blood flow, and drug metabolizing enzymes. Extrapolation from rat pharmacokinetics to human usage will likely require further investigation and careful interpretation.

Glucuronide metabolites of puerarin were also detected in most tissues. The $AUC_{puerarin\ glucuronide}/AUC_{puerarin}$ ratios were 7 after puerarin IV dosing and 30 after puerarin at 10 mg/kg PO (Table 2). Glucuronide metabolites found in biological samples after puerarin administration are formed by UDP glucuronosyltransferases [18]. We found that puerarin was biotransformed to a glucuronide within 5 min in plasma (Fig. 4). These results indicate that glucuronidation occurs rapidly and that most puerarin is converted into glucuronides. This first pass metabolism could reduce the amount of puerarin in the systemic circulation and may account for the relatively low oral bioavailability of puerarin. Sex and interspecies differences of the enzymes responsible for puerarin biotransformation need to be explored for phytopharmaceutical product development [30–32].

The percentage of unchanged puerarin in urine and feces was less than 1% over 72 h after IV or PO dosing, indicating that puerarin is biotransformed to glucuronide metabolites before excretion via the bile or urine. We detected puerarin glucuronide in urine and feces using enzymatic hydrolysis of glucuronidase under optimized conditions. Puerarin was mainly excreted in the form of puerarin glucuronide, and approximately 50% of the administered dose of 1 mg/kg IV was detected in the urine as the glucuronide during the first 24 h. After PO dosing, 1–10% of the administered dose was excreted in urine as the glucuronide. The difference in the percentage recovery between the different routes of administration (IV or PO) might be explained by distinct metabolic pathways. Prasain et al. [19] reported that puerarin can be hydrolyzed to daidzein by microbial metabolism in the GI tract, and then reduced to dihydrodaizein and equol after oral dosing. In this study, we also detected daidzein and equol as minor metabolites in urine and feces at 72 h after dosing. However, the levels of daidzein and equol in urine and feces accounted for only 1–2% of the administered dose (data not shown).

Conclusions

This study showed that puerarin has an oral bioavailability of approximately 7%. For tissue distribution following IV administration, puerarin was widely distributed to several organs including the hippocampus, femur, tibia, and mammary gland. Glucuronides were the major metabolites of puerarin and were mainly excreted in the urine. Further studies in comparative pharmacokinetics of puerarin when administered as a standardized extract compared with pure compound will be required for the phytopharmaceutical product development of *Pueraria mirifica*.

Acknowledgements

The technical language amendment was supervised by Dr. Wanchai Chongcharoen, Dr. Ian Haworth, and Dr. Jessica Lin.

Funding

This study was supported by a Grant for International Research Integration: Chula Research Scholar from the Rachadapisek Sompot Endowment Fund (to S. Malaivijitnond). This research was also supported by Rachadapisek Sompot Fund for Postdoctoral Fellowship, Chulalongkorn University.

Authors' contributions

TA helped to analyze data, reviewed the draft manuscript, responded the reviewers, and edited all revised versions. PP carried out all the in vivo experiments and drafted the manuscript. NH analyzed and interpreted the laboratory data, drafted the manuscript in 'LC-MS/MS analysis' and 'Data analysis' parts of Materials and Methods. RR performed brain and hippocampus tissue collection, drafted the manuscript in 'Animals' and 'Pharmacokinetic studies' parts of Materials and Methods. SM participated in the design of the study, helped draft the manuscript, and supported the chemical (puerarin) and funding. PK contributed to study design, planning and data analysis, and revising the manuscript. All authors have read and approved the final version of the manuscript.

Competing interests

The authors declare that they have no competing interests.

Author details

[1]Department of Pharmacology and Physiology, Faculty of Pharmaceutical Sciences, Chulalongkorn University, Bangkok 10330, Thailand. [2]Department of Biology, Faculty of Science, Chulalongkorn University, Bangkok 10330, Thailand. [3]Preclinical Pharmacokinetics and Interspecies Scaling for Drug Development Research Unit, Chulalongkorn University, Bangkok 10330, Thailand.

References

1. Chandeying V, Sangthawan M. Efficacy comparison of *Pueraria mirifica* (PM) against conjugated equine estrogen (CEE) with/without medroxyprogesterone acetate (MPA) in the treatment of climacteric symptoms in perimenopausal women: phase III study. J Med Assoc Thail. 2007;90:1720–6.
2. Lamlertkittikul S, Chandeying V. Efficacy and safety of *Pueraria mirifica* (Kwao Kruea Khao) for the treatment of vasomotor symptoms in perimenopausal women: phase II study. J Med Assoc Thail. 2004;87:33–40.
3. Suthon S, Jaroenporn S, Charoenphandhu N, Suntornsaratoon P, Malaivijitnond S. Anti-osteoporotic effects of *Pueraria candollei var. mirifica* on bone mineral density and histomorphometry in estrogen-deficient rats. J Nat Med. 2016;70:225–33.
4. Urasopon N, Hamada Y, Asaoka K, Cherdshewasart W, Malaivijitnond S. *Pueraria mirifica*, a phytoestrogen-rich herb, prevents bone loss in orchidectomized rats. Maturitas. 2007;56:322–31.
5. Urasopon N, Hamada Y, Cherdshewasart W, Malaivijitnond S. Preventive effects of *Pueraria mirifica* on bone loss in ovariectomized rats. Maturitas. 2008;59:137–48.
6. Cherdshewasart W, Panriansaen R, Picha P. Pretreatment with phytoestrogen-rich plant decreases breast tumor incidence and exhibits lower profile of mammary ERα and ERβ. Maturitas. 2007;58:174–81.
7. Wattanapitayakul SK, Chularojmontri L, Srichirat S. Effects of *Pueraria mirifica* on vascular function of ovariectomized rabbits. J Med Assoc Thail. 2005; 88(Suppl 1):S21–9.
8. Wong KH, Li GQ, Li KM, Razmovski-Naumovski V, Chan K. Kudzu root: traditional uses and potential medicinal benefits in diabetes and cardiovascular diseases. J Ethnopharmacol. 2011;134:584–607.
9. Woo KS, Yip TWC, Chook P, Kwong SK, Szeto CC, Li JKY, Yu AWY, Cheng WKF, Chan TYK, Fung KP, Leung PC. Cardiovascular protective effects of adjunctive alternative medicine (*Salvia miltiorrhiza* and *Pueraria lobata*) in high-risk hypertension. Evid Based Complement Alternat Med. 2013;2013:1–8.
10. Anukulthanakorn K, Parhar IS, Jaroenporn S, Kitahashi T, Watanbe G, Malaivijitnond S. Neurotherapeutic effects of *Pueraria mirifica* extract in early- and late-stage cognitive impaired rats. Phytother Res. 2016;30:929–39.
11. Cherdshewasart W, Traisup V, Picha P. Determination of the estrogenic activity of wild phytoestrogen-rich *Pueraria mirifica* by MCF-7 proliferation assay. J Reprod Dev. 2008;54:63–7.
12. D-q Q, G-x X, X-g W. Studies on preparation and absolute bioavailability of a self-emulsifying system containing Puerarin. Chem Pharm Bull (Tokyo). 2007; 55:800–3.
13. Li Y, Pan WS, Chen SL, Xu HX, Yang DJ, Chan ASC. Pharmacokinetic, tissue distribution, and excretion of Puerarin and Puerarin-phospholipid complex in rats. Drug Dev Ind Pharm. 2006;32:413–22.
14. Ren F, Jing Q, Shen Y, Ma H, Cui J. Quantitative determination of puerarin in dog plasma by HPLC and study on the relative bioavailability of sustained release tablets. J Pharm Biomed Anal. 2006;41:549–53.
15. Cao L, Pu J, Cao Q-R, Chen B-W, Lee B-J, Cui J-H. Pharmacokinetics of puerarin in pregnant rats at different stages of gestation after oral administration. Fitoterapia. 2013;86:202–7.
16. Liu X, Zhi H, Du F, Ye Z, Wang N, Qin W, Li J. A HPLC-UV method for the determination of puerarin in rat plasma after intravenous administration of PEGylated puerarin conjugate. J Chromatogr B. 2010;878:3297–302.
17. Yu Z, Gao X, Yuan H, Liu T, Ma M, Chen X, Bi K. Simultaneous determination of safflor yellow a, puerarin, daidzein, ginsenosides (Rg1, Rb1, Rd), and notoginsenoside R1 in rat plasma by liquid chromatography–mass spectrometry. J Pharm Biomed Anal. 2007;45:327–36.
18. Luo C-F, Yuan M, Chen M-S, Liu S-M, Zhu L, Huang B-Y, Liu X-W, Xiong W. Pharmacokinetics, tissue distribution and relative bioavailability of puerarin solid lipid nanoparticles following oral administration. Int J Pharm. 2011;410: 138–44.
19. Prasain JK, Jones K, Brissie N, Moore R, Wyss JM, Barnes S. Identification of Puerarin and its metabolites in rats by liquid chromatography–tandem mass spectrometry. J Agric Food Chem. 2004;52:3708–12.
20. Luo C-F, Yuan M, Chen M-S, Liu S-M, Ji H. Metabolites of puerarin identified by liquid chromatography tandem mass spectrometry: similar metabolic profiles in liver and intestine of rats. J Chromatogr B. 2010;878:363–70.
21. Yasuda T, Kano Y, Saito K, Ohsawa K. Urinary and biliary metabolites of Puerarin in rats. Biol Pharm Bull. 1995;18:300–3.
22. Malaivijitnond S, Tungmunnithum D, Gittarasanee S, Kawin K, Limjunyawong N. Puerarin exhibits weak estrogenic activity in female rats. Fitoterapia. 2010;81:569–76.
23. M-y Z, Qiang H, H-q Y, X-q D, K-z W. In vitro and in vivo effects of puerarin on promotion of osteoblast bone formation. Chin J Integr Med. 2012;18:276–82.
24. OECD. Test no. 417: Toxicokinetics. In: OECD guidelines for the testing of chemicals, section 4. Paris: OECD Publishing; 2010. p. 20.
25. Food US, Administration D. Guidance for industry: bioavailability and bioequivalence studies submitted in NDAs or INDs - general considerations. Rockville, MD: Edited by US Department of Health and Human Services; 2014.
26. Prasain JK, Peng N, Acosta E, Moore R, Arabshahi A, Meezan E, Barnes S, Wyss JM. Pharmacokinetic study of puerarin in rat serum by liquid chromatography tandem mass spectrometry. Biomed Chromatogr. 2007;21:410–4.
27. Klincomhum A, Kengkoom K, Ampawong S. Comparison of decalcification methods for adult rat calvarium bone in relation to histomorphological study. In: Proceedings of the 49th Kasetsart University annual conference; February 1st - 4th; Thailand. Kasetsart University; 2011. p. 120–6.
28. Chung HJ, Chung MJ, Houng S-J, Jeun J, Kweon D-K, Choi CH, Park J-T, Park K-H, Lee S-J. Toxicological evaluation of the isoflavone puerarin and its glycosides. Eur Food Res Technol. 2009;230:145–53.
29. Li H, Dong L, Liu Y, Wang G, Wang G, Qiao Y. Biopharmaceutics classification of puerarin and comparison of perfusion approaches in rats. Int J Pharm. 2014;466:133–8.
30. Anakk S, Ku CY, Vore M, Strobel HW. Insights into gender Bias: rat cytochrome P450 3A9. J Pharmacol Exp Ther. 2003;305:703–9.
31. Czerniak R. Gender-based differences in pharmacokinetics in laboratory animal models. Int J Toxicol. 2001;20:161–3.
32. Waxman DJ, Holloway MG. Sex differences in the expression of hepatic drug metabolizing enzymes. Mol Pharmacol. 2009;76:215–28.

5

Prescription opioid dispensing in New South Wales, Australia: spatial and temporal variation

M Mofizul Islam[1*], Ian S. McRae[2], Soumya Mazumdar[3], Paul Simpson[4], Dennis Wollersheim[1], Kaniz Fatema[5,6,7,8] and Tony Butler[4]

Abstract

Background: Patterns of opioid dispensing often exhibit substantial temporal and geographical variability, which has implications for public health policy decisions and interventions. The study examined recent trends in prescription opioid dispensing and identified high dispensing areas and factors associated with the doses dispensed.

Methods: Three years (1 January 2013–31 December 2015) of dispensing data of prescription opioids in local government areas (LGAs) for New South Wales (NSW), Australia's most populous state, were analyzed. The proportion of individuals who were dispensed opioids was computed for four age-groups. A Chi-square test was used to examine trends over time in proportions of the population who were dispensed opioids in four age-groups. The number of prescriptions over time and quantities in daily defined dose/1000 people/day (denoted DDD) were also examined. LGAs with relatively high levels of dispensing were identified and mapped. A multivariate regression model was used to identify factors associated with DDD.

Results: Overall, codeine, oxycodone and tramadol were the main opioids in terms of DDD, number of prescriptions and number of individuals who were dispensed these medications. Quantity (in DDD), and population dispensed to were consistently higher for women than men over time. Proportions of individuals who were dispensed opioids increased significantly over time in all four age-groups. In the multivariate model, age, urbanization, sex and socio-economic indexes for areas were significantly associated with doses dispensed among opioid users. All areas with very high dispensing were outside major metropolitan areas.

Conclusions: Given that over-use of opioids is a major public health problem and that long-term use has substantial side effects including dependence, it is important to understand spatial patterns of opioid prescribing to enable targeted interventions. Nationwide implementation of real-time drug-monitoring programs and access to monitoring databases from both doctor and pharmacy point-of-care sources may potentially reduce excessive and undue use of opioid.

Keywords: Opioid, Dispensing, Prescription opioid, Pain medicine, New South Wales, Australia

Background

Opioids are primarily prescribed for pain relief, and occasionally for reducing coughing and relieving diarrhea. However, these drugs have substantial addictive properties as they produce feelings of euphoria, tranquility, and sedation that may lead to dependence [1, 2]. Rates of nonmedical use, misuse, and fatal poisoning from prescription opioids have increased alongside the medical use of these drugs over recent years [3]. Between 2011 and 2015 in Australia, 3601 people died from opioid-related overdose – a nearly twofold increase from 2001 to 2005 – with Fentanyl being the most common opioid implicated in these deaths [4, 5]. Although the relationship between opioid prescriptions and the risk of overdose and death is widely appreciated [6, 7], opioid prescribing practices, misuse and diversion exhibit substantial geographical variability which may have implications for public health policy decisions and interventions [8–10]. For instance, data show that the

* Correspondence: mofi.islam@latrobe.edu.au
[1]Department of Public Health, La Trobe University, Melbourne, Victoria, Australia
Full list of author information is available at the end of the article

patterns of diversion, misuse and/or unsanctioned use of prescription opioid differ across Australian states and territories [11]. This spatial variation in usage is likely to be influenced by factors such as socio-economic status, age and sex of residents. Studying the relationships between patterns of opioid prescribing, quantity dispensed and population characteristics of those who use opioids at relatively small geographies could be useful for policy development. This information can facilitate understanding of where inappropriate dispensing, prescribing, and prescription opioid-seeking behaviors may occur and offer valuable information for implementation of local-level interventions.

Geographical variation in the prescription of opioids has been widely examined in the United States of America (USA) and found to be helpful in tailoring policy and interventions [9, 12–14]. Federal agencies, such as the Centers for Disease Control and Prevention, and the Drug Enforcement Agency, use a geographical information system (GIS) platform to coordinate efforts to address problematic drug use and supply across the USA. This platform is an infrastructure for the free flow of geographic data between local law enforcement, health agencies, and communities [15]. However, in other countries there have been few geographic studies that explore prescribing patterns at local level. This has been largely attributed to privacy concerns that make it difficult to obtain data for small areas [16]. In Australia, research conducted on prescription opioid utilization mostly relies on national or state level data [17, 18], with little or limited focus on small geographical areas [19]. Identifying locations with relatively high levels of prescription use (defined by unexpectedly high levels of dispensing) on smaller spatial scales is an important first step in describing the use/misuse of prescribed opioids [16]. This study examines (i) trends in prescription opioid dispensing in New South Wales (Australia's most populous state), (ii) variation in the distribution of dispensing in local government areas (LGAs) to identify the areas with relatively high level of dispensing, and (iii) identifies factors associated with the quantity dispensed per person.

Method

Prescription opioid dispensing in Australia

Under Australia's universal healthcare scheme – Medicare – around 80% of all prescription medicines dispensed are subsidized by the Pharmaceutical Benefits Scheme (PBS) [20]. In the PBS the maximum price of a single prescription (i.e. the patient contribution) in 2017 is AU$38.80 for general patients, and $6.30 for those holding government concession cards. There is also a safety net provision on PBS medications such that when a certain threshold (defined as the total patient copayments for a family) is reached in a calendar year, general patients are entitled to PBS medications at the concession price and concessional patients are entitled to PBS medications at no cost – for the remainder of the year. There is also a parallel, albeit small, Repatriation Pharmaceutical Benefits Scheme (RPBS) for military veterans, which is managed and funded by the Department of Veterans' Affairs, that entitles this group to the same copayments as concessional patients. If a medicine is not listed in the PBS schedule (or RPBS), the patient pays the full price as a private prescription and this cannot count towards the safety net threshold [20] and is not included in this data set. A number of PBS items are priced below the maximum co-payment for general patients, and thus patients pay the full cost for those items. This payment contributes to the safety net threshold and these prescriptions are included in this data set.

Analysis

Prescription opioid data on dispensing episodes under the PBS/RPBS were provided by the statistics branch of the Australian Department of Human Services. This study covered data for NSW and the Australian Capital Territory (which was treated as an LGA for the purposes of this study and was included in any reference to NSW data hereafter). The dataset contained information about users' sex and age-groups (0–19 years, 20–44 years, 45-64 years, and 65+ years); generic name, form and strength of opioids; the quantity dispensed; number of prescriptions dispensed; number of persons dispensed; LGA in which the script was dispensed; and scheme (i.e. PBS, RPBS and Under co-payment). The quantity of each drug dispensed was estimated in daily defined dose/1000 people/day (indicated as DDD). The DDD unit was established by the World Health Organization Collaborating Centre for Drug Statistics Methodology [21] and corresponds to an estimated mean daily dose of the drug when used for its main indication in adults. It allows for simple comparisons of medicine use across countries, and across different formulations of the medicine. The DDD is defined by the formula $\frac{N \times M \times Q}{DDD\ factor \times P \times D} \times 1000$ [22]; where N is the number of prescriptions dispensed for a specific drug in a year, M is the mass of each dose (e.g. milligrams or grams, expressed in the same unit as DDD factor), Q is the average dispensed quantity per prescription, P is the population for the year of data collection, D is the number of days in the year [22].

Population data for individual LGAs and Socio-Economic Indexes for Areas (SEIFA) which ranks areas according to relative socio-economic disadvantage were obtained from the Australian Bureau of Statistics. SEIFA data are derived from the information collected in five-yearly national census. Higher scores on the Index of Relative Socio-economic Disadvantage indicate a lower level of disadvantage and lower scores mean a higher level of disadvantage. The proportion of individuals who were dispensed opioids was computed for four age-groups and for individual years from 2013 and 2015. A Chi-square test for trend of proportions was used to determine significant differences over time. LGA urbanization level was determined by the Australian Classification of Local Government, as categorized in 2013 [23].

The differences between "average DDD-quantities dispensed for overall NSW" and "age and sex adjusted DDD-quantities dispensed for individual LGAs" were estimated to identify LGAs with relatively high dispensing rates. LGAs were identified as "normal" if dispensing was less than or equal to the state average; "high" if dispensing was between state average and the third quartile; and "very high" for anything more than that. LGAs of these three categories were then mapped using R software. Trends in dispensing quantities (DDDs) over time were categorized as "increasing", "decreasing" and "mixed".

To examine possible factors associated with the quantity of doses dispensed, a multivariable regression model was developed. As the variable "DDD" was positively skewed we used a logarithmic transformation. To make the coefficients (β) of the regressions easily interpretable they were exponentially transformed and reported as value 'B'. The interpretation of B is that a one unit increase (e.g. from zero to one) of the independent variable would result in a (B-1)*100 percentage change in the quantity of prescription opioids dispensed per person. The index of relative socio-economic disadvantage scores was divided into quartiles for modelling purposes, as a linear relationship does not exist.

STATA SE 14 (StataCorp LP) [24], Microsoft Office Excel 2013 [25] and R [26] were used for analyses. The study received approval from La Trobe University's Ethics Committee (reference number: S17–218). Written informed consent was not required as these are de-identified secondary data.

Results

Opioid dispensing increased in NSW across the study period (1 January 2013–31 December 2015) in terms of number of prescriptions, and number of individuals to whom opioids were dispensed but remained similar in terms of DDD (Fig. 1, Tables 1 and 2). During the three years more than 17 million opioid prescriptions were filled. Codeine and its derivatives dominate the quantity (in DDDs) of individual items dispensed followed by buprenorphine and oxycodone (and derivatives) (Table 1). However, in terms of the number of prescriptions, oxycodone (and derivatives) was the most commonly

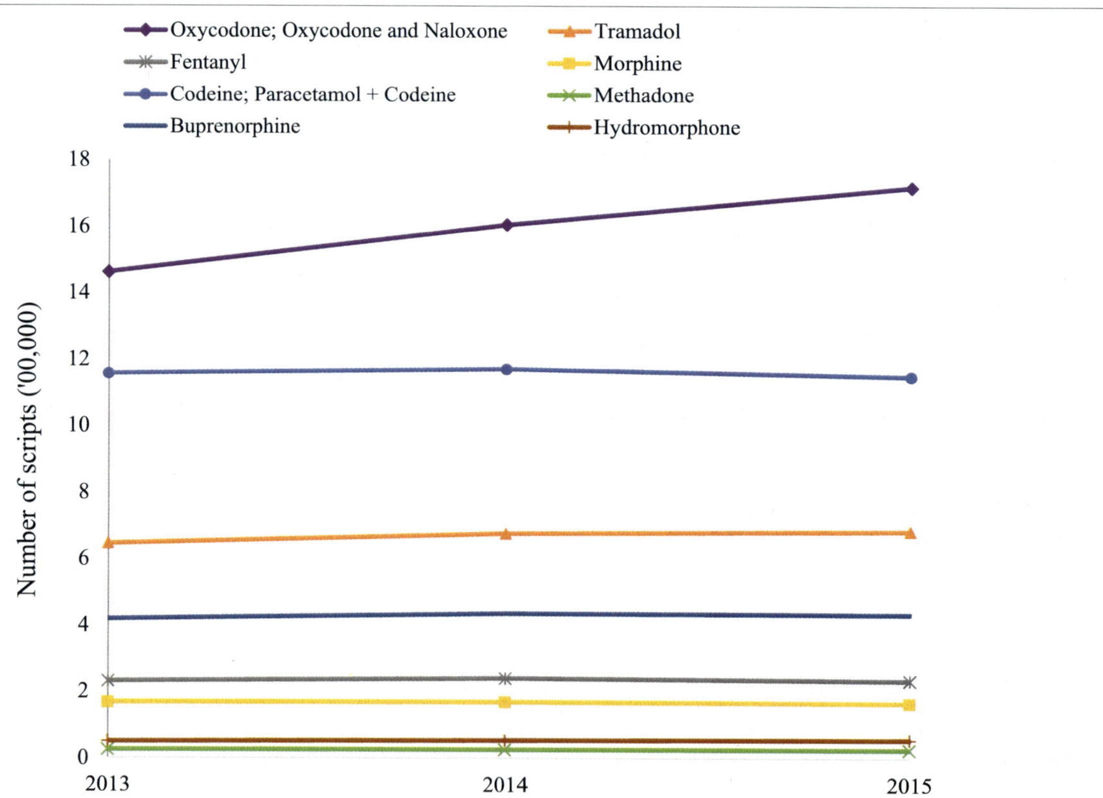

Fig. 1 Annual trends in number of scripts between 2013 and 2015

Table 1 Quantity of major prescription opioids dispensed in PBS/RPBS and under-copayment scheme (in DDD)

Generic drugs	2013	2014	2015
Tramadol	2.53	2.57	2.55
Codeine and derivatives[a]	6.12	6.10	5.86
Oxycodone and derivatives[b]	3.64	3.62	3.56
Fentanyl	1.32	1.36	1.32
Morphine (& derivatives)	0.90	0.86	0.79
Buprenorphine	0.61	0.62	0.61
Hydromorphone	0.36	0.38	0.38
Methadone	0.32	0.31	0.30
Tapentadol[c]	–	0.05	0.26

[a]Codeine and paracetamol combination; [b]Oxycodone and naloxone combination; [c]Tapentadol was listed in Pharmaceutical Benefits Scheme from 2014

prescribed with an increase between 2013 and 2015 (Fig. 1). The rate of increase in the number of individuals dispensed prescription opioids was highest for oxycodone, although more individuals were dispensed codeine (and derivatives) (Table 2). Overall, in all three measures, codeine, oxycodone and tramadol were the main opioids dispensed in NSW.

The quantity of opioids dispensed in terms of DDD was consistently higher for women than men across the years (Table 3). Also, more women were prescribed opioids than men. On average in each year of 2013–2015 around 808, 017 women received prescriptions compared to 659, 880 men. This difference was also reflected in the number of prescriptions per user, which was 37% higher for women than men.

There was a clear age trend in dispensing with consistently highest usage for people aged 65 years or older (Table 4). Almost half (45%) of the total NSW population aged 65 years or older were dispensed opioid. Among the 45–64 age-group around a quarter used opioids across the years. Proportions of individuals who were dispensed opioids increased significantly across 2013 to 2015 for all four age-groups and the rate of increment is similar.

Small differences in DDD quantities across LGAs of low to high SEIFA were observed, although the quantities decreased for very high SEIFA score LGAs (least disadvantaged) (Table 3). Multivariate modelling showed a significant pattern of more opioid use in the least advantaged areas and less use in the most advantaged (Table 5).

Table 3 Opioids dispensed (in DDDs) in PBS/RPBS and under-copayment scheme across four years stratified by SEIFA and Gender

Year	Quantity dispensed in terms of DDD					
	SEIFA				Gender	
	Low	Moderate	High	Very high	Male	Female
2013	19.21	20.05	18.79	9.99	14.56	17.03
2014	19.51	20.21	18.85	10.00	14.65	17.13
2015	19.02	20.05	18.74	9.75	14.32	16.94

Dispensing (in DDDs) was consistently higher in rural areas than in urban areas across the years with a 300% difference in the doses of prescription opioid dispensed between the people in urban areas and the people in rural areas (B = 4.08, CI: 4.00–4.16) (Table 5).

Multivariate regression identified that women were more likely to be dispensed higher quantities of prescription opioids than men. Coefficients increased with age and peaked for the 65+ years age-group (Table 5).

The average quantity of dispensing in DDDs, adjusted for age and sex was mostly similar between 2013 and 2015. Taking all 154 LGAs together, it was estimated that in 2015 on an average 21.17 DDDs were dispensed per LGA (range 5.01 to 45.58, SD = ±9.43). The opioid dispensing (in DDDs) for individual LGAs were "very high" relative to the state average for 39 LGAs, "high" for 38 LGAs and "normal" for the rest of the state's LGAs (Fig. 2), using the definitions outlined in the Methods section. Most areas with "high" or "very high" dispensing were outside of the major metropolitan areas. Quantities (in DDD) dispensed between 2013 and 2015 had mixed trends in different LGAs, increasing for 37 and decreasing for 35 LGAs (Fig. 3).

Discussion

The findings of this study suggest that considerable variation exists in the dispensing of prescription opioids across LGAs in NSW. Overall, there was a slightly increasing trend in the number of scripts written for, and persons prescribed, opioids between 2013 and 2015. However, quantities, expressed in DDDs, were similar during this period. This is likely because the slight increase in prescriptions was mostly for opioids with relatively low DDDs such as hydromorphone and combination of oxycodone with naloxone. Women were more likely to be dispensed opioids than men.

Table 2 Annual trends in terms of number of individuals who were dispensed opioids (in 100,000)

Year	Oxycodone and derivatives[b]	Tramadol	Fentanyl	Morphine (and derivatives)	Codeine and derivatives[a]	Methadone	Buprenorphine	Hydromorphone
2013	4.42	1.86	0.49	0.41	5.93	0.03	0.76	0.12
2014	4.95	1.94	0.49	0.42	6.02	0.03	0.76	0.12
2015	5.28	1.94	0.46	0.42	5.93	0.03	0.73	0.13

[a]Codeine and paracetamol combination; [b]Oxycodone and naloxone combination

Table 4 Dispensing of prescription opioids across the years in four age-groups

	Variable	Age-group			
Year		0–19	20–44	45–64	65+
2013	Population ('00,000)	19.58	27.38	19.26	11.68
	Person used prescription opioids ('00,000)	0.35	3.87	4.54	5.25
	Proportion used prescription opioids (%)	1.78	14.13	23.57	44.95
	Amount of prescription opioids used (DDD)	0.31	8.02	26.23	42.83
2014	Population ('00,000)	19.77	27.73	19.46	12.06
	Person used prescription opioids ('00,000)	0.37	4.01	4.77	5.58
	Proportion used prescription opioids (%)	1.78	14.46	24.51	46.26
	Amount of prescription opioids used (DDD)	0.33	7.89	26.30	43.05
2015	Population ('00,000)	19.95	28.09	19.67	12.43
	Person used prescription opioids ('00,000)	0.37	4.17	4.90	5.75
	Proportion used prescription opioids (%)	1.85	14.84	24.91	46.26
	Amount of prescription opioids used (DDD)	0.31	7.51	25.88	42.45

The proportion of the population dispensed an opioid increased across all age-groups over the study period. Prescriptions for oxycodone plus naloxone (in combination) rose faster than for any other opioid formulation between 2013 and 2015.

Table 5 Multivariate model reflecting factors associated with the DDD dispensed

Variables	B[a]	*p*	95% Confidence Interval
Sex			
Men	1.00	–	–
Women	1.13	< 0.01	1.11–1.15
Age-group (years)			
0–19	1.00	–	–
20–44	4.23	< 0.01	4.06–4.40
45–64	7.98	< 0.01	7.68–8.30
65+	11.39	< 0.01	10.96–11.84
Year			
2013	1.00	–	–
2014	0.97	< 0.01	0.95–0.99
2015	1.02	0.04	1.00–1.04
SEIFA index of disadvantage			
Low	1.00	–	–
Moderate	0.88	< 0.01	0.86–0.90
High	0.85	< 0.01	0.83–0.87
Very high	0.63	< 0.01	0.61–0.64
Urbanization			
Urban	1.00	–	–
Rural	4.08	< 0.01	4.00–4.16
Constant	1.80	< 0.01	1.73–1.88

[a]Exponentiated values of the coefficients estimated in the linear model of the logarithm of quantity of opioids dispensed

Multiple reasons explain the overall increasing trend in the proportion of citizens using prescription opioid in NSW such as an increase in the prevalence and severity of conditions causing chronic pain due to the ageing population [27]. Awareness of pain relief has increased substantially over recent years. Globally, medical, ethical and legal attention and initiatives have emerged suggesting that pain management is a fundamental human right. Such a view acknowledges that failure to treat pain is poor medicine, unethical practice, and contravenes a person's human rights [28]. The cultural precept that "all suffering should be avoided" also encourages patients to seek opioids and the physicians to prescribe them to reduce pain [29]. In most western countries, general practitioners follow the so-called customer service norm rather than a patient care driven practice of medicine. Patients should not be treated only as customers but also as patients and clients. These two views are usually but not always synergetic. An excessive attention to customer satisfaction may encourage the over prescription of opioid-based pain relief [29]. Writing a prescription for opioids is fast and easy, whereas developing a comprehensive pain management plan is complex and seldom financially rewarded in the primary health care setting. Moreover, new products including slow-release formulations have been introduced with aggressive marketing by pharmaceutical companies [30]. Illicit substance users' increasing reliance on prescription opioids may also be implicated in the increasing trend in opioid dispensing [31, 32].

The sharp increase in the number of prescriptions for oxycodone is likely to be due to a mixture of increased prescribing for serious pain relief and increased prescribing for people seeking the medication for non-medical purposes (e.g., recreational use). These changes can be

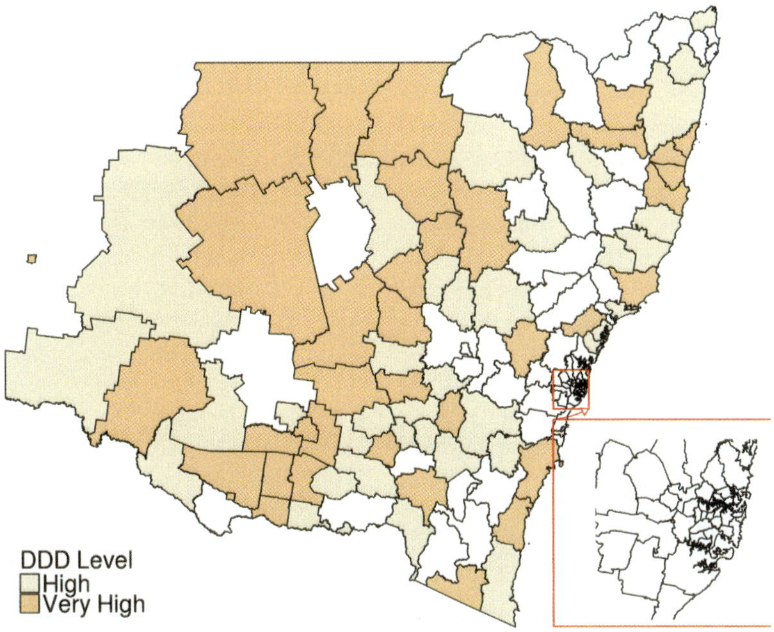

Fig. 2 LGAs with relatively high dispensing of prescription opioid in 2015. (This map has been developed using bioregional assessment source dataset, available under a Creative Commons Attribution license. Australian Bureau of Statistics (2011) Local Government Areas of Australia. Bioregional Assessment Source Dataset)

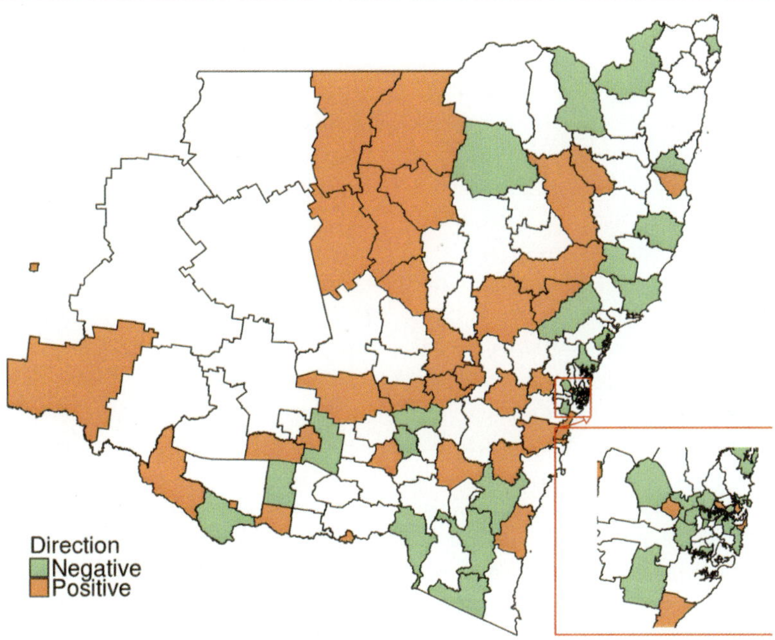

Fig. 3 LGAs with increasing and decreasing trends in quantities (DDD) in year 2013–2015. (This map has been developed using bioregional assessment source dataset, available under a Creative Commons Attribution license. Australian Bureau of Statistics (2011) Local Government Areas of Australia. Bioregional Assessment Source Dataset)

attributed to factors such as formulations with various routes of administration; increased euphoric effects (relative to some other opioid items); illicit substance users' increasing reliance on prescription opioids driven by the relatively low price and easy access [33], and/or a shortage of and price increases in heroin or other more traditional illicit drugs. [34]. Aggressive marketing by pharmaceutical companies also has an impact [30]. Having both immediate release formulations, which work quickly to ease pain, and slow-release formulations, which release oxycodone over several hours to provide a more even pain control could be another reason. Part of this increased dispensing could be attributed to the fact that oxycodone is sometimes used in combination with naloxone, which helps to reduce some of the side-effects of oxycodone such as constipation [35] and makes this formulation more suitable than other generic items.

Our findings suggest that women are more likely than men to be prescribed opioids which is consistent with previous studies [7, 36, 37] and likely due to a greater propensity among women to seek treatment, report symptoms and live longer than men. Although recreational use of prescription opioids by men is much higher than women [38] according to the Centers for Disease Control and Prevention, the likelihood of experiencing pain is higher among women, and so is utilization of pain medications [39]. Also, women use these medications for longer duration and in higher doses than men. A US study found that among opioid users the rate of progression to dependence was quicker among women than men [40], and women experience more craving for opioids. Psychological and or emotional distress among women have been found to be significant risk factors for excessive use of prescription opioid use [41].

Findings from the multivariable model suggest that age was a clear predictor of doses dispensed per person with a clear trend in increased doses with increasing age, peaking for those in the 65+ year age-group. This is likely due to the high prevalence of pain among older people. Interestingly, significantly more quantities (in DDD) were used in LGAs that are categorized as "rural" than in LGAs categorized as "urban". This model also indicates that doses dispensed per person increased with increasing disadvantage. These observations suggest that social determinants which impact on a range of aspects of the health of Australians also affect levels of pharmaceutical drug use [42]. People living in disadvantaged areas are likely to have relatively poor health and well-being. Being in disadvantaged areas also means that they are more likely to have concession cards and enjoy lower copayments under the Australian subsidized medicine program and so may be more likely to access more medications than others [43].

Geographical variations in dispensing were notable – ranging from 5.01 to 45.58 DDDs (in 2015 adjusted for age and sex) – with most of the areas with very high dispensing outside of the major metropolitan cities. This could reflect a lack of alternative treatment/management options for pain in rural and remote locations. It is also possible that prescribing practices among doctors are relatively relaxed in remote areas and possibly reflects the long-term doctor-patient relationship and a socio-cultural approach to healthcare provision in rural areas [44]. Higher levels of dispensing, however, do not necessarily indicate an inappropriate or problematic utilization. Instead, these findings warrant further and area-based research, including qualitative research, to further explore factors leading to higher dispensing in these areas. It is also important to remember that an area being identified as having certain characteristics does not imply all the individuals living in the area possess these characteristics and could represent what has been termed an "ecological fallacy" [45].

This study did not aim to measure the consequences of the growing use of prescription opioids. However, it should be noted that excessive use of prescription opioids and associated harms are a major public health problem in many countries. Dependence and other side effects of long term opioid use and death from overdose have received substantial coverage recently in electronic and print media, prompting policy interventions. Prescription Shopping Information Service is one such intervention, which allows prescribers and suppliers to identify potential prescription shoppers and look at ways to reduce patient need for such shopping [46]. Despite these concerns prescription opioid use has continued to increase in Australia.

Nationwide implementation of a real-time prescription drug-monitoring program (PDMP) and access to the database from both doctors and pharmacists at point-of-care is another measure that may reduce excessive and undue use of opioids [47–50]. Current initiatives of PDMP are taken by the individual states/territories. Tasmania was the first jurisdiction in Australia to implement a program of PDMP. Recently the Victorian state government funded a real-time PDMP [51]. The Australian Government is reported to be interested in rolling out PDMP, and is waiting for each state and territory to commence using it [52]. A nationwide initiative of PDMP is likely to be more effective and sustainable, as interoperability of these state-based systems using different software may be problematic [53]. This will also help prevent the cross-border fraudulent access to opioids. However, the evaluation of PDMP is crucial to ensure therapeutic and social aims of the program can be met and to avoid any unintended consequences such as patients shifting to illicit drugs or other prescription drugs (e.g., benzodiazepines) and overly cautious prescription of drugs when they are clinically indicated.

Limitations

Our study has a number of limitations. Firstly, complete data for only 3 years were available for assessing the temporal trend. Also, opioids dispensed through State Government hospitals or those not listed in the PBS/RPBS schedule were not captured in this dataset. However, overall it should be a small quantity, and is unlikely to have significant impact on our major findings. The DDD metric does not necessarily correspond to the recommended or prescribed daily dose.

Conclusion

Spatial and temporal variations in prescription opioid dispensing were identified for NSW during the study period (1 January 2013–31 December 2015). Very high and high levels of dispensing in terms of DDDs were recorded in a number of LGAs, with most with relatively high dispensing located outside the major cities. Age, sex and neighborhood level disadvantages are three significant factors in doses dispensed. There are likely to be other potential factors which need to be examined further. This study provides a basis for such further investigation. Given that long-term use of opioid has substantial side effects including dependence and given that over-use of opioid is a major public health problem, it is important that research facilitate understanding of behavior in small areas to enable targeted interventions. A real time prescription drug monitoring program may also play a role in reducing problematic use of prescription opioids, however, such programs must be designed well and evaluated rigorously to ensure therapeutic aims are met and unintended consequences are avoided.

Abbreviations

DDD: Daily Defined Dose; LGA: Local Government Area; NSW: New South Wales; PBS: Pharmaceutical Benefit Scheme; PDMP: Prescription Drug Monitoring Programme; RPBS: Repatriation Pharmaceutical Benefits Scheme; SEIFA: Socio-Economic Indexes for Areas

Acknowledgements

We thank Australian Department of Human Services for supplying this dataset.

Funding

This research was funded from the Capacity Building Grants in Population Health and Health Services Research by National Health and Medical Research Council, Australia; Grant number # 533546.

Authors' contributions

MMI conceived this study, analyzed dataset and wrote the first draft of the manuscript. DW and ISM helped in analysis and interpreting the data. DW developed the geospatial pictures. SM, PS, KF and TB interpreted the data and contributed in shaping the manuscript. All authors read and approved the final manuscript.

Competing interests

The authors declare that they have no competing interests.

Author details

[1]Department of Public Health, La Trobe University, Melbourne, Victoria, Australia. [2]Research School of Population Health, ANU College of Health and Medicine, Australian National University, Canberra, Australia. [3]Healthy People and Place Unit, Population Health, Liverpool Hospital, South West Sydney Local Health District, New South Wales Health, Sydney, New South Wales, Australia. [4]The Kirby Institute, University of New South Wales, Sydney, Australia. [5]Centre for Health Equity Training, Research & Evaluation (CHETRE), Sydney, New South Wales, Australia. [6]UNSW Sydney Research Centre for Primary Health Care & Equity, Sydney, New South Wales, Australia. [7]Population Health, South Western Sydney Local Health District, NSW Health, Sydney, New South Wales, Australia. [8]Ingham Institute, Liverpool, New South Wales, Australia.

References

1. Schuckit MA. Treatment of opioid-use disorders. N Engl J Med. 2016;375(4): 357–68.
2. Lembke A. Why doctors prescribe opioids to known opioid abusers. N Engl J Med. 2012;367(17):1580–1.
3. Cicero TJ, Surratt H, Inciardi JA, Munoz A. Relationship between therapeutic use and abuse of opioid analgesics in rural, suburban, and urban locations in the United States. Pharmacoepidemiol Drug Saf. 2007;16(8):827–40.
4. Cohen H, Webb T. During 2011–2015, 3,601 people died from an opioid-related overdose – a nearly twofold increase from 2001–2005: ABC News; 2017. Available at: http://www.abc.net.au/news/2017-11-24/deaths-from-prescription-drug-fentanyl-up-by-1800pc/9184396.
5. The Guardian: Fatal fentanyl overdoses rise as Australians turn to more potent painkillers. 2017, Avialable at: https://www.theguardian.com/australia-news/2017/aug/31/fatal-fentanyl-overdoses-rise-as-australians-turn-to-more-potent-painkillers.
6. Manchikanti L, Kaye AM, Kaye AD. Current state of opioid therapy and abuse. Curr Pain Headache Rep. 2016;20(5):34.
7. Wisniewski AM, Purdy CH, Blondell RD. The epidemiologic association between opioid prescribing, non-medical use, and emergency department visits. J Addict Dis. 2008;27(1):1–11.
8. Webster BS, Cifuentes M, Verma S, Pransky G. Geographic variation in opioid prescribing for acute, work-related, low back pain and associated factors: a multilevel analysis. Am J Ind Med. 2009;52(2):162–71.
9. Gomes T, Juurlink D, Moineddin R, Gozdyra P, Dhalla I, Paterson M, Mamdani M: Geographical variation in opioid prescribing and opioid-related mortality in Ontario. Healthcare Quarterly (Toronto) 2011, 14(1):22–24.
10. Brownstein JS, Green TC, Cassidy TA, Butler SF. Geographic information systems and pharmacoepidemiology: using spatial cluster detection to monitor local patterns of prescription opioid abuse. Pharmacoepidemiol Drug Saf. 2010;19(6):627–37.
11. The Mercury: Morphine addiction woe. Tasmanian has the nation's highest proportion of drug treatment patients seeking help for morphine Addiction. In: The Mercury Tasmania; 2014. p. 2.
12. McDonald DC, Carlson K, Izrael D. Geographic variation in opioid prescribing in the U.S. J Pain. 2012;13(10):988–96.
13. Curtis LH, Stoddard J, Radeva JI, Hutchison S, Dans PE, Wright A, Woosley RL, Schulman KA. Geographic variation in the prescription of schedule II opioid analgesics among outpatients in the United States. Health Serv Res. 2006;41(3 Pt 1):837–55.
14. Painter JT, Crofford LJ, Talbert J. Geographic variation of chronic opioid use in fibromyalgia. Clin Ther. 2013;35(3):303–11.
15. Mapping an Opioid Addiction Community Intervention Plan. Esri Insider. Available at: https://blogs.esri.com/esri/esri-insider/2016/08/31/mapping-an-opioid-addiction-community-intervention-plan/; accessed on 4 Nov 2016.
16. Mazumdar S, McRae IS, Islam MM. How can geographical information systems and spatial analysis inform a response to prescription opioid misuse? A discussion in the context of existing literature. Curr Drug Abuse Rev. 2015;8(2):104–10.
17. Blanch B, Pearson SA, Haber PS. An overview of the patterns of prescription opioid use, costs and related harms in Australia. Br J Clin Pharmacol. 2014; 78(5):1159–66.

18. Islam MM, McRae IS, Mazumdar S, Taplin S, McKetin R. Prescription opioid analgesics for pain management in Australia: twenty years of dispensing. Intern Med J. 2015;46(8):955–63.
19. Degenhardt L, Gisev N, Cama E, Nielsen S, Larance B, Bruno R. The extent and correlates of community-based pharmaceutical opioid utilisation in Australia. Pharmacoepidemiol Drug Saf. 2016;25(5):521–38.
20. Australian Government Department of Health: The Pharmaceutical Benefit Scheme. Available at: http://www.pbs.gov.au/info/about-the-pbs; accessed on 18 August 2016.
21. WHO Collaborating Centre for Drug Statistics Methodology. Guidelines for ATC classification and DDD assignment 2018. Oslo, Norway, 2017. https://www.whocc.no/filearchive/publications/guidelines.pdf.
22. World Health Organization: Daily Defined Dose (DDD): Definition and general considerations. Available at: https://www.whocc.no/ddd/definition_and_general_considera/; accessed on 1 December 2017.
23. Department of Infrastructure and Regional Development (DIRD). Local government national report, 2013–14. Canberra: DIRD; 2015. Available at http://regional.gov.au/local/publications/reports/2013_2014/INFRA2466_LGNR_2013-14.pdf.
24. StataCorp. Stata Statistical Software: Release 14. College Station: StataCorp LP; 2015.
25. Microsoft. Microsoft Excel [computer software]. Redmond, Washington: Microsoft; 2013.
26. R Core Team. R: A language and environment for statistical Computing R Foundation for Statistical Computing. Vienna; 2011. Retrieved from http://www.R-project.org/.
27. Fayaz A, Croft P, Langford RM, Donaldson LJ, Jones GT. Prevalence of chronic pain in the UK: a systematic review and meta-analysis of population studies. BMJ Open. 2016;6(6):e010364.
28. Brennan F, Carr DB, Cousins M. Pain management: a fundamental human right. Anesth Analg. 2007;105(1):205–21.
29. Lembke A. Why doctors prescribe opioids to patients they know are abusing them? SCOPE. Stanford Medicine. Available at: http://scopeblog.stanford.edu/2012/10/25/why-doctors-prescribe-opioids-to-patients-they-know-are-abusing-them/; accessed on 4 November 2016.
30. Van Zee A. The promotion and marketing of oxycontin: commercial triumph, public health tragedy. Am J Public Health. 2009;99(2):221–7.
31. Nielsen S, Bruno R, Degenhardt L, Stoove MA, Fischer JA, Carruthers SJ, Lintzeris N. The sources of pharmaceuticals for problematic users of benzodiazepines and prescription opioids. Med J Aust. 2013;199(10):696–9.
32. Roxburgh A, Bruno R, Larance B, Burns L. Prescription of opioid analgesics and related harms in Australia. Med J Aust. 2011;195:280–4.
33. Stafford J, Burns L. Australian Drug Trends 2012: Findings from the Illicit Drug Reporting System (IDRS). In: Australian Drug Trend Series No 91. Sydney: National Drug and Alcohol Research Centre, University of New South Wales; 2013.
34. Black E, Roxburgh A, Degenhardt L, Bruno R, Campbell G, Bd G, Fetherston J, Kinner S, Moon C, Quinn B, et al. Australian Drug Trends 2007: Findings from the Illicit Drug Reporting System (IDRS) Australian Drug Trend Series No. 1. Sydney: National Drug and Alcohol Research Centre, University of New South Wales; 2008.
35. NPS Medicinewise: Oxycodone-with-naloxone controlled-release tablets (Targin) for chronic severe pain. 2011, Available at: https://www.nps.org.au/radar/articles/oxycodone-with-naloxone-controlled-release-tablets-targin-for-chronic-severe-pain.
36. Sadowski CA, Carrie AG, Grymonpre RE, Metge CJ, St John P. Access and intensity of use of prescription analgesics among older Manitobans. Can J Clin Pharmacol. 2009;16(2):e322–30.
37. Simoni-Wastila L. The use of abusable prescription drugs: the role of gender. J Womens Health Gend Based Med. 2000;9(3):289–97.
38. Back SE, Payne RL, Simpson AN, Brady KT. Gender and prescription opioids: findings from the National Survey on drug use and health. Addict Behav. 2010;35(11):1001–7.
39. Centers for Disease Control and Prevention: Prescription Painkiller Overdoses: A Growing Epidemic, Especially Among Women. 2017, Available at: https://www.cdc.gov/vitalsigns/prescriptionpainkilleroverdoses/index.html; accessed on 18 Nov 2017.
40. Back SE, Payne RL, Wahlquist AH, Carter RE, Stroud Z, Haynes L, Hillhouse M, Brady KT, Ling W. Comparative profiles of men and women with opioid dependence: results from a national multisite effectiveness trial. Am J Drug Alcohol Abuse. 2011;37(5):313–23.
41. Back SE, Lawson KM, Singleton LM, Brady KT. Characteristics and correlates of men and women with prescription opioid dependence. Addict Behav. 2011;36(8):829–34.
42. Galea S, Vlahov D. Social determinants and the health of drug users: socioeconomic status, homelessness, and incarceration. *Public Health Rep.* 2002;117(Suppl 1):S135–45.
43. Allin S, Laporte A. Socioeconomic status and the use of medicines in the Ontario public drug program. Canadian Public Policy. 2011;37(4):563–76.
44. Prunuske JP, St Hill CA, Hager KD, Lemieux AM, Swanoski MT, Anderson GW, Lutfiyya MN. Opioid prescribing patterns for non-malignant chronic pain for rural versus non-rural US adults: a population-based study using 2010 NAMCS data. BMC Health Serv Res. 2014;14:563.
45. Piantadosi S, Byar DP, Green SB. The ecological fallacy. Am J Epidemiol. 1988;127(5):893–904.
46. Australian Government Department of Human Servcies. Prescription Shopping Programme. Available at: https://www.humanservices.gov.au/health-professionals/services/medicare/prescription-shopping-programme; accessed on 1 September 2016.
47. Islam MM, McRae IS. An inevitable wave of prescription drug monitoring programs in the context of prescription opioids: pros, cons and tensions. *BMC Pharmacol Toxicol.* 2014;15(1):46.
48. Nielsen S, Bruno R. Implementing real-time prescription drug monitoring: are we ready? Drug Alcohol Rev. 2014;33(5):463–5.
49. Ogeil RP, Heilbronn C, Lloyd B, Lubman DI. Prescription drug monitoring in Australia: capacity and coverage issues. Med J Aust. 2016;204(4):148.
50. Islam MM, McRae IS. Real-time prescription drug monitoring program in Australia: we should be ready. Drug Alcohol Rev. 2015;34(3):344–5.
51. Victoria State Government: Real-time prescription monitoring initiative FAQ. Available at: https://www2.health.vic.gov.au/public-health/drugs-and-poisons/real-time-prescription-monitoring. 2016.
52. Shand FL, Campbell G, Hall W, Lintzeris N, Cohen M, Degenhardt L. Real-time monitoring of schedule 8 medicines in Australia: evaluation is essential. Med J Aust. 2013;198(2):80–1.
53. Griggs C: 2014–2015 APhA policy committee report. Integrated Nationwide Prescription Drug Monitoring Program Available at: https://www.pharmacist.com/sites/default/files/files/Prescription%20Drug%20Monitoring%20Programs.pdf; Accesson on 26 August 2016.

Proteomic study revealed antipsychotics-induced nuclear protein regulations in B35 cells are similar to the regulations in C6 cells and rat cortex

Tinchou Li[1,2], Mingcheng Lee[3], Fuming Tsai[3,4], Yunhsiang Chen[5], Yiyin Lin[3] and Maoliang Chen[3*]

Abstract

Background: Based on accumulating evidence, the regulation of protein expression by antipsychotic drugs (APDs) might be closely related to the control of psychotic symptoms when these drugs are used to treat mental disorders. The low quantity of nuclear proteins in the cell hinders their detection because signal for rare proteins are masked in most proteomic detection systems.

Methods: Nuclear proteins fractionated from APD-treated B35 cells were labeled with iTRAQ and detected by LC/MS/MS to investigate APD-induced alterations in nuclear protein expression. Western blot, immunofluorescent cell staining, and immunohistochemical staining were applied to validate the findings.

Results: The expression of ADP/ATP translocase 2, heat shock cognate 71 kDa protein, histone H1.2, histone H3.3, histone H4, non-POU domain-containing octamer-binding protein, nucleolin, nucleophosmin, prelamin-A/C, plectin-1, vimentin, and 40S ribosomal protein S3a was regulated by APDs in B35 cells, according to our proteomic data. According to the results of the gene ontology analysis, all these proteins played important roles in biological processes or in molecular functions in cells. Western blot results showing APD-induced alterations in nuclear protein expression in B35 cells were consistent with the LC/MS/MS results. Heat shock cognate 71 kDa protein and vimentin expression in C6 cells were not affected by the three APDs. As shown in the immunofluorescent cell staining, all the three APDs altered protein expression to similar extents. We also examined whether the expression of these proteins was affected by APDs in the prefrontal cortex of rats administered sub-chronic and chronic APD treatments by western blotting and immunohistochemical staining.

Conclusions: The findings of the proteomic analysis of APD-treated B35 cells were recapitulated in the APD-treated rat cortex. The expression of some proteins was altered by APDs in rat prefrontal cortex in a time-dependent manner.

Keywords: Antipsychotic drugs (APDs) - nuclear protein - rat prefrontal cortex - neuronal cell - glial cell

Background

Antipsychotic drugs (APDs) have been proposed to regulate gene and protein expression in the brain [1–3]. Based on accumulating evidence, APDs also ease psychotic symptoms and induce side-effects by regulating gene or protein expression levels [3]. Most psychotic disorders, including schizophrenia, are genetically complex diseases with unclear pathogenic mechanisms. In addition, the complexity of actions of antipsychotic drugs on regulating psychotic symptoms and other drug effects originating from the variety of binding profiles of each APD [4] has hampered our ability to clarify the molecular mechanisms underlying the actions of antipsychotic drugs.

Recently, studies of DNA-methylation, post-translational modifications (PTMs) of histone proteins and non-coding RNA regulated protein translation have suggested that proteins in cell nuclei might play important roles in the epigenetic regulation of cell functions [5, 6]. In addition,

* Correspondence: cater0656@hotmail.com
[3]Department of Research, Taipei Tzu Chi Hospital, Buddhist Tzu Chi Medical Foundation, New Taipei City, Taiwan, Republic of China
Full list of author information is available at the end of the article

proteins' functions related to the regulations of gene and protein expression in cell nuclei are also major targets for studying the mechanism of the actions of APDs and aetiology of mental disorders.

O'Brien and colleagues used 2-dimensional polyacrylamide gel electrophoresis (2D-PAGE) to discover the differential protein expression profiles between the risperidone-treated and control rat striatum and to reveal the possible causes of extrapyramidal symptoms (EPS) induced by antipsychotics [7]. Ji and colleagues also used 2D-PAGE to examine the effects of chlorpromazine, clozapine, quetiapine on rat mitochondria from the rat cerebral cortex and hippocampus and found that abnormal cerebral energy metabolism might be involved in the both the curative effects and side effects of antipsychotics [8]. Kedracka-Krok and colleagues used 2-dimensional difference gel electrophoresis (2D-DIGE) to examine protein expression profiles in the cerebral cortex of rats treated with clozapine or risperidone [9]. Clozapine was shown to regulate proteins related to the cytoskeletal structure and calcium homeostasis.

Liquid chromatography-tandem mass spectrometry (LC/MS/MS) has been widely applied in proteomic studies over the last two decades to identify possible biomarkers for studying various diseases [10–12]. LC/MS/MS separates and detects digested peptides to identify detected proteins utilizing peptide spectrum algorithms in a peptide identification database. It also precedes relative quantification with or without isotope labelling to determine and compare the expression of proteins in different samples [10]. However, the complexity of the sample used for the analysis represents a critical issue in the ability to produce reliable detection results, even when a sensitive and accurate LC/MS/MS platform that has been improved by developing detection techniques is available. Another breakthrough is the use of stable isotope reagents, such as isobaric tags for relative and absolute quantitation (iTRAQ) reagents [13, 14], which were developed for labelling peptides to enable multiplex sample analysis during LC/MS/MS detection processes [15, 16]. These stable isotope reagents enable the identification and quantification of multiple samples in one detection run to reduce the possible bias between batches.

The enrichment of particular types of proteins, such as glycoproteins (glycome) or phosphoproteins (phosphoproteome) [17, 18], is another way to discover the specific low abundance proteins in a crude protein mixture in study of schizophrenia. The fractionation of proteins according to their molecular properties or their location in cells also reduces the sample complexity. In this study, nuclear proteins purified from APD-treated B35 were labelled with iTRAQ reagents and analysed by LC/MS/MS to discover the regulatory effects of APDs on protein expression in nuclei. Differentially expressed nuclear proteins detected by LC/MS/MS were then further validated in APD-treated B35 cells, C6 cells and the rat prefrontal cortex by western blotting, immunofluorescent staining and/or immunohistochemical staining.

Methods

Antibodies

The antibodies included: anti-actin, ab6276 (Abcam, Cambridge, UK); anti-Histone H4 (HIST1H4B), #13919 (Cell Signaling Technology, Danvers, MA, USA); anti-Heat shock cognate 71 kDa protein (HSPA8), #8444 (Cell Signaling Technology); anti-nucleolin (NCL), #12247 (Cell Signaling Technology); anti-nucleophosmin (NPM1), #3542 (Cell Signaling Technology); anti-vimentin (VIM), #3932 (Cell Signaling Technology); anti-plectin-1 (PLEC), #12254 (Cell Signaling Technology). All antibodies were used at the recommended fold dilution described on the manufacture's datasheet.

Cell culture and APD treatments

Risperidone was obtained from Janssen-Pharmaceutica (Beerse, Belgium), and haloperidol and clozapine were obtained from Sigma-Aldrich (St. Louis, MO, USA). C6 and B35 cells were obtained from the Bioresource Collection and Research Center (BCRC) of the Food Industry Research and Development Institute (FRDI), Taiwan. C6 cells were cultured in DMEM high-glucose medium (Invitrogen Life Technologies, Carlsbad, CA, USA) supplemented with 2 mM L-glutamine, 10% horse serum (Invitrogen Life Technologies), and 2% fetal bovine serum (Invitrogen Life Technologies). B35 cells were maintained in MEM medium (Invitrogen Life Technologies) supplemented with 10% fetal bovine serum (Invitrogen Life Technologies). One of the APDs (haloperidol, risperidone, or clozapine) was added to the medium once a day. The concentrations of each APD used in this study were determined based on results from our previous publication. A 1 × PBS solution was added to culture medium to serve as the control supplement. The final concentration of each APD in the culture medium was 4 μg/ml (10 μM) for haloperidol, 4 μg/ml (8 μM) for risperidone, and 2.5 μg/ml (7.65 μM) for clozapine. C6 cells were subcultured when they exhibited a density of approximately 70% confluence to prevent abnormal production of the S100 protein. Cells were harvested when they had reached 60–70% confluence after treatment with APDs for 5 days.

Animals and drug treatment

All experimental procedures used to treat animals in this study were approved by the Institutional Animal Care and Use Committee (IACUC) of Taipei Tzu Chi Hospital, Buddhist Tzu Chi Medical Foundation (101-IACUC-028). Male Sprague-Dawley (SD) rats weighing 120–150 g were housed in a temperature- and humidity-controlled feeding room with a 12-h light/ dark cycle and had free access to water and food for 5 days before the APD treatment. Two independent APD treatment batches were performed in this study. In both batches, rats ($n = 3$ per group) were intraperitoneally injected with haloperidol (1 mg/kg), risperidone (1 mg/kg), clozapine (20 mg/kg), or PBS once daily for 7 days for subchronic APD treatment. For the chronic treatment, two independent APD treatment batches (n = 3 per group in each batch) of SD rats received haloperidol (1 mg/kg), risperidone (1 mg/kg), clozapine (20 mg/kg), or vehicle once daily for 28 days. SD rats were sacrificed by CO_2 asphyxiation 24 h after the last injection. Dissected cerebral cortices were stored in liquid nitrogen or were soaked in 4% paraformaldehyde for 24 h for paraffin embedding.

Nuclear protein extraction

C6 or B35 cells treated with each APD were harvested for nuclear protein extraction using a Nuclear Extraction Kit (Chemicon International Inc., California, USA), according to manufacture's instructions. Briefly, cells were harvested and were resuspended in 1 × Cytoplasmic Lysis Buffer containing 0.5 mM DTT and a Protease Inhibitor Mix (GE Healthcare Bio-Science, Uppsala, Sweden). The mixture was then placed on ice for 15 min and centrifuged at 250×g for 5 min at 4 °C. The cell pellet was resuspended in 1 × Cytoplasmic Lysis Buffer and the cells were disrupted using a syringe with a 27-gauge needle followed by centrifugation at 8000×g for 20 min at 4 °C. The supernatant was collected as the cytoplasmic proteins fraction. The nuclear pellet was washed and lysed with Nuclear Extraction Buffer at 4 °C for 60 min, and the nuclear extract was then centrifuged at 16,000×g for 5 min at 4 °C. The supernatant was transferred to a fresh tube and served as the nuclear protein fraction.

iTRAQ labelling and LC/MS/MS proteomic analysis

Fractionated nuclear proteins from APD-treated B35 cells were labelled with iTRAQ reagents (Applied Biosystems), according to the manufacturer's instructions. Briefly, 10 μg of nuclear proteins from B35 cells were reduced with a reducing reagent at 60 °C for 1 h. Cysteine residues were then blocked with cysteine blocking reagent for 10 min at room temperature, followed by trypsin digestion at 37 °C for 16 h. iTRAQ-4 plex labelling reagents were then added to each peptide sample and the mixtures were further incubated at room temperature for 60 min. Each of the peptide samples was then combined and evaporated in a vacuum dryer at room temperature. The dried residue was dissolved in 50 μl of ddH_2O. Five microliters of iTRAQ-labelled residue were analysed using an HPLC system (Agilent) coupled with a 3200 Q TRAP LC/MS/MS System (MDS SCIEX, Applied Biosystems). The iTRAQ-labelled residue was separated on the reverse-phase C18 column at a flow rate of 10 μl/min. The eluent gradient consisted of buffer A (0.1% formic acid in H_2O) and buffer B (0.1% formic acid in acetonitrile). Peptides were subjected to electrospray ionization followed by tandem mass spectrometry. The collected data were then analysed to identify and quantify the proteins using the ProteinPilot ™ 3.0 (MDS SCIEX) software.

Western blot analysis

Nuclear protein extracts from both cell lines and the rat cerebral cortex were prepared as described above. Approximately 5–20 μg of nuclear proteins were separated on 12.5% sodium dodecyl sulphate polyacrylamide gels. The resolved proteins in the gel were then transferred to polyvinylidene difluoride membranes. After blocking, membranes were incubated with specific primary antibodies for 14 h at 4 °C. After washes with 1 × PBS, membranes were then incubated with horseradish peroxidase-conjugated goat anti-mouse or anti-rabbit antibodies (Cat. # 401215 and # 401315, Calbiochem, Darmstadt, Germany) at room temperature for 1 h. Target protein bands were developed using the Amersham ECL kit (Amersham, Bucks, UK). We examined the lack of GAPDH in the nuclear fraction and the lack of lamin B in the cytosolic fraction to control the quality of nuclear extraction processes. Beta-actin was examined served as a quantification control.

Immunofluorescent staining of C6 and B35 cells

C6 or B35 cells were seeded onto coverslips in a 6-well plate at a density of 5×10^3 cells per well and cultured in medium for 5 days with APDs added daily as described in the drug treatment section above. After APD treatment, coverslips with C6 or B35 cells were transferred to a fresh 6-well plate and washed with 1× PBS. Cells were then fixed by incubating the coverslips in paraformaldehyde for 15 min. Coverslips were then washed with 1× PBS. Cells were further permeabilized with methanol and incubated at − 20 °C for 15 min. After blocking with BSA for 15 min at room temperature, coverslips were incubated with a specific antibody for 1 h at room temperature. Coverslips were washed three times with 0.1% PBST and then incubated with specific secondary antibodies for 1 h at room temperature. Antibodies were removed and the coverslips were washed with 0.1% PBST followed by 4′6-diamidino-2-phenylindole (DAPI) staining for 4 min. Coverslips were then washed with 1 × PBS, mounted on slides with mounting gel, and sealed with nail polish. Quantification of the fluorescent intensity was performed using the image quantification software ImageJ 1.50i obtained from the NIH website (http://imagej.nih.gov/ij/). Areas of interest on the image were selected using the polygon selection method to quantify the immunofluorescent staining. The mean intensities of all areas were then calculated to represent the expression level of the detected protein.

Immunohistochemistry analysis of rat prefrontal cortex

Paraffin-embedded brain samples were sectioned at 5 μm and placed on silane-coated glass slides. Slides containing sections were incubated at 70 °C for 2 h and then immediately immersed in Trilogy solution (Cell Marque, BH, The Hague, NL) to remove the paraffin. Slides were pressure heated in Trilogy solution at 120 °C for 15 min to remove the traces of paraffin and to retrieval the antigen in the samples. After washing the slides twice with ddH_2O, tissue sections were incubated with 3% H_2O_2 in PBS to eliminate endogenous peroxidase activity. Sections were then blocked with 2% BSA in PBS for 20 min and then incubated with a specific antibody for 2 h at 37 °C. Slides were washed twice with PBS and incubated with a specific secondary antibody for 30 min at room temperature. Slides were washed twice with PBS, followed by application of the substrate solution, 3,3′-diaminobenzidine tetrahydrochloride (DAB) to develop the result. The developing reaction was stopped by immersing the slides in ddH_2O twice, followed by the addition of Mayer's haematoxylin for counterstaining (Thermo Fisher Scientific). Slides were then rinsed with ddH_2O three times, cleared in a non-xylene solution, and mounted with coverslips and the slide mounting medium DPX Mountant (Sigma). For determining changes in protein expression in the immunohistochemistry analysis, two independent colleagues were invited to compare the changes in protein expression on images of the immunohistochemical staining.

Total RNA isolation and gene expression assay

Total RNA was extracted from sub-chronic APD-treated C6 or B35 cells using TRIZOL Total RNA Isolation Reagent (Invitrogen Life Technologies), according to the manufacturer's instructions. Briefly, cells were directly lysed and homogenized in 1 ml of TRIZOL denaturing reagent in a 10-cm cell culture dish followed by transfer to 1.5-ml centrifuge tubes. Homogenates were incubated on ice for 5 min, vortexed vigorously, and centrifuged at 12,000 x g for 10 min at 4 °C. Supernatants were then transferred to fresh tubes. Two hundred microliters of chloroform were added to each ml of supernatant, and the samples were then vigorously mixed and incubated on ice for 5 min, followed by centrifugation at 12,000 x g for 10 min at 4 °C. Each aqueous phase was transferred to a fresh tube, and the chloroform extraction procedure was repeated. Each aqueous phase was collected and mixed with 0.7 volume of 2-propanol. The mixtures were incubated at − 20 °C for 1 h and centrifuged at 12,000 x g for 30 min at 4 °C. RNA pellets were washed twice with 75% ethanol, air dried, and dissolved in RNase-free water. Reverse transcription was performed using High Capacity cDNA Reverse Transcription Kits (Applied Biosystems), according to the manufacturer's instructions. Real-time quantitative polymerase chain reactions (RT-QPCR) were performed using an ABI 7900 HT Fast Real-Time PCR System in combination with continuous SYBR Green detection (Applied Biosystems) after the reverse transcription reaction. RT-QPCR was performed in a reaction volume of 20 μl containing 2 μl of diluted cDNAs, 10 μl of SYBR Green PCR Master Mix (Applied Biosystems), 2 μl each of sense and antisense primers (2 mM), and 4 μl of H_2O. The primer sequences for each gene used in this study are listed in Additional file 1: Table S1. The general PCR conditions were: polymerase activation at 95 °C for 10 min followed by 50 cycles of denaturation at 95 °C for 15 s, annealing at 60 °C for 30 s, and extension at 72 °C for 60 s. After amplification, a melting curve was acquired to determine the optimal PCR conditions. The relative standard curve method was used to quantify mRNA expression. The relative gene expression levels in each sample were calculated from the respective standard curves using a linear regression analysis. The mRNA expression levels of each gene were normalized to beta-actin expression. All experiments were performed in duplicate. Differences in the normalized mRNA expression levels of the examined gene between APD-treated and drug-naive C6 or B35 cells were assessed using one-way ANOVA followed by the Dunnett post hoc comparison test. One-way ANOVA and the Dunnett post hoc comparison test were performed with SPSS Statistics 17.0.

Results

LC/MS/MS revealed the regulation of protein expression in the nuclei of APD-treated B35 cells

Nuclear proteins harvested from each of the APDs-treated B35 and control B35 cells were labelled with iTRAQ reagents and were analysed using LC/MS/MS. Three independent batches of nuclear proteins from APD-treated B35 cells were used as biological repeats. Twenty-five proteins were identified by LC/MS/MS. As shown in Table 1, ADP/ATP translocase 2(SLC25A5), heat shock cognate 71 kDa protein (HSPA8), histone H1.2 (HIST1H1C), histone H3.3(H3F3B), histone H4(HIST1H4B), non-POU domain-containing octamer-binding protein(NONO), nucleolin(NCL), nucleophosmin(NPM1), prelamin-A/C(LMNA), plectin-1(PLEC), vimentin(VIM), and 40S ribosomal protein S3a(RPS3A) represent 12 proteins that showed significant changes (p-value< 0.05) in expression in B35 cells treated with at least one of the three APDs. According to the gene ontology analysis, all these proteins played important roles in biological processes in cells (Table 2). Some proteins play roles in molecular functions or as cellular components. HIST1H1C, H3F3B, and HIST1H4B are histone proteins. HSPA8 and NPM1 are chaperone

Table 1 List of proteins identified by LC/MS/MS that were differentially regulated by various APDs in B35 cells

UniProt ID	Name	Fold change compared to control group		
		HAL	RIS	CLO
Q09073	ADP/ATP translocase 2	1.604	1.765	0.967
P63018	Heat shock cognate 71 kDa protein	2.644	3.754	1.414
P15865	Histone H1.2	1.791	1.971	1.182
P84245	Histone H3.3	1.510	1.319	0.539
P62804	Histone H4	1.553	1.235	0.528
Q5FVM4	Non-POU domain-containing octamer-binding protein	1.582	1.428	1.009
P13383	Nucleolin	2.147	2.294	1.527
P13084	Nucleophosmin	2.233	2.651	1.650
P30427	Plectin-1	2.156	2.158	1.230
P48679	Prelamin-A/C	1.775	1.865	1.302
P31000	Vimentin	2.130	2.369	1.593
P49242	40S ribosomal protein S3a	2.238	2.479	1.833

proteins in cells. SLC25A5 and RPS3A are ribosomal proteins that regulate ribosome function. LMNA and VIM are structural proteins and act as intermediate filaments in cells.

Validation of APD-induced regulation of protein expression in the nuclei of B35 and C6 cells

Our previous researches mentioned that APDs might induce differential protein expression regulation in different cell types, such as B35 neuronal cells and C6 glial cells. We then further validated APD-induced regulation of protein expression in the nuclei of B35 and C6 cells. Five proteins were selected for validation using western blotting. Almost all selected targets showed consistent changes in expression in the nuclei of APD-treated B35 cells as measured using LC/MS/MS (Fig. 1(**a**)-(**j**)). Only HIST1H4B expression in B35 nuclei was not affected by risperidone (Fig. 1(**a**) and (**b**)). In C6 nuclei, we found that HSPA8 (Fig. 1(**c**) and (**d**)) and VIM (Fig. 1(**i**) and (**j**)) expression were not affected by any of the three

Table 2 Gene ontology analysis of nuclear proteins identified in APD-treated B35 cells

Name	Protein Class	Function Class
Histone H4 (HIST1H4B)	histone	Biological Process
Histone H3.3 (H3F3B)	histone	Biological Process
ADP/ATP translocase 2 (SLC25A5)	amino acid transportermitochondrial carrier proteintransfer/ carrier proteinribosomal proteincalmodulin	Molecular Function Biological Process Cellular Component
Non-POU domain-containing octamer-binding protein (NONO)	mRNA splicing factor	Molecular Function Biological Process
Histone H1.2 (HIST1H1C)	histone	Biological Process
Plectin-1 (PLEC)	non-motor actin binding protein	Molecular Function Biological Process Cellular Component
Prelamin-A/C (LMNA)	structural protein intermediate filament	Molecular Function Biological Process
Heat shock cognate 71 kDa protein (HSPA8)	Hsp70 family protein chaperone	Biological Process
Nucleolin (NCL)	–	Biological Process
Vimentin (VIM)	structural protein intermediate filament	Molecular Function Biological Process Cellular Component
Nucleophosmin (NPM1)	chaperone	Biological Process
40S ribosomal protein S3a (RPS3A)	ribosomal protein	Molecular Function Biological Process Cellular Component

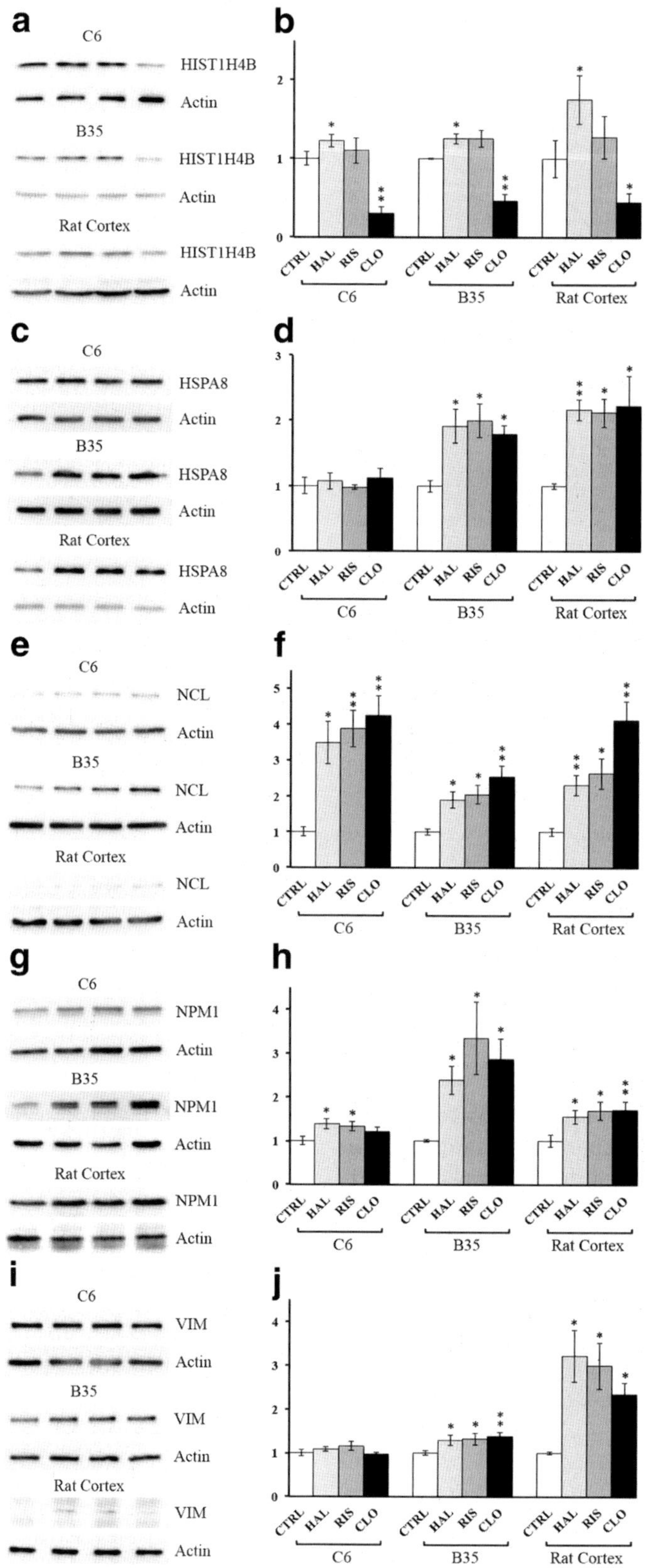

Fig. 1 (See legend on next page.)

(See figure on previous page.)
Fig. 1 Western blot showing APD-induced changes in the expression of the HIST1H4B, HSPA8, NCL, NPM1, and VIM proteins in C6 and B35 cells and the rat cortex. Nuclear protein extracts collected from APD-treated C6 cells, B35 cells and rat cortex were compared. **a** and (**b**), HIST1H4B; (**c**) and (**d**),HSPA8; (**e**) and (**f**), NCL; (**g**) and (**h**), NPM1; (**i**) and (**j**), VIM. Bar charts were constructed from triplicate western blot data obtained from three different batches of APD-treated cells or rat cortices using ANOVA followed by Dunnett's test (*p-value < 0.05; **p-value < 0.01). Haloperidol (HAL), risperidone (RIS), clozapine (CLO), or PBS (control group, CTRL))

APDs. HIST1H4B (Fig. 1(**a**) and (**b**)) and NCL (Fig. 1(**e**) and (**f**)) expression in C6 nuclei were regulated by APDs, similar to APD-treated B35 cells. Haloperidol and risperidone induced NPM1 expression in C6 nuclei (Fig. 1(**g**) and (**h**)). Clozapine did not significantly affect NPM1 expression in C6 nuclei.

Western blots revealed differences in protein expression in the sub-chronic APD-treated rat cortex

We also examined HIST1H4B, HSPA8, NCL, NPM1, and VIM expression in APD-treated rat cortices. As shown in Fig. 1, HSPA8, NCL, NPM1, and VIM expression were upregulated in the rat cortex following treatment with any of the three APDs. HIST1H4B expression in the rat cortex was upregulated by haloperidol but reduced by clozapine (Fig. 1(**a**) and (**b**)). The sub-chronic risperidone treatment did not affect HIST1H4B expression in the rat cortex.

Immunofluorescent staining revealed APD-induced nuclear protein regulation in C6 and B35 cells

Immunofluorescent staining was also used to examine the regulation of protein expression by APD treatments in C6 and B35 cells. In both cell lines, HSPA8, NLC, NPM1, PLEC, and VIM expression were upregulated by each of the three APDs (Additional file 2: Figure S3, Additional file 3: Figure S4, Additional file 4: Figure S5, Additional file 5: Figure S6, Additional file 6: Figure S7, Additional file 7: Figure S8, Additional file 8: Figure S9, Additional file 9: Figure S10, Additional file 10: Figure S11, Additional file 11: Figure S12, Table 3). In contrast to the increase in HIST1H4B expression induced by haloperidol and risperidone, clozapine reduced HIST1H4B expression in both C6 and B35 cells (Additional file 12: Figure S1 and Additional file 13: Figure S2). Moreover, HIST1H4B, NLC, and NPM1 were expressed in cell nuclei. HSPA8 was generally detected throughout cells. The expression of NLM and NPM1 was induced and specifically accumulated in cell nuclei. PLEC and VIM were mainly expressed in cell nuclei, but were also detected in the cell cytoplasm. Furthermore, we also observed accumulation of PLEC and VIM staining on the nuclear membrane of APD-treated cells.

Table 3 Immunofluorescent staining revealed alterations in protein expression in APD-treated C6 and B35 cells

	C6			B35		
	HAL	RIS	CLO	HAL	RIS	CLO
HIST1H4B	↑	↑	↓	↑	↑	↓
HSPA8	↑	↑	↑	↑	↑	↑
NLC	↑	↑	↑	↑	↑	↑
NPM1	↑	↑	↑	↑	↑	↑
PLEC	↑	↑	↑	↑	↑	↑
VIM	↑	↑	↑	↑	↑	↑

"↑" means induction of expression compared to control group; "↓" means reduction of expression compared to control group

Regulation of protein expression in sub-chronic and chronic APD-treated rat cortices

We also compared the regulation of protein expression in sub-chronic and chronic APD-treated rat cortices using immunohistochemistry. As shown in Fig. 2, each of the three APDs induced HSP8A, NLC, NPM1, PLEC, and VIM expression in the cortex of sub-chronic APD-treated rats (Additional file 14: Table S2). Haloperidol and risperidone did not significantly change HIST1H4B expression in the rat cortex. Clozapine reduced HIST1H4B expression in the rat cortex. In the chronic APD-treated rat cortex, NLC, PLEC, and VIM expression were induced by each of the three APDs (Fig. 3, Additional file 14: Table S2). Haloperidol and risperidone did not affect HIST1H4B expression, and clozapine reduced HIST1H4B expression in the chronic APD-treated rat cortex. Moreover, none of the three APDs altered HSPA8 and NPM1 expression in the chronic APD-treated rat cortex.

Real-time quantitative PCR revealed alterations in gene expression in sub-chronic APD-treated C6 and B35 cells

Levels of the HIST1H4B, HSPA8, NCL, NPM1 PLEC and VIM transcripts were measured to investigate the effect of APDs on the expressions of genes encoding the proteins discovered in this study. As shown in Table 4, clozapine, but not haloperidol or risperidone, increased Histlh4b expression in C6 cells. All three APDs decreased Hspa8, Npm1 and Plec expression in C6 cells. Ncl and Vim expression were not significantly affected by the three APDs in C6 cells. In B35 cells, risperidone and clozapine increased Histlh4b expression. None of the three APDs affected Hspa8 and Ncl expression in B35 cells. Npm1 expression was increased by haloperidol and decreased by clozapine treatment in B35 cells. Plec and Vim expression were increased by clozapine in B35 cells.

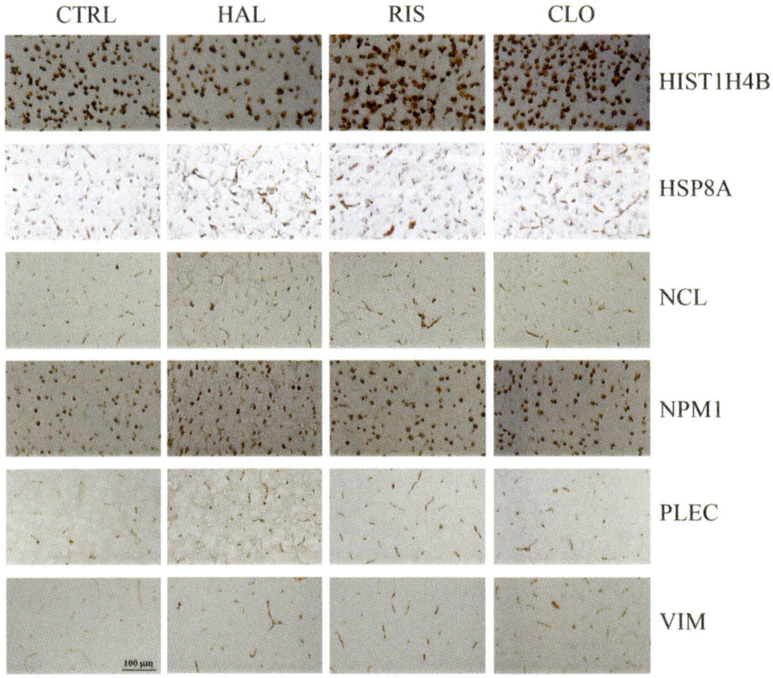

Fig. 2 Immunohistochemical staining of the rat prefrontal cortex following sub-chronic (1 week) treatment with APDs

Discussion

APDs induce nuclear protein regulation in B35 neuronal cells, C6 glial cells and also in the rat cortex. We only identified 25 proteins in this study, even though we used iTRAQ reagent coupled with LC/MS/MS to discover effects on proteins in the nuclei of APD-treated B35 cells. The number of the proteins identified in this study is quite low compared to other LC/MS/MS-based proteomic analyses. In this study, we used a 3200 Q TRAP LC/MS/MS instrument as the detection system to identify iTRAQ labelled peptides. The sensitivity of the equipment we used extremely limited the detection of

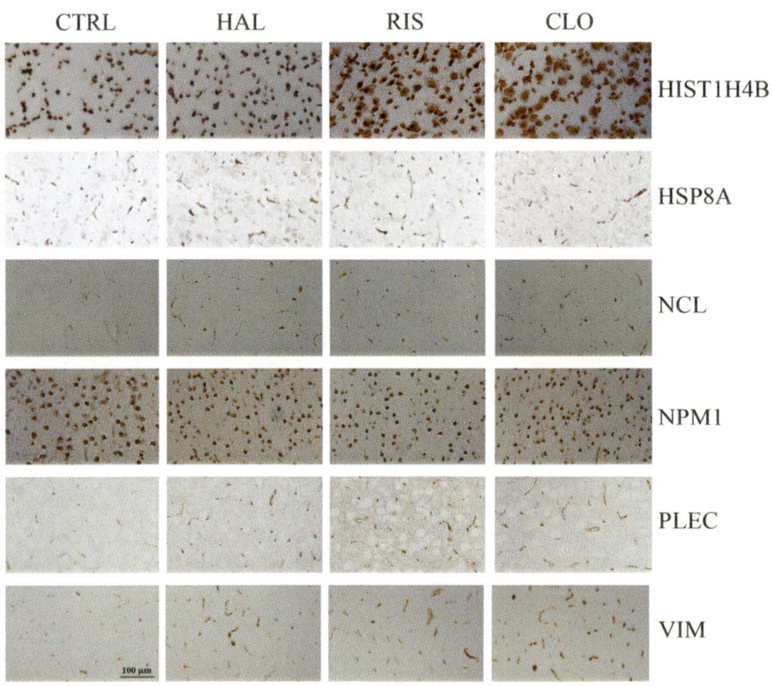

Fig. 3 Immunohistochemical staining of the rat prefrontal cortex following chronic (4-weeks) treatment with APDs

Table 4 Relative expression of Hist1h4b, Hspa8, Ncl, Npm1, Plec, and Vim genes in C6 and B35 cells after sub-chronic treatment by haloperidol, risperidone, or clozapine

		C6						B35					
Gene	Group	Fold Mean ± SD	*p*-valne[a]	MD	*F*	df	ANOVA-*p*	Fold Mean ± SD	*p*-valne	MD	*F*	df	ANOVA-*p*
Hist1h4b	CTRL	1.00 ± 0.183			8.374	12	0.003	1.00 ± 0.199			22.561	12	0.000
	HAL	1.67 ± 0.091	0.764	0.6748				2.23 ± 0.629	0.198	1.2308			
	RIS	0.90 ± 0.811	0.999	−0.0961				3.03 ± 0.778	0.024 [b]	2.0262*			
	CLO	4.56 ± 2.221	0.003[b]	3.5581*				6.17 ± 1.554	0.000 [b]	5.1730*			
Hspa8	CTRL	1.00 ± 0.063			298.9	12	0.000	1.00 ± 0.196			0.690	12	0.575
	HAL	0.13 ± 0.042	0.000 [b]	−0.8703*				0.84 ± 0.196	0.808	− 0.1624			
	RIS	0.08 ± 0.039	0.000 [b]	−0.9187*				1.10 ± 0.514	0.938	0.1023			
	CLO	0.20 ± 0.053	0.000 [b]	−0.8039*				0.84 ± 0.232	0.804	−0.1638			
Ncl	CTRL	1.00 ± 0.183			1.362	12	0.301	1.00 ± 0.420			1.347	12	0.306
	HAL	0.35 ± 0.185	0.162	−0.6501				1.64 ± 0.780	0.197	0.6423			
	RIS	0.74 ± 0.745	0.763	−0.2626				1.36 ± 0.333	0.598	0.3634			
	CLO	0.63 ± 0.481	0.556	−0.3673				1.14 ± 0.204	0.957	0.1374			
Npm1	CTRL	1.00 ± 0.118			4.778	12	0.020	1.00 ± 0.077			17.643	12	0.000
	HAL	0.39 ± 0.235	0.000 [b]	−0.6146*				1.65 ± 0.374	0.005 [b]	0.6497*			
	RIS	0.49 ± 0.381	0.000 [b]	−0.5104*				0.79 ± 0.059	0.467	−0.2109			
	CLO	0.52 ± 0.192	0.000 [b]	−0.4820*				0.49 ± 0.264	0.024 [b]	−0.5105*			
Plec	CTRL	1.00 ± 0.140			44.67	12	0.000	1.00 ± 0.120			27.378	12	0.000
	HAL	0.05 ± 0.040	0.000 [b]	−0.9482*				0.59 ± 0.079	0.052	−0.4090			
	RIS	0.13 ± 0.147	0.000 [b]	−0.8690*				0.99 ± 0.220	1.000	−0.0064			
	CLO	0.14 ± 0.170	0.000 [b]	−0.8556*				1.93 ± 0.347	0.000 [b]	0.9341*			
Vim	CTRL	1.00 ± 0.183			2.002	12	0.167	1.00 ± 0.077			11.822	12	0.001
	HAL	1.36 ± 0.549	0.453	0.36478				1.72 ± 0.365	0.796	0.7236			
	RIS	0.78 ± 0.412	0.769	−0.22386				1.55 ± 0.265	0.891	0.5534			
	CLO	1.33 ± 0.359	0.521	0.3327				6.07 ± 2.688	0.001 [b]	5.0720*			

Data are presented as mean of expression fold change ± SD. All gene expression experiments were performed in biological duplicates. SD = standard deviation; MD = mean difference; df = degree of freedom; ANOVA-*p* = *p*-value from one-way ANOVA analysis. [a]*p*-value = significant value calculated from Dunnett's C-tests that compare each APD-treated group to control group. [b] *p*-value < 0.05. *The mean difference is significant at the 0.05 level in Dunnett's C-tests

protein samples. This limited sensitivity is the major reason why we detected a low number of proteins in this proteomic experiment. Also, the use of nuclear proteins as the restricted sample source to reduce the sample complexity is another reason why we identified few proteins in this study.

Histones are found in eukaryotic cells and package DNA into nucleosomes. Histones also play important roles in DNA condensation and gene regulation. Histone modifications have been suggested to be related to the pathogenesis of schizophrenia. Some previous studies have reported increased histone deacetylase (HDAC1) expression in postmortem brain samples from patients with schizophrenia [19, 20]. Decreased expression of the reelin gene is associated with increased methylation of CpG islands in the reelin promoter [21], and reduced acetylation of histones [22] in NT2 cultures. HDAC inhibition has been proposed to improve neurodegeneration and cognitive function, and to induce neurogenesis in animals [23, 24]. HDAC2 overexpression has been shown to reduce the dendritic spine density, synapse number, and synaptic plasticity of neurons [25]. Some conflicting studies have shown that siRNA- and drug-induced HDAC1 inhibition impairs learning and increases cell death in rats. Moreover, increased HDAC1 expression protects rats from ischemic cell death and DNA damage [26]. In addition, as shown in the study by Akbarian and his colleagues, haloperidol and risperidone induce histone H3 phospho-acetylation, which is reversed by MK-801 [27]. A similar finding was also reported by Alessandra, who showed that haloperidol increased phosphorylation of histone H3 on serine28 (H3S28) [28]. In the present study, haloperidol and risperidone increased HIST1H1C, H3F3B and HIST1H4B expression. Clozapine reduced H3F3B and HIST1H4B expression, but not HIST1H1C expression. Although the results in this study might simply infer that APDs regulate histone expression to further modulate chromatin formation and gene regulation, histone modifications are simply the critical biological processes for mediating chromatin formation. Further examinations should be performed to clarify the relations between APD-induced regulation of histone expression and histone modifications.

HSPA8 and NPM1 are chaperone proteins that were affected by each of the three APDs in both B35 and C6 cells. APD-induced expression of HSPA8 and NPM1 was also observed in the sub-chronic APD-treated rat cortex. According to a recent study, a polymorphism in the HSPA8 gene (rs1136141) in patients with first-episode psychosis served as a risk factor for psychosis development [29]. Proteomic and epigenetic studies of postmortem brains also revealed downregulation of HSPA8 in patients with schizophrenia [10, 30], as well as in patients with Alzheimer's disease (AD) [31]. Another study also revealed downregulation of HSPA8 and NPM1 within layer 2 of the insular cortex, which is closely related to auditory hallucinations and language, in patients with schizophrenia [32]. A microarray study revealed downregulation of NPM1 gene expression in the postmortem cortex of patients with schizophrenia [33]. Based on our data, APD-induced HSP8A and NPM1 expression might be implicated in the possible therapeutic effects of these drugs on treating schizophrenia. As shown in a recent proteomic study, HSPA8 and NPM1 expression are reduced in oligodendrocytes following an acute clozapine treatment and subsequently restored by MK-801 [34]. In our previous research, acute (less than 3 days) APD-induced downregulation of protein expression might be oppositely regulated by a sub-chronic (more than 3 days) APD treatment [35]. This difference might be the reason for the inconsistent APD-induced alternations in the expression of the HSPA8 and NPM1 proteins between the two studies. Interestingly, none of the three APDs modulated HSPA8 and NPM1 expression in the chronic APD-treated rat cortex. This finding is explained by the observation that normal expression levels of HSPA8 or NPM1 should be maintained for these proteins to function as important chaperones in living animals, arguing against chronic APD-induced changes in protein expression. We also propose that living animals may try to maintain the original HSPA8 and NPM1 chaperone functions through various regulatory processes in the brain that prevent changes in protein expression induced by environmental stress.

NPM1 and NCL are multifunctional proteins in cells. NPM and NCL transit to the nucleoplasm in response to stress and participate in the repair of DNA damages [36]. NPM1 and NCL also regulate the expression of proteins related to the MAPK signalling pathway [37], which is abnormally expressed in the anterior cingulate (ACC) and dorsolateral prefrontal cortex (DLPFC) of patients with schizophrenia [38, 39]. We postulate that increased expression of NPM1 and NCL might be implicated in the regulation of proteins related to the MAPK signalling pathway when patients with schizophrenia are treated with certain APDs.

The VIM mRNA levels in superficial, deep, and white matter layers of the anterior cingulate gyrus were not significantly changed in patients with schizophrenia in a previous study [40]. Moreover, VIM expression is not affected by haloperidol or clozapine [41] treatment in rats. In addition, the VIM expression level in postmortem brain samples did not differ between patients with schizophrenia and control groups. VIM interacts with actin filaments through its C-terminal residue and interacts with the actin cytoskeleton through PLEC [42, 43]. In several cell types, PLEC also plays an important role in linking actin microfilaments, microtubules and intermediate filaments [42] to maintain cell morphogenesis and cell plasticity. Schizophrenia has been proposed as a disease with abnormal neuronal plasticity and neuronal regeneration in the brain. APDs were thought to induce plasticity in neuronal cells. All three APDs used in this study increased PLEC and VIM expression in both B35 and C6 cells. We also observed increased expression of PLEC and VIM in the cortex of sub-chronic and chronic APD-treated rats. Several publications have reported a lack of change in VIM expression in patients with schizophrenia. Anchoring of PLEC and VIM on the nuclear membrane is also a critical step in the reorganization ofactin microfilaments, microtubules and intermediate filaments. We also observed an accumulation of PLEC and VIM staining on the nuclear membrane of APD-treated B35 and C6 cells in this study. We propose that APDs-induced modulation of cell plasticity is associated with increased expression of PLEC and VIM. Furthermore, glutamate receptor subunit 3A(NR3A) has been suggested to interact with PLEC to function in intracellular processes, including trafficking and targeting of NR3A-containing receptors and PKC activation [44, 45]. Abnormal NR3A expression has also been observed in patients with various psychiatric disorders, including schizophrenia [46, 47]. Thus, APD-induced PLEC modulation may play important roles in the pathogenesis of schizophrenia by affecting NR3A expression and glutamate receptor function.

In this study, we also examined the regulations of the expression of the Hist1h4b, Hspa8, Ncl Npm1, Plec and Vim genes using real-time quantitative PCR. Compensatory regulation of Hist1h4b expression was observed in clozapine-treated C6 and B35cells. We also revealed compensatory regulation of Hspa8, Npm1 and Plec expression in APD-treated C6 cells. Furthermore, compensatory regulation of Npm1 expression was also investigated in B35 cells treated with clozapine. The compensatory regulation of these genes suggested that the expression of these proteins might not be transcriptionally regulated at the mRNA level in APD-treated cells. Although some proteins whose expression was induced by APDs in this study showed similar trends in gene expression at the transcriptional level, additional examinations should be performed to further verify the relations between APD-induced alterations in protein expression and the regulation of gene expression.

To clarify whether the alterations in protein expression found in this study are APDs specific or not, we examined NCL expression in C6 and B35 cells treated sub-chronically with all-trans retinoic acid (ATRA, 20 μM), H_2O_2 (40 μM), or caffeic acid (CA, 10 μM). As shown in Additional file 15: Figure S13(a), ATRA slightly induced NCL expression while H_2O_2 and CA dramatically induced NCL expression in C6 cells from two independent treatment batches. Moreover, ATRA reduced NCL expression but H_2O_2 and CA slightly induced NCL expression in B35 cells from two independent treatment batches. We also observed induction of VIM expression in ATRA treated C6 (Additional file 15: Figure S13(b)). H_2O_2 and CA did not significantly regulate VIM expression in C6 cells. ATRA, H_2O_2, and CA induce VIM expression in B35 cells. These results suggest that expression changes of NCL induced by APDs in both cells are not APDs specific effects. Also, most of the proteins identified in this study are the downstream proteins in different signaling pathways and to be regulated by various proteins at the same time in cells. We propose that the regulatory effects on these proteins might be similar between APDs but might not be APDs specific.

Based on our LC/MS/MS data, SLC25A5, HIST1H1C, H3F3B, NONO, LMNA and RPS3A expression were regulated in APD-treated B35 cells. HIST1H4B was chosen as a representative of histone protein expression in the follow-up validation experiments. The SLC25A5, NONO, LMNA and RPS3A proteins were not chosen for validation because little information about the relation between schizophrenia and these proteins is available. Although this study is the first to show that APDs (haloperidol, risperidone, and clozapine) regulate the expression of SLC25A5, NONO, LMNA and RPS3A in B35 cells, further studies should be performed to clarify the roles of these proteins in the pathogenesis of schizophrenia and the mechanisms of action of these antipsychotic drugs. As shown in the immunofluorescent staining of B35 and C6 cells, HSPA8 and VIM were expressed in both the cell nucleus and cytoplasm. This distribution might be the reason for the inconsistent results obtained using immunofluorescent staining and western blots in APD-treated C6 cells.

Conclusions

We identified 12 proteins expressed in nuclei of B35 cells that were regulated by the APDs used in this study. We used several experimental methods to validate APD-induced alternation in HIST1H4B, HSPA8, NCL, NPM1, PLEC, and VIM expression in different cell types (B35 and C6 cells) and also in the rat cortex. APD-induced alterations in HSPA8 and VIM expression differed between C6 cells and B35 cells. APD-induced alterations in HSPA8 and PLEC expression varied over time in the rat cortex.

Additional files

Additional file 1: Table S1. Reference sequences and primer sequences used to analyse gene expression in real-time quantitative PCR experiments. (TIFF 983 kb)

Additional file 2: Figure S3. Immunofluorescent staining revealed alterations in HSPA8 expression in APD-treated C6 cells. (TIFF 899 kb)

Additional file 3: Figure S4. Immunofluorescent staining revealed alterations in HSPA8 expression in APD-treated B35 cells. (TIFF 501 kb)

Additional file 4: Figure S5. Immunofluorescent staining revealed alterations in NCL expression in APD-treated C6 cells. (TIFF 666 kb)

Additional file 5: Figure S6. Immunofluorescent staining revealed alterations in NCL expression in APD-treated B35 cells. (DOCX 55 kb)

Additional file 6: Figure S7. Immunofluorescent staining revealed alterations in NPM1 expression in APD-treated C6 cells. (TIFF 554 kb)

Additional file 7: Figure S8. Immunofluorescent staining revealed alterations in NPM1 expression in APD-treated B35 cells. (DOCX 61 kb)

Additional file 8: Figure S9. Immunofluorescent staining revealed alterations in PLEC expression in APD-treated C6 cells. (TIFF 641 kb)

Additional file 9: Figure S10. Immunofluorescent staining revealed alterations in PLEC expression in APD-treated B35 cells. (TIFF 556 kb)

Additional file 10: Figure S11. Immunofluorescent staining revealed alterations in VIM expression in APD-treated C6 cells. (TIFF 732 kb)

Additional file 11: Figure S12. Immunofluorescent staining revealed alterations in VIM expression in APD-treated B35 cells. (TIFF 653 kb)

Additional file 12: Figure S1. Immunofluorescent staining revealed alterations in HIST1H4B expression in APD-treated C6 cells. (TIFF 570 kb)

Additional file 13: Figure S2. Immunofluorescent staining revealed alterations in HIST1H4B expression in APD-treated B35 cells. (TIFF 559 kb)

Additional file 14: Table S2. Immunohistochemical staining revealed alterations in protein expression in the rat prefrontal cortex following sub-chronic (1 week) and chronic (4 week) treatment with APDs. (TIFF 377 kb)

Additional file 15: Figure S13. Western blot showing ATRA-, H2O2-, and CA- induced changes in the expression of the NCL protein in C6 and B35 cells. Samples were collected from two independent batches of ATRA-, H2O2-, and CA- treated C6 and B35 cells. (TIFF 530 kb)

Abbreviation

2D-DIGE: 2-dimensional difference gel electrophoresis; 2D-PAGE: 2-dimensional polyacrylamide gel electrophoresis; ACC: Anterior cingulate; APDs: Antipsychotic drugs; ATRA: All-trans retinoic acid; CA: Caffeic acid; DLPFC: Dorsolateral prefrontal cortex; EPS: Extrapyramidal symptoms; H3F3B: Histone H3.3; H3S28: Histone H3 on serine28; HDAC1: Histone deacetylase; HIST1H1C: Histone H1.2; HIST1H4B: Histone H4; HSPA8: Heat shock cognate 71 kDa protein; iTRAQ: Isobaric tags for relative and absolute quantitation; LC/MS/MS: Liquid chromatography-tandem mass spectrometry; LMNA: Prelamin-A/C; NCL: Nucleolin; NONO: Non-POU domain-containing octamer-binding protein; NPM1: Nucleophosmin; NR3A: Glutamate receptor subunit 3A; PLEC: Plectin-1; PTMs: Post-translational modifications; RPS3A: 40S ribosomal protein S3a; RT-QPCR: Real-time quantitative polymerase chain reaction; SLC25A5: ADP/ATP translocase 2; VIM: Vimentin

Acknowledgments
The author thanks the Core Laboratory of the Taipei Tzu Chi Hospital, Buddhist Tzu Chi Medical Foundation for support.

Funding
This work was supported by grants from the Ministry of Science and Technology, Taiwan (NSC-101-2314-B-303-018-MY3) and Taipei Tzu Chi Hospital, Buddhist Tzu Chi Medical Foundation, New Taipei City, Taiwan (TCRD-TPE-104-37 and TCRD-TPE-105-23). All sponsors or funders play no role in the study design, data collection and analysis, decision to publish, or preparation of the manuscript.

Authors' contributions
MLC designed the study, MCL collected the LC/MS/MS data, YYL collected IHC data, MLC, TCL, FMT and YHC analyzed the data, MLC and TCL prepared the manuscript, and all authors read and approved the final manuscript.

Competing interests
The authors declare that they have no competing interests.

Author details
[1]Division of Neurosurgery, Department of Surgery, Taipei Tzu Chi Hospital, Buddhist Tzu Chi Medical Foundation, New Taipei City, Taiwan, Republic of China. [2]Department of Surgery, School of Medicine, Tzu Chi University, Hualien City, Taiwan, Republic of China. [3]Department of Research, Taipei Tzu Chi Hospital, Buddhist Tzu Chi Medical Foundation, New Taipei City, Taiwan, Republic of China. [4]Department of Microbiology, Soochow University, Shih Lin, Taipei City, Taiwan, Republic of China. [5]Department of Life Science, Fu Jen Catholic University, New Taipei City, Taiwan, Republic of China.

References

1. Girgenti MJ, Nisenbaum LK, Bymaster F, Terwilliger R, Duman RS, Newton SS. Antipsychotic-induced gene regulation in multiple brain regions. J Neurochem. 2010;113:175–87.
2. MacDonald ML, Eaton ME, Dudman JT, Konradi C. Antipsychotic drugs elevate mRNA levels of presynaptic proteins in the frontal cortex of the rat. Biol Psychiatry. 2005;57:1041–51.
3. Lencz T, Malhotra AK. Pharmacogenetics of antipsychotic-induced side effects. Dialogues Clin Neurosci. 2009;11:405–15.
4. Gardner DM, Baldessarini RJ, Waraich P. Modern antipsychotic drugs: a critical overview. Can Med Assoc J. 2005;172:1703–11.
5. Akbarian S. Epigenetic mechanisms in schizophrenia. Dialogues Clin Neurosci. 2014;16:405–17.
6. Dempster E, Viana J, Pidsley R, Mill J. Epigenetic studies of schizophrenia: progress, predicaments, and promises for the future. Schizophr Bull. 2013;39: 11–6.
7. O'Brien E, Dedova I, Duffy L, Cordwell S, Karl T, Matsumoto I. Effects of chronic risperidone treatment on the striatal protein profiles in rats. Brain Res. 2006;1113:24–32.
8. Ji B, La Y, Gao L, Zhu H, Tian N, Zhang M, Yang Y, Zhao X, Tang R, Ma G, et al. A comparative proteomics analysis of rat mitochondria from the cerebral cortex and hippocampus in response to antipsychotic medications. J Proteome Res. 2009;8:3633–41.
9. Kedracka-Krok S, Swiderska B, Jankowska U, Skupien-Rabian B, Solich J, Buczak K, Dziedzicka-Wasylewska M. Clozapine influences cytoskeleton structure and calcium homeostasis in rat cerebral cortex and has a different proteomic profile than risperidone. J Neurochem. 2015;132:657–76.
10. Davalieva K, Maleva Kostovska I, Dwork AJ. Proteomics research in schizophrenia. Front Cell Neurosci. 2016;10:18.
11. Baloyianni N, Tsangaris GT. The audacity of proteomics: a chance to overcome current challenges in schizophrenia research. Exp rev proteomics. 2009;6:661–74.
12. Savino R, Paduano S, Preiano M, Terracciano R. The proteomics big challenge for biomarkers and new drug-targets discovery. Int J Mol Sci. 2012;13:13926–48.
13. Ross PL, Huang YN, Marchese JN, Williamson B, Parker K, Hattan S, Khainovski N, Pillai S, Dey S, Daniels S, et al. Multiplexed protein quantitation in Saccharomyces cerevisiae using amine-reactive isobaric tagging reagents. Mol Cell Proteomics. 2004;3:1154–69.
14. Craft GE, Chen A, Nairn AC. Recent advances in quantitative neuroproteomics. Methods. 2013;61:186–218.
15. Yin HR, Zhang L, Xie LQ, Huang LY, Xu Y, Cai SJ, Yang PY, Lu HJ. Hyperplex-MRM: a hybrid multiple reaction monitoring method using mTRAQ/iTRAQ labeling for multiplex absolute quantification of human colorectal cancer biomarker. J Proteome Res. 2013;12:3912–9.
16. Pottiez G, Wiederin J, Fox HS, Ciborowski P. Comparison of 4-plex to 8-plex iTRAQ quantitative measurements of proteins in human plasma samples. J Proteome Res. 2012;11:3774–81.
17. Saia-Cereda VM, Cassoli JS, Schmitt A, Falkai P, Martins-de-Souza D. Differential proteome and phosphoproteome may impact cell signaling in the corpus callosum of schizophrenia patients. Schizophr Res. 2016;177:70–7.
18. Corena-McLeod M, Walss-Bass C, Oliveros A, Gordillo Villegas A, Ceballos C, Charlesworth CM, Madden B, Linser PJ, Van Ekeris L, Smith K, Richelson E. New model of action for mood stabilizers: phosphoproteome from rat pre-frontal cortex synaptoneurosomal preparations. PLoS One. 2013;8:e52147.
19. Sharma RP, Grayson DR, Gavin DP. Histone deactylase 1 expression is increased in the prefrontal cortex of schizophrenia subjects: analysis of the National Brain Databank microarray collection. Schizophr Res. 2008;98:111–7.
20. Benes FM, Lim B, Matzilevich D, Subburaju S, Walsh JP. Circuitry-based gene expression profiles in GABA cells of the trisynaptic pathway in schizophrenics versus bipolars. Proc Natl Acad Sci U S A. 2008;105:20935–40.
21. Chen Y, Sharma RP, Costa RH, Costa E, Grayson DR. On the epigenetic regulation of the human reelin promoter. Nucleic Acids Res. 2002;30:2930–9.
22. Mitchell CP, Chen Y, Kundakovic M, Costa E, Grayson DR. Histone deacetylase inhibitors decrease reelin promoter methylation in vitro. J Neurochem. 2005;93:483–92.
23. Fischer A, Sananbenesi F, Wang X, Dobbin M, Tsai LH. Recovery of learning and memory is associated with chromatin remodelling. Nature. 2007;447: 178–82.
24. Kim HJ, Leeds P, Chuang DM. The HDAC inhibitor, sodium butyrate, stimulates neurogenesis in the ischemic brain. J Neurochem. 2009;110: 1226–40.
25. Guan JS, Haggarty SJ, Giacometti E, Dannenberg JH, Joseph N, Gao J, Nieland TJ, Zhou Y, Wang X, Mazitschek R, et al. HDAC2 negatively regulates memory formation and synaptic plasticity. Nature. 2009;459:55–60.
26. Kim D, Frank CL, Dobbin MM, Tsunemoto RK, Tu W, Peng PL, Guan JS, Lee BH, Moy LY, Giusti P, et al. Deregulation of HDAC1 by p25/Cdk5 in neurotoxicity. Neuron. 2008;60:803–17.
27. Li J, Guo Y, Schroeder FA, Youngs RM, Schmidt TW, Ferris C, Konradi C, Akbarian S. Dopamine D2-like antagonists induce chromatin remodeling in striatal neurons through cyclic AMP-protein kinase a and NMDA receptor signaling. J Neurochem. 2004;90:1117–31.
28. Bonito-Oliva A, Sodersten E, Spigolon G, Hu X, Hellysaz A, Falconi A, Gomes AL, Broberger C, Hansen K, Fisone G. Differential regulation of the phosphorylation of Trimethyl-lysine27 histone H3 at serine 28 in distinct populations of striatal projection neurons. Neuropharmacology. 2016;107: 89–99.
29. Bozidis P, Hyphantis T, Mantas C, Sotiropoulou M, Antypa N, Andreoulakis E, Serretti A, Mavreas V, Antoniou K. HSP70 polymorphisms in first psychotic episode drug-naive schizophrenic patients. Life Sci. 2014;100:133–7.

30. Focking M, Lopez LM, English JA, Dicker P, Wolff A, Brindley E, Wynne K, Cagney G, Cotter DR. Proteomic and genomic evidence implicates the postsynaptic density in schizophrenia. Mol Psychiatry. 2015;20:424–32.
31. Cacabelos R, Torrellas C. Epigenetics of aging and Alzheimer's disease: implications for pharmacogenomics and drug response. Int J Mol Sci. 2015; 16:30483–543.
32. Pennington K, Dicker P, Dunn MJ, Cotter DR. Proteomic analysis reveals protein changes within layer 2 of the insular cortex in schizophrenia. Proteomics. 2008;8:5097–107.
33. Aston C, Jiang L, Sokolov BP. Microarray analysis of postmortem temporal cortex from patients with schizophrenia. J Neurosci Res. 2004;77:858–66.
34. Cassoli JS, Iwata K, Steiner J, Guest PC, Turck CW, Nascimento JM, Martins-de-Souza D. Effect of MK-801 and clozapine on the proteome of cultured human oligodendrocytes. Front Cell Neurosci. 2016;10:52.
35. Chen ML. Two-dimensional gel electrophoresis revealed antipsychotic drugs induced protein expression modulations in C6 glioma cells. Prog Neuro-Psychopharmacol Biol Psychiatry. 2013;40:1–11.
36. Scott DD, Oeffinger M. Nucleolin and nucleophosmin: nucleolar proteins with multiple functions in DNA repair. Biochem Cell Biol. 2016;94:419–32.
37. Inder KL, Lau C, Loo D, Chaudhary N, Goodall A, Martin S, Jones A, van der Hoeven D, Parton RG, Hill MM, Hancock JF. Nucleophosmin and nucleolin regulate K-Ras plasma membrane interactions and MAPK signal transduction. J Biol Chem. 2009;284:28410–9.
38. Funk AJ, McCullumsmith RE, Haroutunian V, Meador-Woodruff JH. Abnormal activity of the MAPK- and cAMP-associated signaling pathways in frontal cortical areas in postmortem brain in schizophrenia. Neuropsychopharmacology. 2012;37:896–905.
39. Kyosseva SV, Elbein AD, Griffin WS, Mrak RE, Lyon M, Karson CN. Mitogen-activated protein kinases in schizophrenia. Biol Psychiatry. 1999;46:689–96.
40. Katsel P, Byne W, Roussos P, Tan W, Siever L, Haroutunian V. Astrocyte and glutamate markers in the superficial, deep, and white matter layers of the anterior cingulate gyrus in schizophrenia. Neuropsychopharmacology. 2011; 36:1171–7.
41. Feresten AH, Barakauskas V, Ypsilanti A, Barr AM, Beasley CL. Increased expression of glial fibrillary acidic protein in prefrontal cortex in psychotic illness. Schizophr Res. 2013;150:252–7.
42. Svitkina TM, Verkhovsky AB, Borisy GG. Plectin sidearms mediate interaction of intermediate filaments with microtubules and other components of the cytoskeleton. J Cell Biol. 1996;135:991–1007.
43. Wiche G, Osmanagic-Myers S, Castanon MJ. Networking and anchoring through plectin: a key to IF functionality and mechanotransduction. Curr Opin Cell Biol. 2015;32:21–9.
44. Eriksson M, Samuelsson H, Samuelsson EB, Liu L, McKeehan WL, Benedikz E, Sundstrom E. The NMDAR subunit NR3A interacts with microtubule-associated protein 1S in the brain. Biochem Biophys Res Commun. 2007; 361:127–32.
45. Eriksson M, Nilsson A, Samuelsson H, Samuelsson EB, Mo L, Akesson E, Benedikz E, Sundstrom E. On the role of NR3A in human NMDA receptors. Physiol Behav. 2007;92:54–9.
46. Mueller HT, Meador-Woodruff JH. NR3A NMDA receptor subunit mRNA expression in schizophrenia, depression and bipolar disorder. Schizophr Res. 2004;71:361–70.
47. Henson MA, Roberts AC, Salimi K, Vadlamudi S, Hamer RM, Gilmore JH, Jarskog LF, Philpot BD. Developmental regulation of the NMDA receptor subunits, NR3A and NR1, in human prefrontal cortex. Cereb Cortex. 2008;18: 2560–73.

The benefit of combinations of oximes for the ability of antidotal treatment to counteract sarin-induced brain damage in rats

Filip Caisberger[1], Jaroslav Pejchal[2], Jan Misik[2], Jiri Kassa[2], Martin Valis[1] and Kamil Kuca[3,4*]

Abstract

Background: The aim of our study was to compare the ability of two combinations of oximes (HI-6 + trimedoxime and HI-6 + K203) with atropine to counteract acute sarin-induced brain damage with the efficacy of antidotal treatment involving single oxime (HI-6) and atropin using in vivo methods.

Methods: Brain damage and neuroprotective effects of antidotal treatment were evaluated in rats poisoned with sarin at a sublethal dose (108 μg/kg i.m.; 90% LD_{50}) using histopathological, Fluoro-Jade B and Terminal deoxynucleotidyl transferase dUTP nick end labeling (TUNEL) analysis 24 h after sarin administration.

Results: Both combinations of oximes reduce the number of rats that died before the end of experiment compared to non-treated sarin poisoning and sarin poisoning treated with HI-6 and atropine. In the case of treatment of sarin poisoning with HI-6 in combination with K203, all rats survived till the end of experiment. HI-6 with atropine was able to reduce sarin-induced brain damage, however, both combinations were slightly more effective.

Conclusions: The oxime HI-6 in combination with K203 and atropine seems to be the most effective. Thus, both tested oxime combinations bring a small benefit in elimination of acute sarin-induced brain damage compared to single oxime antidotal therapy.

Keywords: Sarin, HI-6, Trimedoxime, K203, Rats, Histopathology, FluoraJadeB, TUNEL

Background

Nerve agents are highly toxic organophosphorus compounds representing potential threats to both military and civilian population. These chemical warfare agents were used in the Iraq-Iran (1980s), in the terrorist attack on the Tokyo subway (1995) and more recently in Syria in the suburbs of Damascus resulting in massive casualties [32, 36]. The basic mechanism of nerve agents´ toxicity lies in irreversible inhibition of acetylcholinesterase (AChE, EC 3.1.1.7) leading to the accumulation of the neurotransmitter acetylcholine at cholinergic synapses and neuromuscular junctions which subsequently results in the cholinergic crisis involving multiple organs. In the central nervous system, nerve agents may induce progressive irreversible damage [4]. The brain damage is associated with the dysfunction of irreversibly inhibited AChE and neuronal excitotoxicity and it seems to be largely responsible for persistent profound neuropsychiatric and neurological impairments in the victims of nerve agent exposure [4, 6].

The standard treatment of nerve agent poisoning usually consists of three types of antidotes – anticholinergic agents, oximes and anticonvulsive drugs. Anticholinergic drugs such as atropine sulphate antagonize the muscarinic overstimulation, anticonvulsants such as diazepam are indicated to prevent centrally mediated seizures and secondary brain damage and the oximes disrupt the covalent bond between nerve agent and AChE and restore the physiological function of this enzyme [8]. Among

* Correspondence: kamil.kuca@uhk.cz
[3]Department of Chemistry, Faculty of Science, University of Hradec Kralove, Hradec Kralove, Czech Republic
[4]Biomedical Research Center, Uiversity Hospital Hradec Kralove, Hradec Kralove, Czech Republic
Full list of author information is available at the end of the article

oximes, monopyridinium oxime pralidoxime and bispyridinium oximes obidoxime, trimedoxime and HI-6 should be mentioned [39]. However, there is no potent broad-spectrum oxime able to sufficiently reactivate AChE inhibited by all nerve agents regardless of their chemical structure. HI-6, for instance, is considered to be a relatively strong reactivator of sarin, soman and cyclosarin inhibited AChE but its ability to reactivate AChE inhibited by tabun and less toxic organophosphorus pesticides is of low to moderate values [7, 17, 21, 26, 39, 41]. Trimedoxime or newly synthesized oxime K203, on the other hand, seem to be effective against tabun and pesticides [22, 24]. Since the effort to develop a potent broad-spectrum reactivator has failed so far, another way how to overcome this issue and possibly to increase the reactivating efficacy of antidotes is to combine the oximes in the antidotal treatment [19, 41].

The main purpose of this study was to compare the neuroprotective efficacy of the oxime HI-6 with two oxime mixtures containing HI-6 and trimedoxime or the oxime K-203 in combination with atropine in sarin-poisoned rats. The neuroprotective potential was evaluated using histopathological examination with the help of Fluoro-Jade B fluorochrome used in neuroscience to label degenerating neurons and terminal deoxynucleotidyl transferase dUTP nick end labeling (TUNEL) assay detecting DNA fragmentation during apoptosis [25, 37].

Methods

Animals

All experiments in this study were approved by the Ethics Committee of the Faculty of Military Health Sciences in Hradec Kralove (Czech Republic) and were conducted in accordance with the Animal Protection Law and Animal Protection Regulations.

Wistar rats (6-week-old, 200–230 g; VELAZ, Unetice, Czech Republic) were kept in an accredited animal facility (22 ± 2 °C, 50 ± 10% relative humidity, 12-h day-night cycle) and allowed access to standard food (Velaz) and tap water ad libitum. The rats were acclimatized for 14 days before starting the experiments. For experiments, they were randomly divided into groups of 8 animals.

Chemicals

Sarin was obtained from Military Technical Institute (Brno, Czech Republic). Its purity (98%) was assayed by acidimetric titration. Trimedoxime (1,1′-propane-1,3--diylbis{4-[(*E*)-(hydroxyimino)methyl]pyridinium} dibromide), HI-6 (1-[[[4(aminocarbonyl)-pyridinio] methoxy] methyl]-2(hydroxyimino)pyridinium dichloride) and the oxime K203 [(E)-1-(4-carbamo-ylpyridinium)-4-(4-hydroxyiminomethylpyridinium)-but-2-ene dibromide] were synthesized earlier at the Department of Toxicology (Faculty of Military Health Sciences, Hradec Kralove, Czech Republic). Their purities (97.5%) were analyzed using high-performance liquid chromatography technique [11]. All other drugs and chemicals of analytical grade were obtained commercially and used without further purification. All substances were administered intramuscularly at a volume of 1 ml/kg of body weight.

In vivo experiments

Animals were divided into 5 groups (8 rats each): 1) a control group (administered with saline), 2) sarin poisoned group (108 μg/kg – 90% LD_{50}), 3) sarin poisoned group treated with atropine sulphate (21 mg/kg) and HI-6 (39 mg/kg), 4) sarin poisoned group treated with atropine sulphate, HI-6 and trimedoxime (7.5 mg/kg), and 5) sarin poisoned group treated with atropine sulphate, HI-6 and K203 (16.3 mg/kg). In order to develop a broad-spectrum mixture, the combinations were selected based on HI-6 being a relatively strong reactivator of sarin, soman and cyclosarin-inhibited AChE, while trimedoxime or K203 are effective against tabun and pesticides. The oximes were administered at equitoxic doses corresponding to 5% of their LD_{50} values. These doses are sufficiently safe. The antidotes were administered 1 min after sarin challenge. Surviving rats were anesthetized by ether vapor 24 h after intoxication and euthanized by decapitation. Their brains were rapidly removed and fixed with a 10% neutral buffered formalin (Chemapol, Prague, Czech Republic). Samples were subsequently embedded into paraffin (Paramix, Holice, Czech Republic) and 6 μm thick coronary brain sections were cut (Microtome model SM2000 R, Leica) at level between 3 mm and 4.2 mm from bregma according to Paxinos stereotactic brain atlas [33]. Three sections for every staining method were evaluated by 2 experts. In a section, damage was scored in 6 regions, including amygdaloid body, cortex, hippocampus, hypothalamus, piriform cortex and thalamus with relevance to sarin-induced neuropathology [13].

Hematoxylin-eosin staining and histopathology evaluation

Selected brain sections were fixed in 10% buffered formalin (Kulich, Hradec Kralove, Czech Republic), processed through conventional histological techniques, and stained with hematoxylin and eosin (both Merck, Kenilworth, NJ, USA). The histological changes were scored using a BX-51 microscope (Olympus, Tokyo, Japan) and following semi-quantitative criteria published previously [20]:

(0) no pathology,
(1) mild damage: 1–2 neurons with nucleus margination, chromatolysis and/or vacuolar degeneration,
(2) moderate damage: ≥ 3 neurons with changes described in (1) and/or ≥ 1 shrunken eosinophilic neurons in 1 nucleus/subregion,
(3) severe damage: focal damage or multiple changes described in (2) present in ≥2 nuclei/subregions and/or hemorrhage
(4) very severe damage: diffuse damage of the region and/or multiple hemorrhages

Fluoro-jade B staining and evaluation

For Fluoro-Jade B staining, paraffin sections were dewaxed and rehydrated through xylene and an alcohol series. Afterwards, the sections were immersed in 0.06% potassium permanganate (Sigma-Aldrich, St. Louis, MO, USA) for 10 min, rinsed in distilled water for 2 min and dyed by 0.0002% solution of the Fluoro-Jade B (Merck) for 20 min in dark. Washed (3 distilled water washes, 1 min each) and dried slides were mounted with DPX (Sigma-Aldrich) in dark. Fluorescent cells were evaluated using a BX-51 microscope (Olympus) with green excitation fluorescence filter and following semi-quantitative criteria published previously [20]:

(0) no fluorescent cells,
(1) 1–2 fluorescent cells in 1 nucleus/subregion,
(2) ≥ 3 in 1 nucleus/subregion or 1–2 fluorescent cells in ≥2 nuclei/subregions,
(3) multiple fluorescent cells in ≥2 nuclei/subregions and/or hemorrhage,
(4) diffuse fluorescent positivity and/or multiple hemorrhages

TUNEL immunostaining and evaluation

TUNEL staining was carried out to identify the apoptotic cells according to the manufacturer's instructions using in situ cell death detection kit (Roche, Mannheim, Germany) as published previously [34]. TUNEL positive cells were evaluated using a BX-51 microscope (Olympus) and following semi-quantitative criteria:

Table 1 Survival of rats following exposure to sarin

group	survival in the time of sample collection (survived/total)	time of death (min)
control	8/8	
GB	5/8	28, 42, 63
GB + A + H	6/8	33, 125
GB + A + H + T	7/8	59
GB + A + H + K	8/8	

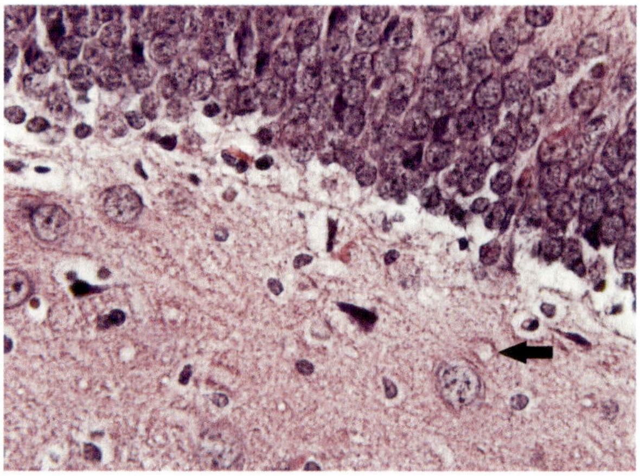

Fig. 1 Sample of dentate gyrus from control group (hematoxylin-eosin, 600fold original magnification). The microphotograph displays a boundary between granular (upper) and polymorphic (lower) layer. The arrow indicates an example of a neuronal vacuole surrounded with condesated cytoplasm

(0) 0–1 TUNEL positive cells in 1 nucleus/subregion
(1) ≥ 2 TUNEL positive cells in 1 nucleus/subregion
(2) multiple TUNEL positive cells in ≥2 nuclei/subregions
(3) diffuse TUNEL positivity

Due to verified false positivity of TUNEL assay and a very slight positivity (1 cell) in all control samples, only 3 levels of damage were recognized compared to the histopathological and Fluoro-Jade B analysis.

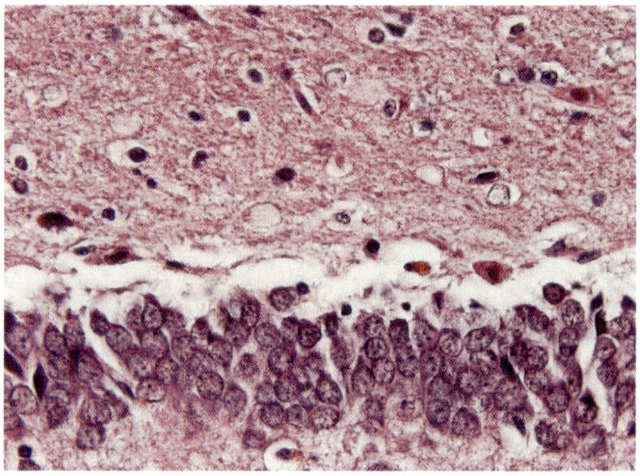

Fig. 2 Sample of dentate gyrus from sarin-poisoned rat receiving no treatement (hematoxylin-eosin, 600fold original magnification). The microphotograph displays a boundary between polymorphic (upper) and granular (lower) layer. Sarin-induced damage dominates in polymorphic layer and includes multiple neuronal vacuoles surrounded with condensated chromatin and red cells with condensated nuclei (acute eosinophilic necrosis)

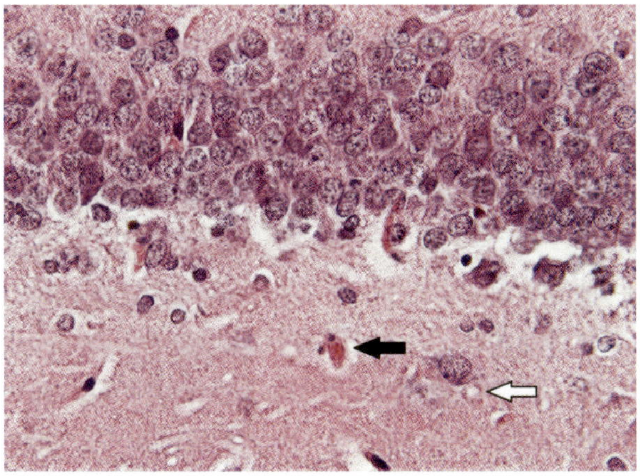

Fig. 3 Sample of dentate gyrus from sarin-poisoned rat treated with HI-6 and trimedoxime (hematoxylin-eosin, 600fold original magnification). The microphotograph displays a boundary between polymorphic (upper) and granular (lower) layer. The treatment significantly reduced the pathological finings in this animal, nevertheless, a red cell with chromatolysis (black arrow) and several neuronal vacuoles (white arrow indicates an example) could be observed

Individual animal brain damage score

Finally, individual animal brain damage scores were calculated representing a sum of histopathological, Fluoro-Jade B and TUNEL scores from all tested brain subregions in one animal.

Data analysis

We used non-parametric Kruskal-Wallis rank sum test with multiple pairwise comparisons to evaluate statistical differences between all groups within particular brain nucleus/subregion, which were considered significant when $p \leq 0.05$. All analyses were performed in IBM SPSS Statistics version 22.0 software (IBM Corp., Armonk, NY, USA).

Results

In the case of sarin poisoning without antidotal treatment, three sarin-poisoned rats did not survive until the end of experiment. Antidotal treatment eliminated or at least reduced the mortality of sarin-poisoned rats. Two rats did not survived till the end of experiment if HI-6 in combination with atropine was used for the antidotal treatment and one rat did not survived till the end of experiment if HI-6 and trimedoxime in combination with atropine were used for the antidotal treatment of sarin poisoning. Only HI-6 and K203 in combination with atropine were able to eliminate sarin-induced death of poisoned animals (Table 1).

Histopathological findings

The most extensive alterations were observed in sarin-poisoned animals receiving no antidotal treatment. Compared to the control group, significantly increased histopathological damage scores were measured in cortex, hypothalamus and piriform cortex ($p = 0.023$, 0.001 and 0.020, respectively). In affected animals, cortex and piriform cortex displayed pseudolaminar necrosis in 1 and 3 cases, respectively. Hemorrhage was present in one case in hypothalamus. Single cell damage characterized by multifocal degenerative/necrotic changes accompanied with oedema was observed in the remaining positively scored rats. Especially, basolateral nucleus of amygdaloid body, the third and fifth layer of cortex (pyramidal cells), neurons in CA1 (> dentate gyrus > CA3 > CA2) zone of hippocampus (Figs. 1 and 2), supramammilary hypothalamic nuclei, the third layer of piriform cortex, and medial and dorsolateral thalamic nuclei were markedly impaired.

Administration of antidotal treatment reduced the extent of damage. Any diffuse changes and/or hemorrhage in all groups treated with antidotes was not observed. However, significantly decreased histopathological scores were found in cortex ($p = 0.009$) of animals administered with atropine and HI-6 and in cortex, hippocampus (Fig. 3), hypothalamus, and piriform cortex ($p = 0.023$, 0.010, 0.009, and 0.020, respectively) in rats treated with atropine, HI-6 and K203 (Table 2).

Table 2 Score of sarin-induced histopathological damage in rat brain and its modulation by different therapeutic approaches

	AMG					CTX					HIPP					HYPOTH					PIRI					TH				
score scale	0	1	2	3	4	0	1	2	3	4	0	1	2	3	4	0	1	2	3	4	0	1	2	3	4	0	1	2	3	4
control	6	1	1	0	0	7	1	0	0	0	5	3	0	0	0	8	0	0	0	0	8	0	0	0	0	6	2	0	0	0
GB	2	0	0	3	0	**1**	**1**	**1**	**1**	**1**	1	1	1	0	2	**0**	**0**	**2**	**3**	**0**	**2**	**0**	**0**	**0**	**3**	1	0	1	3	0
GB + A + H	4	1	1	0	0	***6***	***0***	***0***	***0***	***0***	2	4	0	0	0	3	1	2	0	0	5	1	0	0	0	4	2	0	0	0
GB + A + H + T	5	0	2	0	0	5	2	0	0	0	3	3	0	1	0	4	1	2	0	0	6	0	1	0	0	5	1	1	0	0
GB + A + H + K	6	2	0	0	0	***7***	***1***	***0***	***0***	***0***	***8***	***0***	***0***	***0***	***0***	***6***	***1***	***1***	***0***	***0***	***8***	***0***	***0***	***0***	***0***	5	0	3	0	0

Each number represents a number of animals suffering from particular damage score in the group
Bold: statistically significant compared to control group ($p \leq 0.05$)
Bold Italic: statistically significant compared to sarin-poisoned group ($p \leq 0.05$)
Abbreviations: A atropine, *AMG* amygdaloid body, *CTX* cortex, *GB* sarin, *H* oxime HI-6, *HIPP* hippocampus, *HYPOTH* hypothalamus, *K* oxime K203, *PIRI* piriform cortex, *T* trimedoxime, *TH* thalamus

Fluoro-jade B

Significantly increased Fluoro-Jade B positivity in amygdaloid body, cortex, hypothalamus, piriform cortex, and thalamus ($p = 0.029$, 0.032, < 0.001, 0.032, and 0.029, respectively) was found in non-treated, sarin-poisoned rats. Diffuse fluorescent patterns were present in 3 of 5 surviving rats. In all six regions, maximal Fluoro-Jade B positivity correlated with histopathological findings (Figs. 4 and 5).

The antidotal treatment markedly reduced brain degeneration marked by Fluoro-Jade B. We found significantly decreased Fluoro-Jade B positivity in hippocampus ($p = 0.017$) of atropine and HI-6 treated rats and in amygdaloid body and hippocampus ($p = 0.038$ and 0.026, respectively) of animals administered with atropine, HI-6 and trimedoxime. No hemorrhages were observed in both groups. In atropine, HI-6 and K203 treated group, Fluoro-Jade B fluorescence significantly decreased in cortex, hippocampus (Fig. 6), piriform cortex, and thalamus ($p = 0.032$, < 0.001, 0.032, and 0.029, respectively). On the other hand, a small hemorrhage in the hypothalamic region was found. However, Fluoro-Jade B positivity in this area was scored as 1 (Table 3).

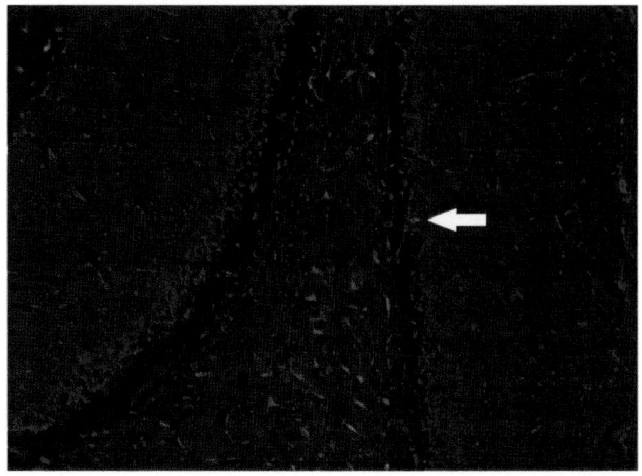

Fig. 5 Sample of dentate gyrus from sarin-poisoned rat receiving no treatement (Fluoro-Jade B and DAPI, 100fold original magnification). Together with autofluorescence of normal red blood cells in capillaries, fluorescence of piramidal and polymorphic cells with dendritic and axonal projections (necrotic neurons) in polymorphic layer could be found. The arrow indicates a necrotic neurone in the granular layer

TUNEL

TUNEL positivity was significantly increased in amygdaloid body, hippocampus and piriform cortex ($p = 0.012$, 0.003 and 0.041, respectively) of sarin-poisoned animals without antidotal treatment. The distribution of TUNEL staining pattern corresponds to the histopathological and Fluoro-Jade B findings except for hippocampal dentate gyrus (Figs. 7 and 8).

Atropine and HI-6 treatment did not significantly influence the outcome of sarin intoxication. In atropine, HI-6 and trimedoxime treated group, a decreased amount of TUNEL positive cells was only observed in amygdaloid body ($p = 0.016$). The combination of atropine, HI-6 and K203 decreased positivity in amygdaloid body, hippocampus (Fig. 9) and piriform cortex ($p = 0.012$, 0.003 and 0.041, respectively) (Table 4).

Individual animal brain damage score

Compared to the control group, a significantly increased individual animal brain damage scores in

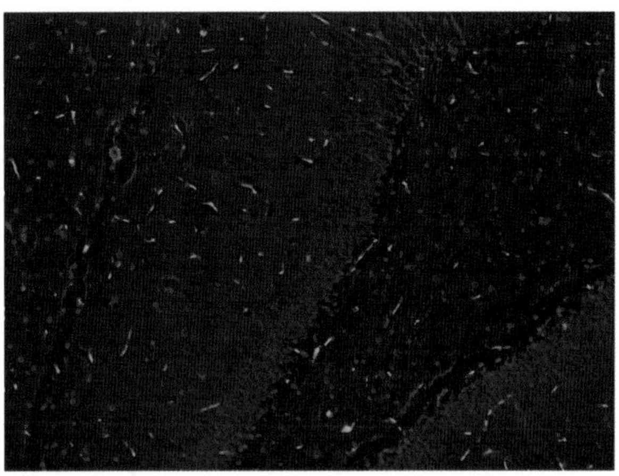

Fig. 4 Sample of dentate gyrus from control group (Fluoro-Jade B and DAPI, 100fold original magnification). Autofluorescence of normal red blood cells in capillaries could be seen in the picture. No pathology was detected

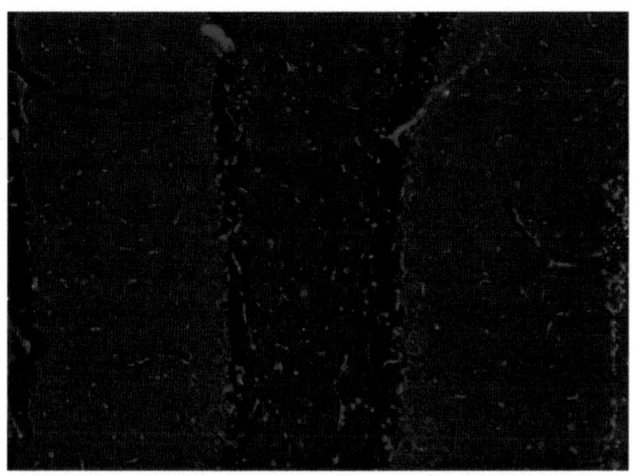

Fig. 6 Sample of dentate gyrus from sarin-poisoned rat treated with HI-6 and K203 (Fluoro-Jade B and DAPI, 100fold original magnification). Only autofluorescence of normal red blood cells in capillaries could be seen in the picture. No pathology was detected

Table 3 Score of sarin-induced degeneration (Fluoro-Jade B positivity) in rat brain and its modulation by different therapeutic approaches

	AMG					CTX					HIPP					HYPOTH					PIRI					TH				
score scale	0	1	2	3	4	0	1	2	3	4	0	1	2	3	4	0	1	2	3	4	0	1	2	3	4	0	1	2	3	4
control	8	0	0	0	0	8	0	0	0	0	8	0	0	0	0	8	0	0	0	0	8	0	0	0	0	8	0	0	0	0
GB	**2**	**0**	**0**	**1**	**2**	**2**	**0**	**0**	**2**	**1**	**0**	**2**	**0**	**1**	**2**	**2**	**0**	**0**	**3**	**0**	**2**	**0**	**0**	**0**	**3**	**2**	**0**	**0**	**2**	**1**
GB + A + H	5	0	0	0	1	5	0	0	0	1	***5***	***0***	***0***	***0***	***1***	5	0	0	1	0	4	1	0	1	0	5	0	0	1	0
GB + A + H + T	***7***	***0***	***0***	***0***	***0***	6	0	1	0	0	***5***	***2***	***0***	***0***	***0***	6	0	0	1	0	***6***	***1***	***0***	***0***	***0***	6	0	0	1	0
GB + A + H + K	7	1	0	0	0	***8***	***0***	***0***	***0***	***0***	***8***	***0***	***0***	***0***	***0***	7	0	0	1	0	***8***	***0***	***0***	***0***	***0***	***8***	***0***	***0***	***0***	***0***

Each number represents a number of animals suffering from particular damage score in the group
Bold: statistically significant compared to control group ($p \leq 0.05$)
Bold Italic: statistically significant compared to sarin-poisoned group ($p \leq 0.05$)
Abbreviations: *A* atropine, *AMG* amygdaloid body, *CTX* cortex, *GB* sarin, *H* oxime HI-6, *HIPP* hippocampus, *HYPOTH* hypothalamus, *K* oxime K203, *PIRI* piriform cortex, *T* trimedoxime, *TH* thalamus

sarin-poisoned group without antidotal treatment was found ($p = < 0.001$). Sarin-induced damage was significantly reduced only in atropine, HI-6 and K203 treated rats ($p = 0.019$) (Table 5).

Discussion

In this study, the neuroprotective effects of single oxime (HI-6) or two oxime mixtures (HI-6 and trimedoxime or oxime K203) in combination with atropine in sarin-poisoned rats was evaluated. The model used in this study follows our previous study, in which the benefit of oxime mixtures for the neuroprotective efficacy of antidotal treatment of nerve agent poisoning was demonstrated using a functional observatory battery [19]. Herein, we focus on structural brain changes using three different approaches, including histopathological, Fluoro-Jade B and TUNEL analysis.

Based on our results, the established scoring system resulted in positivity of histopathological method in 5 (of 8) control animals due to the presence of cytoplasmatic vacuoles. The clinical significance of vacuolation is not known. Neuronal vacuoles can appear spontaneously, especially in aging animals, without having any obvious clinical relevance [23, 40].

After sarin poisoning, a widespread brain damage was observed. The alterations were particularly profound in cholinoceptive subregions and/or subregions sensitive to hypoxic/ischemic stress [3, 27, 29, 35]. This observation is in accordance with generally accepted mechanism of nerve agent-induced acute brain injury and with previously published findings [6, 13, 28]. The distribution of histopathological changes correlated with Fluoro-Jade B and TUNEL staining pattern with one exception. In gyrus dentatus (hippocampus), histopathological findings and Fluoro-Jade B fluorescence showed the highest positivity in the polymorphic layer, whereas TUNEL positivity prevailed in the granular layer. Although both layers display different sensitivity to various stress

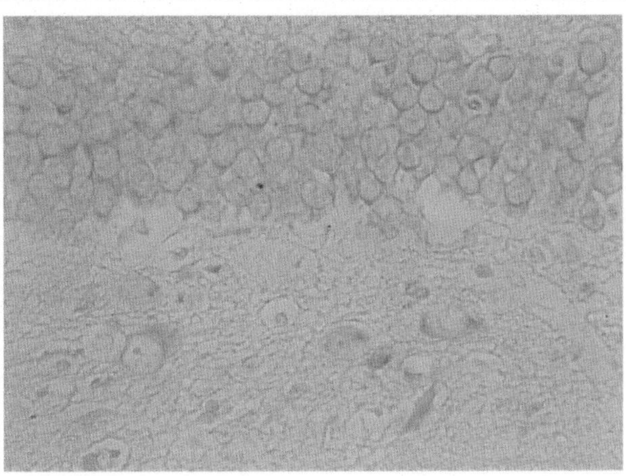

Fig. 7 Sample of dentate gyrus from control group (TUNEL assay counterstained with methyl green, 600fold original magnification). The microphotograph displays a boundary between granular (upper) and polymorphic (lower) layer with no TUNEL positivity

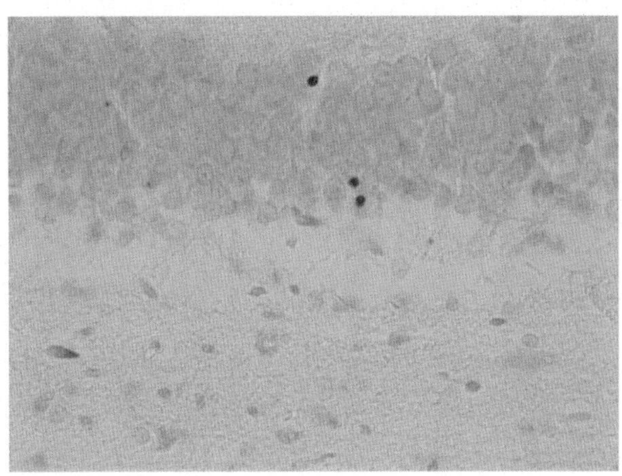

Fig. 8 Sample of dentate gyrus from sarin-poisoned animal receiving no treatement (TUNEL assay counterstained with methyl green, 600fold original magnification). The microphotograph displays a boundary between granular (upper) and polymorphic (lower) layer. Three TUNEL positive cells were detected in the granular layer

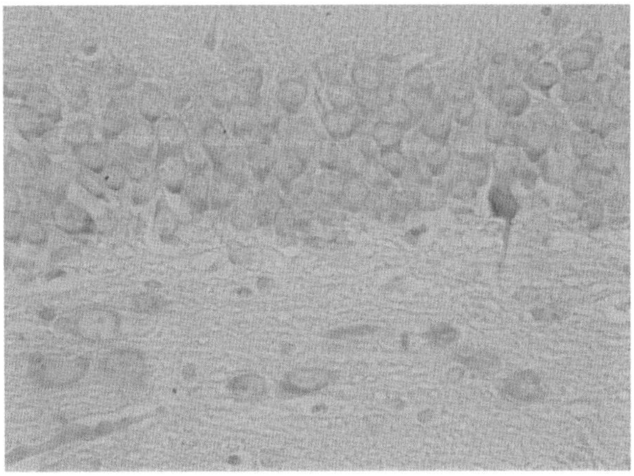

Fig. 9 Sample of dentate gyrus from sarin-poisoned rat treated with HI-6 and K203 (TUNEL assay counterstained with methyl green, 600fold original magnification). The microphotograph displays a boundary between granular (upper) and polymorphic (lower) layer with no TUNEL positivity

stimuli [15, 38], the reason of this discrepancy remains uncertain. An explanation may lie in the limitations of TUNEL method. The method is used to detect DNA fragmentation in apoptotic and necrotic cells [2]. On the other hand, DNA fragmentation occurs also in S phase of cell cycle and the method was reported to produce false positivity in proliferating tissues [9]. Since the subgranular zone of dentate gyrus is considered to be one of the two main neurogenic zones in the adult brain [5], TUNEL positivity observed in this subregion could possibly represent the damage as well as its regeneration.

Antidotal treatment plays a pivotal role in acute phase of nerve agents´ toxicity [6]. In our model, we utilized bispyridinium oximes. Although the bispyridinium oximes poorly penetrate across the blood-brain barrier, they are able to reactivate sarin-inhibited AChE not only at the peripheral compartment but also in the brain when they are administered at equitoxic doses corresponding to 5% of their LD_{50} values at 1 min after the administration of sarin [14, 18, 19]. According to our results, all three therapeutic regimes mitigated the extent of sarin-induced brain injury. Even though we did not find any statistically significant differences among groups treated with oximes, the neuroprotective efficacy of oxime mixtures was slightly higher compared to the group treated with a single oxime. Particularly, the combination of HI-6 and K203 appears to be the most effective to protect experimental animals from acute sarin-induced neuropathological changes in surviving animals. This conclusion corresponds to the previously published results demonstrating the benefit of combinations of oximes for the reactivating and therapeutic efficacy of antidotal treatment of sarin poisoning in rats and mice [18]. Based on the described results, both trimedoxime and K203 do not interfere with HI-6 bioavailability but rather support its action. Therefore, combining the oximes in the antidotal treatment could be a promising step towards a broad-spectrum antidotal treatment of acute nerve agent-exposure regardless of the chemical structure of nerve agent. Such approach may also help to overcome similar issue regarding organophosphorus pesticides. HI-6 has only limited reactivation efficacy towards chlorpyrifos, dichlorvos, methamidophos, and paraoxon [1, 12, 30, 31]. Its combination with trimedoxime or K203 might not only improve these results but may also broaden the spectrum of reactivation towards leptophos-oxon and possibly other pesticides [12]. On the other hand, even in HI-6 and K203 group, animals displayed signs of neuronal damage, which tends to progress overtime [13]. Limited therapeutic efficacy is probably related to low blood-brain barrier (BBB) penetration of bispyridinium oximes [10, 16]. Thus, the development and usage of oxime mixtures with better BBB penetration may further increase their ability to counteract the acute toxicity of organophosphorus compounds.

Table 4 Score of sarin-induced apoptotic activity (TUNEL positivity) in rat brain and its modulation by different therapeutic approaches

	AMG				CTX				HIPP				HYPOTH				PIRI				TH			
score scale	0	1	2	3	0	1	2	3	0	1	2	3	0	1	2	3	0	1	2	3	0	1	2	3
control	8	0	0	0	8	0	0	0	8	0	0	0	8	0	0	0	8	0	0	0	8	0	0	0
GB	**2**	**2**	**1**	**0**	2	2	1	0	**0**	**0**	**5**	**0**	3	1	1	0	**2**	**1**	**2**	**0**	3	0	2	0
GB + A + H	5	1	0	0	4	1	1	0	2	0	4	0	5	0	1	0	4	2	0	0	2	2	2	0
GB + A + H + T	***7***	***0***	***0***	***0***	6	1	0	0	4	0	3	0	5	0	2	0	6	1	0	0	6	0	1	0
GB + A + H + K	***8***	***0***	***0***	***0***	8	0	0	0	***8***	***0***	***0***	***0***	8	0	0	0	***8***	***0***	***0***	***0***	7	1	0	0

Each number represents a number of animals suffering from particular damage score in the group

Bold: statistically significant compared to control group ($p \leq 0.05$)

Bold Italic: statistically significant compared to sarin-poisoned group ($p \leq 0.05$)

Abbreviations: *A* atropine, *AMG* amygdaloid body, *CTX* cortex, *GB* sarin, *H* oxime HI-6, *HIPP* hippocampus, *HYPOTH* hypothalamus, *K* oxime K203, *PIRI* piriform cortex, *T* trimedoxime, *TH* thalamus

Table 5 Individual animal brain damage score

	animal No.							
	1	2	3	4	5	6	7	8
control	0	0	0	1	1	2	2	3
GB	**5**	**10**	**47**	**48**	**51**			
GB + A + H	0	3	5	6	7	36		
GB + A + H + T	0	3	3	4	4	5	28	
GB + A + H + K	***0***	***1***	***1***	***3***	***3***	***3***	***3***	***3***

Each number represents a number of animals suffering from particular damage score in the group
Bold: statistically significant compared to control group ($p \leq 0.05$)
Bold Italic: statistically significant compared to sarin-poisoned group ($p \leq 0.05$)
Abbreviations: *A* atropine, *GB* sarin, *H* oxime HI-6, *K* oxime K203, *T* trimedoxime

Conclusion

Our results show that neuroprotective potency of both oxime combinations (HI-6 with trimedoxime and HI-6 with K203) is slightly higher than using HI-6 alone in sarin poisoned model. Particularly, the oxime HI-6 in combination with K203 seems to be the most effective. Using oxime combinations seems to be an effective approach to develop a potent broad-spectrum reactivator.

Abbreviations

AChE: Acetylcholinesterase; EC: Enzyme commission number; i.m.: Intramuscularly; LD_{50}: Median lethal dose; TUNEL: Terminal deoxynucleotidyl transferase dUTP nick end labeling

Acknowledgements

We would like to express our thanks to Sarka Pruchova and Jana Uhlirova for their skillful technical assistance.

Funding

This work was supported by the Ministry of Defence of the Czech Republic through a Long-term organisation development plan 1011. This work was also supported by Long-term development plans of UHHK and UHK. The funding body did not play any role in the design of the study and collection, analysis, and interpretation of data.

Authors' contributions

FC and JK conceived and planned the experiments. FC, JP and JM carried out the experiments. FC and JP participated in sample evaluation. FC, JP, JM, JK, MV, and KK contributed to the interpretation of the results. FC took the lead in writing the manuscript. All authors provided critical feedback and helped shape the research, analysis and both have read and approved the manuscript.

Competing interests

The authors declare that they have no competing interests.

Author details

[1]Department of Neurology, University Hospital Hradec Kralove, Hradec Kralove, Czech Republic. [2]Department of Toxicology and Military Pharmacy, Faculty of Military Health Sciences, University of Defence, Hradec Kralove, Czech Republic. [3]Department of Chemistry, Faculty of Science, University of Hradec Kralove, Hradec Kralove, Czech Republic. [4]Biomedical Research Center, Uiversity Hospital Hradec Kralove, Hradec Kralove, Czech Republic.

References

1. Antonijevic E, Musilek K, Kuca K, Djukic-Cosic D, Vucinic S, Antonijevic B. Therapeutic and reactivating efficacy of oximes K027 and K203 against a direct acetylcholinesterase inhibitor. Neurotoxicology. 2016;55:33–9.
2. Baille V, Clarke PG, Brochier G, Dorandeu F, Verna JM, Four E, Lallement G, Carpentier P. Soman-induced convulsions: the neuropathology revisited. Toxicology. 2005;215:1–24.
3. Ben-Ari Y, Zigmond RE, Shute CC, Lewis PR. Regional distribution of choline acetyltransferase and acetylcholinesterase within the amygdaloid complex and stria terminalis system. Brain Res. 1977;120:435–44.
4. Brown MA, Brix KA. Review of health consequences from high-, intermediate- and low-level exposure to organophosphorus nerve agents. J Appl Toxicol. 1998;18:393–408.
5. Cayre M, Canoll P, Goldman JE. Cell migration in the normal and pathological postnatal mammalian brain. Prog Neurobiol. 2009;88:41–63.
6. Chen Y. Organophosphate-induced brain damage: mechanisms, neuropsychiatric and neurological consequences, and potential therapeutic strategies. Neurotoxicology. 2012;33:391–400.
7. Clement JG. Central activity of acetylcholinesterase oxime reactivators. Toxicol Appl Pharmacol. 1992;112:104–9.
8. Geoghegan J, Tong JL. Chemical warfare agents. Contin Educ Anaest Crit Care Pain. 2006;6:230–4.
9. Ito Y, Shibata MA, Kusakabe K, Otsuki Y. Method of specific detection of apoptosis using formamide-induced DNA denaturation assay. J Histochem Cytochem. 2006;54:683–92.
10. Joosen MJ, van der Schans MJ, van Dijk CG, Kuijpers WC, Wortelboer HM, van Helden HP. Increasing oxime efficacy by blood-brain barrier modulation. Toxicol Lett. 2011;206:67–71.
11. Jun D, Kuca K, Stodulka P, Koleckar V, Dolezal B, Simon P, Veverka M. HPLC analysis of HI-6 dichloride and dimethanosulfonate – antidotes against nerve agents and organophosphorus pesticides. Anal Lett. 2007;40:2783–7.
12. Jun D, Musilova L, Musilek K, Kuca K. In vitro ability of currently available oximes to reactivate organophosphate pesticide-inhibited human acetylcholinesterase and butyrylcholinesterase. Int J Mol Sci. 2011;12:2077–87.
13. Kadar T, Shapira S, Cohen G, Sahar R, Alkalay D, Raveh L. Sarin-induced neuropathology in rats. Hum Exp Toxicol. 1995;14:252–9.
14. Kalász H, Nurulain SM, Veress G, Antus S, Darvas F, Adeghate E, Adem A, Hashemi F, Tekes K. Mini review on blood-brain barrier penetration of pyridinium aldoximes. J Appl Toxicol. 2015;35:116–23.
15. Kaler S, Dhar P, Bhattacharya A, Mehra RD. Preliminary morphological and immunohistochemical changes in rat hippocampus following postnatal exposure to sodium arsenite. Toxicol Int. 2013;20:160–9.
16. Karasova JZ, Pohanka M, Musilek K, Zemek F, Kuca K. Passive diffusion of acetylcholinesterase oxime reactivators through the blood-brain barrier: influence of molecular structure. Toxicol in Vitro. 2010;24:1838–44.
17. Kassa J, Karasova J, Bajgar J, Kuca K, Musilek K. A comparison of the therapeutic and reactivating efficacy of newly developed bispyridinium compounds (K206, K269) with currently available oximes against tabun in rats and mice. J Enzyme Inhib Med Chem. 2008;23:776–80.
18. Kassa J, Karasova JZ, Sepsova V, Caisberger F. The benefit of combinations of oximes for the reactivating and therapeutic efficacy of antidotal treatment of sarin poisoning in rats and mice. Basic Clin Pharmacol Toxicol. 2011;109:30–4.
19. Kassa J, Kunesova G. The benefit of combination of oximes for the neuroprotective efficacy of antidotal treatment of sarin-poisoned rats. Toxicol Mech Methods. 2012;22:260–7.
20. Kassa J, Misik J, Hatlapatkova J, Zdarova Karasova J, Sepsova V, Caisberger F, Pejchal J. The evaluation of the reactivating and neuroprotective efficacy of two newly prepared Bispyridinium oximes (K305, K307) in Tabun-poisoned rats-a comparison with Trimedoxime and the oxime K203. Molecules. 2017;22:1152.

21. Kassa J, Sepsova V, Matouskova L, Horova A, Musilek K. A comparison of the reactivating and therapeutic efficacy of two novel bispyridinium oximes (K727, K733) with the oxime HI-6 and obidoxime in sarin-poisoned rats and mice. Toxicol Mech Methods. 2015a;25:229–33.
22. Kassa J, Sepsova V, Tumova M, Horova A, Musilek K. A comparison of the reactivating and therapeutic efficacy of two newly developed oximes (k727 and k733) with oxime k203 and trimedoxime in tabun-poisoned rats and mice. Basic Clin Pharmacol Toxicol. 2015b;116:367–71.
23. Krinke GJ. Neuronal vacuolation. Toxicol Pathol. 2011;39:1140.
24. Kuca K, Hrabinova M, Jun D, Musilek K, Penhaker M, Krejcar O, Soukup O. Universality of oxime K203 for reactivation of nerve agent-inhibited AChE. Med Chem. 2015;11:683–6.
25. Labat-Moleur F, Guillermet C, Lorimier P, Robert C, Lantuejoul S, Brambilla E, Negoescu A. TUNEL apoptotic cell detection in tissue sections: critical evaluation and improvement. J Histochem Cytochem. 1998;46:327–34.
26. Lundy PM, Hansen AS, Hand BT, Boulet CA. Comparison of several oximes against poisoning by soman, tabun and GF. Toxicology. 1992;72:99–105.
27. Lysakowski A, Wainer BH, Bruce G, Hersh LB. An atlas of the regional and laminar distribution of choline acetyltransferase immunoreactivity in rat cerebral cortex. Neuroscience. 1989;28:291–336.
28. McDonough JH Jr, Shih TM. Neuropharmacological mechanisms of nerve agent-induced seizure and neuropathology. Neurosci Biobehav Rev. 1997; 21:559–79.
29. Mesulam MM, Mufson EJ, Wainer BH, Levey AI. Central cholinergic pathways in the rat: an overview based on an alternative nomenclature (Ch1-Ch6). Neuroscience. 1983;10:1185–201.
30. Musilek K, Holas O, Jun D, Dohnal V, Gunn-Moore F, Opletalova V, Dolezal M, Kuca K. Monooxime reactivators of acetylcholinesterase with (E)-but-2-ene linker: preparation and reactivation of tabun- and paraoxon-inhibited acetylcholinesterase. Bioorg Med Chem. 2007;15:6733–41.
31. Musilova L, Kuca K, Jung YS, Jun D. In vitro oxime-assisted reactivation of paraoxon-inhibited human acetylcholinesterase and butyrylcholinesterase. Clin Toxicol (Phila). 2009;47:545–50.
32. Okumura T, Seto Y, Fuse A. Countermeasures against chemical terrorism in Japan. Forensic Sci Int. 2013;227:2–6.
33. Paxinos G, Watson C. The rat brain in stereotactic coordinates. 4th ed. San Diego: Academic Press; 2006.
34. Pejchal J, Novotny J, Marak V, Osterreicher J, Tichy A, Vavrova J, Sinkorova Z, Zarybnicka L, Novotna E, Chladek J, Babicova A, Kubelkova K, Kuca K. Activation of p38 MAPK and expression of TGF-ß1 in rat colon enterocytes after whole body γ-irradiation. Int J Radiat Biol. 2012;88:348–58.
35. Riudavets MA, Aronica-Pollak P, Troncoso JC. Pseudolaminar necrosis in cyanide intoxication: a neuropathology case report. Am J Forensic Med Pathol. 2005;26:189–91.
36. Rosman Y, Eisenkraft A, Milk N, Shiyovich A, Ophir N, Shrot S, Kreiss Y, Kassirer M. Lessons learned from the Syrian sarin attack: evaluation of a clinical syndrome through social media. Ann Intern Med. 2014;160: 644–8.
37. Schmued LC, Albertson C, Slikker W Jr. Fluoro-Jade: a novel fluorochrome for the sensitive and reliable histochemical localization of neuronal degeneration. Brain Res. 1997;751:37–46.
38. Valente T, Domínguez MI, Bellmann A, Journot L, Ferrer I, Auladell C. Zac1 is up-regulated in neural cells of the limbic system of mouse brain following seizures that provoke strong cell activation. Neuroscience. 2004;128:323–36.
39. Wilhelm CM, Snider TH, Babin MC, Jett DA, Platoff GE Jr, Yeung DT. A comprehensive evaluation of the efficacy of leading oxime therapies in Guinea pigs exposed to organophosphorus chemical warfare agents or pesticides. Toxicol Appl Pharmacol. 2014;281:254–65.
40. Wohlsein P, Deschl U, Baumgärtner W. Nonlesions, unusual cell types, and postmortem artifacts in the central nervous system of domestic animals. Vet Pathol. 2013;50:122–43.
41. Worek F, Aurbek N, Thiermann H. Reactivation of organophosphate-inhibited human AChE by combinations of obidoxime and HI 6 in vitro. J Appl Toxicol. 2007;27:582–8.

8

Assessment of the state of pharmacovigilance in the South-South zone of Nigeria using WHO pharmacovigilance indicators

Abimbola O. Opadeyi[1,2*], Annie Fourrier-Réglat[3,4,5] and Ambrose O. Isah[1,2,6]

Abstract

Background: WHO pharmacovigilance indicators have been recommended as a useful tool towards improving pharmacovigilance activities. Nigeria with a myriad of medicines related issues is encouraging the growth of pharmacovigilance at peripheral centres. This study evaluated the status of pharmacovigilance in tertiary hospitals in the South-South zone of Nigeria with a view towards improving the pharmacovigilance system in the zone.

Methods: A cross-sectional descriptive survey was conducted in six randomly selected tertiary hospitals in the South-South zone of the country. The data was collected using the WHO core pharmacovigilance indicators. The language of assessment was phrased and adapted in this study for use in a tertiary hospital setting. Data is presented quantitatively and qualitatively.

Results: A total of six hospitals were visited and all institutions had a pharmacovigilance centre, only three could however be described as functional or partially functional. Only one centre had a financial provision for pharmacovigilance activities. Of note was the absence of the national adverse drug reaction reporting form in one of the hospitals. The number of adverse drug reaction reports found in the databases of the centres ranged from none to 26 for the previous year and only one centre had fully committed their reports to the National Pharmacovigilance Centre. There were few documented medicines related admissions ranging from 0.0985/1000 to 1.67/1000 and poor documentation of pharmacovigilance activities characterised all centres.

Conclusion: This study has shown an urgent need to strengthen the pharmacovigilance systems in the South-South zone of Nigeria. Improvement in medical record documentation as well as increased institutionalization of pharmacovigilance may be the first steps to improve pharmacovigilance activities in the tertiary hospitals.

Keywords: Pharmacovigilance, Adverse drug reaction reporting, Nigeria, Tertiary hospitals

Background

Pharmacovigilance in Nigeria commenced in the late 80s and early 90s initially in a tertiary hospital with some preparatory activities at the national level prior to its admission into the WHO program for international drug monitoring (PIDM) in 2004 [1, 2]. It has sustained its activities through active training of healthcare workers, sensitisation campaigns using print and electronic media about medicine safety issues to health care workers and the public [3]. It has also carried out active surveillance through the cohort event monitoring on adverse reactions to antimalarials (artemisinin-based combination therapy) [4]. There has also been the introduction of electronic devices to reduce substandard and falsified medical products which is a major contributor to adverse drug reactions in our setting.

The growth of pharmacovigilance in Nigeria has been propelled by a number of factors including the establishment of the regulatory agency (National Agency for Food

* Correspondence: felabimbola@yahoo.com
[1]Department of Clinical Pharmacology and Therapeutics, University of Benin, Benin-City, Edo State, Nigeria
[2]Department of Medicine, University of Benin Teaching Hospital, Benin-City, Nigeria
Full list of author information is available at the end of the article

and Drug Administration and Control – NAFDAC) by Decree 15 of 1993 (as amended) now cited as Act Cap N1 laws of the Federal Republic of Nigeria 2004, the formulation of the Nigerian National Drug Policy in 2005 [5]. This was further clarified by the introduction of the Nigerian pharmacovigilance policy document in 2012 firmly positing drug safety in national discussion [6]. The actualization of some of these goals has recorded significant progress with the formation of the zonal centres to cover the six geo-political zones in the country in 2012 [7].

Pharmacovigilance has a wide scope with increasing product concerns. The main focus in the Nigeria context has been on adverse drug reactions, substandard and falsified medical products [3, 8–10]. Other areas yet to be fully addressed include medication errors [11], lack of effectiveness reports, acute and chronic poisoning [12, 13], assessing drug related mortality as well as abuse and misuse of medicines [3, 9]. The determination of the burden of these various problems has been poor as the major challenge to the growth of pharmacovigilance in Nigeria has been that of under-reporting as seen worldwide [14–16].

Reporting of drug safety concerns by health-workers in Nigeria is voluntary and the reasons for under-reporting are partly due to fear of litigation, poor understanding of the subject matter, feeling that the "known" Adverse Drug Reactions (ADRs) need not be reported, time constraints and cumbersome reporting processes [17–21]. Lack of appropriate structures and deficient processes at the institutional level may also contribute to the poor reporting rate as found in some studies [17, 21–23].

WHO advocates regional centres as an effective way of enhancing pharmacovigilance activities [24] as observed in some areas of the world where this has been found to improve the number and quality of reports [25, 26].

The aims of the creation of the zonal centres was to decentralize the activities of the National Pharmacovigilance Centre (NPC), e.g. distribution of ADR forms and collection of the Individual Case Safety Reports (ICSRs) from reporters and perform preliminary evaluation with prompt reporting, also transmission of acknowledgements and feedback information to the reporters and dissemination of information from the national centre to the patients and health care workers. Furthermore, they were created to monitor the progress of pharmacovigilance activities at institutional levels as well as support the training and capacity building for pharmacovigilance in the areas of their jurisdiction [6]. These measures would further increase awareness about pharmacovigilance and instil a sense of ownership among the stakeholders regarding pharmacovigilance activities as well as bring closer to the reporters a centre close to their practice.

Currently, the assessment of pharmacovigilance had been largely done at the national level using various tools including evaluating the attainment of minimum requirements for a national centre with interviews of focal persons [27], and recently the use of the Indicator based Pharmacovigilance Assessment Tool (IPAT) indicators [28]. The more recent introduction of the WHO pharmacovigilance indicators provides an opportunity to assess pharmacovigilance activities at the national centres [29]. These indicators targeted at the national centres perform self-evaluation and also identify areas that require intervention. This approach may be applicable to zonal centres and its components which feed data to the national centres. It may also be most appropriate to identify problems at sub-national levels requiring attention [30].

The status of the pharmacovigilance system in the tertiary centres is presently unknown as the WHO indicators and related metrics for evaluating these centres have just been recently released [29] and there is little or no data on the effectiveness and functionality of these centres at this time. Furthermore, the involvement of these centres in this self-appraisal will further facilitate their participation in measures to remedy identified deficiencies with a view towards improving the quantity and quality of adverse drug reaction reports and other areas in pharmacovigilance. This study intends to assess the status of pharmacovigilance structure, processes, outcomes and impact in the South–South zone of Nigeria using the newly introduced WHO pharmacovigilance indicators.

Methods

Study setting and design

This study was carried out in the South-South Zone of Nigeria which is located in the coastal region of Nigeria. It comprises six states namely Akwa-Ibom, Bayelsa, Cross Rivers, Delta, Edo and Rivers with a population of 21,014, 655 million persons (Nigeria national census 2006). Health care professionals in all tiers of hospitals in this zone could send their reports either directly or through the zonal pharmacovigilance centre for onward transmission to the national centre. The South-South zonal pharmacovigilance centre is domiciled in the University of Benin Teaching Hospital, a tertiary hospital for research and learning.

In Nigeria, heath care is delivered at three levels: primary, secondary and tertiary. Tertiary care hospitals provide the highest level of care and serve as referral centres for the secondary and primary centres. Furthermore, there are three main types of tertiary centres. Firstly: the teaching hospitals, which provide teaching (to most cadres in the health professions at undergraduate and postgraduate levels for medical, nursing, pharmacy students etc.) as well as for research and health care services. Secondly: Federal Medical Centres which are mainly for health care services as well as providing residency training in some departments and lastly the specialty hospitals which focuses on particular disease entities of public health importance such as neuro-psychiatric hospitals, orthopaedic hospitals and ophthalmic hospitals among others.

This study was directed at the teaching hospitals because they provide the widest access to all patients with an inclusiveness of all cadres of health care workers. In the South-South zone there are eight teaching hospitals, seven are government owned, and one privately owned.

Eligibility criteria: teaching hospitals were used to ensure inclusiveness of all clinical disciplines and staff complement. All six states in the zone were represented by a teaching hospital. An institutional approval was required from the Chief Medical Director / Management prior to inclusion in the study. The study was subsequently carried out in 6 tertiary health institutions selected through simple random sampling in the various states namely:

- University of Benin Teaching Hospital Benin-City, Edo State, (UBTH).
- Delta State University Teaching Hospital Oghara, Delta State, (DELSUTH).
- Niger Delta University Teaching Hospital Okolobri, Bayelsa State, (NDUTH).
- University of Port Harcourt Teaching Hospital, Port Harcourt, Rivers State, (UPTH).
- University of Uyo Teaching Hospital, Uyo, Akwa-Ibom State, (UUTH).
- University of Calabar Teaching Hospital, Calabar Cross-River State, (UCTH).

Prior to visiting the study sites for data collection, ethical approval was obtained from the research and ethics committee of each of the selected tertiary hospitals. Furthermore, the heads of the institution were contacted for approval and access to the pertinent data. The focal persons in charge of pharmacovigilance in the institution provided answers for the indicator assessments.

Data collection

The data were obtained using a modified WHO data collection form for pharmacovigilance indicators [29] by one of the researchers through interviews of the focal person for pharmacovigilance or the pharmacovigilance committee. The components of this form included *the background information, structural indicators, process indicators, outcome/impact indicators.* The phrasing of the assessment questions was adapted to address the tertiary hospital setting (Additional file 1).

The *background information* collected characteristics of the hospitals: teaching hospital staff strength, i.e. number of post registration health professionals in different categories: doctors, nurses, pharmacists, specialist disposition, average out-patient attendance over the last year, total number of beds in the hospital.

The *structural indicators* assessed the existence of key pharmacovigilance structures, systems and mechanisms in any of the settings studies. It details the basic infrastructure needed to enable good pharmacovigilance activities. It assesses the enabling environment needed for pharmacovigilance activities.

The *process indicators* assessed the degree of pharmacovigilance activities in the various centres. It focussed on the processes that describe the collection, collation, analysis and evaluation of ADR reports. The factors influencing these processes were also considered. These measures were assessed directly or indirectly.

The *outcome/impact indicators* measure the extent of realization of the pharmacovigilance objectives. The hospital records used in assessing the outcome/impact indicators include admission and discharge registers, death registers, International coding of disease registers where available. Other requested details were: the total number of outpatient visits in the previous year, the morbidity and mortality statistics of each institution for the previous year (to include the disease statistics of admitted and deceased persons). Furthermore, to compute the duration of hospital stay, the crude estimates of the duration of admission of patients with serious adverse reactions who were hospitalised was calculated from the adverse drug reaction reports obtained for the previous year.

Data analysis

Analysis was both qualitative and quantitative. All hospitals participating in the study were described according to each indicator. The core Structural indicators are qualitative indicators with categorical data analysed descriptively. The presence or absence of the parameter measured was described for each institution.

Analysis of the core Process and Outcome Indicators are quantitative indicators reflecting rates of reports and actual numbers. They were calculated using frequencies and absolute numbers as dictated by the indicator. The data was analysed with descriptive statistics using Microsoft excel 2007.

Results

All six institutions were visited and the focal Pharmacovigilance persons or committees interviewed following a meeting with the various heads of the institutions. The teaching hospitals in this study are all government owned and serve as referral centres to the primary and secondary tier hospitals. However, they are of varying sizes in terms of bed and staff complement. The demographic characteristics of the institutions at the commencement of the study late January to mid-March 2016 were as follows (Table 1).

Core structural indicators

Responses were obtained from the interviewed personnel for the assessment questions of the 10 structural indicators for all the institutions studied. Three of the 6 institutions had a standardised functional accommodation for pharmacovigilance activities while 1 had non functional rooms and 2 had none. Only one hospital had regular financial provisions for pharmacovigilance. The secretariat in 4 centres had a full time staff to carry out pharmacovigilance activity while 2 had part time staff. Of note was the availability of an institutionalized ADR reporting form in one of the six centres (DELSUTH) while a centre neither had copies of the national nor local forms available. There were no standard forms available which addressed the subset of assessment questions covering the scope of pharmacovigilance in all of the centers (Table 2).

Core process indicators

The absolute number of ADR reports received among the 6 hospitals in the previous year ranged from 0 to 26, two hospitals had no reports for the previous year 2015. Furthermore, the total number of reports in the local database ranged from 0 to 831. Cohort event monitoring of antimalarials (artemisinin-based combination therapy) was carried out and completed in UBTH in the five years preceding the analysis as a form of active surveillance. There were limited numbers of reports on ADRs, medication errors, lack of therapeutic effectiveness etc. in most of the centers. Documentation of feedback and causality assessment carried out on reports in the centers was equally poor in this study (Table 3).

Core outcome/impact indicators

Unusual reports regarding the development of frequent micturition following use of amlodipine besylate was observed in one of the centers and is being evaluated (Table 4). The number of medicine-related hospital admissions per 1000 admissions ranged from 0.00958/1000 to 1.67/1000 and there were no documentations of medicine related deaths in the death registers in the various hospitals. The documentation of pertinent data was inadequate, rendering calculation of other outcome/impact pharmacovigilance indicators in the institutions difficult (Table 4).

Discussion

This is the first published study evaluating the practice of pharmacovigilance in tertiary hospitals of the South-South zone of Nigeria using the WHO indicators. The study has highlighted the strengths and weaknesses of the pharmacovigilance sub-healthcare system in general.

The study revealed that structures were gradually being put in place and there was a general acceptance of the need for pharmacovigilance in all the institutions visited despite institutional challenges. The availability of the newly developed Nigerian national pharmacovigilance policy in some of the centers is a testament to the will of the Nigerian government to institutionalize patient safety through good pharmacovigilance practice.

It was observed that the UBTH performed better than the other hospitals within the zone, this was ascribed to the activities of the pharmacovigilance team and system that started off in the early 90s [2] and has been largely sustained by the commitment of the pharmacovigilance committee, staff and management. It was also observed that despite DELSUTH and NDUTH being relatively smaller hospitals in terms of bed complement, they still performed better than some larger hospitals. This suggests that interest of the key stakeholders in the pharmacovigilance program is needed to sustain the development of the pharmacovigilance system.

Table 1 Characteristics of the tertiary teaching hospitals in the South-South Zone[a]

Characteristic	UCTH	UUTH	UPTH	NDUTH	DELSUTH	UBTH
Number of beds	610	499	782	148	250	701
Approximate number of health care workers (post registration)	1141	739	1028	253	532	1219
Consultant Clinicians	146	86	179	85	65	200
Doctors	359	124	210	53	150	335
Nurses	580	417	600	105	300	660
Pharmacists	56	19	39	10	17	24
Out-patient attendance in the previous year (2015)	81,624	114,523	114,277	32,906	22,540	179,255
Number of in-patient hospital admissions (2015)	7171	9679	10,145	2548	No data	11,324

[a]*UBTH* University of Benin Teaching Hospital Benin-City, Edo State, *UCTH* University of Calabar Teaching Hospital, Calabar Cross-River State. *UPTH* University of Port Harcourt Teaching Hospital, Port Harcourt, Rivers State, *UUTH* University of Uyo Teaching Hospital, Uyo, Akwa- Ibom State. *DELSUTH* Delta State University Teaching Hospital Oghara, Delta State, *NDUTH* Niger Delta University Teaching Hospital Okolobri, Bayelsa State

Table 2 Analysis of WHO Core Pharmacovigilance Structural Indicators of the six tertiary hospitals in the South-South zone of Nigeria

Indicator Item	Assessment	UCTH	UUTH	UPTH	NDUTH	DELSUTH	UBTH	Hospitals with positive answers (n)
CST1	Presence of pharmacovigilance centre/department / unit with a standard accommodation.	Yes	No	No	No	Yes	Yes	3
CST2	Availability of a copy of the Nigerian pharmacovigilance policy	Yes	No	No	Yes	Yes	Yes	4
CST3	Presence of Institutional Drug Therapeutic Committee	Yes	No	No	Yes	Yes	Yes	4
CST4	Availability of regular financial provision for the pharmacovigilance Centre.	No	No	No	No	No	Yes	1
CST5	Availability of human resources to carry out functions of Pharmacovigilance Centre.	Yes	Yes	Yes	Yes	Yes	Yes	6
CST6	Availability of standard ADR reporting form in the institution.	Yes	Yes	No	Yes	Yes	Yes	5
	CP6a-e: Availability of relevant fields in standard ADR reporting form for a) medication error, b) counterfeit/ substandard medicines, c) therapeutic ineffectiveness, d) suspected misuse, abuse, dependence on medicines, e) general public.[a]	No	No	No	No	No	No	0
CST7	A process is in place for collection, recording and analysis of ADR reports	Yes	No	No	No	Yes	Yes	3
CST8	Incorporation of pharmacovigilance into the orientation programme curriculum of newly employed health care professionals	No	No	No	No	No	Yes	1
	CST8a: for Medical doctors	No	No	No	No	No	Yes	1
	CST8b: for Dentists	No	No	No	No	No	Yes	1
	CST8c: for Pharmacists	Yes	No	No	Yes	No	Yes	2
	CST8d: for Nurses/Midwives;	No	No	No	No	No	No	0
CST9	Existence of a newsletter/information bulletin/website as a tool for Pharmacovigilance information dissemination	No	No	No	No	No	Yes	1
CST10	Existence of pharmacovigilance advisory committee or an expert committee in the setting capable of providing advice on medicine safety.	Yes	No	No	Yes	Yes	Yes	4

[a]The items in CST6a-e were all considered separately and the answer was found to be No for each item. *UBTH* University of Benin Teaching Hospital Benin-City, Edo State; *UCTH* University of Calabar Teaching Hospital, Calabar Cross-River State; *UPTH* University of Port Harcourt Teaching Hospital, Port Harcourt, Rivers State; *UUTH* University of Uyo Teaching Hospital, Uyo, Akwa- Ibom State; *DELSUTH* Delta State University Teaching Hospital Oghara, Delta State; *NDUTH* Niger Delta University Teaching Hospital Okolobri, Bayelsa State; *ADR* Adverse Drug Reaction; WHO World Health Organization

Interestingly, one of the centers (DELSUTH) modified the ADR form showing their own hospital logo and domiciling the ADR form to their setting. This showed the willingness of the centre to improve patient safety through a sense of ownership. The inclusion of health facilities in the Nigerian national pharmacovigilance policy was to increase their participation in the pharmacovigilance activities [6]. The study revealed poor budgeting for pharmacovigilance as only a center (UBTH) had financial provision for pharmacovigilance. This was distinct from the finding in Rwanda using the Indicator based pharmacovigilance assessment tool (IPAT) where the hospitals studied had budgetary allocation for pharmacovigilance [31]. The availability of relevant staff and committees are paramount to the development of pharmacovigilance and the hospitals with developed committees and personnel disposition had slightly better reports. It is important to fund pharmacovigilance as development of active pharmacovigilance programs, provision of training, feedback, information dissemination and maintenance of the centers are useful tools in pharmacovigilance that require adequate finances [32]. Capacity development is required for the growth of pharmacovigilance as shown in the review of three countries where insufficient manpower contributed to poor development of pharmacovigilance [27].

The processes and outcomes were however poor in all the facilities probably due to lack of awareness of measuring indices to monitor and evaluate pharmacovigilance. Again, the pharmacovigilance system in this setting is still in their infancy and the requisite culture to ensure effective operations yet to be established. However, it was noted that a cohort event monitoring of antimalarials (artemisinin-based combination therapy)

Table 3 Analysis of WHO Core Pharmacovigilance Process Indicators of the six tertiary hospitals in the South-South zone of Nigeria

Indicator Item	Assessment questions	UCTH	UUTH	UPTH	NDUTH	DELSUTH	UBTH
CP1	Total number of ADR reports received in the previous year	16	0	0	1	9	26
CP2	Reports (current total number) in the local database	41	1	0	12	12	831
CP3	Percentage of total annual reports acknowledged/issued feedback	0	0	0	0	0	0
CP4	Percentage of total reports subjected to causality assessment in the previous year.	0	0	0	0	0	84.6
CP5	Percentage of total annual reports satisfactorily completed and submitted to the local Pharmacovigilance Centre in the previous year.	18.8	0	0	0	77.8	84.6
CP5a	Percentage of reports committed to National Pharmacovigilance Centre database from the local Pharmacovigilance centre	0	0	0	0	0	100
CP6	Percentage of reports of therapeutic ineffectiveness received i n the previous year	0	0	0	0	0	0
CP7	Percentage of reports on medication errors reported in the previous year	0	0	0	0	0	7.7
CP8	Percentage of registered pharmaceutical industries having a functional Pharmacovigilance system? Not applicable in this study.	Only applicable at the level of National Pharmacovigilance Centre					
CP9	Number of active surveillance activities initiated, ongoing or completed in the last five years	0	0	0	0	0	1

UBTH University of Benin Teaching Hospital Benin-City, Edo State; *UCTH* University of Calabar Teaching Hospital, Calabar Cross-River State; *UPTH* University of Port Harcourt Teaching Hospital, Port Harcourt, Rivers State; *UUTH* University of Uyo Teaching Hospital, Uyo, Akwa- Ibom State; *DELSUTH* Delta State University Teaching Hospital Oghara, Delta State; *NDUTH* Niger Delta University Teaching Hospital Okolobri, Bayelsa State; *ADR* Adverse Drug Reaction; *WHO* World Health Organization

was conducted in UBTH as a part of a national program. This active surveillance of medicines used in a disease of public health importance is useful in obtaining better insights into the safety and tolerability pattern in our setting [4]. The need for the indicators could also be seen in a review of three national centers India, Uganda and South Africa using the WHO minimum requirements for a functional pharmacovigilance system by Maigetter et al. [27] which suggested a more efficient and systematic monitoring for pharmacovigilance system. An awareness of regular pharmacovigilance evaluations with pharmacovigilance indicators would translate to better pharmacovigilance processes and outcomes.

Table 4 Analysis of WHO Core Outcome Pharmacovigilance Indicators in six tertiary hospitals in South-South zone of Nigeria[a]

Indicator Item	Assessment questions	UCTH	UUTH	UPTH	NDUTH	DELSUTH	UBTH
CO1	Number of signals generated in the last 5 years	0	0	0	0	0	1[b]
CO2	Number of regulatory notifications issued in the last year	0	0	0	0	0	0
CO3	Number of medicine-related hospital admissions per 1000 admissions[a]	1.67	1.65	0.0985	0.3924	No data	0.97
CO4	Number of medicine-related deaths per 1000 persons served by the hospital per year	Inadequate data	Inadequate data	Inadequate data	Inadequate data	Inadequate data	Inadequate data
CO5	Number of medicine-related deaths per 100,000 persons in the population	Only applicable at the level of National Pharmacovigilance Centre					
CO6	Average cost (US$) of treatment of medicine-related illness	Inadequate data	Inadequate data	Inadequate data	Inadequate data	Inadequate data	Inadequate data
CO7	Average duration (Days) of medicine-related extension of hospital stay	Inadequate data	Inadequate data	Inadequate data	Inadequate data	Inadequate data	5.86 days
CO8	Average cost (US$) of medicine-related hospitalization.	Inadequate data	Inadequate data	Inadequate data	Inadequate data	Inadequate data	Inadequate data

[a]Calculated according to data from Table 1, [b] Frequent micturition following use of amlodipine besylate is being evaluated in the centre
UBTH University of Benin Teaching Hospital Benin-City, Edo State; *UCTH* University of Calabar Teaching Hospital, Calabar Cross-River State, *UPTH* University of Port Harcourt Teaching Hospital, Port Harcourt, Rivers State; *UUTH* University of Uyo Teaching Hospital, Uyo, Akwa- Ibom State; *DELSUTH* Delta State University Teaching Hospital Oghara, Delta State; *NDUTH* Niger Delta University Teaching Hospital Okolobri, Bayelsa State; *ADR* Adverse Drug Reaction

The poor record keeping in all the facilities also made computations of the process and outcomes indicators difficult to achieve. The documentation of medicine related events especially adverse drug reactions were equally poor in this study, this contributed to lack of data even in hospitals where the international coding of diseases was been done. This is not different from what has been reported in other studies about under-recognition of adverse drug reactions and drug related events [33, 34]. It is imperative to inculcate a more articulate approach to routine data gathering and documentation into the healthcare system. Furthermore, planned prospective data collection processes should be put in place to enable evaluation of the outcomes and impact of pharmacovigilance activities.

In the utilization of the WHO pharmacovigilance indicators, it is evident that the scope of reportable incidents by the facilities have been broadened and it is hoped that with the implementation framework of the Nigerian national pharmacovigilance policy, there would be a wider dissemination of the roles that tertiary hospitals are to play in the promotion of pharmacovigilance. The WHO pharmacovigilance indicators would be useful in assessing other tertiary hospitals as it would enable the hospital management develop a strategy towards improving patient safety through pharmacovigilance. It may also help identify areas that need urgent intervention or modification in the health information system management of the tertiary hospitals especially since it is recommended that the indicators be reapplied as needed in the facilities.

Limitations

The WHO indicators have proven to be quite useful in this assessment. However, absence of trained pharmacovigilance personnel hindered the provision of results for the pharmacovigilance process indicators in the centers. Of note is the limitation of the structural pharmacovigilance indicators to fully capture the functionality of the pharmacovigilance system. Furthermore, the overall poor documentation in all centers limited the derivation of the indicators. Again the derivation of the outcome/impact indicator required in-depth survey which young pharmacovigilance systems are unable to execute. There might be a need to develop a scoring system to quantify the indices thus highlighting the deficiencies in numerical terms.

Conclusion

This study has shown an urgent need to strengthen the pharmacovigilance systems in the South-South zone of Nigeria. The WHO pharmacovigilance indicators have been proven to be helpful in assessing the pharmacovigilance system in the zone. Improvement in medical record documentation as well as increased institutionalization of pharmacovigilance may be the first steps to improve pharmacovigilance activities in the tertiary hospitals.

Abbreviations

ADR: Adverse drug reaction; DELSUTH: Delta State University Teaching Hospital Oghara, Delta State; ICSR: Individual case safety report; IPAT: Indicator based Pharmacovigilance Assessment Tool; NAFDAC: National Agency for Food, Drugs Administration and Control, Nigeria; NDUTH: Niger Delta University Teaching Hospital Okolobri, Bayelsa State; NPC: National Pharmacovigilance Centre; UBTH: University of Benin Teaching Hospital Benin-City, Edo State; UCTH: University of Calabar Teaching Hospital, Calabar Cross-River State; UPTH: University of Port Harcourt Teaching Hospital, Port Harcourt, Rivers State; UUTH: University of Uyo Teaching Hospital, Uyo, Akwa-Ibom State; WHO: World Health Organization

Acknowledgements

The authors thank the Chief Medical Directors of the various institutions visited as well as the members of the pharmacovigilance committees, units and staff of the hospitals. We are also grateful to the Director General of the National Agency for Food Drugs Administration and Control (NAFDAC) HQ, Abuja and the South – South Zonal Staff for their kind assistance in carrying out this work.

Funding

The study was self funded.

Authors' contributions

AOO conceptualised the study, modified the data collection tool, collected and analysed data and wrote the initial manuscript. AFR reviewed the protocol, the data collection tool, analysed the data and revised the manuscript. AOI was part of the technical team that drafted the WHO Pharmacovigilance indicators, conceptualised the study, reviewed the study protocol, analysed the data collected and also revised the manuscript. All authors revised and approved the final manuscript.

Competing interests

The authors declare that they have no competing interests.

Author details

[1]Department of Clinical Pharmacology and Therapeutics, University of Benin, Benin-City, Edo State, Nigeria. [2]Department of Medicine, University of Benin Teaching Hospital, Benin-City, Nigeria. [3]Inserm, Bordeaux Population Health Research Center, team, Pharmacoepidemiology, University Bordeaux, UMR 1219, F-33000 Bordeaux, France. [4]Bordeaux PharmacoEpi, INSERM CIC1401, F-33000 Bordeaux, France. [5]CHU de Bordeaux, Pôle de santé publique, Service de Pharmacologie médicale, F-33000 Bordeaux, France. [6]National Drug Safety Advisory Committee, National Agency for Food and Drug Administration and Control, Federal Ministry of Health, Abuja, Nigeria.

References

1. National Pharmacovigilance Centre (NPC) NAFDAC. Safety of medicines in Nigeria: a guide for detecting and reporting adverse drug reactions. NAFDAC-NPC-NIG Lagos, Nigeria: National Pharmacovigilance Centre (NPC), NAFDAC; 2004 I.
2. Isah A, Olowofela A. Clinical pharmacology in Nigeria: the Benin City experience. Pharmacology matters. 2014;7:11–2.
3. Olowofela A, Fourrier-Réglat A, Isah AO. Pharmacovigilance in Nigeria: an overview. Pharmaceut Med. 2016;30:87–94.
4. Bassi PU, Osakwe AI, Isah A, Suku C, Kalat M, Jalo I, et al. Safety of artemisinin-based combination therapies in Nigeria: a cohort event monitoring study. Drug Saf. 2013;36:747–56.

5. Federal Ministry of Health. National drug policy. Abuja, Nigeria: Federal Ministry of Health; 2005.
6. National Agency for Food and Drug Administration And Control {NAFDAC}. National policy and implementation guidleine on pharmacovigilance. Abuja, Nigeria: National Agency for Food and Drug Administration And Control; 2012.
7. National Agency for Food and Drug Administration And Control {NAFDAC}. Directorates. 2013. http://www.nafdac.gov.ng/index.php/about-nafdac/directorates/pharmacovigilance-post-marketing-surveilance. Accessed 29 May 2014.
8. Oshikoya KA, Senbanjo IO, Njokanma OF. Parental reporting of suspected adverse drug reactions in children in Lagos, Nigeria. Arch Dis Child. 2009;94:469–73.
9. Isah AO. Drug safety in emerging countries—a perspective from Nigeria. Clin Ther. 2013;35:e118.
10. Olowofela A, Isah AO. A profile of adverse effects of antihypertensive medicines in a tertiary care clinic in Nigeria. Ann Afr Med. 2017;16:114–9.
11. Ogunleye OO, Oreagba IA, Falade C, Isah A, Enwere O, Olayemi S, et al. Medication errors among health professionals in Nigeria: a national survey. Int J Risk Saf Med. 2016;28:77–91.
12. Okuonghae HO, Ighogboja IS, Lawson JO, Nwana EJ. Diethylene glycol poisoning in Nigerian children. Ann Trop Paediatr. 1992;12:235–8.
13. Ugwu GMI, Okperi BO, Ugwu EN, Okolugbo N. Childhood poisoning in Warri, Niger Delta, Nigeria: a ten year retrospective study. African J Prm Health Care Fam Med. 2012;4 http://www.phcfm.org/index.php/phcfm/article/view/321/406. Accessed 29 May 2018.
14. Moride Y, Haramburu F, Requejo AA, Bégaud B. Under-reporting of adverse drug reactions in general practice. Br J Clin Pharmacol. 1997;43:177–81.
15. Pushkin R, Frassetto L, Tsourounis C, Segal E, Kim S. Improving the reporting of adverse drug reactions in the hospital setting. Postgrad Med. 2010;122:154–64.
16. Isah AO, Pal SN, Olsson S, Dodoo A. Specific features of medicines safety and pharmacovigilance in Africa. Ther Adv Drug Safety. 2012;3:25–34.
17. Ogundele S, Dawodu C, Ogunleye O. Adverse drug reaction reporting among healthcare workers at a Nigerian tertiary hospital: a comparative cross-sectional survey of health care professionals. Glob. Res J Med Sci. 2012;2:32–7.
18. Oreagba A, Ogunleye O, Olayemi S. The knowledge, perceptions and practice of pharmacovigilance amongst community pharmacists in Lagos state, south West Nigeria. Pharmacoepidemiol Drug Saf. 2011;20:30–5.
19. Chinenye JU, Michael OU. Health workers and hospital patients knowledge of pharmacovigilance in Sokoto, north-West Nigeria. Niger J Pharm Sci. 2012;11:31–40.
20. Bello SO, Umar MT. Knowledge and attitudes of physicians relating to reporting of adverse drug reactions in Sokoto, North-Western Nigeria. Ann Afr Med. 2011;10:13–8.
21. Oshikoya KA, Awobusuyi JO. Perceptions of doctors to adverse drug reaction reporting in a teaching hospital in Lagos, Nigeria. BMC Clin Pharmacol. 2009;9:14.
22. Fadare JO, Enwere OO, Afolabi AO, Chedi BAZ, Musa A. Knowledge, attitude and practice of adverse drug reaction reporting among healthcare workers in a tertiary Centre in northern Nigeria. Trop J Pharm Res. 2011;10:235–42.
23. Ali Saleh H, Figueras A, Fourrier-Réglat A. Knowledge, attitude and practice of health professionals towards adverse drug reactions reporting. Eur J Pharm Med Res. 2016;3:12–21.
24. World Health Organization. Safety monitoring of medicinal products: guidelines for setting up and running a pharmacovigilance Centre. Uppsala, Sweden: the Uppsala monitoring Centre (the UMC). In: WHO collaborating Centre for International Drug Monitoring; 2000.
25. Begaud B. Pharmacovigilance in France: a decentralized approach. In: Strom BL, Velo G, editors. Drug epidemiology and post-marketing surveillance. Boston, MA: Springer US; 1992. p. 39–42.
26. Kalaiselvan V, Thota P, Singh GN. Pharmacovigilance Programme of India: recent developments and future perspectives. Indian J Pharmacol. 2016;48:624–8.
27. Maigetter K, Pollock AM, Kadam A, Ward K, Weiss MG. Pharmacovigilance in India, Uganda and South Africa with reference to WHO's minimum requirements. Int J Heal policy Manag. 2015;4:295–305.
28. Strengthening Pharmaceutical Systems (SPS) Program. Safety of Medicines in Sub-Saharan Africa. Assessment of pharmacovigilance systems and their performance. Arlington VA: US Agency for international development; 2011.
29. World Health Organization. WHO pharmacovigilance indicators: A practical manual for the assessment of pharmacovigilance systems WHO. Geneva: World Health Organisation; 2015.
30. Vallano A, Cereza G, Pedròs C, Agustí A, Danés I, Aguilera C, et al. Obstacles and solutions for spontaneous reporting of adverse drug reactions in the hospital. Br J Clin Pharmacol. 2005;60:653–8.
31. Kabore L, Millet P, Fofana S, Berdai D, Adam C, Haramburu F. Pharmacovigilance systems in developing countries: an evaluative case study in Burkina Faso. Drug Saf. 2013;36:349–58.
32. Pimpinella G, Tartaglia L. Pharmacovigilance and the Italian medicines agency. J Pharmacol Pharmacother. 2013;4(Suppl 1):S4–6.
33. Hazell L, Shakir SA. Under-reporting of adverse drug reactions: a systematic review. Drug Saf. 2006;29:385–96.
34. Lopez-Gonzalez E, Herdeiro M, Figueiras A. Determinants of under-reporting of adverse drug reactions. A systematic review. Drug Saf. 2009;32:19–31.

9

Effect of Linagliptin and Voglibose on metabolic profile in patients with Type 2 Diabetes: a randomized, double-blind, placebo-controlled trial

Girish Parthan[1], Shobhit Bhansali[1], Anura V. Kurpad[2], Rama Walia[1], Kishor Bhat[2] and Anil Bhansali[1*]

Abstract

Background: Dipeptidyl peptidase 4 (DPP4) inhibitors improve glycemic control by promoting GLP1-mediated glucose-dependent insulin secretion and suppression of glucagon. Sitagliptin and vildagliptin have been shown to improve insulin sensitivity in patients with type 2 diabetes mellitus (T2DM). However, these patients had uncontrolled blood glucose at inclusion; therefore, the improvement in insulin sensitivity observed in these studies could be attributed to the drug per se and/or reduction in glucotoxicity. This study examines the effect of linagliptin on insulin sensitivity and β-cell function in patients with well-controlled T2DM.

Methods: Thirty patients with T2DM of duration ≤5 years, and having HbA1c < 7.5% were randomized to receive linagliptin, voglibose or placebo ($n = 10$ each), and were followed up for 6 months. Insulin sensitivity was assessed by hyperinsulinemic-euglycemic clamp, and insulin secretory response was measured by basal (M_0) and postprandial (M_1) β-cell function, and area under curve (AUC) for C-peptide during mixed meal tolerance test.

Results: The median HbA1c of the study subjects at inclusion was 6.9% and there was no significant difference among the groups in terms of age, duration of diabetes, body mass index (BMI), HbA1c, insulin sensitivity, AUC of C-peptide and M_0 and M_1 at baseline. At the end of the study, there was a modest reduction in HbA1c (− 0.2%) in the linagliptin group, and a significant decrease (− 0.8%) in the voglibose group, as compared to placebo ($p = 0.038$). However, there were no significant differences in insulin sensitivity, M_0 and M_1 and AUC of C-peptide, within, or among the groups.

Conclusion: Linagliptin modestly improves glycemic profile in patients with well controlled T2DM; however, it may not have an effect on insulin sensitivity in these patients.

Keywords: T2DM, β-cell function, insulin sensitivity, linagliptin, voglibose

Background

The prevalence of diabetes is increasing worldwide and is fast expanding from developed countries to developing countries. As per an estimate by the International Diabetes Federation, 414 million adults were affected with diabetes in 2015, and this number is likely to swell to 642 million by 2040 [1].

* Correspondence: anilbhansaliendocrine@gmail.com
[1]Department of Endocrinology, Post Graduate Institute of Medical Education and Research, Sector- 12, Chandigarh PIN Code-160012, India
Full list of author information is available at the end of the article

Type 2 diabetes mellitus (T2DM) is characterized by two cardinal defects; insulin resistance and insulin deficiency. A plethora of drugs are available for the treatment of T2DM; incretin-based therapies such as dipeptidyl peptidase-4(DPP-4) inhibitors and glucagon like peptide-1(GLP-1) receptor agonists are among the recent additions to the therapeutic armamentarium in T2DM [2].

DPP-4 inhibitors are orally acting drugs that have efficacy similar to sulfonylureas, but without the risk of hypoglycemia or weight gain. DPP-4 inhibitors are commonly used as second-line drugs in the management of T2DM, although they have been found to be useful as monotherapy, as well [3]. These drugs enhance the effect of endogenous GLP-1 by preventing its degradation, and this results in augmentation of glucose-dependent insulin secretion and suppression of glucagon, thereby reducing blood glucose. DPP-4 inhibitors are also known to improve pancreatic β-cell function [4–7]. In addition, DPP-4 has also been shown to be an adipokine, which impairs insulin sensitivity in an autocrine and paracrine fashion [8]; hence, DPP-4 inhibition may improve insulin sensitivity. Previously, few studies have reported an improvement in insulin sensitivity with DPP-4 inhibitors, sitagliptin and vildagliptin [9, 10]. However, these studies included patients with uncontrolled diabetes (HbA1c > 8%) and one of the potential reasons for the improvement in insulin sensitivity observed in these studies could be due to reduction in glucotoxicity, rather than the direct effect of these drugs on peripheral utilization of glucose. Recently, linagliptin has been shown to improve insulin sensitivity in diet-induced obese mice [11].

There are various methods to assess the insulin sensitivity like insulin tolerance test, frequently sampled intravenous glucose tolerance test, quantitative insulin sensitivity check index (QUICKI), mixed meal tolerance test, Matsuda index and homeostasis model assessment-estimated insulin resistance (HOMA–IR) [12]. However, the "gold standard" for the assessment of insulin resistance is hyperinsulinemic euglycemic clamp study [13]. Till date, no study has evaluated the effect of linagliptin on insulin sensitivity in humans by using hyperinsulinemic-euglycemic clamp study. This is a pilot study which aimed to evaluate the effect of linagliptin on insulin sensitivity and β-cell function by using hyperinsulinemic euglycemic clamp and mixed meal tolerance test, respectively, in patients with well controlled T2DM.

Methods

Study design

Patients with T2DM, aged between 30 and 65 years, with duration of diabetes < 5 years, and were on metformin 2 g/day for at least 6 weeks, with HbA1c < 7.5% (< 58.0 mmol/mol) were included in the study. Patients with history of ketoacidosis, abnormal liver function tests (plasma aminotransferase elevations of more than 3 times upper limit of normal), renal failure (serum creatinine more than 1.5 mg/dL), macular edema, coronary artery disease or heart failure, cerebrovascular disease, and those requiring insulin were excluded. Pregnant and lactating women, and those who received any DPP-4 inhibitors in the last 3 months were also excluded. All patients were educated about their disease and were advised life-style modifications. Informed consent was obtained from the study subjects. Institute Ethics Committee approved the study, and the trial was registered at Clinicaltrials.gov (ID number, NCT02097342). Patients were allocated into three groups by random allocation software and received linagliptin 5 mg once daily (OD), placebo OD or voglibose (0.2 mg three times daily), and were followed up for 6 months. Voglibose was used as an active comparator to evaluate the effects of linagliptin on insulin sensitivity independent of alterations in HbA1c. Both patients and physicians were blinded to treatment, but the active comparator group of voglibose was open-labeled, as it was given three times a day.

Baseline evaluation

Baseline evaluation included clinical examination, and biochemical assessment of glycemic control and evaluation for micro- and macrovascular complications.

Fasting plasma glucose (FPG), C-peptide, homeostasis model assessment estimated insulin resistance index (HOMA-IR), homeostasis model assessment β-cell function index (HOMA-β) and hyperinsulinemic euglycemic clamp study were performed at baseline. A mixed meal tolerance study was also done at baseline, after a week of HEC. Laboratory investigations were performed between 8 and 9 am after an overnight fast, and venous blood samples were collected in ethylenediaminetetraacetic acid (EDTA) vacutainer. Glycated hemoglobin (HbA1c) was estimated by an automated high-performance liquid chromatography (HPLC)-based system using ion-exchange cartridge (D-10, Bio-Rad Laboratories, Inc., Hercules, CA, USA). C-peptide estimation was done by electrochemiluminiscence immunoassay (ECLIA) (Elecsys 2010, Roche Diagnostics GmbH, Mannheim, Germany).

Estimation of homeostatic model assessment

The new version of the homeostatic model assessment of insulin resistance (HOMA-IR) and β cell function (HOMA-β) was estimated as per the standard formulae [14, 15].

Hyperinsulinemic-Euglycemic clamp study

Hyperinsulinemic-euglycemic clamp study was performed in all subjects to assess in-vivo insulin sensitivity. Subjects were requested to refrain from vigorous exercise, and reported at 0630 h after an overnight fast of 10 h. An intravenous catheter was inserted into the antecubital vein for infusion of insulin and 25% dextrose solutions, while another catheter was inserted in an anti-flow direction into the dorsal vein of the contralateral hand for arterialized blood sampling. An insulin infusate of 300 mU/ml was prepared from regular human insulin (Eli Lilly & Co. Gurugram, India) in 100 ml isotonic saline and 4 ml of subject's blood. Insulin was infused intravenously based on the surface area at a constant rate (40 mU/m^2/min) to raise the plasma insulin concentration to about 100 μU/mL. The glucose infusion rate was adjusted to maintain a steady state of 4.9 mmol/L. Blood samples for glucose and insulin were collected every 5 and 20 min, respectively. Plasma glucose was analysed by glucose oxidase method on a bedside glucose analyzer (GM9D, Analox instruments, London, UK). M value, a measure of glucose utilization, and M/I, an index of insulin sensitivity were calculated over 40 to 120 min of the clamp study [13].

Mixed meal tolerance test

The mixed meal at a dose of 10 Kcal/Kg, (Ensure, Abbott Nutrition, Abbott Laboratories, India) was dissolved in 500 mL of water and was consumed within 10 min. Medications taken by the subject in the morning were administered 20 min prior to the start of the test meal. C-peptide concentrations were estimated at 0, 30, 60, 90, 120, 150 and 180 min. Total area under curve (AUC) for C-peptide from pre-meal to 180 min was calculated.

Insulin secretion model

Basal β-cell function (BBCF) and postprandial β-cell function (PBCF) were assessed from glucose and C-peptide time-concentration profiles during the MMTT using an insulin secretion model [16]. M_0 is an index of the BBCF and represents the ability of fasting plasma glucose to stimulate the β-cell. M_I is an index of PBCF and represents the ability of postprandial glucose to step up β-cell secretion. It equals the increment in insulin secretion in response to a unit increment in plasma glucose concentration.

Follow-up

All patients were followed up for a period of 6 months. Lifestyle modification advice was reinforced during each visit to all the patients. All concomitant medications were continued throughout the study period without any dose modifications. Biochemical parameters and hyperinsulinemic-euglycemic clamp study and mixed meal tolerance test were repeated after 6 months.

Statistical analysis

All data are expressed as median and interquartile range. Baseline and post-treatment data within the groups were compared using Wilcoxon's signed rank test. The data between the groups were analyzed using the Kruskal Wallis test followed by Mann-Whitney test for two groups (*P* value corrected using Bonferroni procedure). A p value < 0.05 was considered significant. The statistical analysis was carried out using the SPSS version 22 for Windows (SPSS Inc., Chicago, USA).

Results

Study subjects

Twenty-six out of thirty patients completed the study; 10 in the linagliptin group, 9 in the voglibose group and 7 in the placebo group (Fig. 1). One patient in placebo and voglibose group was excluded due to gastrointestinal side-effects, while two patients withdrew their consent for study in the placebo group. The baseline clinical and biochemical characteristics of the three groups were similar (Table 1).

Efficacy

The median HbA1c of the study subjects at baseline was 6.9% and at the end of study it reduced to 6.6%. After 6 months of linagliptin and voglibose therapy reduced the HbA1c from 6.8 to 6.6% ($p = 0.474$) and 7.0 to 6.6%; $p = 0.015$), respectively, whereas in the control group, HbA1c did not change (Table 2, Fig. 2).

Patients treated with linagliptin and voglibose showed a decrease in FPG levels, while FPG increased in the control group. HOMA-IR, HOMA-β, glucose disposal rate, insulin sensitivity, M_0 and M_1 response and AUC for C-peptide did not change significantly in any of the study groups after 6 months (Table 2, Figs. 3 and 4).

Comparison among the groups

Among the groups, there were no significant alterations in clinical parameters at 6 months. HbA1c significantly decreased in the voglibose group as compared to the control group ($p = 0.038$). On mixed meal tolerance test and HEC, there were no significant differences between ΔM_0, ΔM_1, ΔAUC of C-peptide, and Δglucose disposal rate and Δinsulin sensitivity, respectively (Table 3).

Discussion

Our study demonstrated a modest reduction in HbA1c and insignificant alterations in insulin sensitivity indices in patients with well controlled T2DM who were treated with linagliptin. Our study is a pioneer to demonstrate the effect of linagliptin on insulin sensitivity indices, independent of glucotoxicity, as opposed to the previous studies with DPP 4 inhibitors. In addition, this is the first study in the English literature to evaluate the effect of voglibose on insulin sensitivity using HEC.

In the linagliptin group, HbA1c decreased from 6.8 to 6.6%; however, the difference was not statistically significant. The HbA1c reduction with linagliptin in our study was lower than previously reported, and this may be because of lower HbA1c at baseline (6.8%) [17–19]. It is well known that with any anti-diabetic medication, subjects with higher baseline HbA1c exhibit greater reduction in HbA1c, as compared to those with near-normal glycemia. Moreover, the effect of DPP-4 inhibitors is glucose-dependent; hence, in subjects with

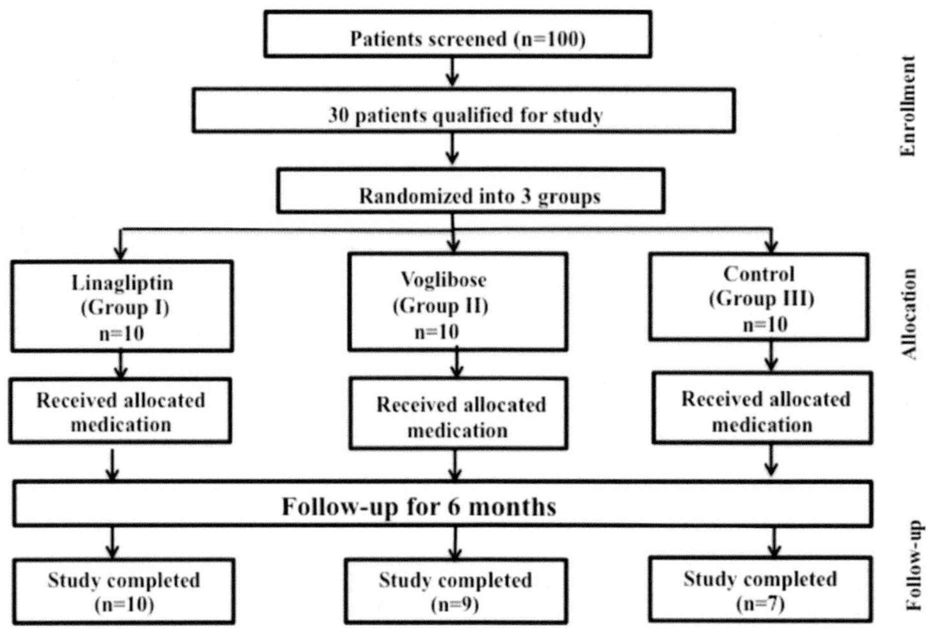

Fig. 1 Schema of the study

near normal HbA1c, their efficacy may be further reduced [20]. There was a significant reduction in HbA1c in the voglibose group at the end of 6 months (from 7.0 to 6.6%). The higher HbA1c reduction observed in our study with voglibose could be due to the dietary habits of the study population, who consume a predominantly carbohydrate-rich diet.

Parameters of insulin resistance assessed by HOMA-IR, glucose disposal rate and insulin sensitivity did not show significant alterations in any of the groups. Improvement in insulin sensitivity with any anti-diabetic agent could be due to its direct insulin sensitizing effect on peripheral tissues or due to reduction in glucotoxicity, or both. Previously, Derosa et al. has shown that both sitagliptin and

Table 1 Baseline clinical and biochemical parameters of the study groups

Parameters	Linagliptin Group ($n = 10$)	Voglibose Group ($n = 9$)	Control Group ($n = 7$)	*P*-value
Age (years)	49.5 (41.5–55.5)	50.0 (45.0–54.0)	54.0 (48.5–59.5)	0.438
Sex (M:F)	5:5	7:2	5:2	
Duration of diabetes (years)	2.5 (1.0–3.0)	2.5 (0.8 to 3.0)	2.0 (0.8–2.8)	0.813
Weight (Kg)	75.3 (69.2–85.3)	60.7 (55.4–71.5)	74.0 (58.7–84.4)	0.071
BMI (Kg/m^2)	25.5 (23.6–31.1)	25.9 (23.8–26.6)	26.4 (23.8–30.5)	0.834
HbA1c (%)	6.8 (6.4–7.1)	7.0 (6.8–7.4)	7.0 (6.8–7.1)	0.350
Fasting Plasma Glucose (mmol/L)	6.5 (5.9–7.3)	6.9 (6.2–7.4)	6.2 (6.1–6.6)	0.287
AUC C-peptide (nmol/L)	473.3 (376.9–567.8)	421.2 (40.9.8–526.9)	595.6 (460.5–623.8)	0.223
$M_0 \times 10^{-8}$ (1/min)	−0.4(− 2.6–0.8)	− 0.5 (− 2.8–1.2)	−2.6(− 5.9–1.2)	0.834
$M_1 \times 10^{-8}$ (1/min)	6.4 (4.5–8.7)	5.7 (3.6–7.6)	7.7 (5.5–10.6)	0.319
Glucose disposal rate (mg/Kg min)	2.7 (2.0–5.5)	3.2 (2.6–3.5)	2.2 (1.8–3.0)	0.297
Insulin sensitivity (mg/(Kgmin)/μU/mL)	4.4 (2.5–8.0)	5.3 (3.6–6.7)	3.2 (2.3–5.1)	0.315
HOMA-IR	2.0 (1.9–2.3)	1.6 (1.3–2.0)	1.9 (1.6–2.1)	0.261
HOMA-β (%)	84.1 (75.1–95.9)	65.0 (52.2–85.7)	92.5 (82.6–102.1)	0.067

All values are expressed as median and interquartile range (1st IQR – 3rd IQR)

AUC Area under curve, M_0 Basal β-cell function, M_1 postprandial β-cell function, *HOMA-IR* Homeostatic model assessment of insulin resistance, and *HOMA-β* Homeostatic model assessment of β cell function

Table 2 Clinical and biochemical parameters within the groups

Parameters	Linagliptin Group Baseline (*n* = 10)	Linagliptin Group 6 months (*n* = 10)	Linagliptin Group *P* value	Voglibose Group Baseline (*n* = 9)	Voglibose Group 6 months (*n* = 9)	Voglibose Group *P* value	Control Group Baseline (*n* = 7)	Control Group 6 months (*n* = 7)	Control Group *P* value
Weight (Kg)	75.3 (69.2–85.3)	73.4(66.3–84.3)	0.066	60.7(55.4–71.5)	56.8(53.5–67.7)	0.208	74.0(58.7–84.4)	75.3(57.9–82.4)	0.612
BMI (kg/m^2)	25.5 (23.6–31.1)	25.0(23.1–30.1)	0.093	25.9(23.8–26.6)	24.4(23.8–25.7)	0.260	26.4(23.8–30.5)	26.6(23.7–30.7)	0.612
HbA1c (%)	6.8 (6.4–7.1)	6.6 (6.3–6.9)	0.474	7.0(6.8–7.4)	6.6 (6.5–6.6)	0.015[a]	7.0(6.8–7.1)	7.0(6.8–7.4)	0.491
Fasting Plasma Glucose (mmol/L)	6.5(5.9–7.3)	6.3(5.6–6.9)	0.308	6.9(6.2–7.4)	6.3(5.8–6.6)	0.058	6.2(6.1–6.6)	6.9(6.2–7.4)	0.310
HOMA-IR	2.0(1.9–2.3)	1.7(1.1–2.1)	0.169	1.6(1.3–2.0)	1.7(1.2–1.9)	0.678	2.4(1.7–3.3)	0.128	0.128
HOMA-β (%)	84.1(75.1–95.9)	81.9(70.8–90.2)	0.285	65.0(52.2–85.7)	78.3(59.9–111.6)	0.374	81.2(69.7–134.8)	0.866	0.866
Mixed Meal Tolerance Test									
AUC C-peptide (nmol/L)	473.3(376.9–567.8)	364.2(301.2–483.1)	0.508	421.2(40.9.8–526.9)	337.6(328.9–353.9)	0.139	595.6(460.5–623.8)	570.6(344.6–697.2)	1.000
$M_0 \times 10^{-8}$ (1/min)	− 0.4(− 2.6–0.8)	2.1(− 0.6–3.3)	0.203	−0.5 (− 2.8–1.2)	2.9(0.5–3.2)	0.214	− 2.6(− 5.9–1.2)	0.1(− 3.7–4.3)	0.176
$M_1 \times 10^{-8}$ (1/min)	6.4(4.5–8.7)	4.6(3.1–5.2)	0.333	5.7(3.6–7.6)	3.3(2.4–4.2)	0.214	7.7(5.5–1.2)	3.8(1.6–8.3)	0.310
Hyperinsulinemic-Euglycemic Clamp Study									
Glucose disposal rate (mg/Kg min)	2.7(2.0–5.5)	2.9(2.7–3.9)	0.508	3.2(2.6–3.5)	3.4(3.1–3.8)	0.173	2.2(1.8–3.0)	2.6(1.8–3.0)	0.866
Insulin sensitivity (mg/(Kgmin)/μU/mL)	4.4(2.5–8.0)	4.0(3.4–5.9)	0.878	5.3(3.6–6.7)	5.6(5.2–6.1)	0.859	3.2(2.3–5.1)	3.4(2.4–4.8)	0.866

All values are expressed as median and interquartile range (1st IQR – 3rd IQR)

AUC Area under curve, M_0 Basal β-cell function, M_1 postprandial β-cell function, *HOMA-IR* Homeostatic model assessment of insulin resistance, and *HOMA-β* Homeostatic model assessment of β cell function

[a]Significant difference from baseline

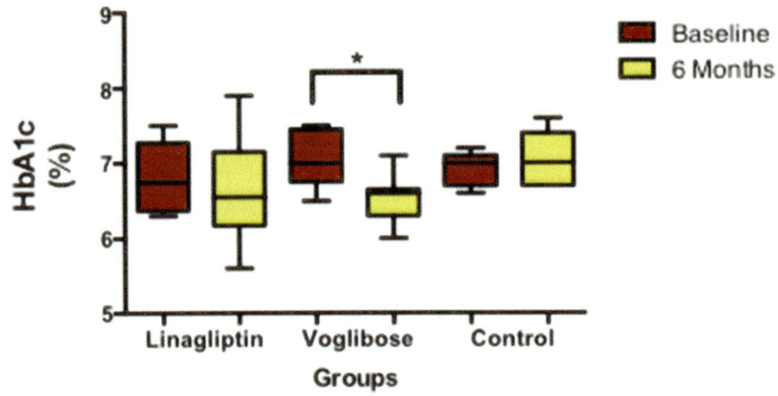

Fig. 2 Change in HbA1c in the study groups. *Means significant difference from baseline

vildagliptin improved insulin sensitivity in patients with T2DM. [9, 10]. However, the impact of reduction of glucotoxicity on improvement in insulin sensitivity could not be ruled out in these studies, as HbA1c reduced from 8.1 to 6.7% and 8.1 to 6.9%, with the use of sitagliptin and vildagliptin, respectively. In the present study, we recruited patients with well controlled diabetes to ameliorate the effect of glucotoxicity on insulin sensitivity. There was no significant effect of linagliptin on indices of insulin sensitivity as assessed by HEC. Moreover, the significant reduction in HbA1c observed in the voglibose group also did not translate into improvement in insulin sensitivity indicating that further reduction in glucotoxicity (< 7%) may not have a considerable influence on insulin sensitivity.

In the present study, we did not observe any significant alterations in β-cell function indices among participants in any of the groups. This is similar to the results of the study by Retankaran et al., where subjects with HbA1c 7.8 ± 0.8% received intensive insulin therapy for 4–8 weeks and then were randomized to receive either placebo or sitagliptin, with a baseline HbA1c of 6.1 and 6.2%, respectively. Sitagliptin did not demonstrate any improvement in β-cell function at the end of the study [21]. As the effect of DPP-4 inhibitors is glucose-dependent, it is quite possible that these drugs may not exert significant beneficial effect on β-cell function in subjects with well-controlled diabetes. On the contrary, a study by Azuma et al., showed that vildagliptin significantly improved both β-cell function and insulin sensitivity in subjects with a baseline HbA1c 7.1% [22]. This raises the possibility that improvement in insulin sensitivity seen with vildagliptin in those with relatively well-controlled diabetes may be a drug-specific effect, rather than a class effect of DPP 4 inhibitors [22].

The strengths of our study include the presence of a placebo arm, active comparator as voglibose and the use of hyperinsulinemic-euglycemic clamp technique to assess insulin sensitivity. Voglibose was chosen as an active comparator because of its unique mechanism of action,

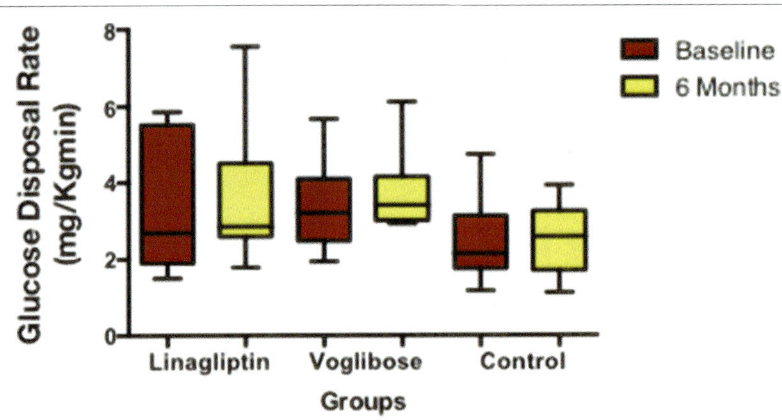

Fig. 3 Change in glucose disposal rate among the study groups

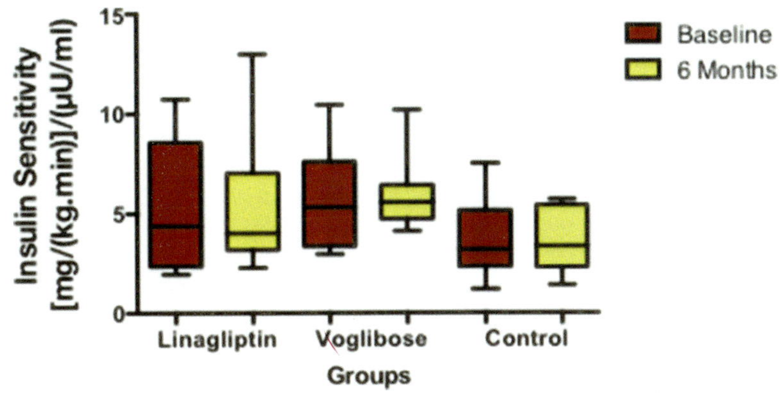

Fig. 4 Change in insulin sensitivity among the study groups

which is insulin-independent, and is not expected to alter insulin sensitivity directly.

There are several limitations in our study. Most importantly, our sample size was small and this prevents us from drawing any meaningful conclusion about the effect of linagliptin on insulin sensitivity. In addition, the duration of study was only 6 months. Since this was a pilot study, we did not calculate the sample size and included 30 patients. Previous studies of DPP 4 inhibitors on insulin sensitivity included larger number of patients and had a follow up of 1 year [9, 10]. However, this was a pilot study to evaluate the effect of linagliptin on insulin sensitivity in patients with well controlled T2DM and more studies involving larger number of patients and longer duration of follow up are needed to conclusively evaluate the effects of linagliptin in patients with well controlled T2DM. We also did not evaluate the presence or severity of nonalcoholic fatty liver disease (NAFLD) in our study subjects, and excluded patients with plasma aminotransferase elevations of more than 3 times upper limit of normal. There is a high prevalence of NAFLD in patients with T2DM [23] .It is well known that NAFLD is closely associated with insulin resistance and subjects with NAFLD have higher insulin resistance as compared to controls [24]. Even though we excluded patients with elevated aminotransferases, NAFLD can be present even in those with normal liver enzymes [25], and this could confound the results of our study. In addition, there was higher number of females in the linagliptin group (5 as compared to 2 in voglibose and placebo groups). Although some studies suggest that women are more insulin resistant as compared to males [26], recent evidence support the fact that women are more insulin sensitive [27, 28]. The higher proportion of females in linagliptin arm could also be a potential confounder in our study. Finally, we used

Table 3 Changes in biochemical parameters among the study groups

Parameters	Linagliptin group ($n = 10$)	Voglibose group ($n = 9$)	Control group ($n = 7$)	*P*-Value Linagliptin V/S Control	*P*-Value Voglibose V/S Control	*P*-Value Voglibose V/S Linagliptin
ΔHbA1c (%)	−0.2(− 0.6 to 0.3)	−0.8 (− 0.9 to − 0.1)	0.1(− 0.1 to 0.3)	0.422	0.038[a]	0.723
Mixed Meal Tolerance Test						
ΔAUC C-pep (nmol/L)	−100.5 (− 174.8 to 75.6)	− 80.3 (− 217.6 to 15.0)	−24.9 (− 153.2184.6)	0.669	0.470	0.780
$\Delta M_0 \times 10^{-8}$ (1/min)	1.5(0.2 to 2.7)	3.5(− 1.4 to 3.9)	3.7(0.6 to 6.7)	0.497	0.918	0.475
$\Delta M_1 \times 10^{-8}$ (1/min)	−2.1 (−3.7 to 0.2)	−3.3(−6.4 to 2.1)	−3.8(− 6.1 to 0.6)	0.842	1.000	0.536
Hyperinsulinemic-Euglycemic Clamp Study						
ΔGlucose disposal rate (mg/Kg min)	0.5(−0.2 to 0.7)	0.2(0.1 to 0.5)	0.1(−0.4 to 0.4)	0.536	0.470	0.842
ΔInsulin sensitivity (mg/(Kgmin)/μU/mL)	0.6(−1.5 to 1.3)	0.2(−0.9 to 0.9)	0.2(−0.8 to 0.7)	0.601	0.905	0.837

All values are expressed as median and interquartile range (1st IQR to 3rd IQR). −Decrease from baseline. [a]Significant difference within the group
ΔAUC Area under curve, ΔM_0 Basal β-cell function, ΔM_1 postprandial β-cell function

mixed meal test to evaluate pancreatic β-cell function and not the gold standard- hyperglycemic clamp study.

Conclusion

Linagliptin modestly improves glycemic profile in patients with well controlled T2DM; however, it may not have an effect on insulin sensitivity in these patients.

Abbreviations

AUC: Area under curve; DPP4: Dipeptidyl peptidase-4; FPG: Fasting plasma glucose; GLP1: Glucagon-like peptide-1; HbA1c: glycated hemoglobin; HEC: Hyperinsulinemic euglycemic clamp; HOMA-IR: Homeostatic model assessment of insulin resistance; HOMA-β: Homeostatic model assessment of β cell function; NAFLD: Nonalcoholic fatty liver disease; OD: Once a day; T2DM: Type 2 diabetes mellitus; TID: Three times a day

Acknowledgements

We acknowledge Ms. Harmanpreet Kaur for her unwavering support and technical assistance during the study. The authors also acknowledge Boehringer Ingelheim, India, for providing study medications.

Authors' contributions

Conceived and designed: AB. Patient's recruitment- GP, AB, RW. Collection and/or assembly of data- GP, SB. Data analysis and interpretation- GP, SB and AB. Data acquisition of clamp and insulin secretion model: AVK, KB. Manuscript writing- GP, SB. Manuscript editing: AB. All authors read and approved the final manuscript.

Competing interests

The authors declare that they have no competing interests.

Author details

[1]Department of Endocrinology, Post Graduate Institute of Medical Education and Research, Sector- 12, Chandigarh PIN Code-160012, India. [2]Department of Physiology, St. John's Medical College, Bangalore, India.

References

1. International Diabetes Federation. IDF diabetes atlas, 6th edn. Brussels. Belgium: International Diabetes Federation; 2013.
2. Drucker DJ, Sherman SI, Gorelick FS, Bergenstal RM, Sherwin RS, Buse JB. Incretin-based therapies for the treatment of type 2 diabetes: evaluation of the risks and benefits. Diabetes Care. 2010;33:428–33.
3. Deacon CF, Lebovitz HE. Comparative review of dipeptidyl peptidase-4 inhibitors and sulphonylureas. Diabetes Obes Metab. 2016;18:333–47.
4. Ahren B, Pacini G, Foley JE, Schweizer A. Improved meal-related beta-cell function and insulin sensitivity by the dipeptidyl peptidase-IV inhibitor vildagliptin in metformin-treated patients with type 2 diabetes over 1 year. Diabetes Care. 2005;28:1936–40.
5. Lyu X, Zhu X, Zhao B, Du L, Chen D, Wang C, et al. Effects of dipeptidyl peptidase-4 inhibitors on beta-cell function and insulin resistance in type 2 diabetes: meta-analysis of randomized controlled trials. Sci Rep. 2017;7:44865.
6. Nonaka K, Kakikawa T, Sato A, Okuyama K, Fujimoto G, Kato N, et al. Efficacy and safety of sitagliptin monotherapy in Japanese patients with type 2 diabetes. Diabetes Res Clin Pract. 2008;79:291–8.
7. van Genugten RE, van Raalte DH, Diamant M. Dipeptidyl peptidase-4 inhibitors and preservation of pancreatic islet-cell function: a critical appraisal of the evidence. Diabetes Obes Metab. 2012;14:101–11.
8. Lamers D, Famulla S, Wronkowitz N, Hartwig S, Lehr S, Ouwens DM, et al. Dipeptidyl peptidase 4 is a novel adipokine potentially linking obesity to the metabolic syndrome. Diabetes. 2011;60:1917–25.
9. Derosa G, Carbone A, Franzetti I, Querci F, Fogari E, Bianchi L, et al. Effects of a combination of sitagliptin plus metformin vs metformin monotherapy on glycemic control, beta-cell function and insulin resistance in type 2 diabetic patients. Diabetes Res Clin Pract. 2012;98:51–60.
10. Derosa G, Ragonesi PD, Carbone A, Fogari E, Bianchi L, Bonaventura A, et al. Vildagliptin added to metformin on beta-cell function after a euglycemic hyperinsulinemic and hyperglycemic clamp in type 2 diabetes patients. Diabetes Technol Ther. 2012;14:475–84.
11. Kern M, Kloting N, Niessen HG, Thomas L, Stiller D, Mark M, et al. Linagliptin improves insulin sensitivity and hepatic steatosis in diet-induced obesity. PLoS One. 2012;7:e38744.
12. Muniyappa R, Lee S, Chen H, Quon MJ. Current approaches for assessing insulin sensitivity and resistance in vivo: advantages, limitations, and appropriate usage. Am J Physiol Endocrinol Metab. 2008;294:E15–26.
13. DeFronzo RA, Tobin JD, Andres R. Glucose clamp technique: a method for quantifying insulin secretion and resistance. Am J Phys. 1979;237:E214–23.
14. Levy JC, Matthews DR, Hermans MP. Correct homeostasis model assessment (HOMA) evaluation uses the computer program. Diabetes Care. 1998;21:2191–2.
15. Matthews DR, Hosker JP, Rudenski AS, Naylor BA, Treacher DF, Turner RC. Homeostasis model assessment: insulin resistance and beta-cell function from fasting plasma glucose and insulin concentrations in man. Diabetologia. 1985;28:412–9.
16. Hovorka R, Chassin L, Luzio SD, Playle R, Owens DR. Pancreatic beta-cell responsiveness during meal tolerance test: model assessment in normal subjects and subjects with newly diagnosed noninsulin-dependent diabetes mellitus. J Clin Endocrinol Metab. 1998;83:744–50.
17. Del Prato S, Barnett AH, Huisman H, Neubacher D, Woerle HJ, Dugi KA. Effect of linagliptin monotherapy on glycaemic control and markers of beta-cell function in patients with inadequately controlled type 2 diabetes: a randomized controlled trial. Diabetes Obes Metab. 2011;13:258–67.
18. Forst T, Uhlig-Laske B, Ring A, Graefe-Mody U, Friedrich C, Herbach K, et al. Linagliptin (BI 1356), a potent and selective DPP-4 inhibitor, is safe and efficacious in combination with metformin in patients with inadequately controlled type 2 diabetes. Diabet Med. 2010;27:1409–19.
19. Taskinen MR, Rosenstock J, Tamminen I, Kubiak R, Patel S, Dugi KA, et al. Safety and efficacy of linagliptin as add-on therapy to metformin in patients with type 2 diabetes: a randomized, double-blind, placebo-controlled study. Diabetes Obes Metab. 2011;13:65–74.
20. Flory JH, Small DS, Cassano PA, Brillon DJ, Mushlin AI, Hennessy S. Comparative effectiveness of oral diabetes drug combinations in reducing glycosylated hemoglobin. J Comp Eff Res. 2014;3:29–39.
21. Retnakaran R, Qi Y, Opsteen C, Vivero E, Zinman B. Initial short-term intensive insulin therapy as a strategy for evaluating the preservation of beta-cell function with oral antidiabetic medications: a pilot study with sitagliptin. Diabetes Obes Metab. 2010;12:909–15.
22. Azuma K, Radikova Z, Mancino J, Toledo FG, Thomas E, Kangani C, et al. Measurements of islet function and glucose metabolism with the dipeptidyl peptidase 4 inhibitor vildagliptin in patients with type 2 diabetes. J Clin Endocrinol Metab. 2008;93:459–64.
23. Dai W, Ye L, Liu A, Wen SW, Deng J, Wu X, et al. Prevalence of nonalcoholic fatty liver disease in patients with type 2 diabetes mellitus: a meta-analysis. Medicine (Baltimore). 2017;96:e8179.
24. Fierbinteanu-Braticevici C, Negreanu L. Tarantino G. Is fatty liver always benign and should not consequently be treated? J Physiol Pharmacol. 2013;64:3–9.
25. Portillo-Sanchez P, Bril F, Maximos M, Lomonaco R, Biernacki D, Orsak B, et al. High prevalence of nonalcoholic fatty liver disease in patients with type 2 diabetes mellitus and normal plasma aminotransferase levels. J Clin Endocrinol Metab. 2015;100:2231–8.
26. Mittendorfer B. Insulin resistance: sex matters. Curr Opin Clin Nutr Metab Care. 2005;8:367–72.
27. Karakelides H, Irving BA, Short KR, O'Brien P, Nair KS. Age, obesity, and sex effects on insulin sensitivity and skeletal muscle mitochondrial function. Diabetes. 2010;59:89–97.
28. Magkos F, Wang X, Mittendorfer B. Metabolic actions of insulin in men and women. Nutrition. 2010;26:686–93.

10

Mineral trioxide aggregate affects cell viability and induces apoptosis of stem cells from human exfoliated deciduous teeth

Chia-Ling Tsai[1], Mu-Chan Ke[1], Yi-Hao Chen[2], Hsi-Kung Kuo[2], Hun-Ju Yu[2], Chueh-Tan Chen[2], Ya-Chi Tseng[2], Pei-Chin Chuang[3,4] and Pei-Chang Wu[2*]

Abstract

Background: Mineral trioxide aggregate (MTA) is widely used for pulp-capping procedures in permanent teeth and as a gold standard material in endodontics. The aim of the study was to investigate the effect of MTA on cell viability and apoptosis when MTA is directly in contact with Stem Cells from Human Exfoliated Deciduous Teeth (SHEDs).

Methods: MTA was mixed and coated in the bottom of a 24-well plate. SHEDs collected and cultured from normal exfoliated human deciduous teeth (passages 3–4) were seeded on square cover glasses. The glasses with seeded SHEDs were incubated in the plates with or without MTA coating. They were divided into four groups: MTA direct contact, direct control, MTA indirect contact, and indirect control. After 1, 2 and 3 days of culturing, cell morphology was observed and cell viability was assessed by the WST-1 cell cytotoxicity assay. TUNEL assay, immunofluorescent labeling and western blot analysis were used to study the effects of MTA on SHEDs apoptosis.

Results: MTA impaired cell viability of SHEDs in 1, 2 and 3 days, and the effect of direct contact was more severe. Cell apoptosis with positive Annexin V and TUNEL staining was noted when there was direct contact with MTA. Western blot analysis revealed that Bcl-2 and Bcl-xL decreased after SHEDs were in contact with MTA.

Conclusions: This study shows that direct contact with 1 week post-set MTA significantly decreases the viability of SHEDs and induced cell apoptosis. The results suggest that there is a possible cytotoxic effect of pulp tissue when there is direct contact with MTA. Different responses would be expected due to the strong alkaline characteristics of fresh mixed MTA.

Keywords: Stem cells, Human exfoliated deciduous teeth, Apoptosis, Cytotoxicity, Mineral trioxide aggregate

Background

Dental pulp capping is indicated for teeth that have had pulp exposure. It can offer an alternative to root canal therapy when pulp is exposed with reversible injury or without signs of inflammation, thereby offering a more conservative approach. Ultimately, the goal of treating the exposed pulp with an appropriate pulp-capping material is to promote the dentinogenic potential of the pulpal cells. Mineral trioxide aggregate (MTA) is widely used for pulp-capping procedures in permanent teeth and as a gold standard material in endodontics [1]. It has been investigated for endodontic applications since the early 1990s and became commercially available as ProRoot MTA (Tulsa Dental Products, Tulsa, USA) in 1998. MTA was broadly used in endodontics for various applications such as root-end filling, root perforation and reabsorption repair, apexification, pulp capping and

* Correspondence: wpc@adm.cgmh.org.tw
[2]Department of Ophthalmology, Kaohsiung Chang Gung Memorial Hospital and Chang Gung University College of Medicine, 123, Da-Pi Road, Niao-Sung District, Kaohsiung 88301, Taiwan, Republic of China
Full list of author information is available at the end of the article

dressing for pulpotomy in primary and permanent teeth [2]. This widespread implementation is explained by MTA's beneficial properties, including its antimicrobial action [3], insolubility in oral fluids and radiopacity [4], good sealing ability [5], and especially its biocompatibility [6, 7] and bioactivity [8].

Theoretically, set MTA contains calcium hydroxide in a silicate matrix which is what attributes the high pH to MTA [9]. MTA maintains its high pH throughout a period of more than 2 months [10]. According to a study of the responses of cells to pH changes, when the pH was raised from 7.3 to 8.9, a marked contraction and detachment of cells occurred [11]. It may be inferred that the cells should express similar unfavorability in cell culture with MTA. Diametrically, a number of investigations have shown that MTA is one of the least cytotoxic dental materials by using various cell culture systems [12]. Many biocompatibility studies have been conducted in vitro and have shown favorable biological properties of MTA in terms of absence of cytotoxicity, lack of genotoxicity, lack of reactive oxygen species production [7], promotion of bone cell adhesion [13, 14], and a slight increase in cell proliferation [6, 15, 16]. It has been demonstrated that MTA induces repair and/or regeneration of mineralized tissues in vivo [17]. Osteogenesis has been observed when MTA implants were placed in intraosseous sites in rats, suggesting an osteoconductive behavior of the endodontic cement [18].

The responses of pulp in primary teeth to MTA pulpotomies and pulp capping were also favorable from clinical and radiographic perspectives [19]. However, a variety of histological responses, including normal or irregular odontoblasts, intra- pulpal calcifications, internal resorption, and inflammatory infiltrate or pulp necrosis were noted [20]. More cytological support is necessary for the use of MTA as a pulp capping material in primary teeth [21]. Some of these studies used human dental pulp stem cells from permanent teeth for in vitro assays [22–25], but few of them used dental pulp stem cells from primary teeth [26, 27]. Meanwhile, most of the studies evaluated the materials by culturing cells with diluted eluates from the MTA, which is distinctly different from the clinical application of MTA that was mixed and directly dressed on the exposed pulp tissue.

The dental mesenchymal stem cells (MSCs) play a role in tooth development as well as in tooth homeostasis and repair [28]. There are many kinds of dental MSCs, such as dental pulp stem cells (DPSC), stem cells from exfoliated deciduous teeth (SHED), periodontal ligament stem cells (PDLSC), stem cells from apical papilla (SCAP) and stem cells from dental follicle (DFSC) [29]. The discovery of stem cells from human exfoliated deciduous teeth (SHED) has offered a potentially noninvasive source of dental stem cells [30]. SHEDs are multipotent cells with high differentiation potential, osteogenic and chondrogenic potential, and express pluripotent stem cell markers [31]. They demonstrated differences from DPSCs of permanent teeth in terms of growth, differentiation characteristics, and gene expression profile [32]. Several studies have demonstrated that many growth factors and stress can induce differentiation from dental pulp cells [33–35]. The MTA-induced odontoblastic differentiation of human DPSCs was investigated [36]. However, the detail of the direct interaction of MTA with SHEDs is still not known. In this study, we want to clarify if there was any overlooked cytotoxic and possible apoptosis effect of MTA when in direct contact with SHEDs.

Apoptosis is known as type I programmed cell death. It is a tightly controlled process crucial for tissue homeostasis. Apoptosis can be triggered by extracellular or intracellular stimuli with extrinsic or intrinsic pathway activation [37]. The B cell lymphoma 2 (BCL-2) gene family encodes more than 20 proteins that regulate the intrinsic apoptotic pathway and the balance of cell survival and death [38, 39]. BCL-2, BCL-XL, BCL-W, MCL1 and BCL-2A1 are anti-apoptotic proteins and they inhibit the essential apoptosis effectors including BAK and BAX [40].

The aim of the present study was to investigate the effects of MTA on cell viability and apoptosis when in direct contact with SHEDs.

Methods

SHED primary culture and identification

The experimental protocols involving human tissue and cells were approved by the Institute Review Board of Chang Gung Memorial Hospital (#100-4678B). Dental pulp was extracted from normal exfoliated human deciduous teeth of 5 to 7-year-old children (8 patients) under local anesthetics at the Outpatient Department of Pediatric Dentistry. Written informed consent was obtained from the patients' guardians. The pulp separated from a remnant crown was digested in a solution of 2 mg/ml collagenase type I (Millipore, Temecula, CA) and 4 mg/ml dispase (Gibco, NY, USA) for 1 h at 37 °C. Cells were seeded into 3 cm plates (Corning incorporated, NY, USA) with the culture medium and then incubated at 37 °C in 5% CO_2 for the primary culture. The culture medium was Minimum Essential Medium Alpha Medium (Gibco, NY, USA) supplemented with 15% FBS (Gibco, NY, USA), 100 μM L-ascorbic acid 2-phosphate (Sigma-Aldrich, MO, USA), 2 mM L-glutamine(Gibco, NY, USA), and 100 units of Antibiotic-Antimycotic (Gibco, NY, USA). The cell colonies that showed containing over 90% CD105, CD90, CD73, CD44 and CD29 surface antigens confirmed by flow cytometry were considered as SHEDs in this study.

MTA Preparation

Under sterile conditions, 1 g PROROOT MTA was mixed(Dentsply Tulsa dental, TN, USA) with 5 ml dd H_2O (w/p ratio is 5:1) using a mixing stick for about 1 min to ensure all the powder was hydrated. The bottom of 24-well plates was coated (Corning incorporated, NY, USA) with 400ul creamy mixed MTA in each well. The bottom area of the 24-well plate is 200 mm^2.

The plates with MTA coating wells were set for 1 week at 37 °C in a humidified 5% CO_2 and 95% air atmosphere for further cell study.

SHEDs cultured with MTA

To evaluate the reaction of SHEDs when in direct or indirect contact with MTA, SHEDs (passages 3–4) were seeded at an initial density of a 2×10^4 cell/ a piece of 12 mm square cover glass (Deckgläser, laudakönigshofen, Gemany) for 24 h with culture medium (the same medium as used to grow the cells). Then, the cover glasses with SHEDs were moved and incubated with 1 ml fresh culture medium in the plates with or without MTA coating for 1, 2, or 3 days. The SHEDs were divided into four groups: MTA direct contact, direct control, MTA indirect contact, and indirect control. In the MTA direct contact group, the cover glass with SHEDs was inversely placed onto the MTA-coated well and the surface of MTA was in direct contact with the SHEDs. In the direct control group, the cover glass with SHEDs was also inversely placed into the well without MTA coating. In the MTA indirect contact group, the cover glass with SHEDs was placed upright and inside the MTA-coated well and SHEDs were not in contact with the MTA. In the indirect control group, the cover glass with SHEDs was also placed upward into the well without MTA coating (Fig. 1). Each group was studied in triplicate experiments. During the incubation period of 3 days, the cell morphology was examined every day under a phase-contrast microscope (CK40 Culture Microscope; Olympus American Inc., Melville, NY) and photographed.

Cell viability and proliferation assay

The cell viability and proliferation assay was measured by the Cell Proliferation Reagent WST-1 (Roche, Mannheim, Germany). The cells were cultured with or without MTA for 1, 2, or 3 days, and the Wst-1 assay was performed according to the manufacturer's protocol. At the end of the culture period, the medium was discarded and the wells, including the square glasses, inside were washed with PBS. Each well was filled with a 1:9 solution of Wst-1 in fresh medium and incubated at 37 °C for 30 min. The solution in each well was transferred to a new 96-well plate. The spectrophotometric absorbance at 450 nm was then measured using an ELISA analyzer. All experiments were performed at least 3 times. Differences between the 2 groups were analyzed using the Student's t-test.

In situ cell death detection

To detect the dead cells, the in situ cell death detection kit (Roche,Mannheim, Germany) based on the TdT-mediated dUTP nick end labeling (TUNEL) to detect DNA fragmentation was used. The cells that were cultured in 1 U/ul of DNase I (Zymo Research, CA, USA) for 4 h at room temperature were used as a positive control. In the permeabilization step, samples were treated with 0.1% Triton X-100 (Sigma-Aldrich, MO, USA) in 0.1% sodium citrate (Sigma-Aldrich, MO, USA) for 10 min at 20 °C. After the TUNEL reaction, samples were counterstained with DAPI and then directly analyzed using fluorescence microscopy (Leica DMI3000B, Wetzlar, Germany).

Detection of apoptosis and/or necrosis by Annexin V/7-AAD staining

To detect apoptosis and/or necrosis, the Dual Detection Reagent (Enzo Life Sciences, NY, USA) containing an apoptosis detection reagent (Annexin VEnzoGold) and a necrosis detection reagent (7-AAD) was used. The cells were fixed with 2% formaldehyde. The cover glasses with cells were washed with diluted phosphate buffered saline and then reacted with 50 mL of Dual Detection Reagent containing the apoptosis detection reagent in 1× binding

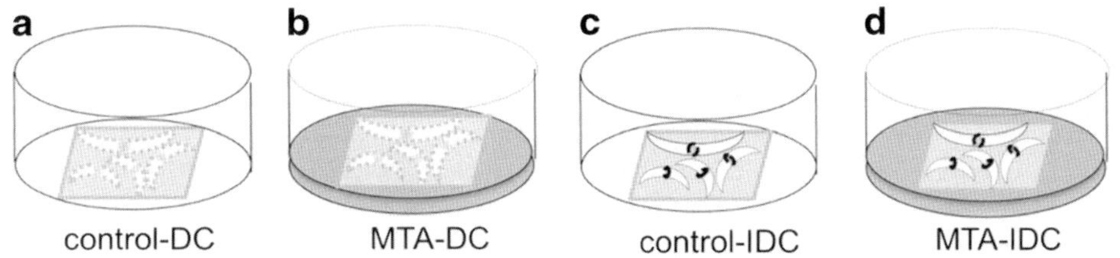

Fig. 1 The control groups (**a** and **c**): no MTA coating on the bottom of the wells. The experimental groups (**b** and **d**): MTA coating on the bottom of the wells. The SHEDs cells were seeded on the square cover glasses. In the direct contact (DC) groups (**a** and **b**), the surface of square glass with seeded cells faced downward and toward the bottom of the well. In the indirect contact (IDC) groups (**c** and **d**), the surface of square glass with seeded cells faced upward

buffer. The samples were incubated at room temperature for 15 min in the dark. After staining, the cells were washed with binding buffer and covered. The stained cells were observed under a fluorescence microscope (Leica DMI3000B, Wetzlar, Germany) with a filter set for Annexin V-EnzoGold (Ex/Em: 550/570 nm) and 7-AAD (Ex/Em: 546/647 nm).

Western blot analysis

A 2× Laemmli sample buffer (BIO-RAD, CA, USA) containing 65.8 mM Tris-HCl, pH 6.8, 2.1% SDS, 26.3% (*w/v*) glycerol, and 0.01% bromophenol blue was used to extract protein samples which were then loaded onto a 10% sodium dodecyl sulfate-polyacrylamide gel (BIO-RAD, CA, USA). Electrophoresis was performed and proteins were then transferred onto nitrocellulose membranes. The membranes were blocked using 5% skim milk (Sigma-Aldrich, MO, USA) in TBS (Sigma-Aldrich, MO, USA) containing 0.05% Tween-20 (Sigma-Aldrich, MO, USA) for 1 h at room temperature, after which they were incubated overnight at 4 °C with the specific primary antibodies. The anti-GAPDH antibody (Millipore, Temecula, CA) was used to ensure equal protein loading. After incubation, the membranes were washed and incubated with HRP-conjugated secondary antibodies. Chemiluminescence was used to detect the protein bands. Antibodies used in this study included rabbit monoclonal anti-Bcl2 (Cell signaling, MA, USA), anti-Bcl-X_L (Cell signaling, MA, USA), rabbit polyclonal anti-Bax (Cell signaling, MA, USA), secondary anti-rabbit IgG HRP-linked antibodies (Cell signaling, MA, USA) and secondary anti-mouse IgG, HRP-linked antibodies (Cell signaling, MA, USA).

Results

SHEDs confirmed by flow cytometry

According to the flow cytometry, more than 90% of the 3rd passage SHEDs expressed mesenchymal stem cell markers including CD105, CD90, CD73, CD44 and CD29 on their surfaces. The hematopoietic surface markers CD14 and CD34 only expressed 0.1 and 0.2%.

Worse cell adhesion in MTA groups

In the direct and indirect contact groups with MTA, sparse shrinkage spindle-shaped cells and worse cell adhesion compared to the control groups were observed. On day 1, many cells detached from the glass slip and floated in the culture medium. In the first 3 days, the number of attached cells clearly decreased (Fig. 2).

Direct contact with MTA decreases cell viability

The cell viability of SHEDs in contact with MTA was evaluated by the WST-1 assay for 1, 2, or 3 days. The existence of MTA significantly inhibited cell proliferation compared with the control groups. When MTA was present, direct or indirect contact also influenced cell viability significantly. However, the cell viability in the indirect contact groups was not significantly different with or without MTA in day 2 (Fig. 3).

Identification of DNA fragmentation by fluorescent TUNEL assay

To study the effects of MTA on SHEDs apoptosis, we exposed SHEDs to MTA for 2 days, and performed the TUNEL assay to detect DNA ends. Because apoptosis is characterized by DNA fragmentation, increased staining in the nucleus (TUNEL-positive cells) indicates apoptosis. Negative results were seen in the Control_DC or Control_IDC groups, whereas the MTA_DC group showed positive stains. However, the MTA_IDC group also showed positive stains, but not as obviously (Fig. 4).

Apoptosis assessment using Annexin V/7-AAD staining assay

Fluorescence imaging was conducted to visualize the difference between apoptosis induced and necrotic cell death. After incubation of SHED cells with MTA for 2 days, the number of cells in MTA groups that remained as an adherent monolayer was greatly decreased compared to the control. In addition, floating cells showed morphological changes, with characteristics similar to apoptosis or necrosis. We co-incubated cells with Annexin V EnzoGold (enhanced cyanine), an early marker of phosphatidylserine externalization at the cell membrane, and red emitting dye 7-AAD, a marker of late apoptosis or necrosis at the nucleus. SHED cells in direct contact with MTA for 2 days were positively stained by Annexin V (Fig. 5). The results suggested that direct contact with MTA induced marked early apoptosis in SHED cells.

MTA-triggered apoptosis involves Bcl-2 and Bcl-xL decreasing

To determine whether Bcl-2 protein families are majorly involved in MTA-induced apoptotic cell death, the Bcl-2, Bcl-xL and Bax activities were examined using a Western blot assay. Our results demonstrated that anti-apoptotic proteins (Bcl-2, Bcl-xL) were decreased significantly compared with the control following 2 days of exposure to MTA. Although the pro-apoptotic protein (Bax) was slightly increased within MTA groups, there was no significant difference when compared with the control (Fig. 6).

Discussion

To mimic the clinical application of tamping material on the dental pulp tissue, the present study designed an environment in which cells were challenged by

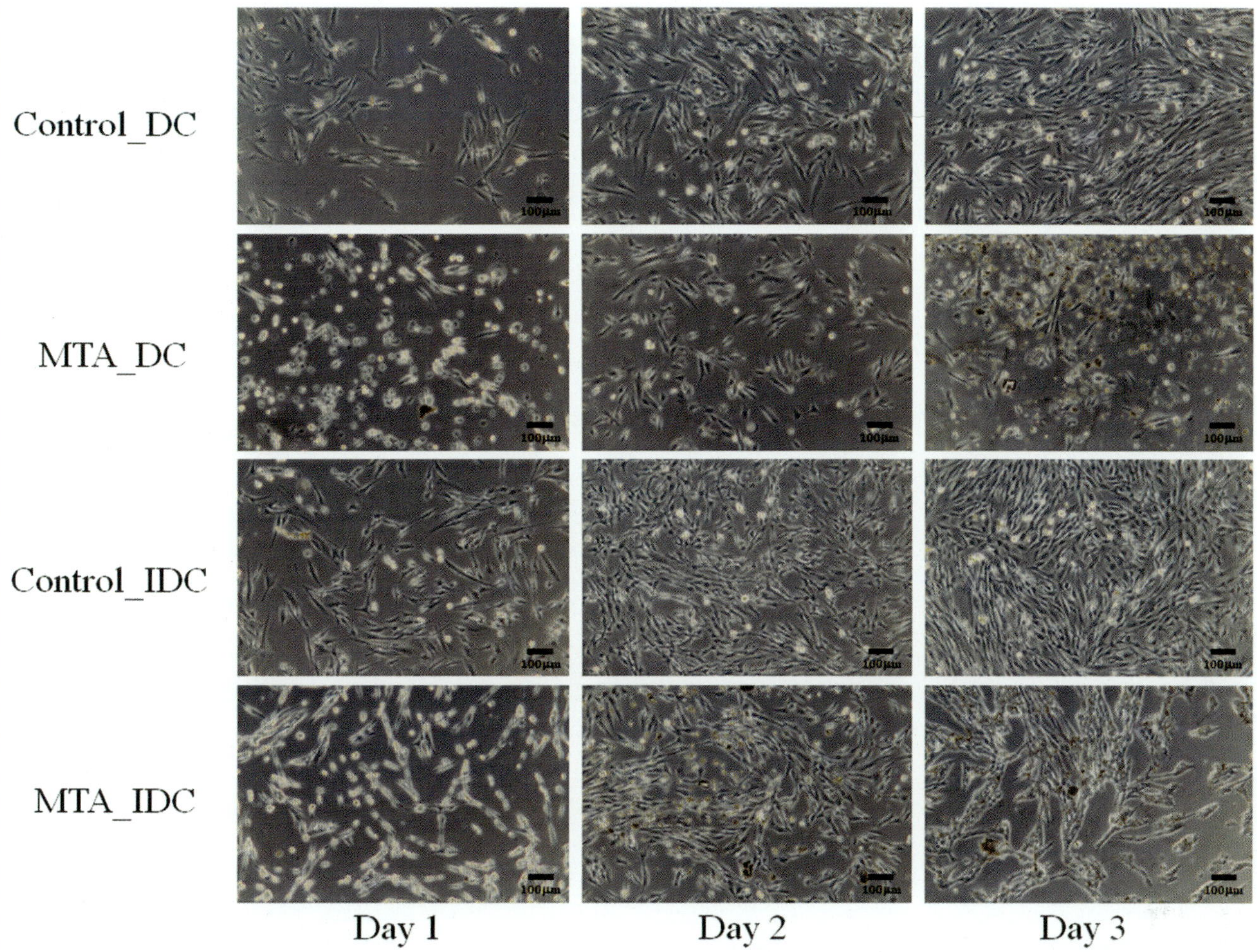

Fig. 2 Representative morphology of SHED cells in contact with MTA or not for 1, 2, and 3 days. In the MTA_DC and MTA_IDC groups, sparse shrinkage spindle-shaped cells and worse cell adhesion compared with the control groups were observed. On day 1, many cells detached from the glass slip and floated in the culture medium. The dispersed cells in the groups in which MTA existed showed a poignant contrast to the control. Black bar, 100μm

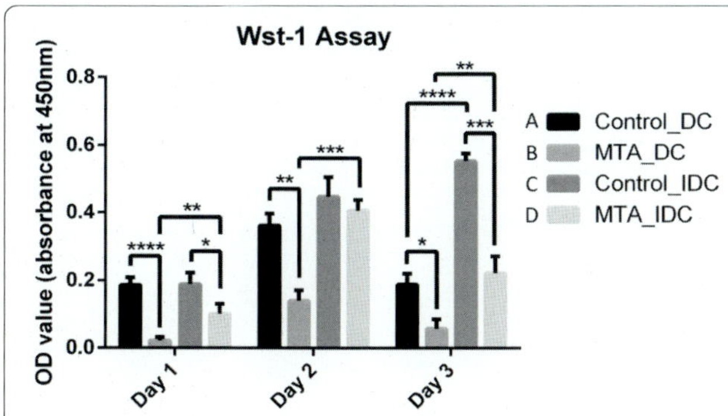

Fig. 3 Wst-1 assay was used for cell viability evaluation. Except for the Day 2 IDC pairs, the existence of MTA significantly inhibited cell proliferation compared with the control groups. (A vs. B, C vs. D) When MTA existed, direct or indirect contact also influences cell viability significantly. Comparing B and D in Day 1, 2, or 3, direct contact with MTA significantly inhibited cell proliferation. Data represent mean values (±SD) of triplicate samples per condition. Graphs are representative of results obtained in three independent experiments. * represents for $p < 0.05$, ** for $p < 0.01$, *** for $p < 0.001$ and **** for $p < 0.0001$

pressure and MTA-contact. The study used the novel method that can check the attached cells' reaction after direct contact with MTA. This study showed that 1 week post-set MTA impaired cell viability of SHEDs and the effect of direct contact was more severe. Cell apoptosis was noted especially when SHEDs were in direct contact with MTA.

The present study revealed that post-set MTA inhibits viability of SHEDs in the culture of the first 3 days. It seems that the results from the present in vitro assay challenge the biocompatible image of MTA. Actually, cell culture studies on MTA show that the cell response to the material depends on many factors such as the cell types and the choice of study duration, use of a fresh or cured material, frequency of changing the medium, the use of direct contact or extracts of MTA, and the concentration of the material in the cell culture media [12]. Conclusions drawn from in previous vitro studies are limited

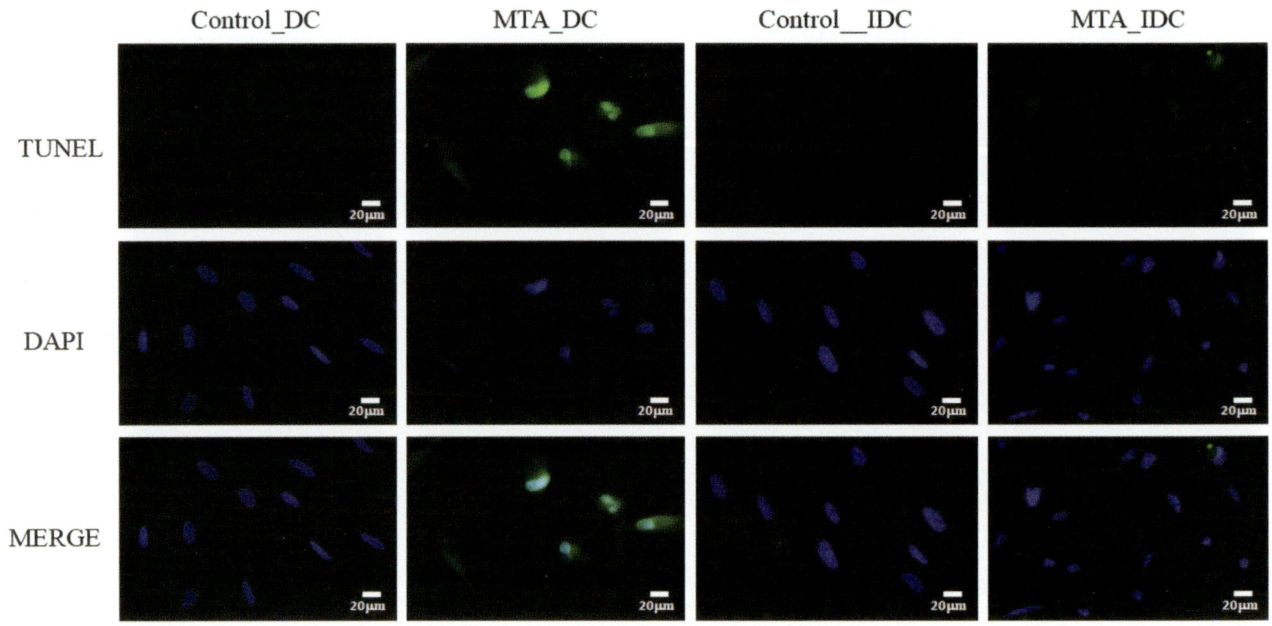

Fig. 4 Images of SHED cells with fragmented DNA marked using a TUNEL assay (In situ cell death detection kit, AP, Roche) at 2 days incubated with direct or indirect MTA contact. Positive cells show a bright green nucleus. DAPI staining was used to check the location of the nucleus. Apoptosis was indicated by TUNEL-positive cells. MTA_DC specimens showed positive staining, whereas the MTA_IDC specimen also showed positive staining, but not as obviously. White bar, 20μm

due to the use of monolayer cultures exposed to the eluate of the test materials [24].

In clinical practice, fresh mixed MTA is directly applied to the surface of dental pulp and sets thereafter. Set MTA contains calcium hydroxide in a silicate matrix; the presence of calcium hydroxide is what attributes the high pH to MTA [41]. The pH value of MTA is 10.2 after mixing. This value rises to 12.5 at 3 h [3] MTA kept its high pH value that ranged between 11.00 and 12.00 throughout the course of a long-term (78 day) study [10]. MTA acts as a "calcium hydroxide-releasing material" [8], but it does not cause as much caustic

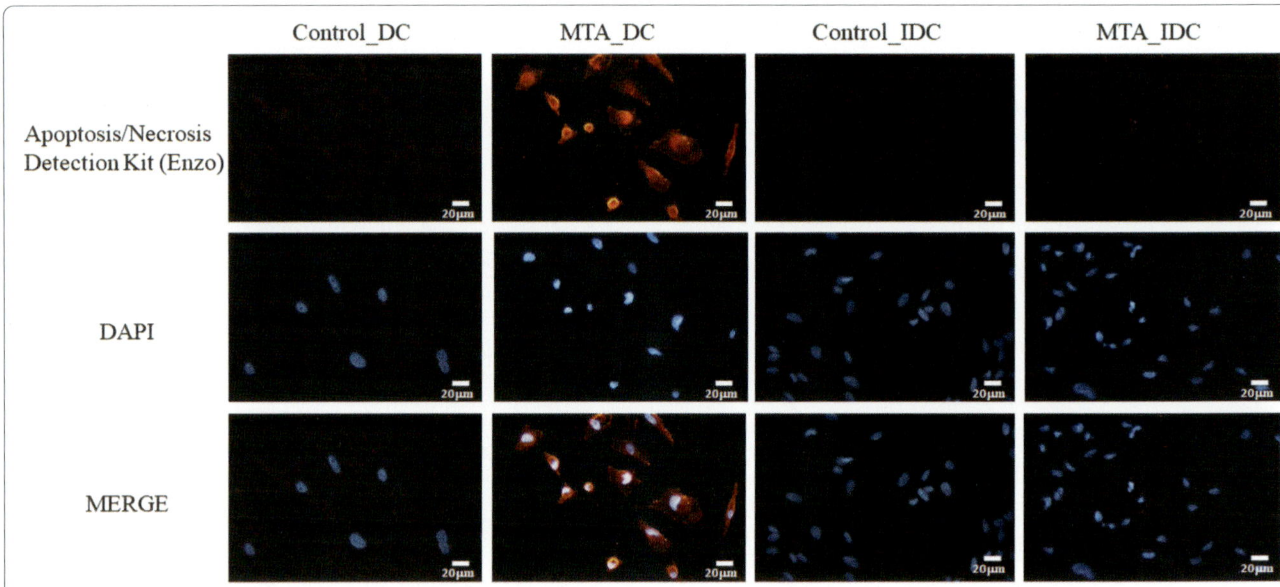

Fig. 5 Apoptosis assessment using Annexin V/7-AAD staining Fluorescent microscopic analysis of SHED cells stained with Annexin V/7-AAD. Yellow and red indicates early and late apoptotic cells, respectively. Shown are representative images of three independent experiments. SHED cells in direct contact with MTA for 2 days were positively stained by Annexin V. White bar, 20μm

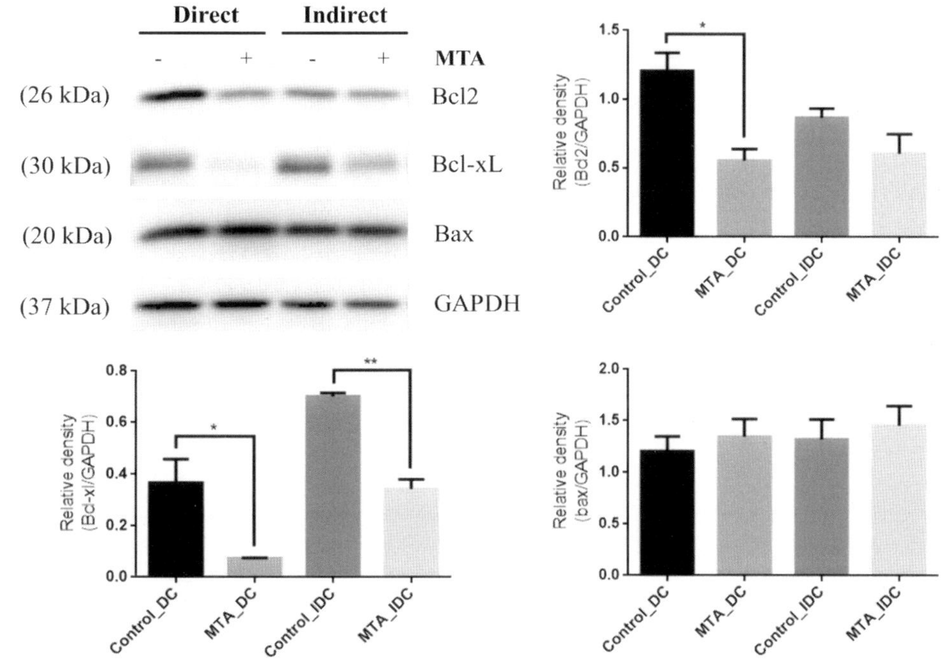

Fig. 6 The Bcl-2 family of proteins consists of members that either promote or inhibit apoptosis, and control apoptosis by governing mitochondrial outer membrane permeabilization. The Bcl-2, Bcl-xL and Bax activities were examined using a Western blot assay. The results demonstrated that anti-apoptotic proteins (Bcl-2, Bcl-xL) were significantly decreased compared to the control following 2 days of direct contact with MTA. When the SHEDs were incubated in the environment with the existence of MTA (MTA_IDC), the anti-apoptotic protein BcL-xL was significantly decreased. There was no significant difference between groups in the amount of pro-apoptotic protein (Bax)

injury as pure calcium hydroxide when in contact with tissue [42, 43]. Investigations have shown that it can conduct and induct hard tissue formation [21]. Previously, pure calcium hydroxide itself has been used in pulp therapies for decades [44, 45]. Due to its alkalinity, it induces a superficial necrosis and a moderate inflammatory response in adjacent pulp tissue. Healing is initiated by the resolution of inflammation, recruitment, and differentiation of stem cells, and is completed with the formation of tertiary dentin at the cell-material interface [24, 46]. The formation of reparative dentine in response to calcium hydroxide may not be due to the bioinductive capacity of the material, and instead due to the result of a defense mechanism by the pulp induced by the irritant nature of calcium hydroxide [7, 47]. If one of the successful mechanisms of MTA is the steady releasing of calcium hydroxide, we think that the pulp reaction to the MTA dressing might be a reparative reaction during the healing process.

According to an experiment of cell and tissue reactions to mineral trioxide aggregate, Saidon et al. found that freshly mixed ProRoot MTA caused denaturation of adjacent cells and medium proteins because of the high surface pH. As the materials set with the medium changed every day, the pH changes and the cell injuries subside [48]. In contrast, tissue reaction to post-set ProRoot MTA was well tolerated with a minimal inflammatory response inside the bone [48]. From the above, it suggested that fresh mixed MTA might cause serious cell damage in the soft tissue rather than hard tissue. In another in vitro study comparing the cytotoxicity of Biodentine, MTA Angelus, TheraCal LC and IRM, the researchers found that cell viability was significantly affected and decreased in the presence of materials ($P < 0.001$) in the first 2 cycle periods. At the same time, a significant decrease in the percentage of healthy, non-apoptotic, and non-necrotic cells was detected among the hDPSCs exposed to the above materials ($P < 0.001$). The cytotoxic effects of these materials on hDPSCs were noted [22]. Their direct evaluation method is similar to our indirect contact method. The inhibition in cell growth after stimulation with MTA could be caused by the release of calcium hydroxide from the material and the induced increase in pH [49]. This condition has also been shown with similar materials such as Biodentine [50].

The Alpha MEM, the base of the culture medium, contains 2.2 g/L sodium bicarbonate ($NaHCO_3$), 140 mg/L Sodium Phosphate monobasic (NaH_2PO_4-H_2O). It is optimized for 5% CO_2 in the incubator for proper buffering. We checked the pH of the culture medium changed after being placed onto the MTA. Out of incubator and in absence of CO_2, the pH of culture medium is 7.8. After MTA was in the culture medium for 3 days, the pH elevated to 8.4. When we cultured SHEDs without MTA for 3 days, the pH was about 8.09. After cultured SHEDs were with MTA for 3 days, the pH was about 8.35. As for the concentration of calcium ions, it was 9.1, > 15, 9.5 and 7.5 mg/dL in culture medium only, culture medium with MTA, SHEDs in culture medium, and SHEDs in culture medium with MTA. The change of pH and concentration of calcium ion in the study is interesting. SHEDs Culturing would mildly lower the high pH and the concentration of calcium ions that related to MTA existing. Besides the bicarbonate and the phosphate system, the culture medium is also composed of 15% FBS that may provide protein buffer system. Although the exact pH level should be lower in the incubator with 5% CO_2, the buffer system in the culture medium could not stabilize the pH when MTA was existed in this study. The strength of buffers is not exactly as the same as the serum. Further associated study is warranted.

The clinically high success rate for MTA pulp capping or pulpotomy may be due to tissue homeostasis in vivo, and is likewise able to reduce the initially high concentrations of calcium hydroxide and thus alkalinity [8, 51]. This is essential to overcome the dose-dependent toxic effect of calcium silicate-based materials on dental pulp stem cells [52]. A dose effect of MTA on cell viability has previously investigated that concentrations larger than 2 mg/ml of MTA extract were found to have a toxic effect on cells. However, when MTA was prepared at concentrations ranging from 0.1 to 2 mg/ml by a leaching method, the dental pulp stem cells' (DPSCs) viability increased and DPSCs were able to differentiate into odontoblasts [36]. In clinical practice, the application of fresh mixed MTA into pulp tissue might induce more severe tissue damage in superficial pulp and less in the deeper tissue according to the gradient concentration of calcium hydroxide from MTA.

One study focused on the differentiation of human dental pulp cells (DPCs) after direct contact with MTA. Their results showed that MTA does not influence cell proliferation, but direct contact with MTA is necessary to help differentiate into odontoblast-like cells [53]. Another study about the effect of MTA on mesenchymal stem cells (MSC) claimed that MTA was able to assist MSC adhesion, growth, and migration. However, their morphologic observation of marked MSC under laser scanning microscopy showed worse adhesion to the MTA compared with the control [54]. In contrast, the results of our study are different. Direct contact with MTA significantly decreased cell viability when compared to groups without direct contact. Tunnel and Annexin V/7-AAD staining assay proved that the lower cell viability is due to apoptosis of the cells. More studies including in vivo studies are warranted.

The present study confirms the positive stain of apoptosis cells after direct contact with MTA. In a previous in vitro study about the effect of MTA on pulp cell lines, the authors concluded that MTA induced proliferation, and not apoptosis [6]. The major difference compared to our study is that their indirect contact of MTA with the permeable membrane insert was only for 1 day. The other study showed that when the materials are placed in close proximity to the cells for 3 days, the flow cytometry study for the distribution of vital, early apoptosis, late apoptosis, and necrotic cells revealed that MTA or biodentine treated hDPSCs were significantly less healthy [22]. Collado-Gonzalez, M. et al. tested several materials on SHEDs by their eluates, and the 2 days' results revealed that MTA and Biodentin did not induce apoptosis [27]. To sum up the results of the above studies, direct contact with MTA may be the key factor for apoptosis of the tested cells.

In the present study, the pressure from the cover slip was also a factor that influences cell viability and proliferation. The pressure from the applicator must be taken into consideration during the studies. However, the control-group setting may control this factor. On the other hand, the pressure did not induce an apoptosis reaction. The shortcoming of this study was that the cell number decreased when in contact with MTA and there was not enough to do a quantitative analysis of the flow cytometry for apoptosis detection. Instead, a qualitative analysis of TUNEL and Annexin V/7-AAD staining was performed in the present study.

Conclusion

Direct contact with 1-week post-set MTA significantly decreases the viability of SHEDs and induces cell apoptosis. The results suggest that there is a possible cytotoxic effect of pulp tissue when in direct contact with MTA. Further in vivo studies are warranted because different responses would be expected due to the strong alkaline characteristic of fresh mixed MTA.

Abbreviations

CH: Calcium hydroxide; DAPI: 4′6-diamidino-2-phenylindole; DC: Direct contact; DPSCs: Dental pulp stem cells; FBS: Fetal bovine serum; hDPSCs: Human dental pulp stem cells; IDC: Indirect contact; MSCs: Mesenchymal stem cells; MTA: Mineral trioxide aggregate; SDS: Sodium dodecyl sulfate; SHEDs: Stem Cells from Human Exfoliated Deciduous Teeth; TUMEL: Terminal deoxynucleotidyl transferase (TdT) dUTP nick end labeling

Acknowledgements

This work was supported by the Stem Cell Research Core Laboratory and a grant from Kaohsiung Chang Gung Memorial Hospital, Taiwan (CMRPG8B0791). The authors thank the Stem Cell Research Core Laboratory in Kaohsiung Chang Gung Memorial Hospital for supporting this work.

Funding

This study was supported by the Kaohsiung Chang Gung Memorial Hospital, Taiwan (CMRPG8B0791).

Authors' contributions

CLT, PCW and MCK designed the study, developed the methodology, analyzed the data and wrote the manuscript. YHC and HKK analyzed the result of the experiments, revised the manuscript and contributed to the writing. HJY and CTC helped technical supports and revising the manuscript. YCT and PCC supplied critical support in the experiments and revision of manuscript. All authors read and approved the final manuscript.

Competing interests

The authors declare that they have no competing interests.

Author details

[1]Department of Dentistry, Kaohsiung Chang Gung Memorial Hospital and Chang Gung University College of Medicine, Kaohsiung, Taiwan. [2]Department of Ophthalmology, Kaohsiung Chang Gung Memorial Hospital and Chang Gung University College of Medicine, 123, Da-Pi Road, Niao-Sung District, Kaohsiung 88301, Taiwan, Republic of China. [3]Department of Medical Research, Kaohsiung Chang Gung Memorial Hospital, and Chang Gung University College of Medicine, Kaohsiung, Taiwan. [4]Center for Translational Research in Biomedical Sciences, Kaohsiung Chang Gung Memorial Hospital, Kaohsiung, Taiwan.

References

1. Asl Aminabadi N, Satrab S, Najafpour E, Samiei M, Jamali Z, Shirazi S. A randomized trial of direct pulp capping in primary molars using MTA compared to 3Mixtatin: a novel pulp capping biomaterial. Int J Paediatr Dent. 2016;26:281–90.
2. Roberts HW, Toth JM, Berzins DW, Charlton DG. Mineral trioxide aggregate material use in endodontic treatment: a review of the literature. Dent Mater. 2008;24:149–64.
3. Torabinejad M, Hong CU, McDonald F, Pitt Ford TR. Physical and chemical properties of a new root-end filling material. J Endod. 1995;21:349–53.
4. Danesh G, Dammaschke T, Gerth HU, Zandbiglari T, Schafer E. A comparative study of selected properties of ProRoot mineral trioxide aggregate and two Portland cements. Int Endod J. 2006;39:213–9.
5. Torabinejad M, Watson TF, Pitt Ford TR. Sealing ability of a mineral trioxide aggregate when used as a root end filling material. J Endod. 1993;19:591–5.
6. Moghaddame-Jafari S, Mantellini MG, Botero TM, McDonald NJ, Nor JE. Effect of ProRoot MTA on pulp cell apoptosis and proliferation in vitro. J Endod. 2005;31:387–91.
7. Camargo SE, Camargo CH, Hiller KA, Rode SM, Schweikl H, Schmalz G. Cytotoxicity and genotoxicity of pulp capping materials in two cell lines. Int Endod J. 2009;42:227–37.
8. Okiji T, Yoshiba K. Reparative dentinogenesis induced by mineral trioxide aggregate: a review from the biological and physicochemical points of view. International journal of dentistry. 2009;2009:464280.
9. Camilleri J. Characterization of hydration products of mineral trioxide aggregate. Int Endod J. 2008;41:408–17.
10. Fridland M, Rosado R. MTA solubility: a long term study. J Endod. 2005;31:376–9.
11. Taylor AC. Responses of cells to pH changes in the medium. J Cell Biol. 1962;15:201–9.
12. Torabinejad M, Parirokh M. Mineral trioxide aggregate: a comprehensive literature review–part II: leakage and biocompatibility investigations. J Endod. 2010;36:190–202.
13. Al-Rabeah E, Perinpanayagam H, MacFarland D. Human alveolar bone cells interact with ProRoot and tooth-colored MTA. J Endod. 2006;32:872–5.
14. Zhu Q, Haglund R, Safavi KE, Spangberg LS. Adhesion of human osteoblasts on root-end filling materials. J Endod. 2000;26:404–6.
15. Takita T, Hayashi M, Takeichi O, Ogiso B, Suzuki N, Otsuka K, Ito K. Effect of mineral trioxide aggregate on proliferation of cultured human dental pulp cells. Int Endod J. 2006;39:415–22.
16. Oviir T, Pagoria D, Ibarra G, Geurtsen W. Effects of gray and white mineral trioxide aggregate on the proliferation of oral keratinocytes and cementoblasts. J Endod. 2006;32:210–3.
17. Main C, Mirzayan N, Shabahang S, Torabinejad M. Repair of root perforations using mineral trioxide aggregate: a long-term study. J Endod. 2004;30:80–3.
18. Moretton TR, Brown CE Jr, Legan JJ, Kafrawy AH. Tissue reactions after subcutaneous and intraosseous implantation of mineral trioxide aggregate and ethoxybenzoic acid cement. J Biomed Mater Res. 2000;52:528–33.
19. Tuna D, Olmez A. Clinical long-term evaluation of MTA as a direct pulp capping material in primary teeth. Int Endod J. 2008;41:273–8.
20. Caicedo R, Abbott PV, Alongi DJ, Alarcon MY. Clinical, radiographic and histological analysis of the effects of mineral trioxide aggregate used in direct pulp capping and pulpotomies of primary teeth. Aust Dent J. 2006;51:297–305.
21. Parirokh M, Torabinejad M. Mineral trioxide aggregate: a comprehensive literature review–part III: clinical applications, drawbacks, and mechanism of action. J Endod. 2010;36:400–13.
22. Bortoluzzi EA, Niu LN, Palani CD, El-Awady AR, Hammond BD, Pei DD, Tian FC, Cutler CW, Pashley DH, Tay FR. Cytotoxicity and osteogenic potential of silicate calcium cements as potential protective materials for pulpal revascularization. Dent Mater. 2015;31:1510–22.
23. Seo MS, Hwang KG, Lee J, Kim H, Baek SH. The effect of mineral trioxide aggregate on odontogenic differentiation in dental pulp stem cells. J Endod. 2013;39:242–8.
24. Widbiller M, Lindner SR, Buchalla W, Eidt A, Hiller KA, Schmalz G, Galler KM. Three-dimensional culture of dental pulp stem cells in direct contact to tricalcium silicate cements. Clin Oral Investig. 2016;20:237–46.
25. Kulan P, Karabiyik O, Kose GT, Kargul B. Biocompatibility of accelerated mineral trioxide aggregate on stem cells derived from human dental pulp. J Endod. 2016;42:276–9.
26. Ong RM, Luddin N, Ahmed HM, Omar NS. Cytotoxicity of accelerated white MTA and Malaysian white Portland cement on stem cells from human exfoliated deciduous teeth (SHED): an in vitro study. Singap Dent J. 2012;33:19–23.
27. Collado-Gonzalez M, Garcia-Bernal D, Onate-Sanchez RE, Ortolani-Seltenerich PS, Alvarez Muro T, Lozano A, Forner L, Llena C, Moraleda JM, Rodriguez-Lozano FJ. Cytotoxicity and bioactivity of various pulpotomy materials on stem cells from human exfoliated primary teeth. International endodontic journal. 2017;50(Suppl 2):e19–30.
28. Sharpe PT. Dental mesenchymal stem cells. Development. 2016;143: 2273–80.
29. Saito MT, Silverio KG, Casati MZ, Sallum EA, Nociti FH Jr. Tooth-derived stem cells: update and perspectives. World journal of stem cells. 2015;7:399–407.
30. Miura M, Gronthos S, Zhao M, Lu B, Fisher LW, Robey PG, Shi S. SHED: stem cells from human exfoliated deciduous teeth. Proc Natl Acad Sci U S A. 2003;100:5807–12.
31. Kerkis I, Caplan AI. Stem cells in dental pulp of deciduous teeth. Tissue Eng B Rev. 2012;18:129–38.
32. Wang X, Sha XJ, Li GH, Yang FS, Ji K, Wen LY, Liu SY, Chen L, Ding Y, Xuan K. Comparative characterization of stem cells from human exfoliated deciduous teeth and dental pulp stem cells. Arch Oral Biol. 2012;57:1231–40.
33. Yu V, Damek-Poprawa M, Nicoll SB, Akintoye SO. Dynamic hydrostatic pressure promotes differentiation of human dental pulp stem cells. Biochem Biophys Res Commun. 2009;386:661–5.
34. Yongchaitrakul T, Pavasant P. Transforming growth factor-beta1 up-regulates the expression of nerve growth factor through mitogen-activated protein kinase signaling pathways in dental pulp cells. Eur J Oral Sci. 2007;115:57–63.
35. Wang FM, Hu T, Tan H, Zhou XD. p38 mitogen-activated protein kinase affects transforming growth factor-beta/Smad signaling in human dental pulp cells. Mol Cell Biochem. 2006;291:49–54.
36. Zhao X, He W, Song Z, Tong Z, Li S, Ni L. Mineral trioxide aggregate promotes odontoblastic differentiation via mitogen-activated protein kinase pathway in human dental pulp stem cells. Mol Biol Rep. 2012;39:215–20.
37. Jin Z, El-Deiry WS. Overview of cell death signaling pathways. Cancer biology & therapy. 2005;4:139–63.
38. Czabotar PE, Lessene G, Strasser A, Adams JM. Control of apoptosis by the BCL-2 protein family: implications for physiology and therapy. Nat Rev Mol Cell Biol. 2014;15:49–63.
39. Ashkenazi A, Fairbrother WJ, Leverson JD, Souers AJ. From basic apoptosis discoveries to advanced selective BCL-2 family inhibitors. Nat Rev Drug Discov. 2017;16:273–84.
40. O'Neill KL, Huang K, Zhang J, Chen Y, Luo X. Inactivation of prosurvival Bcl-2

proteins activates Bax/Bak through the outer mitochondrial membrane. Genes Dev. 2016;30:973–88.
41. Camilleri J, Montesin FE, Brady K, Sweeney R, Curtis RV, Ford TR. The constitution of mineral trioxide aggregate. Dent Mater. 2005;21:297–303.
42. Aeinehchi M, Eslami B, Ghanbariha M, Saffar AS. Mineral trioxide aggregate (MTA) and calcium hydroxide as pulp-capping agents in human teeth: a preliminary report. Int Endod J. 2003;36:225–31.
43. Hargreaves KMG. In: Goodis HE, Tay FR, editors. Seltzer and Bender's dental pulp. Chicago: Quintessence Publishing Company; 2012.
44. Fuks AB. Current concepts in vital primary pulp therapy. Eur J Paediatr Dent. 2002;3:115–20.
45. Schroder U. Effects of calcium hydroxide-containing pulp-capping agents on pulp cell migration, proliferation, and differentiation. Journal of dental research. 1985;64:541–8.
46. Holland R, de Mello W, Nery MJ, de Souza V, Bernabe PF, Otoboni Filho JA. Healing process of dog dental pulp after pulpotomy and pulp covering with calcium hydroxide in powder or paste form. Acta de odontologia pediatrica. 1981;2:47–51.
47. Goldberg M, Six N, Decup F, Lasfargues JJ, Salih E, Tompkins K, Veis A. Bioactive molecules and the future of pulp therapy. Am J Dent. 2003;16:66–76.
48. Saidon J, He J, Zhu Q, Safavi K, Spangberg LS. Cell and tissue reactions to mineral trioxide aggregate and Portland cement. Oral Surg Oral Med Oral Pathol Oral Radiol Endod. 2003;95:483–9.
49. Haglund R, He J, Jarvis J, Safavi KE, Spangberg LS, Zhu Q. Effects of root-end filling materials on fibroblasts and macrophages in vitro. Oral Surg Oral Med Oral Pathol Oral Radiol Endod. 2003;95:739–45.
50. Zanini M, Sautier JM, Berdal A, Simon S. Biodentine induces immortalized murine pulp cell differentiation into odontoblast-like cells and stimulates biomineralization. J Endod. 2012;38:1220–6.
51. Darvell BW, Wu RC. "MTA"-an hydraulic silicate cement: review update and setting reaction. Dent Mater. 2011;27:407–22.
52. Zhou HM, Shen Y, Wang ZJ, Li L, Zheng YF, Hakkinen L, Haapasalo M. In vitro cytotoxicity evaluation of a novel root repair material. J Endod. 2013; 39:478–83.
53. Paranjpe A, Smoot T, Zhang H, Johnson JD. Direct contact with mineral trioxide aggregate activates and differentiates human dental pulp cells. J Endod. 2011;37:1691–5.
54. D'Anto V, Di Caprio MP, Ametrano G, Simeone M, Rengo S, Spagnuolo G. Effect of mineral trioxide aggregate on mesenchymal stem cells. J Endod. 2010;36:1839–43.

11

A newly developed oxime K203 is the most effective reactivator of tabun-inhibited acetylcholinesterase

Kamil Kuca[1,2*], Kamil Musilek[1,2], Daniel Jun[1,3], Jana Zdarova-Karasova[1,3], Eugenie Nepovimova[1,2], Ondrej Soukup[1,3], Martina Hrabinova[1,3], John Mikler[4], Tanos C. C. Franca[5,6], Elaine F. F. Da Cunha[7], Alexandre A. De Castro[7], Martin Valis[8] and Teodorico C. Ramalho[5,7]

Abstract

Background: Based on in vitro and in vivo rat experiments, the newly developed acetylcholinesterase (AChE) reactivator, K203, appears to be much more effective in the treatment of tabun poisonings than currently fielded oximes.

Methods: To determine if this reactivating efficacy would extend to humans, studies were conducted in vitro using human brain homogenate as the source of AChE. The efficacy of K203 was compared with commercially available oximes; pralidoxime, obidoxime and asoxime (HI-6).

Results: Reactivation studies showed that K203 was the most effective reactivator with a second order kinetic constant (k_r) of 2142 min^{-1}. M^{-1}, which was 51 times higher than that obtained for obidoxime (k_r = 42 min^{-1}. M^{-1}). Both pralidoxime and asoxime (HI-6) failed to significantly reactivate tabun-inhibited human AChE.

Discussion: According to these results and previous studies, using K203, it appears that oxime K203 is the most effective reactivator of tabun-inhibited cholinesterase in several species including humans and should be considered as a possible medical countermeasure to tabun exposure.

Keywords: Antidotes, Chemical warfare agents, Poisoning, Treatment, Reactivator, Oxime

Background

Organophosphorus nerve agents comprise a group of the most toxic chemicals ever synthesized. [1] There is currently a lack of sufficiently effective antidotes against the entire spectrum of these compounds [2, 3]. Tabun (Fig. 1), is considered one of the most toxic compounds within this group; especially considering that there are very few fielded cholinesterase-reactivators able to treat tabun intoxications [4–6]. Tabun's extraordinary toxicity and resistance to current medical countermeasures appear to be the result of inhibition of acetylcholinesterase (AChE), which is difficult to reactivate due to the presence of a lone electron pair on the amidic group [7]. This novel enzyme inhibition mechanism was presented by Ekstrom et al. using a theoretical binding site model [8]. However, from a treatment point of view, if the efficacy of cholinesterase-reactivation directly correlates to the effectiveness of treatment, there are several reactivators with low to moderate potency to treat tabun intoxications.

Among these reactivators trimedoxime and obidoxime, symmetrical bispyridinium bis-oximes, are considered the best of the commercially available acetylcholinesterase (AChE) reactivators [4, 9, 10]. Unfortunately their use has been associated with adverse effects [11, 12]. Consequently novel reactivators with higher reactivation activity and lower toxicity should be developed [13]. In 2003, two new oximes aimed at the reactivation of tabun-intoxications, K027 and K048 were developed [14, 15]. They differ from the chemical structure of trimedoxime and obidoxime, which are symmetric compounds, and a carbamoyl group was introduced into their structure to

* Correspondence: kamil.kuca@uhk.cz
[1]Biomedical Research Center, University Hospital Hradec Kralove, Hradec Kralove, Czech Republic
[2]Department of Chemistry, Faculty of Science, University of Hradec Kralove, Hradec Kralove, Czech Republic
Full list of author information is available at the end of the article

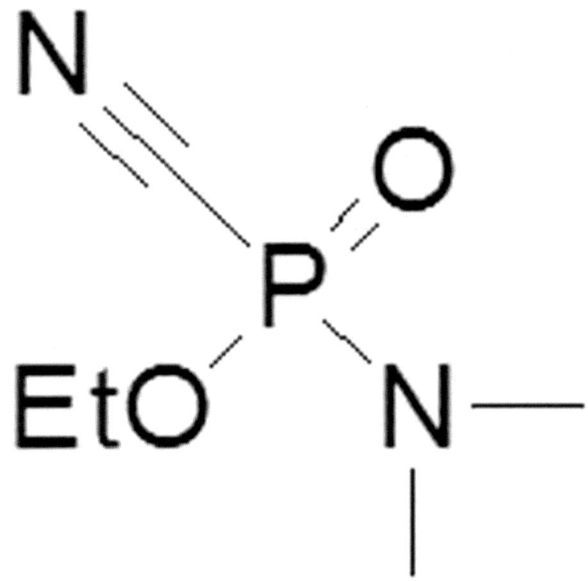

Fig. 1 Chemical structure of tabun

decrease their toxicity. Their in vitro and in vivo properties were shown to be promising [5, 16–21]. Two additional oximes were synthesized – K074 and K075 – differing from trimedoxime and obidoxime by the linker between the two heteroarenium rings [22, 23]. Although these oximes achieved higher reactivation potency, they were more toxic than the original compounds [24, 25].

Recently a new low-toxic oxime with high reactivation potency was developed, K203 [26, 27] (Fig. 2). When compared with other oximes K203 has been shown to have the best reactivation activity and toxicity. All previous studies with K203 have been conducted in rodents and therefore we were interested in determining its in vitro reactivation of human brain AChE. As is known, differences in reactivation are observed depending on the species used [22, 23, 28, 29]. This raises the intriguing question of how to improve the action of drugs. Firstly, one way is to identify structural and electronic determinants of drug sensitivity by mean of experimental data as well as theoretical calculations, which in turn provide important clues about the active site of the molecular targets and its interaction with inhibitors. Thus, in the current work, to rationalize the electronic and steric features that modulate the oxime action, molecular modeling techniques were employed. In this line, the the current study demonstrates the efficacy of K203 reactivation of tabun-inhibited AChE in human brain homogenate. Commercially available pralidoxime, obidoxime, asoxime (HI-6) were used in this study as the standards for comparison.

Methods

Chemicals

K203 ((*E*)-1-(4-carbamoylpyridinium)-4-(4-hydroxyimino-methylpyridinium)-but-2-ene dibromide) was prepared at the Toxicology Department according to the published method [26]. The structure of K203 and structure of oximes tested for comparison (pralidoxime, obidoxime, asoxime (HI-6)) are shown in Fig. 3. Purity of all tested reactivators was measured using TLC (DC-Alufolien Cellulose F; Merck, Germany; mobile phase BuOH-CH_3COOH-H_2O 5–1-2; detection by solution of Dragendorff reagent), HPLC (P200 gradient pump Spectra-Physics Analytical, Fremont, USA; a 7125 injection valve – 10 ul loop, Rheodyne, Cotati, USA; an UV1000 detector, Spectra-Physics Analytical, Fremont, USA) and melting point determination (Micro heating stage PHMK 05; VEB Kombinat Nagema, Radebeul, Germany) [30, 31].

Tabun (GA; *O*-ethyl-*N,N*-dimethyl phosphoramidocyanidate) was obtained from the Military Facility Brno and was shown to have a purity of at least 97% purity. All other chemicals used were of reagent grade (Sigma-Aldrich, Czech Republic).

Source of human brain cholinesterase

The nucleus caudatus was obtained from autopsy patient material (male) aged 68 and 70, who died by accident (Department of Forensic Medicine, Faculty of Medicine in Hradec Kralove, Charles University In Prague). The brain parts were directly frozen. Ex tempore, 1–2 g of defrosted human brain tissue macroscopically free from white matter was taken and homogenized by Ultra-Turrax apparatus in saline solution (1/10, wet weight/volume of 0.9% saline solution). Experiments were approved in compliance with relevant laws and institutional guidelines and were approved by the Ethics Committee of the Faculty of Military Health Sciences in Hradec Kralove (Czech Republic).

Cholinesterase assay

Cholinesterase activity was measured using the procedures previously published by Kuca and Kassa [16]. Briefly, reactivation efficacy of the oximes was evaluated in an in vitro model of brain cholinesterases inhibited by tabun using the standard reactivation method with electrometric instrumentation. The human brain homogenate (0.5 ml) was mixed with 0.01 μM isopropanol tabun solution (0.5 ml) and then incubated for 30 min at room temperature to reach approximately 95% AChE inhibition. Tabun-inhibited AChE was incubated for 10 min with an oxime solution (1 ml) at various oxime concentrations. Following incubation, 3 M sodium chloride solution (2.5 ml) was added, along with distilled water, to a constant volume (23 ml). Finally, 0.02 M acetylcholine iodide (2 ml) was added and the enzyme activity was measured titrimetrically at pH 7.6 and 25 °C on an Autotitrator RTS 822 (Radiometer, Denmark).

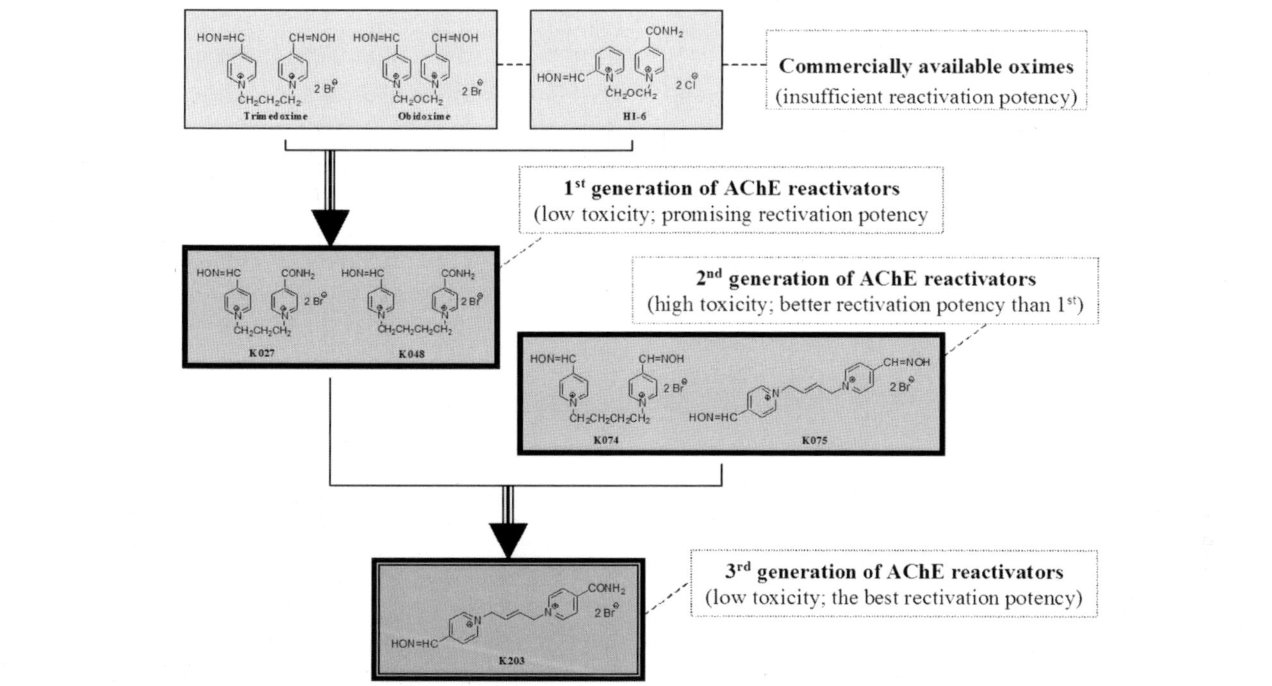

Fig. 2 Developmental strategy of the AChE reactivator K203

Computational details

Docking procedure

Firstly, the molecular docking technique was performed using the reactivators K203 and Obidoxime to perform the docking methodology with the non-aged form of *Mus musculus* Acetylcholinesterase (*Mm*AChE) inhibited by tabun (PDB code 3DL4; resolution = 2.50 Å) [32], and with the human enzyme, also inhibited by this nerve agent, being a model of *Hss*AChE already used in other works [33–35]. The oximes structures were constructed by using the PC Spartan Pro® software [36], with a subsequent optimization at the DFT level, with the Gaussian 09 package [37], using B3LYP density functional and 6-31 g (d, p) basis set. The partial charges of the atoms were elucidated via the Chelpg method [34]. The ligands were docked within the crystallographic structure of both AChE species by employing the Molegro Virtual Docker software (MVD®) [38], considering the same procedures previously employed [39–41]. For the docking procedure, within a radius of 8 Å, water molecules and amino acid residues were considered as flexible. Due to the essence of the molecular docking methodology, the calculations were performed giving rise to 50 different conformations (poses) for the reactivators. The most significant

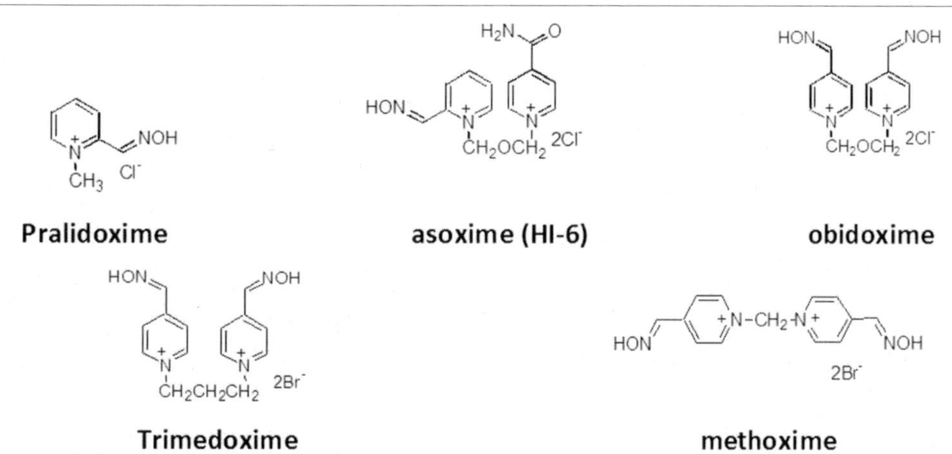

Fig. 3 Currently commercially available oximes

conformation for each ligand was chosen taking into account the most promising interaction energy within the enzyme active site, always searching for appropriate accommodations in the site, beyond the potent conformations for the reactivation mechanism.

The MolDock scoring function employed in the MVD software has its origin on the piecewise linear potential (PLP), a reduced potential whose settings are adjusted to enzyme-ligand complexes [42]. The docking scoring function values, E_{score}, are defined by Eq. 1:

$$E_{score} = E_{inter} + E_{intra} \quad (1)$$

Where:

$$E_{Einter} = \sum_{i\varepsilon ligand} \sum_{j\varepsilon protein} \left[E_{PLP}(r_{ij}) + 332.0 \frac{qiqj}{4r_{ij}^2} \right] \quad (2)$$

E_{PLP} stands for "piecewise linear potential", which consists in the use of two different parameter sets, as described as follows: one employed for approach of the steric term among atoms (Van der Waals), and the other for the hydrogen bonding. The second term is associated to electrostatic interactions in relation to overloaded atoms. It consists of a Coulomb potential, presenting a dielectric constant dependent on the range (D(r) = 4r). The numeric amount of 332.0 is important, given that the electrostatic energy unit can be provided in kilocalories per molecule [38]. E_{intra} is associated to the inner energy of the ligand:

$$E_{intra} = \sum_{i\varepsilon ligand} \sum_{j\varepsilon ligand} E_{PLP}(r_{ij}) + \sum_{flexiblebonds} A[1 - \cos(m.\theta - \theta_0)] + E_{clash} \quad (3)$$

The first portion of the equation (double addition) is related to all pairs of atoms in the ligand, ruling out those that are linked by two bonds. The second term qualifies the torsional energy, where θ is the torsional angle of the bond. If several torsions are capable of being resolved, each torsional energy is important and an average in relation to them is employed. The last measure, E_{clash}, attributes a penalty equals to 1000 in the situation of distances less than 2.0 Å among heavy atoms, not considering impracticable ligand conformations [38]. The search algorithm in MVD combines the differential evolution optimization method with a cavity forecast algorithm, throughout the search process, thus allowing a rapid and precise recognition of potential binding modes (poses) [38, 43, 44].

Reaction mechanism and QM/MM methodology

From the structures selected with the docking methodology, the hybrid QM/MM was carried out to evaluate the energetic barrier (activation energy) for the mechanism in the reactivation pathway of the rat and human AChE inhibited by tabun. QM/MM techniques allow the modeling of larger systems, like reactions within enzymes, by combining the electronic degrees of a quantum chemical approach with the MM methods, increasing performance and decreasing computational demand [45]. Thus, in this study, hybrid quantum and molecular mechanics (QM/MM) associated with molecular docking methods have been carried out to determine the reactivation reaction pathway for the inhibited AChE, using different reactivators. Actually, this theoretical strategy has been previously applied in other occasions [35, 46–48]. With the purpose of getting more accurate results, capturing electronic effects, QM calculations were performed at the density functional theory (DFT) level with the Gaussian 09 package [37]. DFT techniques have shown a significant performance for large systems, such as biomolecules [49–51]. This relationship between functional and basis sets has been tested for similar systems. [44, 52]

The QM systems were constituted of amino acid residues, water molecules, reactivators and Ser203-tabun complex, for both AChE species. In the reaction mechanism simulation, all transition states were calculated and characterized identifying imaginary frequencies [53, 54]. Each system was fully optimized at DFT level, with conjugate gradient and quasi-Newton-Raphson algorithms. The final geometries were obtained with B3LYP functional density [43], using 6-31 g (d, p) basis set.

Results

In vitro results obtained in this study are summarized in Table 1 and Fig. 4. The reactivation process is characterized by several constants. Constant K_R represents the affinity of the AChE reactivator to the inhibited enzyme. k_R is the first order kinetic constant characterizing the splitting of the bond between enzyme and inhibitor. And finally, k_r is the second order kinetic constant characterizing the entire reactivation process.

From the results obtained, only obidoxime and K203 were able to reactivate tabun-inhibited human brain cholinesterases. When they were directly compared, K203 surpassed obidoxime in all parameters including a 25-times higher affinity towards the inhibited enzyme. K203 was also able to disrupt the inhibitor-enzyme complex at twice the rate of obidoxime. Based on these two parameters the overall second order kinetic constant characterizing the whole reactivation process (k_r) favored K203 for reactivation of tabun-inhibited AChE. If the reactivation curves were compared, K203 surpasses all other reactivators tested in this study. K203 reactivated over 60% of

Table 1 Tabun-inhibited acetylcholinesterase reactivation constants

	HUMAN			RAT	
Constants Oxime	K_R [μM]	k_R [min^{-1}]	k_r [min^{-1}. M^{-1}]	k_r^c [min^{-1}. M^{-1}]	Species Difference ratio
Pralidoxime	-[a]	-[a]	-[a]	10	-[b]
Obidoxime	1412	0.060	42	6250	149
Asoxime (HI-6)	-[a]	-[a]	-[a]	1111	-[b]
K203	56	0.120	2142	16,000	7.5

[a, b]Unable to estimate the appropriate constants due to lack of reactivated AChE by this oxime
[c]Rat brain homogenate results published by Musilek et al. J. Med. Chem. (2007)

cholinesterase activity at human attainable concentrations. Obidoxime was the second most efficient oxime with 33% reactivation, but at concentrations between 10^{-2} and 10^{-3} M that are supposed to be not attainable in plasma after i.v. or i.m. administration. Other oximes did not appreciably reactivate tabun-inhibited human AChE.

Discussion

This study is the first to compare the effectiveness of four oximes in reactivating tabun-inhibited acetylcholinesterase (AChE) in human brain homogenate. Only five oximes are currently clinicaly available worldwide for the treatment of organophosphorus nerve agent or pesticide poisoning, pralidoxime, trimedoxime, obidoxime, methoxime and asoxime (HI-6). Asoxime (HI-6) has been the most extensively investigated as a broad-spectrum antidote but has been shown to be a very weak reactivator of tabun-inhibited AChE in several rodent species [9, 10, 22, 23, 55, 56]. The ineffectiveness of asoxime (HI-6) has also been reported in in vivo and in vitro studies conducted in rats [26, 57]. Of the commercially available oximes, only trimedoxime and obidoxime are able to reactivate tabun-inhibited AChE, however, their reactivation potency is less than ideal [4, 5]. K203 has been previously shown to be the most effective reactivator of tabun-inhibited AChE in both in vitro and in vivo rodent studies [57]. This study was the first to evaluate the efficacy of K203 on real human brain AChE and as was observed in the rodent study, K203 is more effective in reactivating tabun-inhibited enzyme than obidoxime. At therapeutic concentrations, K203 was able to reactivate over 60% of tabun-inhibited AChE, while obidoxime reactivated only 33% of its activity at supra-pharmacological doses (Fig. 4). When the overall reaction rate constant (k_r) of human tissue is compared (Table 1), the constant for K203 was 51-times higher than that of obidoxime but only 2.5-times higher when the rat tissue was tested [26]. However when k_r ratios are compared between human and rat enzymes, obidoxime results decrease 149-times while K203 decreases only 7.5-times. These results suggest that a direct correlation in oxime-mediated reactivation between species does not exist and that comparative studies in one species may not truly reflect the reactivation effects in humans.

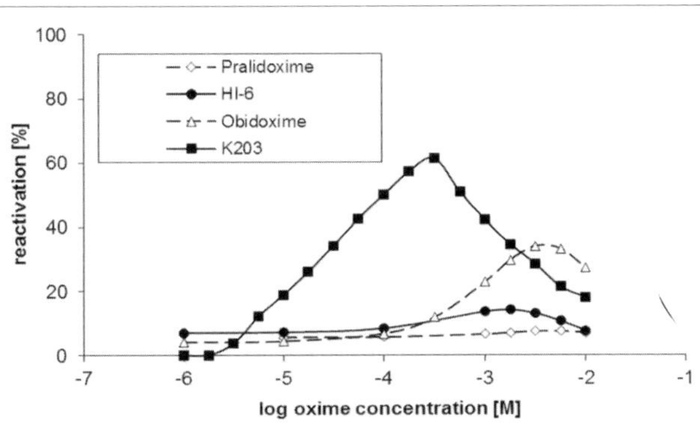

Fig. 4 The effectiveness of oximes at varying concentrations to reactivate tabun-inhibited human cholinesterase. Cholinesterase activity measured in human brain homogenate is shown as a percentage of control activity. Tabun was incubated with brain homogenate for 30 min prior to the addition of the oxime. Reactivation was carried out for 10 min. All experiments were carried out at pH 7.6 and 25 °C. Each point represents the mean±SEM for 2 measurements

The better reactivation efficacy of K203 was expected based on structure-activity relationship requirements [4, 58]. K203 meets four main requirements; two quaternary pyridinium rings, one nucleophilic oxime group, oxime at position four on the pyridinium ring and four carbon linkages between pyridinium rings (Fig. 5). Hundreds of compounds have been synthesized over the last decade to develop an effective reactivator of tabun-inhibited AChE. Of these compounds, K027, K048, K074 and K075 have yielded promising results against other organophosphorus compounds and are currently being evaluated by several laboratories worldwide [5, 19, 21, 59–64]. However, K203 appears to be the most effective reactivator following tabun exposure and it has also been reported to have a lower acute toxicity than trimedoxime and obidoxime [26]. The efficacy and toxicity profile of K203 supports the continued efforts in developing this compound as a medical countermeasure against.

Molecular affinity: Docking studies

At the first scenario, molecular docking calculations have been used in order to look into the association/

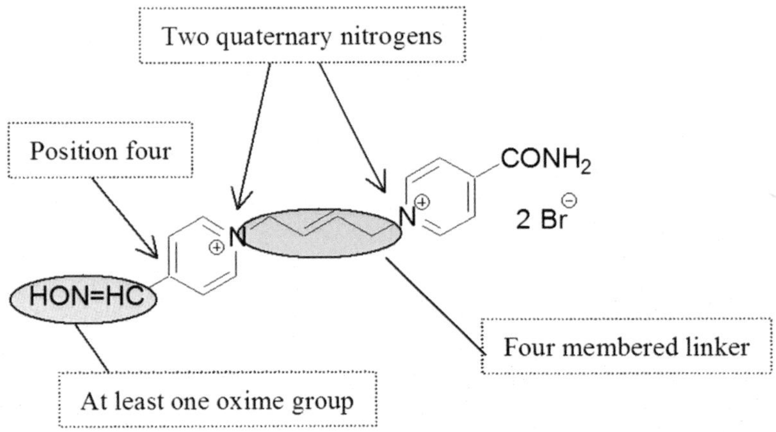

Fig. 5 Structural requirements for reactivators of tabun-inhibited AChE

affinity between oxime and inhibited AChE. A cavity forecast algorithm, which is based on a 3D box was employed to bring forth binding sites in the enzymes, and for this, the Molegro Virtual Docker program was quite helpful. [38] The oximes were docked in a cavity whose volume was 115,200 Å [3] in *Mm*AChE and 282,112 Å [3] in *Hss*AChE. The respective energy values acquired from the oximes-AChE interactions were determined to have a better understanding the binding modes of each ligand, thus investigating the structural aspects that modulate the biological activity in the enzyme reactivation. Table 2 shows the intermolecular interaction energy values of the most appropriate pose of K203, selected for the subsequent mechanistic studies in both enzymes. By observing Table 2, it is easy to notice that K203 interacted better with the human enzyme, *Hss*AChE, with an intermolecular interaction energy value of – 101.94 $kcal.mol^{-1}$, and an energy difference of 12.16 $kcal.mol^{-1}$ in relation to the rat enzyme, *Mm*AChE. K203 has shown itself to have a high stability in the *Mm*AChE, experimenting hydrogen bonds with two water molecules as well as two amino acid residues, Thr238 and Gly234. Interestingly the fact that this oxime presented much more hydrogen bonds in the *Hss*AChE active site, where it also presented a good intermolecular interaction energy, – 89.78 $kcal.mol^{-1}$. In the human enzyme, K203 showed several interactions with amino acid residues and water, more precisely, six water molecules and two amino acid residues, Tyr120 and Gly117. Besides those interactions in the *Hss*AChE active site, K203 showed a better energy value when docked in the *Mm*AChE active site, and with this event, one can suppose that there are other important features that assist the good stabilization of this oxime in the enzyme active site, such as structural aspects, i.e., *Mm*AChE interacts better with K203 in relation to *Hss*AChE.

The docking methodology provides a good start to understand the performance of these oximes in the inhibited AChE active site. It is important to keep in mind that diverse interactions are responsible for the better accommodation and affinity of these reactivators within the active site. Among these interactions, the hydrogen bonds are the most common (H-bonds), but it is noteworthy to cite electrostatic interactions as well as hydrophobic interactions, which could even have a great contribution to the conformation and orientation adopted by the reactivators in the active site. The H-bonds performed by this oxime, in both enzymes, are shown in Fig. 6.

Both enzymes (*Mm*AChE and *Hss*AChE) were evaluated in order to have a deeper understanding of their main aspects and hydrophobic and electrostatic parameters. All these features, including the flexibility effect on the residues in a significant radius of the active site, contributed to simulate the interaction of these reactivators with the inhibited enzymes, producing a good starting point for the reaction mechanism calculations. The

Table 2 Intermolecular interaction energy (ΔE) values and hydrogen bonds between K203 and both AChE species

AChE	Interaction Energy ($kcal.mol^{-1}$)	H-Bonds	H-bond Strength ($kcal.mol^{-1}$)
Human	−89.78	H_2O	– 4.92
		H_2O	−2.50
		H_2O	−1.47
		H_2O	−1.39
		H_2O	−4.73
		H_2O	−4.79
		Tyr120	−0.66
		Gly117	−1.34
Rat	−101.94	H_2O	−3.89
		H_2O	−2.41
		Thr238	−6.12
		Gly234	−5.00

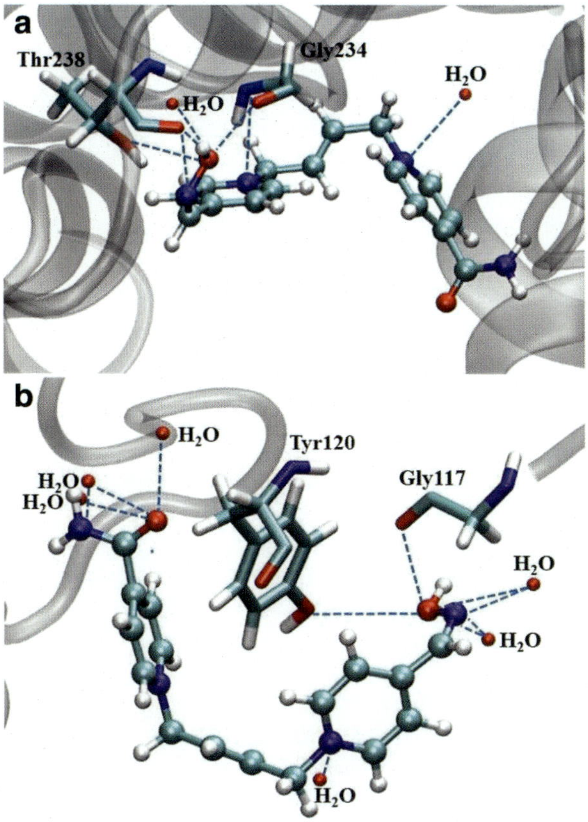

Fig. 6 Interactions performed by K203 in the *Mm*AChE (**a**) and *Hss*AChE (**b**) active site

theoretical methodologies employed here are quite important in the design of new drugs. Other docking calculations were also carried out with Obidoxime. These results are presented in Table 3.

From the theoretical calculations, the docking results for Obidoxime are shown in Table 3. Those findings indicate that Obidoxime presented higher stability when docked in the *Hss*AChE active site, with an intermolecular interaction energy of – 107.98 kcal.mol^{-1}. On the other hand, this oxime also interacted very favorably with the rat enzyme, with an energy value of – 91.88 kcal.mol^{-1}. For Obidoxime, the energy difference was 16.10 kcal.mol^{-1} between both enzymes. Obidoxime performed several hydrogen bonds in the *Hss*AChE active site, being four water molecules and three amino acid residues, Ser294, Glu281 and Gly117, which are important for the stabilization of this reactivator in the site. Meanwhile, this oxime also presented many interactions in the *Mm*AChE active site, being three water molecules and many amino acid residues (Thr238, Gly234, Glu313, Asn533 and Gln369), thus showing the great affinity of the rat enzyme with this antidote. These interactions are shown in Fig. 7. Our docking calculations are in good agreement to K_R values, which represent the affinity of the AChE reactivator to the inhibited enzyme.

Chemical reactivity: Quantum studies in the rat and human AChE active site

For the reactivation process, it is necessary to take into account the steric and electronic effects in the reaction as well as the preferential binding modes of the reactivators. In this context, the QM/MM techniques could be employed for the understanding of the binding modes between the oximes K203 and Obidoxime in the AChE

Table 3 Intermolecular interaction energy (ΔE) values and hydrogen bonds between Obidoxime and both AChE species

AChE	Interaction Energy (kcal.mol^{-1})	H-Bonds	H-bond Strength (kcal.mol^{-1})
Human	−107.98	H_2O	−2.43
		H_2O	−4.17
		H_2O	−2.50
		H_2O	−5.00
		Ser294	−2.24
		Glu281	−2.50
		Gly117	−1.69
Rat	−91.88	H_2O	−1.18
		H_2O	−3.46
		H_2O	−5.00
		Thr238	−7.52
		Gly234	−1.18
		Glu313	−2.24
		Asn533	−0.72
		Gln369	−0.96

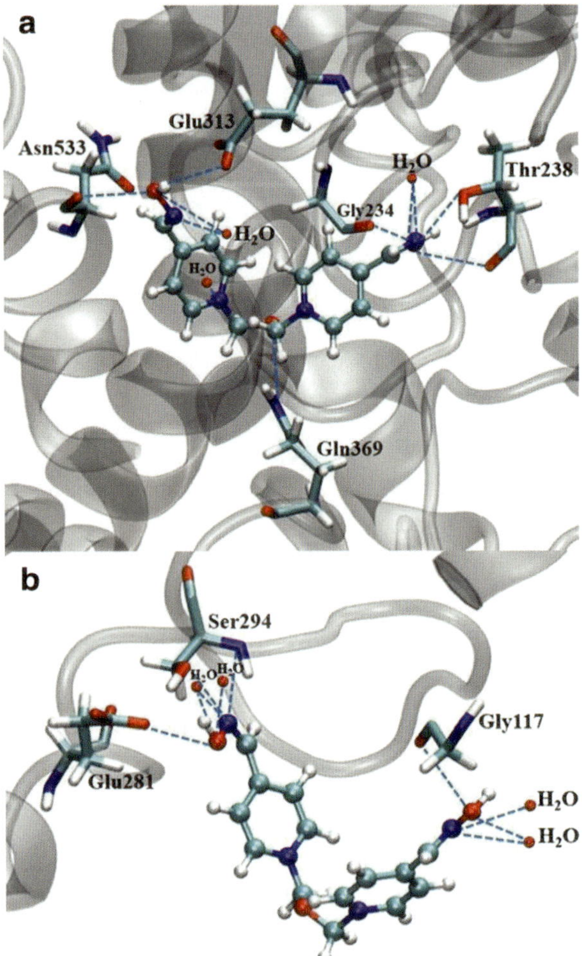

Fig. 7 Interactions performed by Obidoxime in the *Mm*AChE (**a**) and *Hss*AChE (**b**) active site

active site, for both human and rat species. During the reactivation mechanism simulation, the energetic barriers for the reaction process (activation energy) were obtained and the values described in Table 4.

According to Table 4, the oximes K203 and Obidoxime are most reactive in the rat enzyme than in the human AChE. These quantum theoretical results corroborate our experimental rate constant (k_r) values very well. K203 has shown itself to be very efficient in reactivating the inhibited *Mm*AChE, revealing an energetic barrier of 38.81 kcal.mol^{-1} lower than the value obtained for the human enzyme, which is in a good agreement with the experimental results, wherein k_r is 16,000 min^{-1}.M^{-1} for the rat enzyme. This fact leads us to believe that the transition state is better stabilized in the reactivation pathway of *Mm*AChE than *Hss*AChE, allowing the oxime to interact stronger with the nerve agent.

Table 4 Relative activation energy values ($\Delta\Delta E^{\#}$) obtained for the reaction mechanism in the reactivation process and experimental results

Oxime/Enzyme	$\Delta\Delta E^{\#}$	k_r [min^{-1}. M^{-1}]
K203		
Rat	0.00	16,000
Human	38.81	2142
Obidoxime		
Rat	0.00	6250
Human	54.42	42

This trend also corroborates to the intermolecular interaction energies from molecular docking calculations (Table 2), which have shown the best interaction and stability of K203 in *Mm*AChE. From the experimental side (Table 1), there is good agreement between binding constant (K_R) and ΔE values. It should be kept in mind, however, that the mechanistic studies with Obidoxime are also in a good agreement with the experimental results. By observing the k_r values for the oxime mediated reactivation, the difference between the rat and human enzyme is significant, and as expected, the reaction mechanism simulation has also shown this result. Obidoxime interacted much more in the rat enzyme, with a large difference between the values found for the energetic barrier in the reaction pathway, being 54.42 kcal.-mol^{-1} in relation to *Hss*AChE. From the docking results, in contrast to K203, Obidoxime showed a slightly better interaction energy value for *Hss*AChE, but during the simulation, there must be intermediate species which are better stabilized, thus leading to lower global activation energy during the full process.

Conclusions

We have applied computational chemistry methods in order to evaluate the high reactivity of the oximes K203 and Obidoxime for different AChE species. Our theoretical results showed that these oximes are more effective towards the rat enzyme. The reactivation process for *Mm*AChE takes place more easily by both oximes investigated. This result was confirmed by DFT calculations, being the lowest activation energy barrier for the rat enzyme, corroborating our experimental results. From molecular docking results, both reactivators are well stabilized in both AChE species, mainly due to the hydrogen bonds with the amino acid residues Ser, Glu and Gly performed in the active site.

Abbreviations

AChE: Acetylcholinesterase; HPLC: High-performance liquid chromatography; QM/MM: Quantum and molecular mechanics; TLC: Thin-layer chromatography

Acknowledgements

No.

Funding

Authors are grateful to the Grant agency of the Czech Republic for the financial support (No. 15-16701S). This work was also supported by the long term development plan UHHK and UHK and the Brazilian agencies FAPEMIG, CAPES, and CNPq.

Authors' contributions

Writing of the manuscript (KK, KM. DJ, JM, TF, MV, TR), synthesis of compounds (EN, KM, KK, MH), purity evaluation (JZK, DJ, OS), in vitro evaluation (KK, MH, OS, DJ), computational chemistry (TF, EDC, ADC, TR). All authors read and approved the final manuscript.

Competing interests

The authors declare that they have no competing interests.

Author details

[1]Biomedical Research Center, University Hospital Hradec Kralove, Hradec Kralove, Czech Republic. [2]Department of Chemistry, Faculty of Science, University of Hradec Kralove, Hradec Kralove, Czech Republic. [3]Faculty of Military Health Sciences, University of Defence, Hradec Kralove, Czech Republic. [4]Defence Research and Development Canada - Suffield Research Centre, Department of National Defence, Suffield, Alberta, Canada. [5]Center for Basic and Applied Research, Faculty of Informatics and Management, University of Hradec Kralove, Hradec Kralove, Czech Republic. [6]Department of Chemical Engineering, Military Institute of Engineering, Rio de Janeiro, RJ 22290-270, Brazil. [7]Department of Chemistry, Federal University of Lavras, Lavras/MG, Brazil. [8]Neurology Clinic, University Hospital Hradec Kralove, Hradec Kralove, Czech Republic.

References

1. Marrs TC. Organophosphate poisoning. Pharmacol Ther. 1993;58:51–66.
2. Bajgar J. Organophosphates/nerve agent poisoning: mechanism of action, diagnosis, prophylaxis, and treatment. Adv Clin Chem. 2004;38:151–216.
3. Jokanovic M, Stojiljkovic MP. Current understanding of the application of pyridinium oximes ascholinesterase reactivators in treatment of organophosphate poisoning. Eur J Pharmacol. 2006;553:10–7.
4. Cabal J, Kuca K, Kassa J. Specification of the structure of oximes able to reactivate tabun inhibited acetylcholinesterase. Basic Clin Pharmacol Toxicol. 2004;95(2):81–6.
5. Calic M, Lucic VA, Radic B, Jelic D, Jun D, Kuca K, Kovarik Z. In vitro and in vivo evaluation of pyridinium oximes: mode of interaction with acetylcholinesterase, effect on tabun- and soman-poisoned mice and their cytotoxicity. Toxicol. 2006;219(1-3):85–96.
6. Koplovitz I, Stewart JR. A comparison of the efficacy of HI-6 and 2-PAM against soman, tabun, sarin and VX in the rabbit. Toxicol Lett. 1994;70:169–79.
7. Wilson IB, Sondheimer F. A specific antidote against lethal alkyl phosphate intoxication. V. Antidotal properties. Arch Biochem Biophys. 1957;69:468–74.
8. Ekstrom F, Akfur C, Tunemalm AK, Lundberg S. Structural changes of phenylalanine 338 and histidine 447 revealed by the crystal structures of tabun-inhibited murine acetylcholinesterase. Biochem. 2006;45:74–81.
9. Puu G, Artursson E, Bucht G. Reactivation of nerve agent inhibited acetylcholinesterases by HI-6 and obidoxime. Biochem Pharmacol. 1986;35:1505–10.
10. Clement JG, Shiloff JD, Gennings C. Efficacy of a combination of acetylcholinesterase reactivators, HI-6 and obidoxime, against tabun and soman poisoning in mice. Arch Toxicol. 1987;61:70–5.
11. Jun D, Kuca K, Hronek M, Opletal L. Effect of some acetylcholinesterase reactivators on human platelet aggregation *in vitro*. J App Toxicol. 2006; 26(3):262–8.
12. Balali-Mood M, Shariat M. Treatment of organophosphate poisoning. Experience of nerve agents and acute pesticide poisoning on the effects of oximes. J Physiol (Paris). 1998;92:375–8.
13. Musilek K, Kuca K, Jun D, Dohnal V, Dolezal M. Synthesis of the novel series of bispyridinium compounds bearing (*E*)-but-2-ene linker and evaluation of their reactivation activity against chlorpyrifos-inhibited acetylcholinesterase. Bioorg Med Chem Lett. 2006;16(3):622–7.
14. Kuca K, Bielavský J, Cabal J, Bielavská M. Synthesis of a potential reactivator of acetylcholinesterase 1-(4-hydroxyiminomethylpyridinium)-3-(carbamoylpyridinium)-propane dibromide. Tetrahedron Lett. 2003;44:3123–5.
15. Kuca K, Bielavský J, Cabal J, Kassa J. Synthesis of a new reactivator of tabun inhibited acetylcholinesterase. Bioorg Med Chem Lett. 2003b;13:3545–7.
16. Kuca K, Kassa J. A Comparison of the Ability of a New Bispyridinium Oxime–1-(4-hydroxyiminomethylpyridinium)-4-(4-carbamoylpyridinium)butane Dibromide and Currently used Oximes to Reactivate Nerve Agent-inhibited Rat Brain Acetylcholinesterase by In Vitro Methods. J Enzym Inhib Med Chem. 2003;18:529–35.
17. Kuca K, Kassa J. In vitro reactivation of acetylcholinesterase using of the oxime K027. Veterinary and Human Toxicology. 2004a;46:15–8.
18. Kuca K, Kassa J. Oximes-induced reactivation of rat brain acetylcholinesterase inhibited by VX agent. Hum Exp Toxicol. 2004b;23(4):167–71.
19. da Silva AP, Farina M, Franco JL, Dafre AL, Kassa J, Kuca K. Temporal effects of newly developed oximes (K027, K048) on malathion-induced acetylcholinesterase inhibition and lipid peroxidation in mouse prefrontal cortex. NeuroToxicology. 2008;29(1):184–9.
20. Kassa J, Kuca K, Cabal J, Paar M. A comparison of the efficacy of new asymmetric bispyridinium oximes (K027, K048) with currently available oximes against tabun by in vitro and in vivo methods. J Toxicol Environ Health. 2006;69(20):1875–82.
21. Lucić-Vrdoljak A, Čalić M, Radić B, Berend S, Kuca K, Kovarik Z. Pre-treatment with pyridinium oximes improves antidotal therapy against tabun poisoning. Toxicology. 2006;228(1):41–50.
22. Kuca K, Cabal J, Kassa J. In vitro reactivation of sarin-inhibited brain acetylcholinesterase from various species by various oximes. J Enzym Inhib Med Chem. 2005;20(3):227–32.
23. Kuca K, Cabal J, Musilek K, Jun D, Bajgar J. Effective bisquaternary reactivators of tabun-inhibited AChE. J Appl Toxicol. 2005;25(6):491–5.
24. Kassa J, Jun D, Kuca K. A comparison of reactivating efficacy of newly developed oximes (K074, K075) and currently available oximes (obidoxime, HI-6) in cyclosarin and tabun-poisoned rats. J Enzym Inhib Med Chem. 2007; 22(3):297–300.
25. Kuca K, Cabal J, Jun D, Musilek K. In vitro reactivation potency of acetylcholinesterase reactivators – K074 and K075 – to reactivate tabun inhibited human brain cholinesterases. Neurotoxicity Res. 2007;11(2):101–6.
26. Musilek K, Jun D, Cabal J, Kassa J, Gunn-Moore F, Kuca K. Design of a Potent Reactivator of Tabun-Inhibited Acetylcholinesterase - Synthesis and evaluation of (*E*)-1-(4-carbamoylpyridinium)-4-(4-hydroxyiminomethylpyridinium)-but-2-ene Dibromide (K203). J Med Chem. 2007;50(22):5514–8.
27. Kassa J, Karasova J, Musilek K, Kuca K. An evaluation of therapeutic and reactivating effects of newly developed oximes (K156, K203) and commonly used oximes (obidoxime, trimedoxime, HI-6) in tabun-poisoned rats and mice. Toxicology. 2008;243(3):311–6.
28. Worek F, Reiter G, Eyer P, Szinicz L. Reactivation kinetics of acetylcholinesterase from different species inhibited by highly toxic organophosphates. Arch Toxicol. 2002;76:523–9.
29. Wiesner J, Kriz Z, Kuca K, Jun D, Koca J. Acetylcholinesterases – the structural similarities and differences. J Enzym Inhib Med Chem. 2007;22(4): 417–24.
30. Jun D, Stodulka P, Kuca K, Koleckar V, Dolezal B, Simon P, Veverka M. HPLC analysis of HI-6 dichloride and dimethanesulfonate – antidotes against nerve agents and organophosphorus pesticides. Anal Lett. 2007;40(14): 2783–7.
31. Jun D, Stodulka P, Kuca K, Koleckar V, Dolezal B, Simon P, Veverka M. TLC analysis of intermediates arising during the preparation of oxime HI-6 dimethanesulfonate. J Chromatogr Sci. 2008;46(4):316–9.
32. Carletti E, Li H, Li B, Ekstroem F, Nicolet Y, Loiodice M, Gillon E, Froment MT, Lockridge O, Schopfer LM, Masson P, Nachon F. Aging of cholinesterases phosphylated by tabun proceeds through O-dealkylation. J Am Chem Soc. 2008;130:16011–20.
33. Goncalves AS, Franca TCC, Wilter A, Figueroa-Villar JD. Molecular Dynamics of the Interaction of Pralidoxime and Deazapralidoxime with Acetylcholinesterase Inhibited by the Neurotoxic Agent Tabun. J Braz Chem Soc. 2006;17:968–75.
34. Gonçalves AS, França TCC, Figueroa-Villar JD, Pascutti PG. Molecular Dynamics Simulations and QM/MM Studies of the Reactivation by 2-Pam of Tabun Inhibited Human Acethylcolinesterase. J Braz Chem Soc. 2011;22: 155–65.

35. Hehre WJ, Deppmeier BJ, Klunzinger PE. PC SPARTAN Plus TUTORIAL version 2.0. Irvine, CA: Wavefunction, Inc.; 1999.
36. Frisch, M.J., Trucks, G.W., Schlegel, H.B., Scuseria, G.E., Robb, M.A., Cheeseman, J.R., Montgomery, J.A. Jr., Vreven, T., Kudin, K.N., Burant, J.C., Millam, J.M., Iyengar, S.S., Tomasi, J., Barone, V., Mennucci, B., Cossi, M., Scalmani, G., Rega, N., Petersson, G.A., Nakatsuji, H., Hada, M., Ehara, M., Toyota, K., Fukuda, R., Hasegawa, J., Ishida, M., Nakajima, T., Honda, Y., Kitao, O., Nakai, H., Klene, M., Li, X., Knox, J.E., Hratchian, H.P., Cross, J.B., Adamo, C., Jaramillo, J., Gomperts, R., Stratmann, R.E., Yazyev, O., Austin, A.J., Cammi, R., Pomelli, C., Ochterski, J.W., Ayala, P.Y., Morokuma, K., Voth, G.A., Salvador, P., Dannenberg, J.J., Zakrzewski, V.G., Dapprich, S., Daniels, A.D., Strain, M.C., Farkas, O., Malick, D.K., Rabuck, A.D., Raghavachari, K., Foresman, J.B., Ortiz, J. V., Cui, Q., Baboul, A.G., Clifford, S., Cioslowski, J., Stefanov, B.B., Liu, G., Liashenko, A., Piskorz, P., Komaromi, I., Martin, R.L., Fox, D.J., Keith, T., Al-Laham, M.A., Peng, C.Y., Nanayakkara, A., Challacombe, M., Gill, P.M.W., Johnson, B., Chen, W., Wong, M.W., Gonzalez, C., Pople, J.A.: Gaussian 03, Revision C.02. Gaussian, Inc., Wallingford, Connecticut (2004)
37. Thomsen R, Christensen MH. MolDock: A new technique for high-accuracy molecular docking. J Med Chem. 2006;49:3315–21.
38. Silva MC, Torres JA, Castro AA, da Cunha EF. Alves de Oliveira LC., Corrêa AD., Ramalho TC. Combined experimental and theoretical study on the removal of pollutant compounds by peroxidases: affinity and reactivity toward a bioremediation catalyst. J Biomol Struct Dyn. 2016;34(9):1839–48.
39. Guimarães AP, França TCC, Ramalho TC, Rennó MN, Ferreira da Cunha EF, Matos KS, Mancini DT, Kuča K. Docking studies and effects of. syn-anti isomery of oximes derived from pyridine. imidazol bicycled systems as potential human. acetylcholinesterase reactivators. J Appl Biomed. 2011;9: 163–71.
40. Matos KS, Mancini DT, da Cunha EF, Kuca K, França TC, Ramalho TC. Molecular aspects of the reactivation process of acetylcholinesterase inhibited by cyclosarin. J Braz Chem Soc. 2011;22:1999–2004.
41. Ramalho TC, Caetano MS, da Cunha EF, Souza TC, Rocha MV. Construction and assessment of reaction models of class I EPSP synthase: molecular docking and density functional theoretical calculations. J Biomol Struct Dyn. 2009;27(2):195–207.
42. da Cunha EF, Ramalho TC, Reynolds RC. Binding mode analysis of 2,4-diamino-5-methyl-5-deaza-6-substituted pteridines with Mycobacterium tuberculosis and human dihydrofolate reductases. J Biomol Struct Dyn. 2008;25(4):377–85.
43. da Cunha EE, Barbosa EF, Oliveira AA, Ramalho TC. Molecular modeling of Mycobacterium tuberculosis DNA gyrase and its molecular docking study with gatifloxacin inhibitors. J Biomol Struct Dyn. 2010 Apr;27(5):619–25.
44. Borman SA. Much to do about enzyme mechanism. Chem Eng News. 2004; 8:35–9.
45. Heyden A, Lin H, Truhlar DG. Adaptive partitioning in combined quantum mechanical and molecular mechanical calculations of potential energy functions for multiscale simulations. J Phys Chem B. 2007;111:2231–41.
46. Ramalho TC, Da Cunha EFF, De Alencastro RB. Solvent effects on 13 C and 15 N shielding tensors of nitroimidazoles in the condensed phase: a sequential molecular dynamics/quantum mechanics study. J Phys Condens Matter. 2004;16:6159–70.
47. Matos KS, da Cunha EFF, Abagyan R, Ramalho TC. Computational evidence for the reactivation process of human acetylcholinesterase inhibited by carbamates. Comb.Chem. High Throughput Screen. 2014;17(6):554–64.
48. Singh UC. Kollman PA An approach to computing electro-. static charges for molecules. J Comput Chem. 1984;5:129–34.
49. Besler BH, Merz KM, Kollman PA. Atomic charges derived from semiempirical methods. J Comput Chem. 1990;11:431–9.
50. Gustin DJ, Mattei P, Kast P, Wiest O, Lee L, Cleland WW, Hilvert D. Heavy atom isotope effects reveal a highly polarized. transition state for chorismate mutase. J Am Chem Soc. 1999;121:1756–65.
51. Rutkowska-Zbik D, Witko M. Following nature-theoretical studies on factors modulating catalytic activity of porphyrins. J Mol Catal Chem. 2006;258(1-2): 376–80.
52. Giacoppo JOS, França TCC, Kuca K, da Cunha EFF, Abagyan R, Mancini DT, Ramalho TC. Molecular modeling and in vitro reactivation study between the oxime BI-6 and acetyl- cholinesterase inhibited by different nerve agents. J Biomol Struct Dyn. 2015;33:2048–58.
53. Li R, Liu Y, Zhang J, Chen K, Li S, Jiang J. An isofenphos-. methyl hydrolase (Imh) capable of hydrolyzing the P–O–Z moiety. of organophosphorus pesticides containing an aryl or heterocyclic group. Appl Microbiol Biotechnol. 2012;94(6):1553–64.
54. Gorecki L, Korabecny J, Musilek K, Malinak D, Nepovimova E, Dolezal R, Jun D, Soukup O. Kuca K.¨ SAR study to find optimal cholinesterase reactivator against organophosphorous nerve agents and pesticides. Arch Toxicol. 2016;90(12):2831–59.
55. Nepovimova E, Korabecny J, Dolezal R, Nguyen TD, Jun D, Soukup O, Pasdiorova M, Jost P, Muckova L, Malinak D, Gorecki L, Musilek K, Kuca K. A 7-methoxytacrine–4-pyridinealdoxime hybrid as a novel prophylactic agent with reactivation properties in organophosphate. Toxicol res. 2016;4(5): 1012–6.
56. Kuca K, Cabal J. Evaluation of newly synthesized reactivators of the brain cholinesterase inhibited by sarin nerve agent. Toxicol Mech Methods. 2005; 15(4):247–52.
57. Kuca K, Jun D, Musilek K. Structural requirements of acetylcholinesterase reactivators. Mini Rev Med Chem. 2006;6(3):269–77.
58. Kalász H, Hasan MY, Sheen R, Kuca K, Petroianu GA, Ludány K, Gergely A, Tekes K. HPLC Analysis of K-48 concentration in plasma. Anal Bioanal Chem. 2006;385(6):1062–7.
59. Tekes K, Hasan MY, Sheen R, Kuca K, Petroianu G, Ludányi K, Kalász H. HPLC determination of the serum concentration of K-27, a novel oxime-type cholinesterase reactivator. J Chromatogr A. 2006;1122(1-2):84–7.
60. Petroianu GA, Arafat K, Nurulain SM, Kuca K, Kassa J. In vitro oxime reactivation of red blood cell acetylcholinesterase inhibited by methyl-paraoxon. J Appl Toxicol. 2007;27(2):168–75.
61. Petroianu GA, Nurulain SM, Nagelkerke N, Shafiullah M, Kassa J, Kuca K. Five oximes (K-27, K-48, obidoxime, HI-6 and trimedoxime) in comparison with pralidoxime: survival in rats exposed to methyl-paraoxon. J Appl Toxicol. 2007;27(5):453–7.
62. Kovarik Z, Lucić VA, Berend S, Katalinić M, Kuca K, Musilek K, Radić B. Evaluation of oxime K203 as antidote in tabun poisoning. Arhiv za Higijenu Rada i Toksikologiju. 2009;60(1):19–26.
63. Lorke DE, Hasan MY, Nurulain SM, Sheen R, Kuca K, Petroianu GA. Entry of two new asymmetric bispyridinium oximes (K-27 and K-48) into the rat brain: comparison with obidoxime. J Appl Toxicol. 2007;27(5):482–90.
64. Petroianu GA, Arafat K, Kuca K, Kassa J. Five oximes (K-27, K-33, K-48, BI-6 and methoxime) in comparison with pralidoxime: in vitro reactivation of red blood cell acetylcholinesterase inhibited by paraoxon. J Appl Toxicol. 2006; 26(1):64–71.

12

Cationic liposomes induce cytotoxicity in HepG2 via regulation of lipid metabolism based on whole-transcriptome sequencing analysis

Ying Li[1†], Xiu-Liang Cui[3,4†], Qing-Shan Chen[1†], Jing Yu[1], Hai Zhang[5], Jie Gao[6], Du-Xin Sun[2*] and Guo-Qing Zhang[1*]

Abstract

Backgroud: Cationic liposomes (CLs) can be used as non-viral vectors in gene transfer and drug delivery. However, the underlying molecular mechanism of its cytotoxicity has not been well elucidated yet.

Methods: We herein report a systems biology approach based on whole-transcriptome sequencing coupled with computational method to identify the predominant genes and pathways involved in the cytotoxicity of CLs in HepG2 cell line.

Results: Firstly, we validated the concentration-dependent cytotoxicity of CLs with an IC_{50} of 120 μg/ml in HepG2 exposed for 24 h. Subsequently, we used whole-transcriptome sequencing to identify 220 (77 up- and 143 down-regulated) differentially expressed genes (DEGs). Gene ontology (GO) and pathway analysis showed that these DEGs were mainly related to cholesterol, steroid, lipid biosynthetic and metabolic processes. Additionally, "key regulatory" genes were identified using gene act, pathway act and co-expression network analysis, and expression levels of 11 interested altered genes were confirmed by quantitative real time PCR. Interestingly, no cell cycle arrest was observed through flow cytometry.

Conclusions: These data are expected to provide deep insights into the molecular mechanism of CLs cytotoxicity.

Keywords: Cationic liposomes, Nanoparticle, Cytotoxicity, RNA-seq, Lipid metabolism

Background

Gene therapy is a promising approach for the prevention and treatment of severe human diseases such as cancer and AIDs. One of the major obstacles to the clinical success of gene therapy is the lack of effective gene transfer vectors. Offering numerous advantages for gene transfection and drug delivery, nanomaterials are considered as promising diagnostic and therapeutic candidates in medicine [1]. Synthetic vectors, though generally not as efficient as viral vectors, have the potential advantages of being non-immunogenic, versatile and easier to produce. Moreover, synthetic vectors such as cationic liposomes (CLs) can protect drugs from being degraded in the body before they reach their target, and allow for better control over the timing and distribution of drugs to tumor tissue [2]. For example, CLs have a high affinity to the endothelial cells of tumor blood vessels, thus allowing for selective targeting and delivery of paclitaxel to the tumor microenvironment [3]. To date, liposomes have been the most used nanovectors for drug delivery, of which liposomal doxorubicin and amphotericin B received accelerated approval as early as 1995 [4] followed by liposomal daunorubicin in 1996 [5]. More liposomes are currently undergoing advanced clinical trials [6]. Additionally, CLs have also been verified to protect siRNA from RNase degradation efficiently [7]. With more CLs put into clinical use, their cytotoxicity has become a vital concern. CLs present the unique properties

* Correspondence: duxins@umich.edu; gqzhang@smmu.edu.cn
[†]Ying Li, Xiu-Liang Cui and Qing-Shan Chen contributed equally to this work.
[2]Department of Pharmaceutical Science, College of Pharmacy, University of Michigan, Ann Arbor, MI 48109, USA
[1]Department of Pharmacy, Eastern Hepatobiliary Surgery Hospital, Second Military Medical University, Shanghai 200438, China
Full list of author information is available at the end of the article

of nanoparticles, such as surface and interface effect, small size effect, and quantum size effect, which lead to their specific distribution and accumulation in organs and tissues in vivo. Moreover, due to high concentrations of negatively charged plasma proteins including glycosaminoglycan, glycoprotein and apolipoproteins, CLs could aggregate into micelles and cause cytotoxicity [8]. In a word, CLs may exert their effect on cell function through various ways.

The liver is considered to be the main organ of metabolic clearance for most drugs and xenobiotics. Previous studies have shown that nanoparticles are preferentially deposited in the liver under systemic exposure, resulting in prolonged retention within the organ and some instances that are significantly hepatoxic [9, 10]. Therapeutic or toxicological studies showed that when nanoparticles doses overwhelmed the hepatic biodegradation capacity, the excess would accumulate in the organ over a long period of time [11]. In this study, we chose human liver-derived hepatoma cells (HepG2) to carry out our research. Additionally, HepG2 cells have been used for studying delivery and cytotoxicity of CLs [12, 13].

It was reported that oxidative stress, autophagy, and certain physicochemical properties could induce cytotoxicity of nanoparticles. High reactive oxygen species (ROS) induced by nanoparticles may damage cells by peroxidizing lipids, disrupting DNA [14, 15], interfering with signaling functions, and modulating gene transcription [16]. Other studies demonstrated that inhibition of autophagy reversed cell death caused by cationic PAMAM dendrimers, indicating the cytotoxic role of autophagy [17, 18]. It was reported that some nanoparticles caused the unfolding of fibrinogen [19] and elevation of proinflammatory cytokines [20]. However, the CLs biological activities are complicated and mechanism of CLs cytotoxicity remains ambiguous.

Additionally, there were few studies to identify key genes and pathways involved in cytotoxicity of CLs. Spurred on by the development of deep sequencing technology, we are allowed to investigate the mechanisms of CLs cytotoxicity at the whole-transcriptome level. In the present study, we used high-throughput RNA-seq technology to explore the potential mechanism underlying CLs cytotoxicity at whole-transcriptome level by analyzing changes in the global gene expression profile in HepG2 cells after CLs exposure for the first time. The purpose of this study is to obtain transcriptome information of HepG2 cells exposed to CLs and preliminarily investigate molecular mechanism regarding the relationship between levels of genes expression and cytotoxicity of CLs. In this study, differentially expressed genes (DEGs), related gene ontology (GO) and pathways were determined. Subsequently, gene act, pathway act and co-expression network were constructed to further explore the role of the related genes and pathways.

Methods

Preparation of CLs

CLs were prepared by using the thin-film dispersion method as described previously with minor modification [21]. Briefly, 27.97 mg 1,2-dioleoyl-3-trimethylammonium-propane (DOTAP) (Avanti Polar Lipids, 890890P, USA), 11 mg cholesterol (Sigma-Aldrich, C8667, USA) and 10.48 mg DSPE-mPEG 2000 (Avanti Polar Lipids, 880120P, USA) in chloroform solutions were mixed in a round-bottomed flask for 45 min-1 h to form dry film. Then the lipid film was rehydrated with 10 ml 10 mM phosphate-buffered saline (PBS, PH 7.4) using a rotary evaporator (Senco, China, Shanghai). After the liposome film hydration in PBS, the liposome dispersion was ultrasonicated for 10 min. Subsequently, CLs were downsized by a high-pressure hand-held extrusion through 400 nm, 200 nm, and 100 nm polycarbonate and polyester membranes (Whatman, UK) at 65 °C using a liposome extruder LF-1 (Avestin, Canada). The obtained CLs in PBS were stored as stock solution at 4 °C.

Dynamic light scattering (DLS)

Mean diameter, polydispersity index (PDI), and zeta-potential of CLs were performed by using Malvern Zetasizer ZS90 (Malvern instruments Ltd., UK) according to the standard operation protocol. CLs were diluted 1:10 in Milli-QH_2O, and all the operations were detected after room temperature balance for 10 min. Each assay was performed in three replications.

Cell viability assay

HepG2 cells (American Type Culture Collection, HB-8065) were cultured in Dulbecco's Modified Eagle Medium (DMEM, Invitrogen) containing 10% fetal bovine serum (FBS, Hyclone), 100 U/ml penicillin and 100 μg/ml streptomycin (Corning, USA) and maintained at 37 °C in a humidified 5% carbon dioxide (CO_2) atmosphere. Cell viability was assessed by the Cell Counting Kit-8 (CCK-8) kit (Dojindo, Japan) according to the instruction. 100 μg/ml ZnO nanoparticles (IBU-tec, Germany) were used as a positive control. Briefly, HepG2 cells were seeded in 96-well plate at a density of 3000/well and incubated for 24 h. The cells were then exposed to a series of concentrations of CLs (25, 50, 100, 200, 400, 800, 1600, 3200 μg/ml) for another 24 h. Added 10 μl of the CCK-8 solution to each well of the plate, incubated the plate for 2 h in the incubator, and measured the absorbance the 450 nm using a microplate reader (Thermo Scientific Multiskan MK3). The data was normalized to the blank, and six independent experiments were conducted. Half-maximum inhibitory concentration (IC_{50}) value of CLs was determined by GraphPad Prism 5.

RNA extraction and RNA-sequencing (RNA-seq)

Total RNA was extracted using Trizol Reagent (Invitrogen, USA) according to the manufacturer's instruction. RNA quantity and RNA integrity number (RIN) were assessed by Agilent 2200 bioanalyzer. Sample RNA with the RIN value below 6.4 was discarded [22]. The complementary DNA (cDNA) libraries for single-end sequencing were prepared using Ion Total RNA-seq Kit v2.0 (Life technologies, USA) according to the protocol provided by the manufacturer.

Filtering raw reads and mapping statistics

We applied Fast-QC (http://www.bioinformatics.babraham.ac.uk/projects/fastqc/) software to assess the quality of data, including the distribution of the base quality value, content of GC, proportion of PCR duplication, and frequency of kmers. MapSplice v2.1.8 software was used for RNA-seq read mapping analysis, whose core program is Bowtie. It has been approved a highly accurate algorithm for the alignment of RNA-seq reads to splice junctions [23]. We calculated the mapping rate for filtered clean reads and the distribution of genes on chromosomes.

Identification of differentially expressed genes (DEGs)

To quantify the expression levels of the transcripts, the RNA-seq data normalization was carried out to obtain an RPKM value [24]. We applied EBSeq to filter the DEGs. After the statistical analysis, we screened the DEGs by the following criteria: fold change>1.50 or fold change<0.67, FDR<0.05.

Functional analysis of DEGs

Gene ontology (GO) analysis

The enriched biological processes were identified using Fisher's exact test and χ^2 test, and the false discovery rate (FDR) was calculated to correct the *P*-value. Within the significant category, the enrichment Re was given by $Re = (n_f/n)/(N_f/N)$, where n_f is the number of DEGs within the particular category, n is the total number of genes with the same category, N_f is the number of DEGs, and N is the total number of genes. Only categories that had a significance of *P*-value< 0.05 and FDR<0.05 were reported. GO terms were organized as a directed acyclic graph (DAG), and we performed GO tree analysis to investigate the internal relationship between the enriched GO terms.

Pathway analysis

Fisher's exact test and χ^2 test were used to identify the significantly enriched pathways of the DEGs, and the threshold of significance was defined by P-value and FDR [25]. Pathway categories with P-value<0.05 and FDR<0.05 were reported.

Network analysis of DEGs

Network analysis was performed to trace the interactions among DEGs (*p*-value<0.01). Gene interaction and co-expression networks were constructed, and Cytoscape was used for graphical representation [26]. The gene interaction network was built using KEGG pathways as a background network, which provided information about the relationship among the genes, proteins and compounds [27, 28].

The co-expression network was built according to the normalized signal intensity of their expression levels. For each pair of genes, we calculated the Pearson's correlation and chose the significant correlation pairs to construct the network [29]. Degree centrality and K-core were two widely used topological importance indicators [30, 31]. In our analysis, "key regulatory" genes were determined by the degree and k-core differences between control and CLs-treated groups.

Quantitative real-time reverse transcription-PCR (qRT-PCR) assay

A 2-step method for qRT-PCR was used to determine mRNA expression level. Briefly, cDNA was synthesized using oligo (dT) primers with PrimeScript™ II 1st strand cDNA synthesis Kit (Takara Biotechnology, China) according to the manufacturer's protocol. qRT-PCR was performed using Applied Biosystems StepOne™ Real-Time PCR System (Applied Biosystems, USA) and SYBR Premix Ex Taq™ (Tli RNaseH Plus) kit (Takara Biotechnology, China). The primers of these detected genes were shown in Table 5 and primers for endogenous reference gene GAPDH applied a commercial product (Sangon Biotech, China). The expression levels were measured in terms of the cycle threshold (Ct) and were normalized to GAPDH expression using the $2^{-\Delta\Delta Ct}$ method [32].

Cell cycle analysis

Cell cycle was analyzed using flow cytometry (FCM). The concentration of 120 μM and exposure of 24 h was applied in CLs-treated group and 25 μM resveratrol was adopted as a positive control group. HepG2 cells were harvested, washed once in PBS, and then fixed in 75% pre-cold ethanol for 6 h at 4 °C. Staining for DNA content was performed with 50 μg/ml propidium iodide (PI) and 1 mg/ml RNase (BD Biosciences, USA) for 15 min

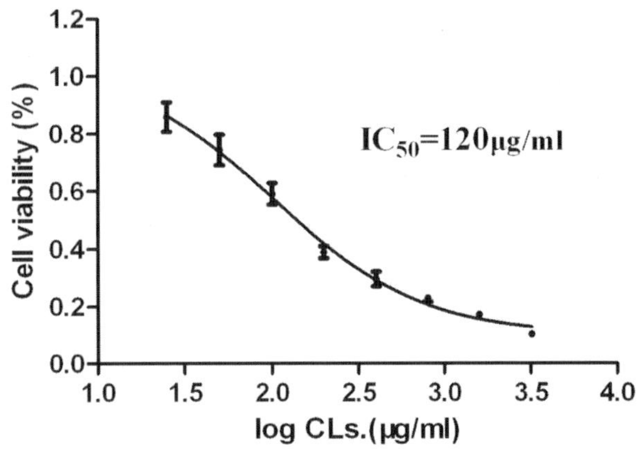

Fig. 1 HepG2 cytotoxicity of CLs at a series of concentrations (exposure for 24 h)

at room temperature. Stained cells were analyzed by cell cycle distribution on MACS Quant Analyzer (Germany).

Results

Synthesis, characterization and concentration-dependent cytotoxicity of CLs

CLs were successfully synthesized using the thin-film dispersion method. Subsequently, CLs were characterized using DLS to determine their mean diameter and size distribution. All the data represented the mean of three independent experiments. DLS revealed that their mean diameter size was 158 nm and they were well-distributed (PDI = 0.13). The zeta potential of CLs was + 22.1 mV.

In CCK-8 test, morphological alteration was observed under the microscope. Then, the concentration-dependency of cytotoxicity was investigated with an IC_{50} of 120 μg/ml via a cell viability assay, as shown in Fig. 1. It showed 14% inhibition of cell viability and no obvious cytotoxicity at the concentration of 25 μg/ml. However, at the highest concentration (3200 μg/ml), the inhibition increased to approximately 90% after 24 h of CLs exposure, suggesting that the high dose of CLs showed significant cell toxicity. In summary, CLs could induce obvious morphological alteration and significant cell viability reduction in HepG2 cells, which indicated the cytotoxic effect of CLs.

DEGs identification between control and CLs-treated groups

RNA-seq was employed to investigate the potential mechanism of cytotoxicity of CLs. The concentrations of 6 extracted RNAs were between 0.65–1.22 mg/ml and they had an average RIN value of 8.0 ± 0.6 (average ± standard error). The RNA sequencing generated approximately 12 gigabases (Gb) of raw data that were uploaded in NCBI with GEO accession number GSE89701. The filtered data set comprised approximately 15 million total reads that were distributed almost evenly between the six samples (Table 1), yielding a high sequencing depth (14.71–19.16 million raw data reads per sample). The average GC content was approximately 51% for each sample. Approximately 13.60 ± 1.17 million reads (83.4–87.3%) were mapped to the human genome sequence in the 6 independent samples and 13.00 ± 1.08 million reads were uniquely aligned to the human genome. The RNA-seq data normalization was carried out to determine the RPKM value [24].

To characterize the gene expression changes induced by CLs, the EBSeq algorithm was conducted and the criteria of screening DEGs was as follows: fold change>1.50 or fold change<0.67, FDR<0.05. There were 77 genes up-regulated and 143 genes down-regulated (Fig. 2a). Some of the DEGs were involved in primary and secondary metabolism including PLA2G3, SLC27A6, HOGA1, TM7SF2, DHCR7, LSS, SRD5A3, AKR1C4 and PDK4 and 6 among these were involved in the lipid metabolic process. Besides, there were 4 DEGs including NFKBIZ, DRAM1, DAPK1 and HMOX, respectively involved in inflammatory, autophagy, cell death, and antioxidant response (Table 2).

GO and pathway analysis

Of these DEGs, 61 up- and 88 down-regulated, respectively, could be annotated with gene ontology categories. GO analysis indicated that 10 GO terms were enriched ($P < 0.05$, FDR < 0.05). DEGs were mainly involved in multiple metabolic biological processes, including steroid metabolic process, cholesterol biosynthetic process, cholesterol metabolic process, steroid biosynthetic process, small molecule metabolic process, sterol biosynthetic process, and lipid metabolic process (Fig. 2b).

Table 1 Mapping statistics, reads distribution and quantification of RNA-seq

Sample ID	Raw reads (million)	Unmapped reads (million)	Mapped reads (million)	Mapped ratio (%)	Uniquely mapped ratio (%)
Control-1	15.20	1.94	13.26	87.2	83.5
Control-2	15.25	2.09	13.16	86.3	82.7
Control-3	15.15	1.93	13.23	87.3	83.5
CLs-1	19.16	3.18	15.98	83.4	79.2
CLs-2	15.11	1.98	13.13	86.9	83.0
CLs-3	14.72	1.87	12.85	87.3	83.5

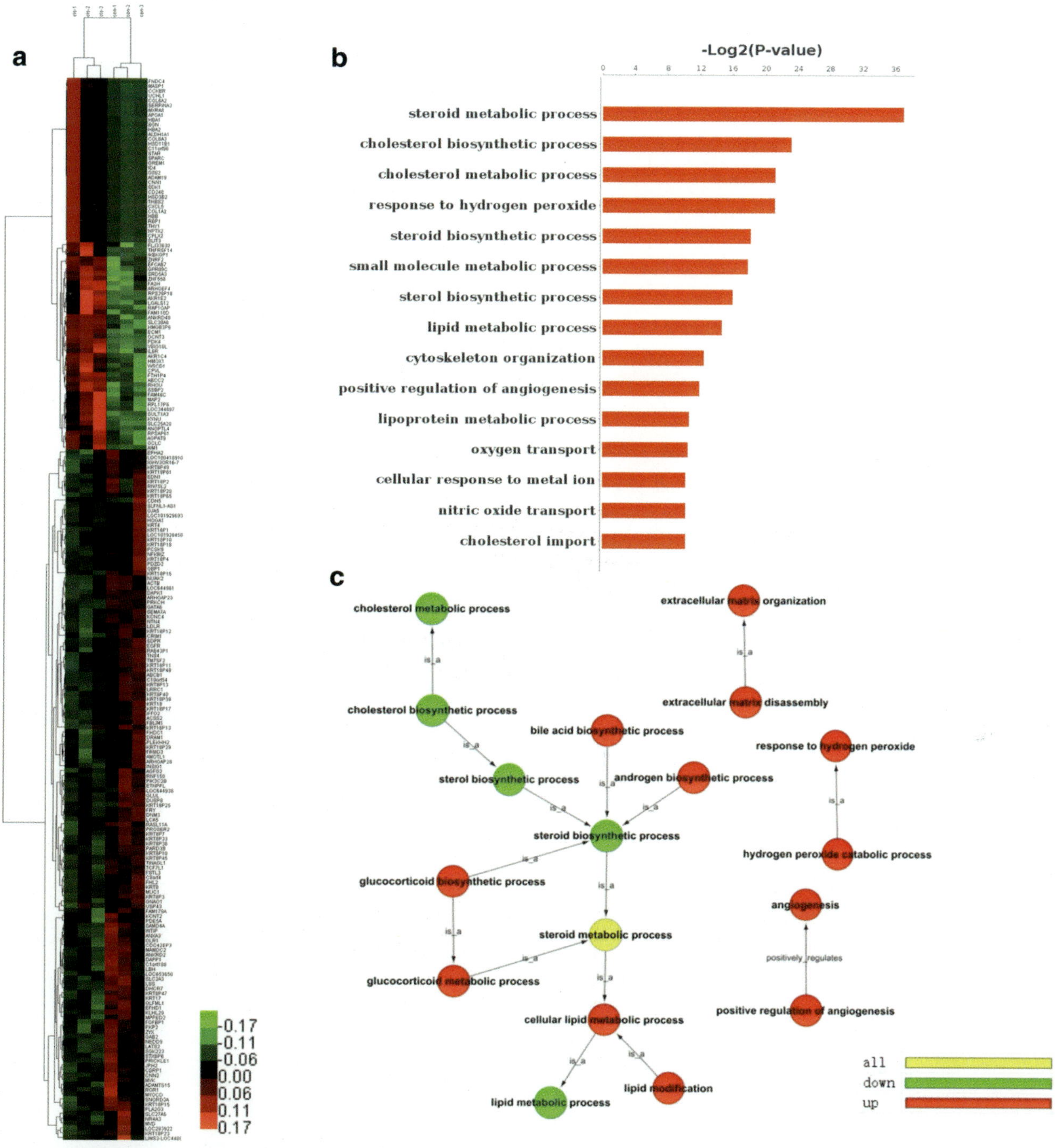

Fig. 2 a Expression profile heat map of DEGs in HepG2 cells following exposure to CLs. A total of 77 up-regulated and 143 down-regulated genes are shown. **b** GO analysis of DEGs. **c** GO tree analysis of enriched GO terms. Red circles represent up-regulated genes; Green circles represent down-regulated genes; Yellow circles represent ambiguous-regulated genes

Notably, the GO category for "steroid metabolic process" encompassing 15 genes ($p<10^{-12}$) was the most strongly changed category, and Hydroxy-delta-5-steroid dehydrogenase gene HSD3B2, Corticosteroid 11-beta-dehydrogenase isozyme 1 gene HSD11B1 and Steroidogenic acute regulatory protein gene STAR were among the most affected genes in this category. Among the 149 DEGs, there were 34 genes participating in the small molecule metabolic process (Table 3). In addition to the above categories, we found other GO terms are also involved in response to hydrogen peroxide, cytoskeleton organization and positive regulation of

Table 2 Gene regulated by cationic liposomes in the HepG2 cell

Gene ID	Gene Symbol	Description	Log_2FC	FDR
50,487	PLA2G3	Group 3 secretory phospholipase A2	−3.02	2.88E-02
28,965	SLC27A6	cDNA, FLJ94000, highly similar to *Homo sapiens* solute carrier family 27 (fatty acid transporter), member 6 (SLC27A6), mRNA	−1.47	7.5E-03
112,817	HOGA1	4-hydroxy-2-oxoglutarate aldolase, mitochondrial	−1.23	3.6E-03
1612	DAPK1	Death-associated protein kinase beta	−1.20	0
64,332	NFKBIZ	NF-kappa-B inhibitor zeta	−1.04	1E-05
7108	TM7SF2	Transmembrane 7 superfamily member 2, isoform CRA_a	−0.95	9.9E-03
1717	DHCR7	7-dehydrocholesterol reductase, isoform CRA_a	−0.82	5.18E-11
4047	LSS	cDNA, FLJ92849, highly similar to Homo sapiens lanosterol synthase (2,3-oxidosqualene-lanosterolcyclase) (LSS), mRNA	−0.66	1.59E-05
55,332	DRAM1	DNA damage-regulated autophagy modulator protein 1	−0.60	4.44E-02
79,644	SRD5A3	Polyprenolreductase	0.75	2.75E-04
1109	AKR1C4	Aldo-ketoreductase family 1 member C4	1.00	6.59E-07
3162	HMOX1	Heme oxygenase 1	1.21	3.12E-03
5166	PDK4	Pyruvate dehydrogenase kinase, isoenzyme 4	2.54	0

angiogenesis (Fig. 2b). GO tree can help us to make certain the relationship of the enriched GO terms. As shown in Fig. 2c, the biosynthetic process of cholesterol and steroid is in the term of their metabolic process, respectively. In addition, the term "cholesterol biosynthetic process" is in the term "steroid biosynthetic process" which is included in the most significant category "steroid metabolic process" and all the above are in the category "lipid metabolic process". Down-regulation of genes mainly occurs under the GO terms of cholesterol biosynthetic process, cholesterol metabolic process, sterol biosynthetic process, steroid biosynthetic process,

Table 3 Gene Ontology (GO) categories of differentially expressed genes (DEGs)

GO ID	Term	Total	Significant	Genes	P-value
GO: 0008202	steroid metabolic process	122	15	INSIG1, DHCR7, AKR1C4, SRD5A3, PCSK9, MVD, APOA1, LDLR, MVK, HSD3B2, HSD11B1, STAR, TM7SF2, LSS, SULT1A3	6.79E-12
GO: 0006695	cholesterol biosynthetic process	34	7	INSIG1, DHCR7, MVD, APOA1, MVK, TM7SF2, LSS	1.08E-07
GO: 0008203	cholesterol metabolic process	89	9	INSIG1, DHCR7, PCSK9, MVD, APOA1, LDLR, MVK, STAR, TM7SF2	4.28E-07
GO: 0042542	response to hydrogen peroxide	43	7	OLR1, GNAO1, HMOX1, HBA1, HBB, STAR,	4.43E-07
GO: 0006694	steroid biosynthetic process	60	7	DHCR7, MVD, MVK, HSD3B2, STAR, TM7SF2, LSS	3.35E-06
GO: 0044281	small molecule metabolic process	1410	34	ANGPTL4, PIK3C2B, ABCB1, INSIG1, FHL2, KYNU, ALDH1A1, DHCR7, HMOX1, HBA2, HBA1, PLA2G3, GPAT3, ACSS2, AKR1C4, HBB, SRD5A3, GLUL, SLC25A20, MVD, PDK4, APOA1, G0S2, LDLR, MVK, HSD3B2, GCLC, BGN, SLC2A3, HSD11B1, STAR, TM7SF2, LSS, SULT1A3	4.28E-06
GO: 0016126	sterol biosynthetic process	29	5	INSIG1, DHCR7, MVD, MVK, TM7SF2,	1.55E-05
GO: 0006629	lipid metabolic process	490	16	INSIG1, DHCR7, FA2H, PLA2G3, AGPAT9, SRD5A3, PCSK9, MVD, APOA1, LDLR, SLC27A6, MVK, HSD11B1, TM7SF2, LSS, SULT1A3	3.91E-05
GO: 0007010	cytoskeleton organization	7	117	KRT4, NEDD9, THY1, WTIP, RHOU, KRT8, CNN2	1.80E-04
GO: 0045766	positive regulation of angiogenesis	6	88	ANGPTL4, ECM1, HMOX1, GREM1, GATA6, ANXA3	2.65E-04

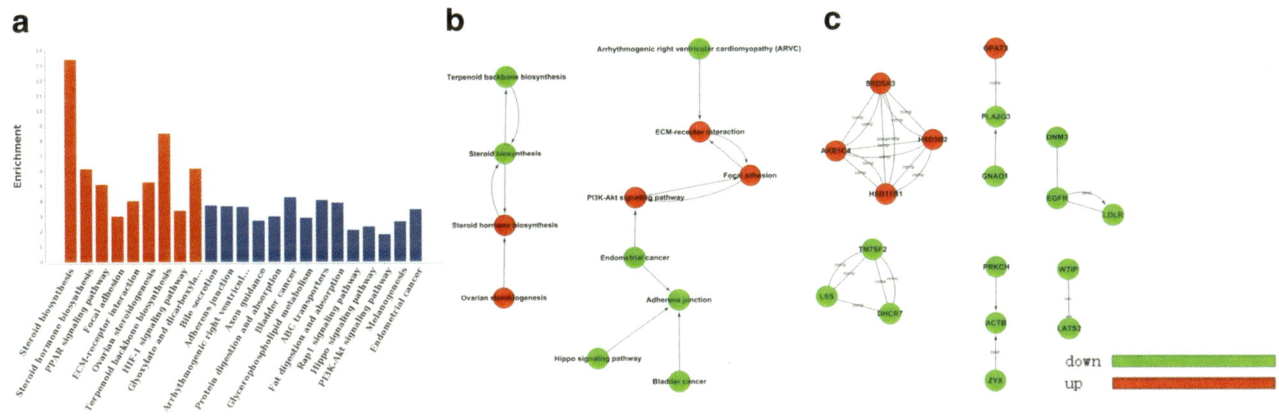

Fig. 3 **a** Pathway analysis of DEGs. Red represents the significant pathway. **b** Pathway act network. **c** Gene act network

and lipid metabolic process, while a majority of other terms consist of up-regulated genes. Taken together, we showed that CLs altered genes that were strongly correlated to the lipid metabolic process.

The pathway analysis showed the DEGs were associated with steroid biosynthesis, steroid hormone biosynthesis, PPAR signaling pathway, focal adhesion, ECM-receptor interaction, ovarian steroidogenesis, Terpenoid backbone biosynthesis, HIF-1 signaling pathway and glyoxylate, dicarboxylate metabolism ($P < 0.05$) (Fig. 3a). Among them, 5 pathways were involved in metabolism. We built the pathways act network to perform deep analysis (Fig. 3b). It was obvious that steroid biosynthesis and focal adhesion followed by steroid hormone biosynthesis, ECM-receptor interaction and PI3K-Akt signal pathway were the most important pathways involved, and these pathways were located at the centers of each cluster and showed more interactions with their surrounding pathways.

Network analysis

To illustrate the biological effect of CLs, we built the network of DEGs using the KEGG database. An important network module including HSB11B1, AKR1C4, SRD5A3 and HSD3B2 was identified (Fig. 3c). Interestingly, these genes were all involved in the most significant GO category steroid metabolic process.

In co-expression network analysis, "key regulatory" factors were determined by the degree and k-core differences between the control and CLs-treated groups. As shown in Fig. 4 and Table 4, HSD11B1, HSD3B2, G0S2, and CXCL5 followed STAR possessed the

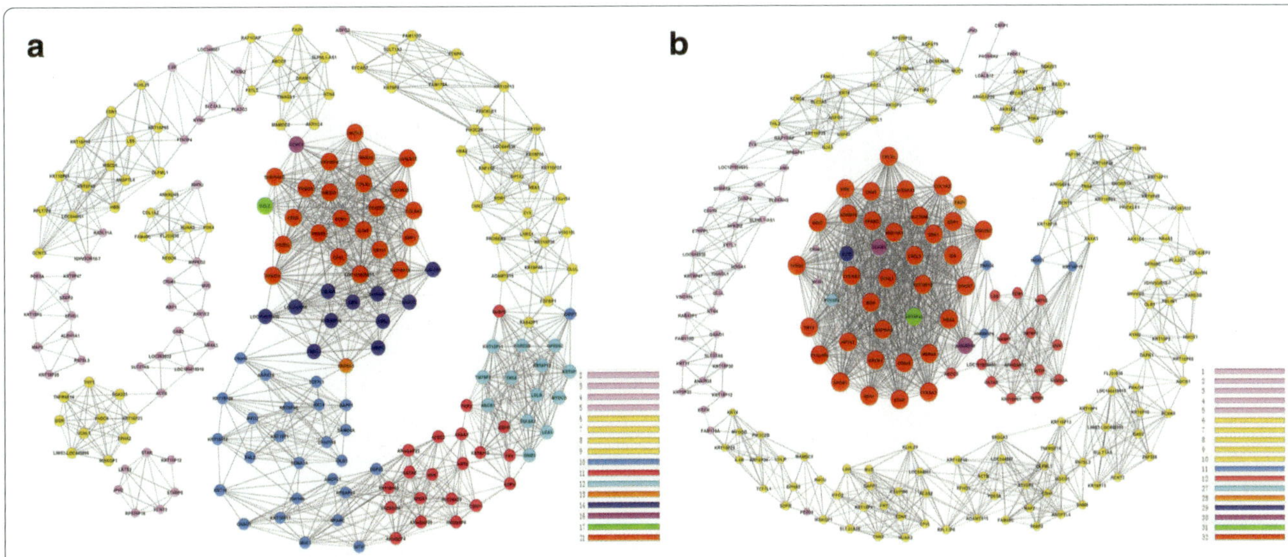

Fig. 4 Co-expression network of DEGs in the control (**a**) and CLs-treated (**b**) groups. Solid lines represent positive correlation, and dashed lines represent negatively correlation. The size and color of the nodes correspond to their co-expression ability. The greater the size of the node, the greater the number of its direct neighbors

Table 4 Intersection of DEGs between control and CLs-treated groups

Gene	Degree		K-core		Dif Degree	Dif K-core
	control	CLs-treated	control	CLs-treated		
G0S2	0	38	0	32	38	32
HSD11B1	0	38	0	32	38	32
HSD3B2	0	38	0	32	38	32
CXCL5	0	38	0	32	38	32
STAR	6	37	4	32	31	28
FA2H	9	31	7	28	22	21
DHCR7	23	38	21	32	15	11

biggest degree differences. HSD11B1, HSD3B2, STAR, FA2H and DHCR7 were members of steroid metabolic process. G0/G1 switch gene 2 (G0S2) is an important negative regulator of the rate-limiting lipolytic enzyme adipose triglyceride lipase-mediated lipolysis [33]. Chemokine C-X-C motif ligand 5 (CXCL5) is manifested to participate in the inflammatory process for nanotoxicology [34].

qRT-PCR and cell cycle analysis

qRT-PCR was performed to validate the relative gene expression of the 11 selected genes. As shown in Fig. 5a and b, the mRNA expression levels of 8 up-regulated and 3 down-regulated genes measured by qRT-PCR were almost comparable to the RNA-seq results. We analyzed the fold change of the gene expression ratios between RNA-seq and qRT-PCR by linear regression, the overall correlation coefficient was 0.9808, indicating the reliability of the RNA-seq data.

FCM analysis was applied to detect whether cell cycle arrest was induced. Resveratrol is well known as a positive compound to trigger accumulation of cells in S-phase of the cell cycle. As shown in Fig. 5c, no significant differences in cell cycle progression could be observed between control and CLs-treated groups. However, resveratrol triggered retention of HepG2 cells in S-phase, showing that these cells were not resistant to cell cycle arrest (Fig. 5c).

Discussion

Using whole-transcriptome sequencing and computational approaches, we showed herein that CLs caused changes in gene expression in HepG2 cells and that gene categories related to lipid metabolism were the most significantly affected categories. In the previous studies, CLs were reported to interact with negatively charged cellular components (opsonin, serum protein and enzyme) resulting in hemolysis, impairment of mitochondrial function and membrane integrity in vitro [12, 35]. In vivo, hepatotoxicity and weight loss have also been observed in mice after systemic administration of cationic siRNA nanoparticles [36]. In our study, the cytotoxicity of CLs in HepG2 was studied with a CCK-8 test after 24 h exposure. Morphological alteration under the

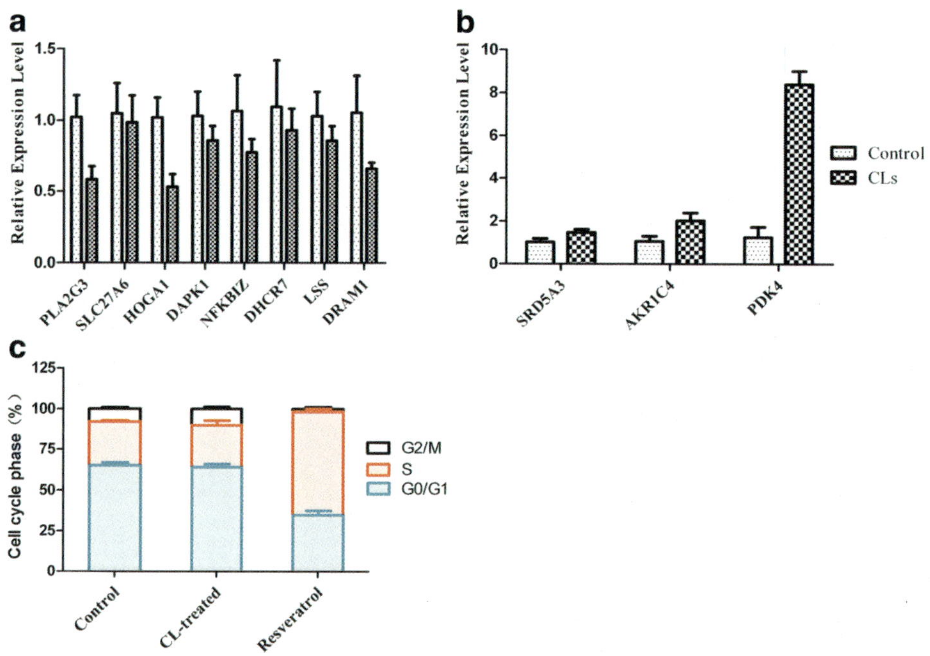

Fig. 5 **a**, **b** qRT-PCR verification of selected DEGs including 8 down-regulated and 3 up-regulated genes. The relative expression levels of these genes were normalized to GAPDH. **c** HepG2 cell cycle analysis was performed by flow cytometry. The percent of cells in each phase of the cell cycle was shown

microscope and concentration-dependency of cytotoxicity with IC_{50} of 120 μg/ml via a cell viability assay indicated the cytotoxic effect of CLs. To more clearly and exactly identify the changed level of DEGs, the concentration of IC_{50} (120 μg/ml) and exposure time of 24 h were chosen for subsequent experiments.

In the transcriptome sequencing, there were several DEGs involved in primary and secondary metabolism. Remarkably, 6 DEGs including PLA2G3, SLC27A6, TM7SF2, DHCR7, LSS and SRD5A3 were involved in the lipid metabolic process (Table 2). In addition, in the down-regulated genes, NFKBIZ, NF-kappa-B inhibitor zeta, is a member of the ankyrin-repeat family. The C-terminal portion of the encoded product shares high sequence similarity with the I kappa B family of proteins. The latter are known to play a role in inflammatory responses. DRAM1, DNA damage regulated autophagy modulator 1, was reported to increase autophagy flux through promoting lysosomal acidification and protease activation [37]. It was found that DRAM1 knockdown inhibited autophagy flux and aggravated cell injury in Neuro-2a cells [38]. A recent study has shown that CLs induced cell necrosis involved in late-stage autophagic flux inhibition [39]. DAPK1, death-associated protein kinase 1, is an important regulator of cell death and autophagy [40]. Additionally, it is a mediator of pro-apoptotic pathways and is involved in multiple cell death processes induced by various internal and external apoptotic stimulants [41]. In the up-regulated genes, HMOX1, Hemeoxygenase 1, is a gene for the antioxidant response and is considered to be a marker of oxidative stress. In a previous study, the expression of HMOX1 was increased in liver tissue after 7 days of repeated doses of CLs in rat [42]. In summary, apart from cellular metabolism process, the DEGs were also involved in inflammatory, autophagy, cell death, and antioxidant response.

In GO enriched terms, DEGs were mainly involved in multiple metabolic biological processes, including steroid metabolic process, cholesterol biosynthetic process, cholesterol metabolic process, steroid biosynthetic process, small molecule metabolic process, sterol biosynthetic process, and lipid metabolic process (Table 3). Moreover, to make certain the relationship of the enriched GO terms, we constructed the GO tree graph. The biosynthetic process of cholesterol and steroid is in the term of their metabolic process, respectively. In addition, the term "cholesterol biosynthetic process" is in the term "steroid biosynthetic process" which is included in the most significant category "steroid metabolic process" and all the above are in the category "lipid metabolic process" (Fig. 2c). At present, it is well accepted that cellular energy metabolism disturbance is one of the most important mediators of disease occurrence. Dysregulation of cellular energy is one of the hallmarks of cancer, and metabolic reprogramming is attracting increased attention in cancer research [43]. Many mechanisms for cytotoxicity of nanoparticles have been explained but little has been reported on the energy metabolism response. A previous study has shown that excessive exposure to certain metal nanoparticles can cause cellular metabolic turbulence [44]. Lipid metabolism is an important resource for cellular energy. In our study, GO results revealed that cytotoxicity of CLs mainly correlates with lipid metabolism, in addition to a response to hydrogen peroxide and dysfunction of angiogenesis.

In pathway analysis, 5 of the enriched 9 pathways including steroid biosynthesis, steroid hormone biosynthesis, Glyoxylate and dicarboxylate metabolism were involved in metabolism. Additionally, the PPARs are a group of nuclear receptors that are activated by fatty acids and their derivatives. Each of the three distinct subtypes is encoded by a separate gene and binds fatty acids and eicosanoids. Their activation leads to interruption of cell metabolism, cell growth and stress response [45]. Some reports suggested PPAR modulation by either agonist or antagonist might be a potential treatment for metabolic diseases [46]. Focal adhesion, transmembrane junctions between the extracellular matrix and the cytoskeleton, consists of a large number of both cytoskeletal and signal transduction (adapter) proteins and are rich in tyrosine phosphorylated proteins [47]. In cell biology,

Table 5 Primer sequences for quantitative Real-time reverse transcription-PCR (qRT-PCR) assay

Gene	Primer sequences (5'-3')
PLA2G3	Forward:AGAGAGGATGGACCATGCCT Reverse:GTTCCCGGCAACAGAGATCA
SLC27A6	Forward: TCCTGTGGGCTTTTGGTTGT Reverse: AAGTGGCACCCAACTCAACA
HOGA1	Forward: GGATCCCAGGGCTGAAGAAA Reverse: CTGGTGAAATCCATGCGCAG
DAPK1	Forward: AAGATCAAGTGCTGCCTGCT Reverse: GGCTGGTAGATCATGACGGG
NFKBIZ	Forward: GCCCAGTTGCCTGTCTTTTG Reverse: TTCCTCATCAACAGGCGGAC
DHCR7	Forward: CCAGGTGCTTCTGTACACGT Reverse: ACTTGTTCACAACCCCTGCA
LSS	Forward: GAGCGGCGTTATTTGCAGAG Reverse: AGACACCGGACTCCTCTCTC
DRAM1	Forward: CATCTCTGCCGTTTCTTGCG Reverse: AAACCAAAGGCCACTGTCCA
SRD5A3	Forward: CGAGTGCCTCTACGTCAGTG Reverse: ATCCATTGGCACTTGGCTCA
AKR1C4	Forward: CTCTCAAGCCAGGTGAGACG Reverse: AGTTTGACACCCCGATGGAC
PDK4	Forward: AGAGGTGGAGCATTTCTCGC Reverse: ATGTTGGCGAGTCTCACAGG

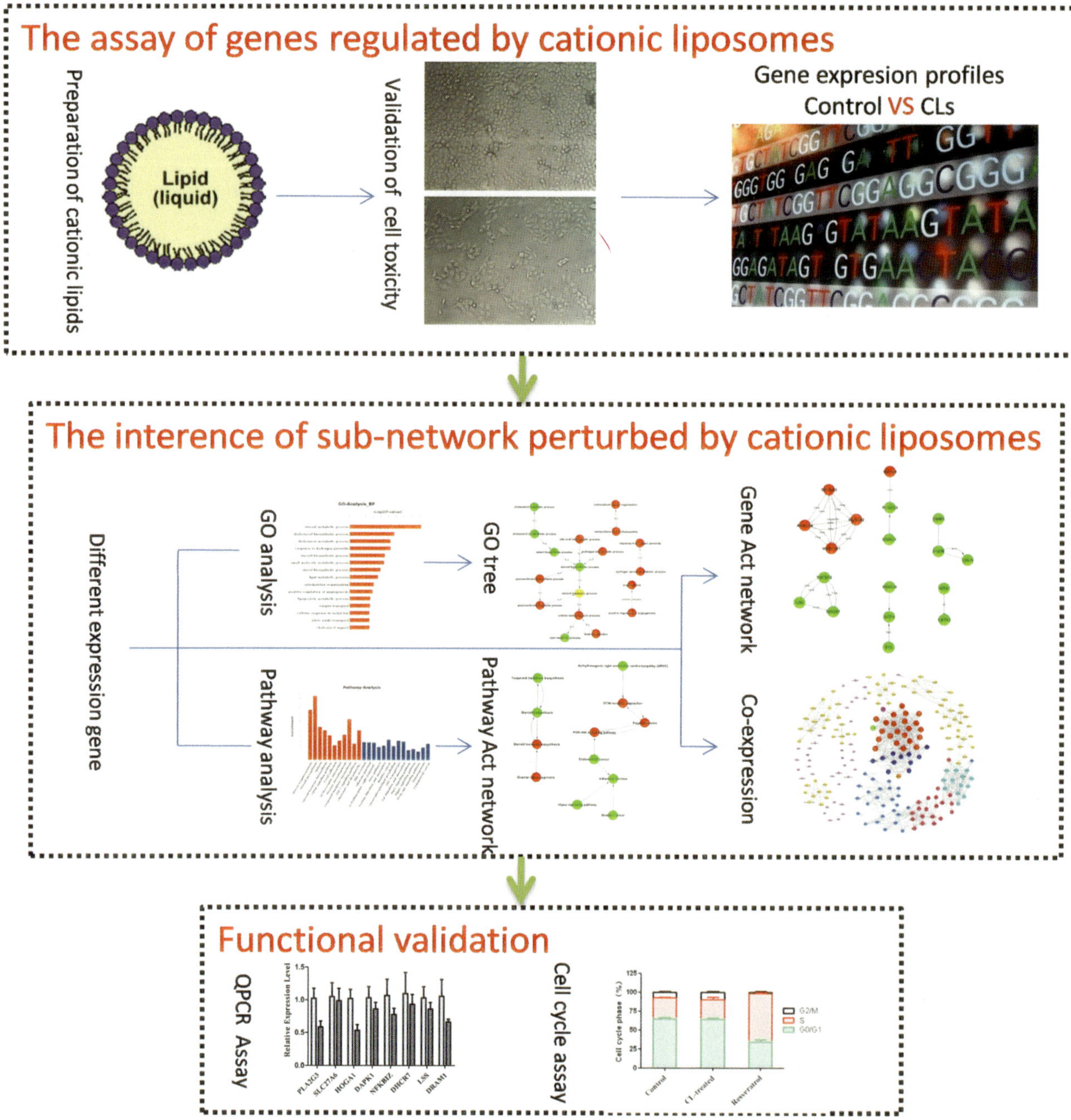

Fig. 6 The schematic diagram of this study. The procedure included three steps. Firstly, the cytotoxicity of cationic liposomes (CLs) was detected in HepG2 cell and DEGs in the CLs group comparing with control were identified through next generation RNA-seq technology. Then, functional analysis and bioinformatics computing were employed to explore the key genes and pathways. Finally, expression levels of these genes were confirmed by qPCR, and the cell cycle was assessed by flow cytometry

focal adhesions are large macromolecular assemblies that serve as the mechanical linkages to the ECM and as a biochemical-signaling hub to concentrate and direct numerous signaling proteins. Activation of the PI3K/AKT signaling pathway is implicated in the regulation of cell proliferation, death and metastasis [48]. Pathway results indicated that down-regulation of steroid biosynthesis and dysfunction of focal adhesion through PI3K/AKT signaling may be the key biological events after CLs exposure and the dominant elements involved in cytotoxicity in HepG2. Combining the results of GO and pathway analysis, we concluded that during the process of CLs entering into the cells, HepG2 cells produced a series of cellular responses such as a disorder of energy metabolism, regulation of microvascular function, dysfunction of focal adhesion and response to oxidative stress. Collectively, steroid biosynthesis was highly correlated to cytotoxicity induced by CLs.

To explore the potential relationship between the 220 DEGs involved in CLs cytotoxicity, we constructed co-expression networks for the control group and CLs-treated group. The key genes HSD11B1, HSD3B2, STAR, FA2H and DHCR7 indicated cytotoxicity of CLs mainly related to lipid metabolism. Previous studies have suggested that the size, shape and surface charge could affect the therapeutic effect and cytotoxicity of nanoparticles [49, 50]. Our results revealed the toxicity of CLs in HepG2 was mainly related to lipid metabolic process, which was possibly because of the materials of the nanoparticles. It indicates that in addition to the size and surface charge, the materials of nanoparticles may play an important role in their cytotoxicity and further studies are needed to conclusively explain their toxicity mechanism.

To confirm the accuracy and reproducibility of the transcriptome analysis results, 11 genes were selected from the list in Table 5 in our further study, and qRT-PCR was performed to validate the relative gene expression of these genes. Of these, 8 genes were in the following GO categories: steroid metabolic process, cholesterol biosynthetic process, cholesterol metabolic process, steroid biosynthetic process, and lipid metabolic process. 2 genes including DAPK1 and DRAM1 are related to apoptosis and autophagy. NFKBIZ is a well-known factor associated with the inflammatory response.

Several studies have shown that cytotoxicity may involve in the cell cycle, checkpoint control and DNA damage responses [51]. To evaluate whether cell cycle arrest was induced by CLs, the cell cycle was analyzed using FCM after treatment with the same concentration and exposure time via PI staining. These data suggest that cell cycle arrest is not obviously involved in the cytotoxicity of CLs in the HepG2 cell line, while the positive control resveratrol triggered retention of HepG2 cells in S-phase.

Conclusions

CLs have been extensively applied for gene and drug delivery as a means of protecting siRNA against enzymatic degradation, facilitating tumor cell uptake, and promoting escape from the endosomal compartment, resulting in effective cytoplasmic delivery. The increasing use of CLs in research and medical products has aroused global concern regarding their fate in biological systems, resulting in a demand for parallel risk assessment. Currently, CLs have only modest success as a delivery vehicle for gene therapy, primarily due to issues with toxicity. The objective of this work was to explore the mechanism of cytotoxicity induced by CLs. According to the previous report [8], the toxicity of cationic liposomes (CLs) is mainly related with their electrical property. Herein, we employed the common used DOTAP CLs in our study. As Fig. 6 shown, we initially successfully synthesized and characterized CLs, and then validated their cytotoxicity in HepG2 cells after 24 h exposure via a CCK-8 assay. The result demonstrated a concentration-dependent cytotoxicity with an IC_{50} of 120 μg/ml. Subsequently, we presented a systems biology approach based on next-generation whole transcriptome sequencing coupled with computational methods, including GO enrichment, pathway and co-expression analysis to reveal key roles involved in cellular responses to CLs. It revealed that cytotoxicity of CLs was mainly related to cholesterol, steroid and lipid biosynthetic and metabolic processes. qRT-PCR was performed to validate the RNA-seq results and FCM indicated the cell cycle arrest was not involved. Fortunately, recent studies have reported that modification to CLs have enabled better, long term transfection capability and low toxicity result in therapeutic efficacy. Our study may provide useful clue for further studies for preventing cytotoxicity. Collectively, CLs could become a promising tool for gene and drug delivery with low toxicity in the future.

Abbreviations

CLs: Cationic liposomes; DEGs: Differentially expressed genes; FCM: Flow cytometry; GO: Gene ontology; qRT-PCR: quantitative real time PCR; RNA-seq: RNA-sequencing

Acknowledgements

This work was supported by Science and Technology Commission of Shanghai Municipality. We would like to thank the study participants for providing response.

Authors' contribution

GQZ and DXS conceived the study. GQZ, DXS and JG designed and supervised the study, and made a substantial contribution of the local implementation of the study. GQZ, DXS, JG and HZ were accountable for aspects of the work and contributed to the formation of experimental concept. YL, QSC and YJ performed the experiments including cell viability assay, flow cytometer and quantitative real time PCR and contributed to acquisition of data. YL and HZ contributed to analysis of data. YL and XLC contributed the work of bioinformatics analysis and wrote the paper. All authors read and approved the final manuscript.

Funding

This work was supported by Science and Technology Commission of Shanghai Municipality [Grant number 15540723500].

Competing interests

The authors declare that they have no competing interests.

Author details
[1]Department of Pharmacy, Eastern Hepatobiliary Surgery Hospital, Second Military Medical University, Shanghai 200438, China. [2]Department of Pharmaceutical Science, College of Pharmacy, University of Michigan, Ann Arbor, MI 48109, USA. [3]National Center for Liver Cancer, Shanghai 201805, China. [4]The International Cooperation Laboratory on Signal Transduction, Eastern Hepatobiliary Surgery Hospital, Shanghai 200438, China. [5]Department of Pharmacy, Shanghai First Maternity and Infant Hospital, Tongji University School of Medicine, Shanghai 201204, China. [6]Department of Pharmaceutical Sciences, Second Military Medical University, 325 Guohe Road, Shanghai 200433, China.

References

1. Kargul J, Irminger-Finger ILaurent GJ, *Nanomedicine: Application of nanoparticles in clinical therapies and diagnostics[J].* International Journal of Biochemistry & Cell Biology. 2016;**75**(140-.
2. Hsueh CT, Selim JH, CT TJYH. Nanovectors for anti-cancer drug delivery in the treatment of advanced pancreatic adenocarcinoma[J]. World J Gastroenterol. 2016;22(31):7080–90.
3. Schmitt-Sody M, Strieth S, Krasnici S, Sauer B, Schulze B, Teifel M, Michaelis U, Naujoks KDellian M. Neovascular targeting therapy: paclitaxel encapsulated in cationic liposomes improves antitumoral efficacy[J]. Clin Cancer Res. 2003;9(6):2335–41.
4. Baker R. Early approval for two lipid-based drugs[J]. BETA. 1995;4
5. *FDA approves DaunoXome as first-line therapy for Kaposi's sarcoma. Food and Drug Administration[J].* J Int Assoc Physicians AIDS Care. 1996;2(5):50–1.
6. Marchal S, El Hor A, Millard M, Gillon VBezdetnaya L. Anticancer drug delivery: an update on clinically applied Nanotherapeutics[J]. Drugs. 2015; 75(14):1601–11.
7. Chen YC, Wu JJ, Huang L. Nanoparticles targeted with NGR motif deliver c-myc siRNA and doxorubicin for anticancer therapy[J]. Mol Ther. 2010;18(4): 828–34.
8. Obata Y, Tajima STakeoka S. Evaluation of pH-responsive liposomes containing amino acid-based zwitterionic lipids for improving intracellular drug delivery in vitro and in vivo[J]. J Control Release. 2010;142(2):267–76.
9. Abdelhalim MA, Jarrar BM, *Gold nanoparticles administration induced prominent inflammatory, central vein intima disruption, fatty change and Kupffer cells hyperplasia[J].* Lipids in Health and Disease. 2011;10.
10. Esmaeillou M, Moharamnejad M, Hsankhani R, Tehrani AA, Maadi H. Toxicity of ZnO nanoparticles in healthy adult mice[J]. Environ Toxicol Pharmacol. 2013;35(1):67–71.
11. Wang B, He X, Zhang Z, Zhao YFeng W. Metabolism of nanomaterials in vivo: blood circulation and organ clearance[J]. Acc Chem Res. 2013;46(3): 761–9.
12. Roursgaard M, Knudsen KB, Northeved H, Persson M, Christensen T, Kumar PEK, Permin A, Andresen TL, Gjetting T, Lykkesfeldt J, Vesterdal LK, Loft SMoller P, *In vitro toxicity of cationic micelles and liposomes in cultured human hepatocyte (HepG2) and lung epithelial (A549) cell lines[J].* Toxicology in Vitro. 2016;36(164–71.
13. Naicker K, Ariatti MSingh M, *PEGylated galactosylated cationic liposomes for hepatocytic gene delivery[J].* Colloids and Surfaces B-Biointerfaces. 2014; 122(482–90.
14. Sharifi S, Behzadi S, Laurent S, Forrest ML, Stroeve PMahmoudi M. Toxicity of nanomaterials[J]. Chem Soc Rev. 2012;41(6):2323–43.
15. Petersen EJ, Nelson BC. Mechanisms and measurements of nanomaterial-induced oxidative damage to DNA[J]. Anal Bioanal Chem. 2010;398(2): 613–50.
16. Oberdoester G, *Nanotoxicology: An Emerging Discipline Evolving from Studies of Ultrafine Particles (vol 113, pg 823, 2005)[J].* Environmental Health Perspectives. 2010;118(9):A380-A.
17. Mishra AR, Zheng JW, Tang XGoering PL. Silver nanoparticle-induced Autophagic-lysosomal disruption and NLRP3-Inflammasome activation in HepG2 cells is size-dependent[J]. Toxicol Sci. 2016;150(2):473–87.
18. Tzeng CW, Tzeng WS, Lin LT, Lee CW, Yen FL, Lin CC. Enhanced autophagic activity of artocarpin in human hepatocellular carcinoma cells through improving its solubility by a nanoparticle system[J]. Phytomedicine. 2016; 23(5):528–40.
19. Deng ZJ, Liang MT, Monteiro M, Toth IMinchin RF. Nanoparticle-induced unfolding of fibrinogen promotes mac-1 receptor activation and inflammation[J]. Nat Nanotechnol. 2011;6(1):39–44.
20. Lonez C, Vandenbranden M, Elouahabi ARuysschaert JM. Cationic lipid/DNA complexes induce TNF-alpha secretion in splenic macrophages[J]. Eur J Pharm Biopharm. 2008;69(3):817–23.
21. Gao J, Chen HW, Yu YS, Song JJ, Song H, Su X, Li W, Tong X, Qian WZ, Wang H, Dai JX, Guo YJ. Inhibition of hepatocellular carcinoma growth using immunoliposomes for co-delivery of adriamycin and ribonucleotide reductase M2 siRNA[J]. Biomaterials. 2013;34(38):10084–98.
22. Romero IG, Pai AA, Tung JGilad Y, *RNA-seq: impact of RNA degradation on transcript quantification[J].* Bmc Biology. 2014;12.
23. Wang K, Singh D, Zeng Z, Coleman SJ, Huang Y, Savich GL, He XP, Mieczkowski P, Grimm SA, Perou CM, MacLeod JN, Chiang DY, Prins JF, Liu JZ, *MapSplice: Accurate mapping of RNA-seq reads for splice junction discovery[J].* Nucleic Acids Research. 2010;38(18):
24. Mortazavi A, Williams BA, McCue K, Schaeffer L, Wold B. Mapping and quantifying mammalian transcriptomes by RNA-Seq[J]. Nat Methods. 2008; 5(7):621–8.
25. Draghici S, Khatri P, Tarca AL, Amin K, Done A, Voichita C, Georgescu CRomero R. A systems biology approach for pathway level analysis[J]. Genome Res. 2007;17(10):1537–45.
26. Smoot ME, Ono K, Ruscheinski J, Wang PL, Ideker T. Cytoscape 2.8: new features for data integration and network visualization[J]. Bioinformatics. 2011;27(3):431–2.
27. Li CLi H. Network-constrained regularization and variable selection for analysis of genomic data[J]. Bioinformatics. 2008;24(9):1175–82.
28. Wang M, Verdier J, Benedito VA, Tang Y, Murray JD, Ge Y, Becker JD, Carvalho H, Rogers C, Udvardi MHe J. LegumeGRN: a gene regulatory network prediction server for functional and comparative studies[J]. PLoS One. 2013;8(7):e67434.
29. Prieto C, Risueno A, Fontanillo C, De las Rivas J. *Human gene coexpression landscape: confident network derived from tissue transcriptomic profiles[J].* PLoS One. 2008;3(12):e3911.
30. Barabasi AL, Oltvai ZN. Network biology: understanding the cell's functional organization[J]. Nat Rev Genet. 2004;5(2):101–13.
31. Carlson MR, Zhang B, Fang Z, Mischel PS, Horvath SNelson SF, *Gene connectivity, function, and sequence conservation: predictions from modular yeast co-expression networks[J].* BMC Genomics. 2006;7(40.
32. Schmittgen TD, Livak KJ. Analyzing real-time PCR data by the comparative C(T) method[J]. Nat Protoc. 2008;3(6):1101–8.
33. Zhao NQ, Wang L, Guo N, *alpha-Linolenic acid increases the G(0)/G(1) switch gene 2 mRNA expression in peripheral blood mononuclear cells from obese patients: a pilot study[J].* Lipids in Health and Disease. 2016;15.
34. Leppanen M, Korpi A, Mikkonen S, Yli-Pirila P, Lehto M, Pylkkanen L, Wolff H, Kosma VM, Alenius H, Joutsensaari JPasanen P. Inhaled silica-coated TiO2 nanoparticles induced airway irritation, airflow limitation and inflammation in mice[J]. Nanotoxicology. 2015;9(2):210–8.
35. Senior JH, Trimble KR, Maskiewicz R. Interaction of positively-charged liposomes with blood: implications for their application in vivo[J]. Biochim Biophys Acta. 1991;1070(1):173–9.
36. Kedmi R, Ben-Arie N, Peer D. The systemic toxicity of positively charged lipid nanoparticles and the role of toll-like receptor 4 in immune activation[J]. Biomaterials. 2010;31(26):6867–75.
37. Zhang XD, Qi L, Wu JC, Qin ZH, *DRAM1 Regulates Autophagy Flux through Lysosomes[J].* Plos One. 2013;8(5):
38. Yu MQ, Jiang YG, Feng QL, Ouyang YA, Gan J. DRAM1 protects neuroblastoma cells from oxygen-glucose deprivation/reperfusion-induced injury via autophagy[J]. Int J Mol Sci. 2014;15(10):19253–64.
39. Yang K, Lu Y, Xie F, Zou H, Fan X, Li B, Li W, Zhang W, Mei L, Feng SS, Yin Y, Liu Y, Zhang H, Yin C, Zhong YGao J. Cationic liposomes induce cell necrosis through lysosomal dysfunction and late-stage autophagic flux inhibition[J]. Nanomedicine (Lond). 2016;11(23):3117–37.
40. Gade P, Manjegowda SB, Nallar SC, Maachani UB, Cross AS, Kalvakolanu DV. Regulation of the death-associated protein kinase 1 expression and autophagy via ATF6 requires apoptosis signal-regulating kinase 1[J]. Mol Cell Biol. 2014;34(21):4033–48.

41. Celik S, Akcora D, Ozkan T, Varol N, Aydos SSunguroglu A. Methylation analysis of the DAPK1 gene in imatinib-resistant chronic myeloid leukemia patients[J]. Oncol Lett. 2015;9(1):399–404.
42. Knudsen KB, Northeved H, Kumar PEK, Permin A, Gjetting T, Andresen TL, Larsen S, Wegener KM, Lykkesfeldt J, Jantzen K, Loft S, Moller PRoursgaard M. In vivo toxicity of cationic micelles and liposomes[J]. Nanomedicine-Nanotechnology Biology and Medicine. 2015;11(2):467–77.
43. Hanahan D, Weinberg RA. Hallmarks of cancer: the next generation[J]. Cell. 2011;144(5):646–74.
44. Wang J, Deng X, Zhang F, Chen D, Ding W. ZnO nanoparticle-induced oxidative stress triggers apoptosis by activating JNK signaling pathway in cultured primary astrocytes[J]. Nanoscale Res Lett. 2014;9(1):117.
45. Wang G, Cao R, Wang Y, Qian G, Dan HC, Jiang W, Ju L, Wu M, Xiao Y, Wang X, *Simvastatin induces cell cycle arrest and inhibits proliferation of bladder cancer cells via PPARgamma signalling pathway[J].* Sci Rep. 2016; 6(35783.
46. Langle Y, Lodillinsky C, Belgorosky D, Sandes EO, Eijan AM. Role of peroxisome proliferator activated receptor-gamma in bacillus Calmette-Guerin bladder cancer therapy[J]. J Urol. 2012;188(6):2384–90.
47. Alderliesten M, de Graauw M, Oldenampsen J, Qin Y, Pont C, van Buren L, van de Water B. Extracellular signal-regulated kinase activation during renal ischemia/reperfusion mediates focal adhesion dissolution and renal injury[J]. Am J Pathol. 2007;171(2):452–62.
48. Li B, Cheung PY, Wang X, Tsao SW, Ling MT, Wong YC, Cheung AL. Id-1 activation of PI3K/Akt/NFkappaB signaling pathway and its significance in promoting survival of esophageal cancer cells[J]. Carcinogenesis. 2007; 28(11):2313–20.
49. Jo DH, Kim JH, Lee TG, Kim JH. Size, surface charge, and shape determine therapeutic effects of nanoparticles on brain and retinal diseases[J]. Nanomedicine-Nanotechnology Biology and Medicine. 2015;11(7):1603–11.
50. Park YH, Bae HC, Jang Y, Jeong SH, Lee HN, Ryu WI, Yoo MG, Kim YR, Kim MK, Lee JK, Jeong JSon SW. Effect of the size and surface charge of silica nanoparticles on cutaneous toxicity[J]. Molecular & Cellular Toxicology. 2013;9(1):67–74.
51. Feliu N, Kohonen P, Ji J, Zhang Y, Karlsson HL, Palmberg L, Nystrom AFadeel B. Next-generation sequencing reveals low-dose effects of cationic dendrimers in primary human bronchial epithelial cells[J]. ACS Nano. 2015; 9(1):146–63.

13

Grifolic acid induces GH3 adenoma cell death by inhibiting ATP production through a GPR120-independent mechanism

Yufeng Zhao[1†], Lei Zhang[2†], Aili Yan[1], Di Chen[1], Rong Xie[1], Yingguang Liu[1], Xiangyan Liang[1], Yanyan Zhao[1], Lanlan Wei[1], Jun Yu[3], Xi Xu[1*] and Xingli Su[1*]

Abstract

Background: Grifolic acid is a derivative of grifolin, an antitumor natural compound, and it was reported as an agonist of free fatty acid receptor GPR120. Little is known about its antitumor effects and the involvement of GPR120.

Methods: GH3 cells, the rat anterior pituitary adenoma cells, were cultured and the cell death was measured by MTT assay and Annexin V/PI staining. The mitochondrial membrane potential (MMP) of GH3 cells was measured by JC-1 staining. Cellular ATP levels and the intracellular NAD/NADH ratio were measured. GPR120 expression in GH3 cells was observed by RT-PCR and Western Blot, and siRNA was used to inhibit GPR120 expression in GH3 cells.

Results: Grifolic acid dose- and time-dependently induced the necrosis of GH3 cells. Grifolic acid significantly reduced the mitochondrial membrane potential (MMP) and decreased cellular ATP levels in GH3 cells. In contrast, the MMP of isolated mitochondria was not decreased by grifolic acid. The intracellular NAD/NADH ratio was significantly increased by grifolic acid. GPR120 is expressed in GH3 cells, but GPR120 agonists such as EPA, GW9508 and TUG891 did not affect the viability of GH3 cells. Moreover, GPR120 siRNA knockdown showed no significant influence on grifolic acid-induced GH3 cell death.

Conclusion: Grifolic acid induces GH3 cell death by decreasing MMP and inhibiting ATP production, which may be due to the inhibition of NADH production through a GPR120-independent mechanism.

Keywords: Grifolic acid, GH3 cells, Mitochondria, Cell death

Background

Some natural compounds, which are isolated from botany, fungi and marine organism, are putative candidates for antitumor drugs [1]. It is well known that grifolin, one of the natural compounds isolated from the fresh fruiting bodies of the mushroom *Albatrellus confluens* [2], exhibits antitumor effects on nasopharyngeal carcinoma, osteosarcoma, and gastric tumor cells [3–5]. Grifolic acid (the structure in Additional file 1) is a derivative of grifolin, but its effects on tumor cells are not well established. Some reports showed that grifolic acid was an agonist of free fatty acid receptor GPR120 [6], and grifolic acid was able to activate extracellular regulated protein kinases (ERK1/2), causing increased secretion of glucose-dependent insulinotropic polypeptide (GIP) from GPR120-expressing enteroendocrine cells [7]. It was also showed that GPR120 activation might produce protective effects on murine enteroendocrine cell line STC-1 cells [8]. The effects of grifolic acid on tumor cells and the involvement of GPR120 warrants further study.

Anterior pituitary adenomas, one of the common intracranial tumors, is increasingly diagnosed due to the advances in neuroimaging technology [9]. Besides transsphenoidal surgery, medical therapies are important treatments for anterior pituitary adenomas [10]. New

* Correspondence: 511685623@qq.com; xingli_su@163.com
†Yufeng Zhao and Lei Zhang contributed equally to this work.
[1]The institute of Basic Medical Sciences, Xi'an Medical University, Xi'an 710021, China
Full list of author information is available at the end of the article

effective antitumor drugs may significantly improve the therapy of anterior pituitary adenomas. In this study, we observed the effects of grifolic acid on the viability of GH3 cells, the rat anterior pituitary adenoma cells that secret growth hormone and prolactin [11].

The death of tumor cells is often related to the dysfunction of mitochondria. Mitochondria are essential to produce ATP and play a dominant role in cellular viability, apoptosis and death [12]. Intracellular ATP at the normal level is required for cell survival, and the reduction of ATP level results in the apoptosis or necrosis of living cells [13, 14]. Mitochondrial membrane potential (MMP), which is generated during the procedure of redox energy transfer from NADH to oxygen via the electron transport chain in mitochondria, represents the function of mitochondria and is critical for ATP production. The actions of grifolic acid on mitochondria function such as MMP and ATP production were also investigated in this study. In addition, we found GPR120 expression in GH3 cells, and the role of GPR120 in the effects of grifolic acid on GH3 cells was studied.

Methods

Chemicals

Grifolic acid and TUG891 were obtained from R&D Inc. (Minnneapolis, USA). GW9508, EPA, GPR120 polyclonal antibody, MTT and Cellular ATP assay kits were bought from Sigma-Aldrich (St. Louis, USA). Annexin V-FITC/PI staining kits were the products of BD Pharmingen (San Jose, USA). Rat GPR120 siRNA, lipofectamine RANiMAX, DMEM, FBS, JC-1 and Mitochondria Isolation Kit for Culture Cells were obtained from Thermo Fisher Scientific (Waltham, USA). NAD/NADH Assay Kits were the products of Abcam (Cambridge, UK). Protein extraction kits were bought from Bio-Rad (Hercules, USA). RNA isolation kits, reverse transcription kits and PCR kits were the products of Takara Biotechnology (Dalian, China).

Cell culture

GH3 cells were obtained from American Type Culture Collection (ATCC Number: CCL-82.1™) and cultured in DMEM containing 10% FBS, 100 U/ml penicillin and 100 μg/ml streptomycin. The media were changed every 2 days, and GH3 cells were sub-cultured after 80% confluence and seeded to plates or dishes for the following measurements.

Cell viability assay

GH3 cells grew up to 90% confluence in 96-well plates and then were changed to serum-free medium with regent treatment including grifolic acid, EPA, GW9508 and TUG891. At the end of treatment, MTT was added into media at a final concentration of 0.5 mg/ml. Four hours later, the media were discarded and 100 μl isopropanol with 0.01 mol/L HCl was added to each well. After the formazan crystals were fully solubilized, the absorbance values at 560 nm were measured by ELISA reader (Thermo Fisher, USA). The background absorbance values at 630 nm were also measured and subtracted from that of 560 nm. Then the absorbance values were used for statistical analysis. The experiments were performed in triplicate.

Flow cytometry analysis of cell death

After being treated by grifolic acid in serum-free medium, GH3 cells were detached from the dishes by 0.05% trypsin/EDTA and stained using AnnexinV-FITC/PI staining kits [15]. Briefly, the cells were re-suspended into the binding buffer at 1×10^6 cells/ml, and AnnexinV-FITC/PI was added to cell suspension in a dilution of 1:20. The cells were gently mixed and incubated for 15 min at room temperature in the dark. Finally, the cells were diluted into binding buffer and went through the flow cytometry to measure AnnexinV- and PI-staining positive cells (BD Biosciences, USA). The experiments were performed in triplicate.

Cellular ATP measurement

Cellular ATP levels in GH3 cells were measured using ATP detection assay kits [16]. Briefly, GH3 cells after being treated by grifolic acid in serum-free medium were lyzed by detergent under shaking at 700 rpm for 5 min. The constituted substrate solutions were added for incubation for 5 min in a dark place. Then the luminescence of each sample was recorded using the luminescence plate reader (Thermo Fisher, USA). The standard curves were constructed and the ATP level of each sample was calculated. The total protein levels were quantified by BCA assay and used to correct the cellular ATP levels for data analysis. The experiments were performed in triplicate.

NAD/NADH measurement

GH3 cells (4×10^5 cells per sample) were washed in cold PBS and treated with NAD/NADH Extraction Buffer. The buffer was centrifuged at 12,000 g for 5 min at 4 °C and the supernatants were collected for NAD/NADH assay [17]. As indicated by the instruction, each sample was divided into two parts for NADt (total NAD including NAD and NADH) assay and NADH assay respectively. The samples were mixed with Reaction Mix firstly and incubated for 5 min at room temperature. Then NADH Developer was added to incubate for 4 h. The OD value of each sample was read at 450 nm. NAD/NADH ratio was calculated as: NAD/NADH ratio = (NADt-NADH) / NADH. The experiments were performed in triplicate.

MMP measurement

GH3 cells were stained with JC-1 (a final concentration of 5 μg/ml) in the serum-free medium for 15 min at 37 °C in a humidified 5% CO_2 incubator. Then the cells were washed with the serum-free medium and put onto the stage of confocal microscope (Leica TCS SP8). The fluorescence intensity was recorded every 5 min before and after the treatment with grifolic acid. The red fluorescence (excitation wavelength at 560 nm and emission wavelength at 600 nm) and green fluorescence (excitation wavelength at 488 nm and emission wavelength at 535 nm) were measured synchronously, and the ratio of fluorescent intensity (red/green) for each cell was analyzed using the LAS LITE software [18]. The experiments were performed in triplicate.

Mitochondria isolation

The mitochondria were extracted from GH3 cells using the Mitochondria Isolation Kit for the Culture Cells under the instruction [19]. GH3 cells (1×10^7 cells per sample) were loaded with JC-1 firstly and then were harvested to isolate mitochondria. Mitochondria isolation reagent A was added to incubate on ice for 2 min, followed by the adding of mitochondria isolation reagent B and C. Then the mixtures were centrifuged at 700 g for 10 min at 4 °C. The supernatants were collected and centrifuged at 12,000 g for 15 min at 4 °C, and the pellets were collected and incubated in mitochondria isolation reagent C for MMP measurement.

GPR120 siRNA transfection

GH3 cells grew to 70% confluent at the time of transfection. The transfection complexes for rat GPR120 Silencer Select siRNA (siRNA ID: S148233, Invitrogen) and Lipofectamine RNAiMAX were prepared by mixture of siRNA (100 pmol in 50 μl of Opti-MEM medium) and Lipofectamine RNAiMAX (1 μl in 50 μl of Opti-MEM medium). The complexes were added to the medium at a dilution of 1:4. The cells were cultured for 48 h and then GPR120 knockdown was measured by Western blot. The cells with transfection were used to measure cell death, cellular ATP levels and MMP.

Western blot

In brief, GH3 cells were homogenized and total protein was extracted using ReadyPrep protein extraction kits and quantified by BCA assay. The protein (40 μg) was analyzed by SDS-PAGE on a 10% Peptide Criterion Gel and transferred to nitrocellulose membranes using a Trans-Blot SD semi-dry electrophoresis transfer cell (Bio-Rad). The membranes were then probed with rabbit-anti GPR120 antibody (1:1000) and the blot was developed with the chemiluminescent reagents. The luminescence of the membranes was imaged by the ChemiDoc MP gel imaging analysis system. The experiments were performed in triplicate.

RT-PCR

The total RNA from GH3 cells were extracted and reverse transcription was performed using the kits from Takara. cDNA was used to run PCR with rat GPR120 primers. The forward primer is 5′- GCA TAG GAG AAA TCT CAT GG-3′ and the reverse primer is 5′-GAG TTG GCA AAC GTG AAG GC-3′. The PCR product size was 340 bp. The reaction mixture was denatured for 5 min at 94 °C for 30 s, and then it went to 30 cycles of denaturing at 94 °C for 30 s, annealing at 58 °C for 15 s and extending at 72 °C for 15 s. PCR products were analyzed by electrophoresis on 1.4% agarose gel with ethidium bromide. The experiments were performed in triplicate.

Data analysis

The data were expressed as Mean ± S.EM. D'Agostino-Pearson omnibus test was used to test the normality of data distribution. For the normal distribution data, comparisons of means of multiple groups with each other or against one control group were analyzed with one way ANOVA followed by the appropriate *post-hoc* tests. For the abnormal distribution data, Kruskal-Wallis H test was used to analyze the significance of groups. $P < 0.05$ was considered to be significantly different.

Results

Effects of grifolic acid on GH3 cell viability

Grifolic acid (20 μmol/L) inhibited the viability of GH3 cells after 1 h incubation and resulted in total cell death 6 h later. It showed a dose- and time-dependent inhibition of GH3 cell viability from 2.5 μmol/L to 20 μmol/L in 24 h incubation (Fig. 1). The IC50 of grifolic acid at 24 h treatment was 4.25 μmol/L. AnnexinV/PI staining and the flow cytometry analysis was also used to observe the death of GH3 cells. The percentage of Annexin V and PI-positive GH3 cells in control was 2.45% ± 0.83%, and it increased to 42.51% ± 7.86% after treatment with grifolic acid (10 μmol/L) for 6 h. The represent analysis results were shown in Fig. 2a and b. GH3 cells in control showed normal shape (Fig. 2c), but they were significantly swollen and mostly broken after grifolic acid treatment (Fig. 2d).

Effects of grifolic acid on MMP and ATP production in GH3 cells

MMP was indicated by JC-1 fluorescence [20]. JC-1 exhibited membrane potential-dependent accumulation in mitochondria, showing the shift of emission wavelength from green to red. Mitochondrial depolarization was indicated by a decrease in the red/green fluorescence intensity

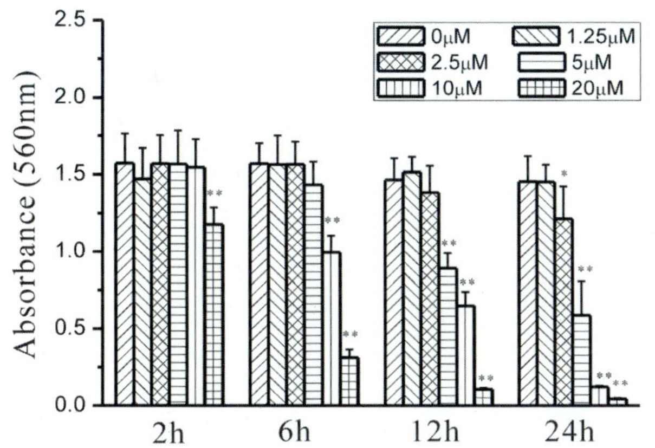

Fig. 1 Grifolic acid reduces GH3 cells viability. GH3 cells in serum-free medium were treated by grifolic acid for different time, and then MTT assay was used to measure cell viability. The absorbance values of MTT assay at 560 nm were analyzed. * means $P < 0.05$ vs control. ** means $P < 0.01$ vs control, $n = 16$

ratio [21]. We found that grifolic acid resulted in a significant decrease in the red/green fluorescence intensity ratio in a dose-dependent and time-dependent manner. Grifolic acid (20 μmol/L) significantly attenuated MMP after 5 min incubation and caused the maximal effect in 20 min. Grifolic acid (10 μmol/L) also took effects in 10 min and achieved maximal effect in 40 min. Grifolic acid at the concentration of 5 μmol/L and 2.5 μmol/L also attenuated MMP in a longer 60 min. Grifolic acid at the concentration of 1.25 μmol/L did not attenuate MMP in 60 min compared to control (Fig. 3).

The cellular ATP levels were then measured. The cellular ATP level was 38.18 ± 4.23 nmol/mg protein in control GH3 cells, and it began to significantly drop after the treatment with 20 μmol/L grifolic acid for 0.5 h and dropped to 17.76 ± 3.23 nmol/mg protein in 2 h (Fig. 4a). Grifolic acid at concentration of 10μmol/L also significantly resulted in the decrease in cellular ATP levels from 37.67 ± 4.89 nmol/mg protein in control to 22.56 ± 2.49 nmol/mg protein after 2 h of the treatment and to 8.15 ± 2.03 nmol/mg protein after 6 h (Fig. 4b).

Role of GPR120 in grifolic acid-induced GH3 cell death

As shown in Fig. 5a, RT-PCR showed the expression of GPR120 in GH3 cells. The negative control using RNA without reverse transcription did not show the amplification of GPR120 gene, confirming the specificity of RT-PCR. In accordant to it, western blot showed that the proteins from GH3 cells were stained positively by GPR120 antibody and the molecular size of the stained band was 41KDa, the exact molecular size of rat GPR120 (Fig. 5b). GPR120 agonists including EPA (20 μmol/L), GW9508 (20 μmol/L) and TUG891 (20 μmol/L) did not show significant effects on the viability of GH3 cells after the incubation for 24 h. In contrast,

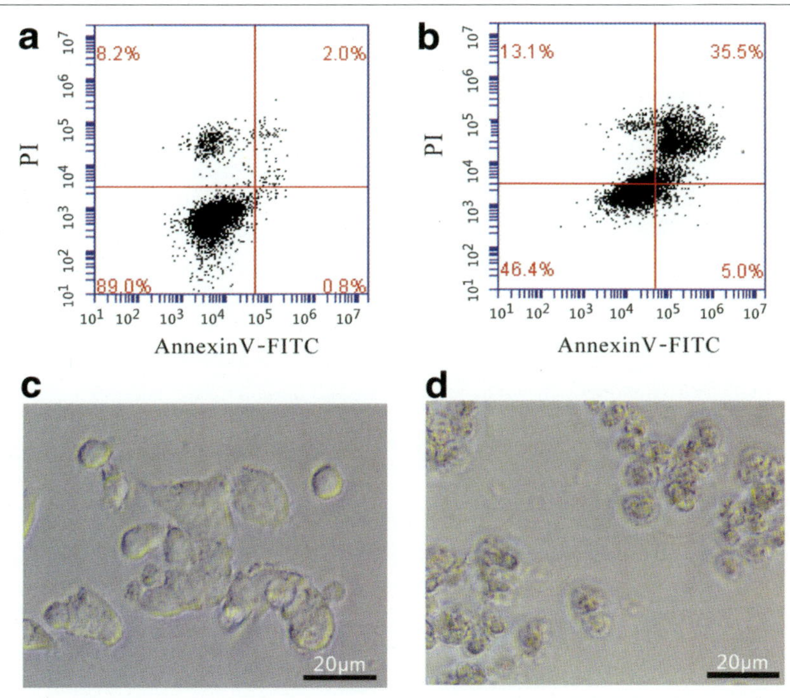

Fig. 2 Grifolic acid induces cell death of GH3 cells. **a** Flow cytometry measurement showed that GH3 cells in control had low level of cell death as indicated by low staining of Annexin V and PI; **b** GH3 cell after grifolic acid treatment (10 μmol/L for 6 h) showed a significant increase in cell necrosis as indicated by high percentage of Annexin V and PI-positive staining cells; **c** The normal shape of GH3 cells in control; **d** GH3 cells showed swelling and broken after grifolic acid treatment. The photos were representative results of 3 independent experiments

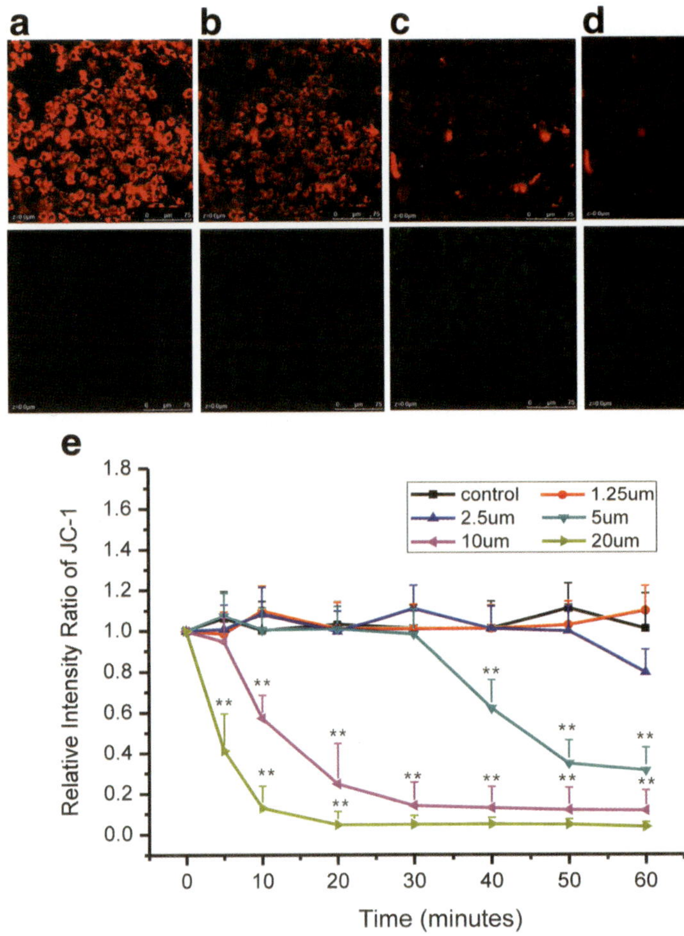

Fig. 3 Grifolic acid diminishes MMP of GH3 cells. The fluorescent intensity of MMP indicator JC-1 in control (**a**) and after 20 μmol/L grifolic acid treatment for 5 min (**b**), 10 min (**c**) and 20 min (**d**). The statistical analysis of fluorescent intensity ratio of JC-1 in each cell was shown in (**e**) to reflect MMP levels. ** $P < 0.01$ vs control, $n = 80$

grifolic acid (20 μmol/L) had a significant inhibitory effect on the viability of GH3 cells (Fig. 5c).

A significant reduction of GPR120 protein level was achieved in GH3 cells with GPR120 siRNA transfection compared to the control (Fig. 6a). GPR120 knockdown did not significantly influence grifolic acid-induced inhibition of the GH3 cell viability (Fig. 6b). In addition, the decrease in ATP levels and MMP by grifolic acid treatment was not significantly influenced by GPR120 knockdown too (Fig. 6c and d).

Effects of grifolic acid on electron transport chain of mitochondria and NADH production

The mitochondria from GH3 cells were stained with JC-1. JC-1 intensity of mitochondrial sample that was extracted from GH3 cells remained stable during the measurement. The uncoupler carbonyl cyanide 3-chlorophenylhydrazone (CCCP) significantly reduced JC-1 intensity of the isolated mitochondria to 25.67 ± 4.81% of the control. This result indicated that the isolated mitochondria in the experiments maintained normal MMP during the measurement. Although grifolic acid inhibited MMP in the whole cells, it did not induce any change in MMP in the isolated cell-free mitochondria during the incubation for 20 min (Fig. 7a). It is suggested that grifolic acid-induced decrease in MMP in GH3 cells is initiated by the changes prior to electron transport chain inside mitochondria.

In the next, NAD/NADH ratio in GH3 cells was measured. The NAD/NADH ratio was significantly increased after 5 min of the grifolic acid treatment and reached a higher level after 20 min, indicating that the reduction of NADH may be the reason for the decreased MMP in GH3 cells after grifolic acid treatment (Fig. 7b).

Discussion

Grifolic acid is a farnesyl phenolic compound first isolated from the mushroom *Albatrellus confluens* and can be totally synthesized now [2]. It has been shown that grifolin, an analog of grifolic acid, has inhibitory effects

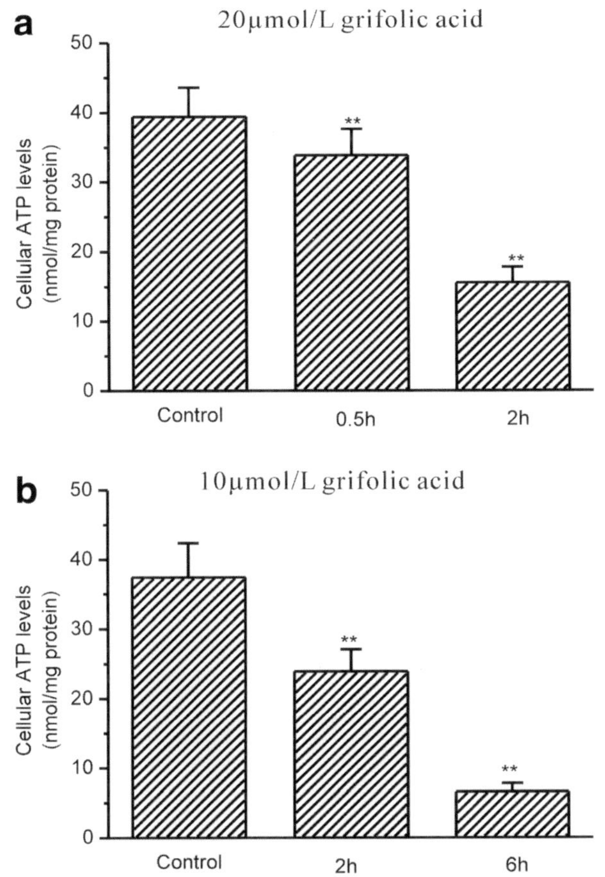

Fig. 4 Grifolic acid reduces cellular ATP levels in GH3 cells. **a** The cellular ATP levels of GH3 cells being treated by 20 μmol/L grifolic acid; **b** The cellular ATP levels of GH3 cells being treated by 10 μmol/L grifolic acid. ** means P < 0.01 vs control, $n = 12$

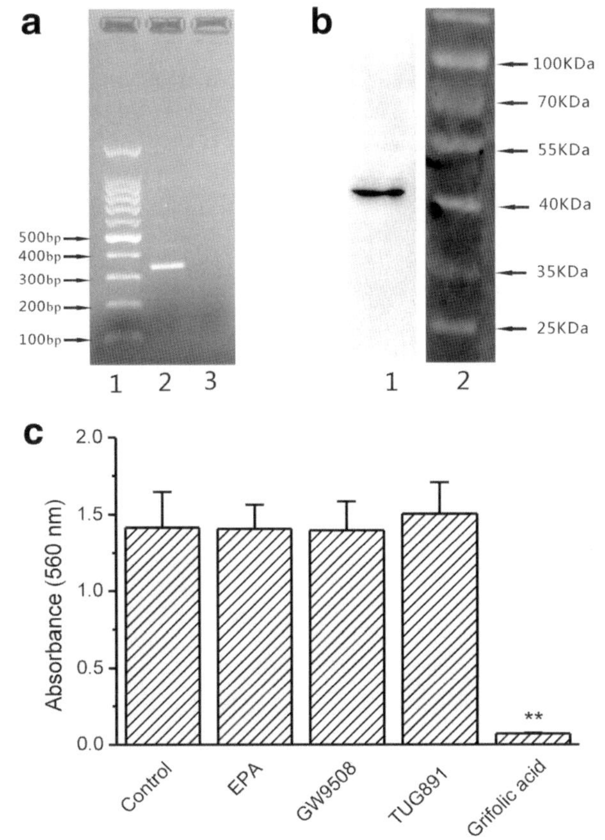

Fig. 5 GPR120 is expressed in GH3 cells and did not influence GH3 cell viability. **a**: GPR120 transcription in GH3 cells was shown by RT-PCR. Lanes 1-3 were cDNA marker, GPR120 amplification products from GH3 cells and negative control, respectively. The size of PCR product is 340 bp. **b**: The protein expression of GPR120 in GH3 cells was shown by western blot. Lane 1 was the immunostaining of GPR120 and lane 2 was the protein marker. **c**: MTT assay of GH3 cell viability in response to GPR120 agonists and grifolic acid. ** means $P < 0.01$ vs control, $n = 12$

on variety of tumor cells [4, 22–24]. In this study, we demonstrated that grifolic acid induced the death of GH3 pituitary adenoma cells in a dose- and time-dependent manner. Grifolic acid in concentration of 20 μmol/L induced total death of GH3 cells after 6 h treatment. In contrast, grifolin in concentration of 50 μmol/L induced only 15% of cell death after the incubation for 6 h on U2OS and MG63 osteosarcoma cells [3]. The discrepancy may result from the difference in the cell types and the culture conditions. In this study, GH3 cells were treated with grifolic acid in the serum-free medium to exclude the influence of serum ingredients. Serum-free medium may increase the sensitivity of GH3 cells to grifolic acid treatment.

It was indicated that PI3K/Akt, ERK1/2 and p53 were the possible intracellular signaling molecules that mediated the antitumor effects of grifolin in different types of tumor cells [3, 22, 24]. Although PI3K, ERK1/2 and p53 were involved in the regulation of cell viability and growth in many tumor cell types, the inhibition of PI3K, ERK1/2 and p53 did not acutely induce cell death [11, 25–28]. We also found that PI3K inhibitor Wortmannin, ERK1/2 inhibitor U-0126, and p53 inactivator cyclic pifithrin-α, p-nitro, respectively did not induce cell death in GH3 cells (Additional file 2). Therefore, it is suggested that grifolic acid-induced GH3 cell death may not be mediated by PI3K, ERK1/2 and p53.

The cellular ATP level is a critical factor maintaining cellular viability. The reduction rate of ATP production determines the cell death types [13, 29, 30]. Rapid falling of intracellular ATP leads to cell death through necrosis pathways such as oncosis [31]. Grifolic acid at 10 μmol/L induced a significant increase in the number of Annexin V and PI -positive cells, indicating that GH3 cells died mainly through necrosis. Grifolic acid also resulted in a significant and fast decrease in the cellular ATP levels in GH3 cells. The rapid deprivation of ATP may be responsible to the necrosis of GH3 cells.

Mitochondria are vital to cellular viability, with its dominant role in the production of ATP as cell energy

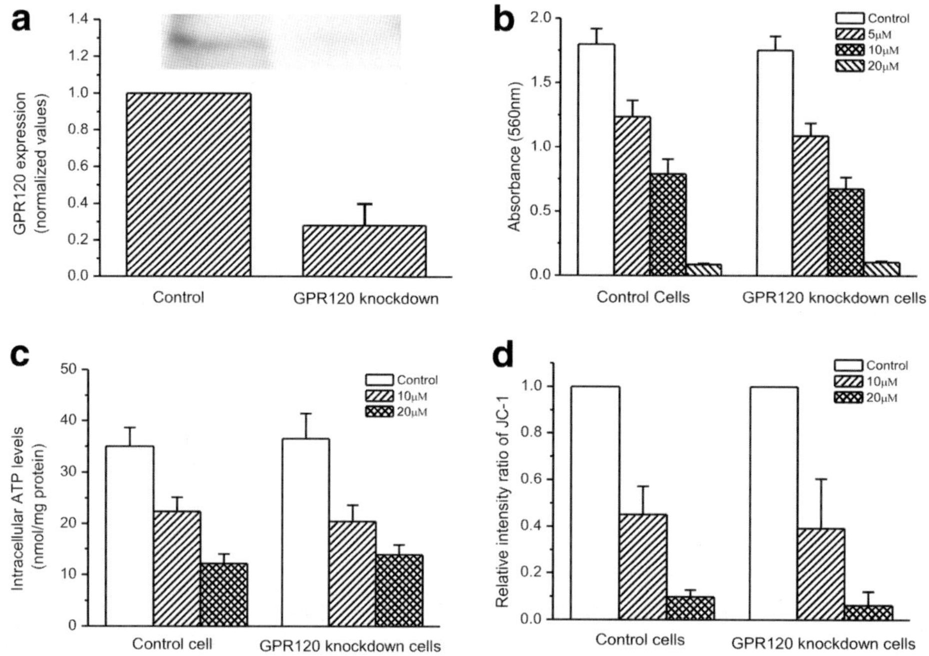

Fig. 6 GPR120 does not mediate the effects of grifolic acid on GH3 cell viability. **a** The inhibition of GPR120 expression was achieved by siRNA transfection for 48 h; **b** Grifolic acid-induced cell death was not affected by GPR120 knockdown; **c** Grifolic acid-induced decrease in ATP production was not affected by GPR120 knockdown; **d** Grifolic acid-induced attenuation of MMP was not affected by GPR120 knockdown

source [32, 33]. The fuel energy is mainly transported to NADH during oxidation, and the redox energy from NADH is transferred to oxygen via the electron transport chain in mitochondria. This procedure generates MMP, which drives the protons into mitochondrial matrix through ATP synthase to produce ATP or through uncoupling proteins to produce energy. Mitochondria dysfunction may be the reason for grifolic acid-induced decrease in cellular ATP levels. We then investigated the effects of grifolic acid on mitochondrial function. MMP is usually measured using JC-1 because it accumulates in mitochondria driven by MMP to emit red fluorescence in the mitochondria and emits green fluorescence when it releases into the cytoplasm under the condition of MMP reduction [34, 35]. Grifolic acid induced a fast decrease in the red/green intensity ratio of JC-1 in GH3 cells, indicating MMP reduction or less JC-1 kept within mitochondria. Accordingly, the ATP levels in GH3 cells significantly decreased after the grifolic acid treatment. The direct action of grifolic acid on mitochondria was then studied. In the isolated mitochondria, the uncoupler CCCP, which leads to proton leak and MMP reduction [36, 37], significantly diminished MMP as expected, indicating that the isolated mitochondria may function well. Grifolic acid, however, did not reduce MMP in the isolated mitochondria of GH3 cells. It indicated that grifolic acid did not act directly on the electron transport chain of mitochondria. The MMP reduction observed in the cells may be due to the deficiency of NADH and consequent rundown of proton pump. As expected, it was found that the cellular NADH levels decreased and NAD/NADH ratio increased acutely after the grifolic acid treatment. Therefore, it is concluded that grifolic acid blocks fuel metabolism and NADH production, which in turn decreases MMP and ATP production and leads to GH3 cell death. Because fuel metabolism is executed by a series of complex enzyme reactions, the accurate targets of grifolic acid need to be further clarified in detail.

It was reported that grifolic acid is an agonist of GPR120 [7, 19, 38]. GPR120 is considered to be a promising pharmaceutical target for the treatment of metabolic diseases [39]. Recently, several non-FFA agonists of GPR120 including GW9508, TUG891, and grifolic acid have been discovered [38, 40, 41]. In this study, the mRNA and protein expression of GPR120 in GH3 cells was confirmed by RT-PCR and western blot. To our knowledge, this is the first report of GPR120 expression in GH3 cells. It was reported that GPR120 activation protects mouse enteroendocrine cell line STC-1 cells against serum deprivation-induced apoptosis [8], showing protective effects of GPR120 on cellular viability. However, we found that grifolic acid induced cell death of GH3 cells in serum-free culture condition. To clarify the role of GPR120 in the action of grifolic acid on GH3 cells, we tested the effects of the other putative GPR120

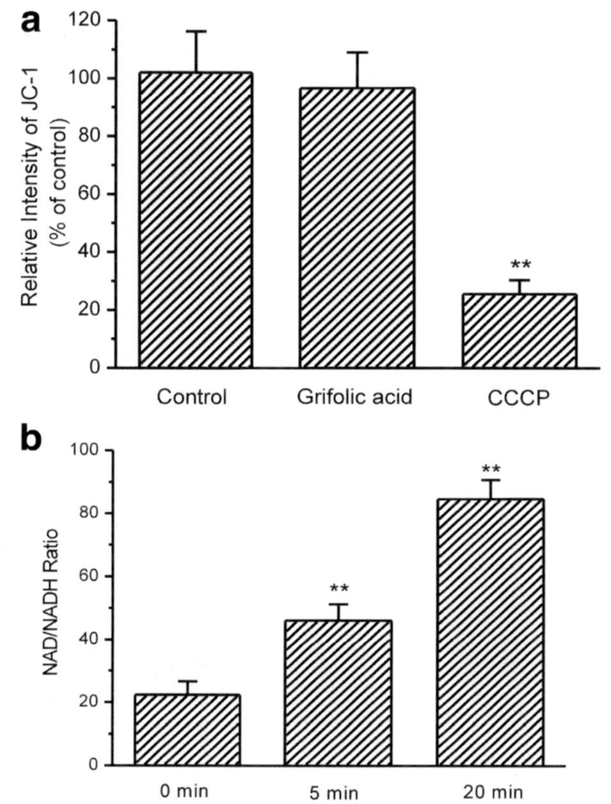

Fig. 7 Grifolic acid does not reduce MMP of isolated mitochondria but reduces cellular NAD/NADH ratio in GH3 cells. **a** MMP of isolated mitochondria from GH3 cells was represented by JC-1 intensity. Grifolic acid (20 μmol/L) did not decrease MMP of isolated mitochondria in 20 min incubation. The uncoupler CCCP significantly inhibited MMP; **b** Grifolic acid (20 μmol/L) acutely induced a significant increase in NAD/NADH ratio in GH3 cells. ** $P < 0.01$, $n = 6$

agonists on the viability of GH3 cells. Applications of EPA, GW9508 and TUG891 did not show any cytotoxic effects on GH3 cells under same conditions. In addition, GPR120 knockdown in GH3 cells did not affect the cytotoxic effects of grifolic acid. Taken together, GPR120 is not involved in the action of grifolic acid on GH3 cells. Grifolic acid was used within a range of 10-100 μmol/L in other studies to activate GPR120 [7, 19, 42, 43]. Considering that the concentration of grifolic acid used in this study is within the same range, it is more likely that grifolic acid is not a pure GPR120 agonist and have other acting targets.

Conclusions

Grifolic acid induces GH3 cell death by inhibiting ATP production. Inhibition of mitochondrial fuel metabolism and NADH production may be the reason for the inhibition of ATP production. GPR120 is not the target of grifolic acid in GH3 cells to induce cell death and the exact signaling molecules for grifolic acid to inhibit cell viability remain to be further elucidated.

Abbreviations

Cyclic pifithrin-α-p-nitro: 2-(4-Nitrophenyl) imidazo[2,1-b]-5,6,7,8-tetrahydrobenzothiazole)ATCCAmerican Type Culture Collection; ATP: Adenosine triphosphate; CCCP: Carbonyl cyanide 3-chlorophenylhydrazone; ELISA: Enzyme linked immunosorbent assay; EPA: Eicosapentaenoic acid; ERK1/2: Extracellular regulated protein kinases; FBS: Fetal bovine serum; GIP: Glucose-dependent insulinotropic polypeptide; GPR120: G protein-coupled receptor 120; JC-1: 5,5′,6,6′-tetrachloro-1,1′,3,3′-tetraethylbenzimi- dazolylcarbocyanine iodide; MMP: Mitochondrial membrane potential; MTT: 3-(4,5-dimethyl-2-thiazolyl)-2,5-diphenyl-2-H-tetrazolium bromide; NADH: Nicotinamide adenine dinucleotide; PBS: Phosphate buffered solution; TUG891: 3-(4-((4-fluoro-49-methyl-[1,19-biphenyl]-2-yl)methoxy)phenyl) propanoic acid

Funding

This work was supported in by the grant from Shaanxi Province (2015KTCQ03-03) and Xi'an Medical University (2015RCYJ02).

Authors' contributions

YZ and LZ designed the study, analyzed the data and drafted the manuscript. AY, DC, RX and YL contributed to acquisition of data, analysis of data and critical revision of the manuscript. XL, YZ, LW and JY designed the experiment for mitochondrial membrane potential assay and flow cytometry and did the work of data analysis and manuscript writing. XX and XS were accountable for all aspects of the work and contributed to the formation of experimental concept and the final approval of the manuscript for publication. All authors gave the final approval of the version to be published.

Competing interests

The authors declare that they have no competing interests.

Author details

[1]The institute of Basic Medical Sciences, Xi'an Medical University, Xi'an 710021, China. [2]Department of Gerontological Surgery, The First Affiliated Hospital, Xi'an Medical University, Xi'an 710061, China. [3]Medical Research Center, The Second Affiliated Hospital, Xi'an Medical University, Xi'an 710038, China.

References

1. Gerhauser C. Cancer chemoprevention and nutriepigenetics: state of the art and future challenges. Top Curr Chem. 2013;329:73–132.
2. Grabovyi GA, Mohr JT. Total synthesis of Grifolin, Grifolic acid, LL-Z1272alpha, LL-Z1272beta, and Ilicicolinic acid a. Org Lett. 2016;18:5010–3.
3. Jin S, Pang RP, Shen JN, Huang G, Wang J, Zhou JG. Grifolin induces apoptosis via inhibition of PI3K/AKT signalling pathway in human osteosarcoma cells. Apoptosis. 2007;12:1317–26.
4. Wu Z, Li Y. Grifolin exhibits anti-cancer activity by inhibiting the development and invasion of gastric tumor cells. Oncotarget. 2017;8:21454–60.
5. Luo XJ, Li LL, Deng QP, Yu XF, Yang LF, Luo FJ, Xiao LB, Chen XY, Ye M, Liu JK, Cao Y. Grifolin, a potent antitumour natural product upregulates death-associated protein kinase 1 DAPK1 via p53 in nasopharyngeal carcinoma cells. Eur J Cancer. 2011;47:316–25. (Oxford, England : 1990)
6. Hara T, Hirasawa A, Sun Q, Sadakane K, Itsubo C, Iga T, Adachi T, Koshimizu TA, Hashimoto T, Asakawa Y, Tsujimoto G. Novel selective ligands for free fatty acid receptors GPR120 and GPR40. Naunyn Schmiedeberg's Arch Pharmacol. 2009;380:247–55.
7. Iwasaki K, Harada N, Sasaki K, Yamane S, Iida K, Suzuki K, Hamasaki A, Nasteska D, Shibue K, Joo E, Harada T, Hashimoto T, Asakawa Y, Hirasawa A, Inagaki N. Free fatty acid receptor GPR120 is highly expressed in enteroendocrine K cells of the upper small intestine and has a critical role in GIP secretion after fat ingestion. Endocrinology. 2015;156:837–46.
8. Hirasawa A, Tsumaya K, Awaji T, Katsuma S, Adachi T, Yamada M, Sugimoto Y, Miyazaki S, Tsujimoto G. Free fatty acids regulate gut incretin glucagon-like peptide-1 secretion through GPR120. Nat Med. 2005;11:90–4.

9. Mehta GU, Lonser RR. Management of hormone-secreting pituitary adenomas. Neuro-Oncology. 2016;
10. Molitch ME. Diagnosis and treatment of pituitary adenomas: a review. JAMA. 2017;317:516–24.
11. Secondo A, De Mizio M, Zirpoli L, Santillo M, Mondola P. The cu-Zn superoxide dismutase (SOD1) inhibits ERK phosphorylation by muscarinic receptor modulation in rat pituitary GH3 cells. Biochem Biophys Res Commun. 2008;376:143–7.
12. Seppet E, Gruno M, Peetsalu A, Gizatullina Z, Nguyen HP, Vielhaber S, Wussling MH, Trumbeckaite S, Arandarcikaite O, Jerzembeck D, Sonnabend M, Jegorov K, Zierz S, Striggow F, Gellerich FN. Mitochondria and energetic depression in cell pathophysiology. Int J Mol Sci. 2009;10:2252–303.
13. Eguchi Y, Shimizu S, Tsujimoto Y. Intracellular ATP levels determine cell death fate by apoptosis or necrosis. Cancer Res. 1997;57:1835–40.
14. Gonzalez VM, Fuertes MA, Alonso C, Perez JM. Is cisplatin-induced cell death always produced by apoptosis? Mol Pharmacol. 2001;59:657–63.
15. van Engeland M, Ramaekers FC, Schutte B, Reutelingsperger CP. A novel assay to measure loss of plasma membrane asymmetry during apoptosis of adherent cells in culture. Cytometry. 1996;24:131–9.
16. Jana S, Sinha M, Chanda D, Roy T, Banerjee K, Munshi S, Patro BS, Chakrabarti S. Mitochondrial dysfunction mediated by quinone oxidation products of dopamine: implications in dopamine cytotoxicity and pathogenesis of Parkinson's disease. Biochim Biophys Acta. 1812;2011:663–73.
17. Yu JH, Song SJ, Kim A, Choi Y, Seok JW, Kim HJ, Lee YJ, Lee KS, Kim JW. Suppression of PPARgamma-mediated monoacylglycerol O-acyltransferase 1 expression ameliorates alcoholic hepatic steatosis. Sci Rep. 2016;6:29352.
18. Zhang X, Yeung ED, Wang J, Panzhinskiy EE, Tong C, Li W, Li J. Isoliquiritigenin, a natural anti-oxidant, selectively inhibits the proliferation of prostate cancer cells. Clin Exp Pharmacol Physiol. 2010;37:841–7.
19. Chen W, Paradkar PN, Li L, Pierce EL, Langer NB, Takahashi-Makise N, Hyde BB, Shirihai OS, Ward DM, Kaplan J, Paw BH. Abcb10 physically interacts with mitoferrin-1 (Slc25a37) to enhance its stability and function in the erythroid mitochondria. Proc Natl Acad Sci U S A. 2009;106:16263–8.
20. Salvioli S, Ardizzoni A, Franceschi C, Cossarizza A. JC-1, but not DiOC6(3) or rhodamine 123, is a reliable fluorescent probe to assess delta psi changes in intact cells: implications for studies on mitochondrial functionality during apoptosis. FEBS Lett. 1997;411:77–82.
21. Perelman A, Wachtel C, Cohen M, Haupt S, Shapiro H, Tzur A. JC-1: alternative excitation wavelengths facilitate mitochondrial membrane potential cytometry. Cell Death Dis. 2012;3:e430.
22. Holliday ND, Watson SJ, Brown AJ. Drug discovery opportunities and challenges at g protein coupled receptors for long chain free fatty acids. Front Endocrinol. 2011;2:112.
23. Che X, Yan H, Sun H, Dongol S, Wang Y, Lv Q, Jiang J. Grifolin induces autophagic cell death by inhibiting the Akt/mTOR/S6K pathway in human ovarian cancer cells. Oncol Rep. 2016;36:1041–7.
24. Anbazhagan AN, Priyamvada S, Gujral T, Bhattacharyya S, Alrefai WA, Dudeja PK, Borthakur A. A novel anti-inflammatory role of GPR120 in intestinal epithelial cells. Am J Physiol Cell physiol. 2016;310:C612–21.
25. Bavelloni A, Faenza I, Aluigi M, Ferri A, Toker A, Maraldi NM, Marmiroli S. Inhibition of phosphoinositide 3-kinase impairs pre-commitment cell cycle traverse and prevents differentiation in erythroleukaemia cells. Cell Death Differ. 2000;7:112–7.
26. Chattopadhyay C, Grimm EA, Woodman SE. Simultaneous inhibition of the HGF/MET and Erk1/2 pathways affect uveal melanoma cell growth and migration. PLoS One. 2014;9:e83957.
27. Huang HC, Chang TM, Chang YJ, Wen HY. UVB irradiation regulates ERK1/2- and p53-dependent thrombomodulin expression in human keratinocytes. PLoS One. 2013;8:e67632.
28. Yea SS, So L, Mallya S, Lee J, Rajasekaran K, Malarkannan S, Fruman DA. Effects of novel isoform-selective phosphoinositide 3-kinase inhibitors on natural killer cell function. PLoS One. 2014;9:e99486.
29. Leist M, Single B, Castoldi AF, Kuhnle S, Nicotera P. Intracellular adenosine triphosphate (ATP) concentration: a switch in the decision between apoptosis and necrosis. J Exp Med. 1997;185:1481–6.
30. Ferrari D, Stepczynska A, Los M, Wesselborg S, Schulze-Osthoff K. Differential regulation and ATP requirement for caspase-8 and caspase-3 activation during CD95- and anticancer drug-induced apoptosis. J Exp Med. 1998;188:979–84.
31. Nicotera P, Leist M, Ferrando-May E. Intracellular ATP, a switch in the decision between apoptosis and necrosis. Toxicol Lett. 1998;102-103:139–42.
32. Newmeyer DD, Ferguson-Miller S. Mitochondria: releasing power for life and unleashing the machineries of death. Cell. 2003;112:481–90.
33. Garcia-Souza LF, Oliveira MF. Mitochondria: biological roles in platelet physiology and pathology. Int J Biochem Cell Biol. 2014;50:156–60.
34. Reers M, Smith TW, Chen LB. J-aggregate formation of a carbocyanine as a quantitative fluorescent indicator of membrane potential. Biochemistry. 1991;30:4480–6.
35. Smiley ST, Reers M, Mottola-Hartshorn C, Lin M, Chen A, Smith TW, Steele GD Jr, Chen LB. Intracellular heterogeneity in mitochondrial membrane potentials revealed by a J-aggregate-forming lipophilic cation JC-1. Proc Natl Acad Sci U S A. 1991;88:3671–5.
36. Sureda FX, Escubedo E, Gabriel C, Comas J, Camarasa J, Camins A. Mitochondrial membrane potential measurement in rat cerebellar neurons by flow cytometry. Cytometry. 1997;28:74–80.
37. Wang MX, Ren LM. Growth inhibitory effect and apoptosis induced by extracellular ATP and adenosine on human gastric carcinoma cells: involvement of intracellular uptake of adenosine. Acta Pharmacol Sin. 2006;27:1085–92.
38. Sun Q, Hirasawa A, Hara T, Kimura I, Adachi T, Awaji T, Ishiguro M, Suzuki T, Miyata N, Tsujimoto G. Structure-activity relationships of GPR120 agonists based on a docking simulation. Mol Pharmacol. 2010;78:804–10.
39. Yonezawa T, Kurata R, Yoshida K, Murayama MA, Cui X, Hasegawa A. Free fatty acids-sensing G protein-coupled receptors in drug targeting and therapeutics. Curr Med Chem. 2013;20:3855–71.
40. Briscoe CP, Peat AJ, McKeown SC, Corbett DF, Goetz AS, Littleton TR, McCoy DC, Kenakin TP, Andrews JL, Ammala C, Fornwald JA, Ignar DM, Jenkinson S. Pharmacological regulation of insulin secretion in MIN6 cells through the fatty acid receptor GPR40: identification of agonist and antagonist small molecules. Br J Pharmacol. 2006;148:619–28.
41. Hudson BD, Shimpukade B, Mackenzie AE, Butcher AJ, Pediani JD, Christiansen E, Heathcote H, Tobin AB, Ulven T, Milligan G. The pharmacology of TUG-891, a potent and selective agonist of the free fatty acid receptor 4 (FFA4/GPR120), demonstrates both potential opportunity and possible challenges to therapeutic agonism. Mol Pharmacol. 2013;84:710–25.
42. Janssen S, Laermans J, Iwakura H, Tack J, Depoortere I. Sensing of fatty acids for octanoylation of ghrelin involves a gustatory G-protein. PLoS One. 2012;7:e40168.
43. Murase R, Sato H, Yamamoto K, Ushida A, Nishito Y, Ikeda K, Kobayashi T, Yamamoto T, Taketomi Y, Murakami M. Group X Secreted phospholipase A2 releases omega3 polyunsaturated fatty acids, suppresses colitis, and promotes sperm fertility. J Biol Chem. 2016;291:6895–911.

14

Self-medication practice and associated factors among adult household members

Aster Desalew Kassie[1], Berhanu Boru Bifftu[2] and Habtamu Sewunet Mekonnen[2*]

Abstract

Background: Self-medication practice (SMP) is the use of medication without the prescription of health care professionals. The major problems associated with self-medication practice have been drug resistance, drug side effects, wastage of resources, and serious health hazards including death. Thus, the main purpose of this study was to assess the prevalence of self-medication practice and its associated factors among adult household members in Meket District, Northeast Ethiopia.

Methods: A community based cross-sectional study was conducted among 722 adult household members in Meket District, from April 5 to May 5, 2017. The systematic random sampling method was used to select study participants. A pre-tested, structured questionnaire was used for data collection using an interviewer-administered technique. Epi-info version and SPSS version 22 were utilized for data entry and analysis, respectively. Univariate and multivariate logistic regression was used to identify association factors.

Results: The overall prevalence of self-medication was found to be 35.9%. Unmarried status (AOR = 2.17, 95% CI = 1.18, 4.01), previous experience of self-medication (AOR = 1.78, 95% CI = 1.22, 2.61), accessibility of pharmacies (AOR = 3.71, 95% CI = 1.31, 10.51), peer/family pressure (AOR = 2.88, 95% CI = 1.98, 4.18) and presence of medication at home (AOR = 1.80, 95% CI = 1.11, 2.92) were factors associated with self-medication practices.

Conclusion: More than one-third of the study participants practiced self-medication. Thus, strengthening communities awareness on drug side effects and integrated efforts of individuals, communities, health facilities, and regulatory bodies are highly necessary.

Keywords: Adult, Northeast Ethiopia, Self-medication practice

Background

Self-medication practice (SMP), as one element of self-care, is the use of medication without the prescription of health care professionals (e.g. resubmitting old prescriptions, sharing medication with relatives/family members or using leftover medications) for the treatment of self--recognized illnesses [1]. Globally, the prevalence of SMP is inconsistent ranging from 32.5 to 81.5% [2–4]. In Ethiopia, the prevalence of self-medication practice ranges from 12.8% to 77.1% [5].

Essential medications are planned to be available in-appropriately functioning health systems at intended times, in sufficient amounts, in the proper dosage forms, in assured quality and adequate information, and at prices the individual and the community can afford [6]. However, self-medication practice influences health care seeking behavior of individuals. It leads to wastage of resources, delay in diagnosis of problems and appropriate treatments. Can also lead to serious health hazards and adverse drug reactions [6, 7].

People may practice self medication for a variety of reasons, like the urge for self-care, sympathy for family members in sickness, lack of health services, poverty, ignorance, misbelief, excessive advertisements of drugs,

* Correspondence: habtsew@ymail.com
[2]University of Gondar, College of Medicine and Health Science, School of Nursing, Gondar, Ethiopia
Full list of author information is available at the end of the article

and availability of drugs in establishments other than pharmacies [8].

Self-medication has an important role in health care and in the continued improvement of public education [9]. Despite this studies found out that medical and health science students are the most prone groups to practice self-medication recurrently. The studies done in India in two phases showed that the prevalence of self-medication practices among students were 74.6% and 69.4%, respectively. Oral antibacterial and anti-inflammatory agents and antipyretics were the most common group of drugs used in both phases of the study [10]. Other studies which examined the prevalence of self medication, for example, on students in Belgrade, Serbia [11], three institutes in Nagara, Mandya district, Karnataka [12], South India [13], Jiangsu University, eastern China [14], in Brazil [15], at a tertiary care medical college, West Bengal [16] and Mekele University, Ethiopia [17], reported 79.9%, 92.39%, 78.6%, 47.9%, 56.0%,43.24%, respectively.

Still other studies in primary health care centers in Erbil City (52.6%) [18], a public health care system in Tabuk City (83.3%) [19], Dental patients in Bangalore (100%) [20], at four hospitals in Dar es Salaam, Tanzania (88.6%) [21] and among diabetic patients in Southeast Iran (80.7%) [22], reported the prevalence of self medication practice.

According to such studies, level of education, pervious experience of self-medication, occupation, lack of medical insurance, lack of time to visit physicians, low income [23–25], female sex [26], urban residece [27], youth age [28] and men [29, 30] were factors associated with SMP. Despite the negative consequences of self-medication and its high spread, studies on its prevalence and associated factors in this study area are limited. Therefore, the aim of this study was to assess the prevalence of self-medication practice and associated factors among adult household members in Meket District, Northeast Ethiopia.

Methods

Study design and period

A community-based cross sectional study design was used to conduct the study from April, 5 to May, 5, 2017.

Study area

The study was conducted in Meket district found in North Wollo Zone, Amhara Region Northeast Ethiopia. It is located at 1015 km from Addis Ababa the capital of Ethiopia. This district has 36 kebeles (lowest administrative units) and total of 273,617 inhabitants. Of these, 137,629 (50.3%) were females. In addition to eight government health centers, the district has four clinics and two pharmacies owned privately.

Source population

All people in Meket district, Northeast Ethiopia.

Study population

All adults, (age ≥ 18 years) in Meket district, Northeast Ethiopia.

Sampling frame

The official records were used as frames to determine sample kebeles and households.

Inclusion criteria

All people aged ≥18 years and had live in for at least six months in the district.

Exclusion criteria

People who were seriously ill and incapable of hearing and speaking at the time of data collection were excluded.

Sample size and sampling procedure

The sample size was calculated by using the single population proportion formula ($n = [(Z\alpha/2)2 \times P\ (1\text{-}P)]/D2$), by assumptioning, a prevalence of self-medication practice as 32.55% [31], 95% CI =1.96, margin of error 5%, design effect of 2 and plus 10% non-response rate, the final sample size was 744. In accordance with the multistage stratified sampling method, seven kebeles were selected by using the lottery method. Then, the total sample was proportionally allocated to each kebeles. Finally, participants were selected by the systematic random sampling method.

Data collection tool and procedure

For the assessment of the theme of the research, a questionnaire which included socio- demographic factors, history of illness in the month preceding the study, and self-medication practice was prepared. The data were collected by 14 health extension workers supervised by seven BSc degree graduate nurses.

Data were collected in a face-to- face interview on a structured questionnaire. Whenever selected houses were found closed or missing adult members, they were revisited continuously for three subsequent days in order to collect data. For house-holds which were missing adult members, the nearest houses were selected, while houses which were found closed during the three subsequent days were considered as non-response cases. When multiple adults were preset in the same household, lottery was used to select a single adult. The required data were collected after written informed consents were obtained (Additional file 1).

Data quality control

The questionnaire prepared in English was translated into the local language, Amharic and then to ensure consistency, it was retranslated to English. A pre-test was conducted on 38 participants in non-selected kebeles two weeks prior to the actual data collection

Table 1 Socio-emographic characteristics of respondents, Meket district, Northeast Ethiopia, 2017 (*n* = 722)

Variables	Category	Frequency	Percent
Sex	Female	384	53.2
	Male	338	46.8
Age in year	18–24	92	12.8
	25–34	180	24.9
	35–44	180	24.9
	45–54	113	15.7
	> 55	157	21.7
Marital statues	Married	450	62.3
	Unmarried	105	14.5
	Divorced	102	14.1
	Widowed	65	9.0
Occupation	Farmer	329	45.6
	Housewife	136	18.8
	Civil servant	107	14.8
	Student	71	9.8
	Merchant	65	9.1
	Daily workers	14	1.9
Average monthly household income	< 150 birr	58	8.1
	150–500 birr	292	40.4
	501–1000 birr	143	19.8
	> 1000 birr	229	31.7
Place of residence	Rural	525	72.7
	Urban	197	27.3
Level of education	Unable to read and write	303	42.0
	Only able to read and write	137	19.0
	1–8 grades	105	14.5
	9–12 grades	63	8.7
	Diploma and above	114	15.8
Religion	Orthodox	649	89.9
	Muslim	70	9.7
	Protestant	3	0.4
Ethnicity	Amhara	705	97.6
	Tigray	17	2.4
Number of family	< 5	576	79.8
	5 and above	146	20.2
Relationship with family	Father	283	39.2
	Mother	310	42.9
	Child	115	15.9
	Relative	14	1.9

date. A one day training was given to data collectors and supervisors about the questionnaire and data collection techniques.

Table 2 Environmental and personal characteristics of participants, Meket district Northeast Ethiopia, 2017 (*n* = 722)

Variable	Category	Frequency	Percent
Distance of health institution	< 1 h	100	13.9
	≥ 1 h	622	86.2
Accessibility of pharmacy	Yes	198	27.4
	No	524	72.6
Presence of health profession in the family	Yes	56	7.2
	No	666	92.8
Presence of medication at home	Yes	105	14.5
	No	617	85.5
Previous experience of SMP	Yes	402	55.7
	No	320	44.3
Peer/family pressure	Yes	226	31.3
	No	496	68.7
Member of health insurance	Yes	448	62.0
	No	274	38.0

Operational definition

In this study, self-medication practice was defined as any use of medications without the prescribtions of health care professionals (such as physicians, nurses, health officers and other who have government license to prescribe drugs) for the treatment of self- recognized illnesses in the last one month [32].

Data processing and analysis

Data were cheeked for completeness and consistency before entry. Coded data were entered into EPI-info version 7 and exported to Statistical Package for Social Science (SPSS) version 22 for analysis. Descriptive statistics like, frequency, percentage, mean, standardization, and median were used for data presentation. Univariate and multivariate logistic regression was fitted to identify associated factors with 95% CI using *p*-value < 0.05 as a cutoff point.

Results

Socio-demographic characteristics of respondents

In this study, 744 participants were enrolled with a response rate of 722 (97%). The mean age of the respondents was 40.51 years (standard deviation ±14. 6). More than half (53.2%) of the participants were female 450 (62.3%) of whom were married. Three hundred and twenty-nine (45.6%) were farmers by occupation. The majority of the respondents 649, (89. 9%), were Orthodox Christians and 705 (97.6%) of whom were Amhara by ethnicity. Regarding educational level, 303 (42.0%) were unable to read and write (Table 1).

Table 3 Reasons of participants for self-medication practice, Meket district, Northeast Ethiopia, April to May, 2017, ($n = 259$)

Reasons	Frequency	Percent
Perceive illness as mild	130	50.2
Similarity of symptoms with past illness	36	13.9
Need quick relive	20	7.7
Unable to afford the health care fee	33	12.7
Dissatisfaction by health care system service	17	6.6
Long waiting time	23	8.9

Environmental and personal characteristics of participants

In this study, the majority of the participants, 622 (86. 15%), traveled over one hour to reach health institutions, while 524 (72.58%) had access to pharmacies. On the whole, 617 (85.46%) had medication at home (Table 2).

Reasons of participants for self-medication practice

Perceptions of illness as mild 130 (50.19%), similarity of symptoms with previous illnesses 36 (13.9%) and inability to afford health care fee 33 (12.74%) were the major reasons for self-medication practice (Table 3).

Symptoms' of illnesses and utilized groups of medications

Among the total 722 study participants, 435 (60.2%) complained about illnesses in the last one month. Headache/fever 217 (30.06%) and analgesics/antipyretics 113 (40.79%) were the common symptom and utilized self-medications (Fig. 1).

Prevalence of self-medication practice

In this study, the prevalence of self-medication practice was found to be 259 (35.9%) (95% Cl: 32.7, 39.2).

Factors associated with self-medication practice

According to the multivariate logistic regression analysis, unmarried status, previous experience of self-medication, accessibility of pharmacy, peer/family pressure, and the presence of medication at home were factors associated with self-medication practice. Unmarried respondents were 2 times (AOR = 2.17, 95% CI = 1.18, 4.01) more likely to practice self-medication compared to married respondents.

Previous experience of SMP was nearly two times (AOR = 1.78, 95% CI = 1.22, 2.61) more likely experienced self-medication practice than their counter respondents. Accessibility of pharmacy were nearly four times (AOR = 3.71, 95% CI = 1.31, 10.51) more likely experienced self-medication practice compared to those inaccessibility. Respondents who had medication at home were nearly 2 times (AOR = 1.80, 95% CI = 1.11, 2.92) more likely to practice self-medication compared to those who had not such access. The odds ratio of self medication practice among respondents who had peer/family pressure was almost 3 times (AOR = 2.88, 95% Cl = 1.98, 4.18) more likely practice self medication compared to those who had not peer pressure (Table 4).

Discussion

In this study, the overall prevalence of self-medication practice was found to be 35.9% (95% Cl; 32.70, 39.20). This finding is in-line with other studies of carried out in different parts of Ethiopia such as Nekemte (36.7%) [33], DireDawa (41%) and Koladiba [31]. This result is also similar with study carried out in South India (35.9%) [34].

The current finding is higher than those of the studies done in Bahir Dar (23,3%) [35], Sire town (27.16%) [36], Silte zone (24.40%) [37] and Brazil (16%) [26]. On the

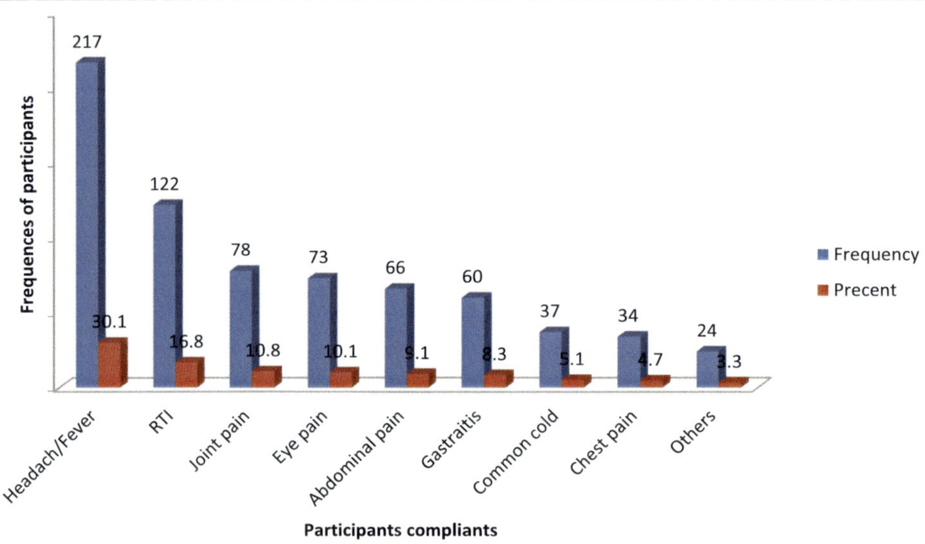

Fig. 1 Participants complaints for self medication practice, Meket District, Northeast Ethiopia, 2017, ($n = 435$)

Table 4 Univariate and multivariate logistic regression analysis of self medication practice among participants, Meket district, Northeast Ethiopia, 2017($n = 722$)

Variables	Category	Self medication practice		COR (95% CI)	AOR (95% CI)
		Yes	No		
Sex	Female	153	231	1.45(1.07, 1.97)*	1.11(0.76, 1.63)
	Male	106	232	1	1
Age in year	18–24	32	60	1	1
	25–34	51	129	0.74(0.43, 1.27)	0.86(0.45, 1.66)
	35–44	60	120	0.94 (0.58, 1.52)	1.29(0.62, 2.69)
	45–54	44	69	1.2(0.68, 2.12)	1.42(0.64, 3.17)
	> 55	72	85	1.54(0.93, 2.79)	1.73(0.80, 3.75)
Marital status	Married	140	310	1	1
	Unmarried	42	63	1.48(0.95, 2.29)	2.17(1.18, 4.01)**
	Divorced	44	58	1.68(1.08, 2.61)*	1.28(0.76, 2.14)
	Widowed	33	32	2.28(1.35, 3.86)*	1.32(0.704, 2.48)
Level of education	Unable to read and write	124	179	1	1
	Only able to read and write	41	96	0.62(0.40, 0.95)	0.73(0.45, 1.20)
	1-8grade	34	71	0.69(0.43, 1.10)	0.82(0.45, 1.48)
	9-12grade	20	43	0.67(0.38, 1.2)	0.55(0.25, 1.23)
	Diploma and above	40	74	0.78(0.50, 1.23)	0.85(0.42, 1.71)
Average household monthly income	<150birr	27	31	1.62(0.91, 2.91)	1.28(0.62, 2.66)
	150-500birr	109	183	1.11(0.77, 1.59)	1.22(0.75, 2.01)
	501–1000 birr	43	100	0.80(0.51, 1.26)	0.91(0.52, 1.58)
	> 1000 birr	80	149	1	1
Place of residence	Urban	82	115	1	1
	Rural	117	348	0.47(0.51, 0.99)*	1.97(0.69, 5.64)
Accessibility of pharmacy	Yes	89	108	1.72(1.23, 2.41)*	3.71(1.31, 10.51)**
	No	170	355	1	1
Presence of medication at home	Yes	58	47	2.56(1.68, 3.69)*	1.80(1.11, 2.92)**
	No	201	416	1	1
Previous experience of SMP	Yes	185	217	2.83(2.05, 3.93)*	1.78(1.22, 2.61)**
	No	74	246	1	1
Peer/family pressure	Yes	128	98	3.64(2.62, 5.06)*	2.88(1.98, 4.13)**
	No	131	365	1	1
Due to lack of time	Yes	32	31	1.96(1.17, 3.30)*	1.61(0.90, 2.89)
	No	227	432	1	1
Distance of health institution	< 1 h	27	73	1	1
	≥ 1 h	232	390	1.61(1.01, 2.57)*	1.45(0.85, 2.47)

*Variables those were significant during univariate logistic analysis at P value < = 0.05
**Variables that was found to have significant association during multivariate analysis at p value < = 0.05

other hand, the prevalence of SMP in this study is lower than those of conducted in Pakistan (61.20%) [38], India (55%) [30], and Italy (69.20%) [32]. This may be due to the differences in socio-demographic factors and sample sizes. In the Pakistan study the sample size was 500 from which health professionals who were found in the community were excluded from the study. In the Indian study, the sample size was 260, and the study participants were only urban residents. Regarding associated factors, unmarried participants were two times (AOR 2.17, 95% Cl; 1.18, 4.01) more likely to utilize self medication compared to married respondents. This is consistent with the study finding in India [34]. The possible explanation could be that unmarried respondents are more influenced by peer pressure than married ones.

Those participants who had access to pharmacies were nearly 4 times (AOR 3.71, 95% Cl; 1.31, 10.51) more likely to utiliz self medication compared to those who hadn't. This result is consistent with those of studies carried out in China [39], India [34], and Nigeria [40]. This might be due to lack of income and time to consult health care professionals. This is supported by finding in that inability to afford health care fees is noted as the reason for self-medication practice. Previous experience of SMP was nearly 2 times (AOR 1.78, 95% Cl; 1.22, 2. 61) more likely to lead to self-medication compared to those who hadn't previous experience. This study is similar with the study finding in Jimma [41], Uganda [42], Nigeria [40] and Congo [43]. The possible explanation could be that those who had experience may have some awareness about treatment which encourage them, to use self medication rather than taking other actions.

Participants who had peer/family pressure were nearly 3 times (AOR 2.88, 95%Cl; 1.98, 4.18) more likely to use self-medication compared to those who hadn't. The current result is consistent with those of studies carried out in China [39] and Uganda [42]. The possible explanation may be that friends/families were the common sources of information about medication.

Participants who had medication at home were nearly 2 times (AOR 1.80, 95% Cl; 1.11, 2.92) more likely to use self medication than who hadn't. This finding is consistent with that of the studies in South India [34] and Egypt [44]. This is due to the fact that participants who store medication mostly for the purpose of emergency in cases of similar illnesses in the future would have the possibility to use it. In the current study, 105 (14.5%) participants had medication at home, and 55.2% of them used self-medication.

The category of medication mostly used in this study included analgesics/antipyretics, antibiotics, GI medications, and eye medication, while headaches, fever, respiratory tract infection, gastrointestinal diseases and eye diseases were the conditions for which self-medication was used. These findings are consistent with other studies [31, 36, 37, 45] as well as studies in Nigeria [40] and India [46].

The most common reasons why respondents practiced self-medication were perceiving illnesses as mild 68 (26. 3%), the similarity of illnesses with the past 26 (10.%) and unable to afford health care fee 20 (7.7%).This is similar with studies done in Sire town [36], Jimma town [29] and Iran [47].

As to the limitation; this study was intended to assess modern self-medication practice, which does not include the traditional medications. So, the prevalence of SMP might be under estimated. This imposed the generalization of the findings to all types of medications.

Conclusion

More than one-third of the study participants practiced self-medication. Factors like being unmarried, presence of medication at home, accessibility of pharmacies, peer pressure and previous experience of SMP were the predictors of self-medication practice. Strengthening of the communities awarness on the side effects of self medication practice and regulation of pharmacies are very important mechanisms to decrease the practice. Thus, integrated efforts of individuals, communities, health facilities, and the regulatory bodies are highly important.

Abbreviations

AOR: Adjusted odd ratio; COR: Crude odd ratio; POM: Prescription only medication; SMP: Self medication practice; SPSS: Statistical Package for Social Sciences; WHO: World Health Organization

Acknowledgements

Authors would like to express our gratitude to University of Gondar College of Medicine and Health Science School of Nursing for the ethical clearance approval and Amhara Regional State Health Bureau for financial support. The authors also would like to thank supervisors and data collectors for their effort and the study participants for their participation.

Authors' contribution

ADK wrote the proposal, participated in data collection, analyzed and drafted the manuscript. BBB and HSM participated in data analysis and review of the manuscript. All authors read and approved the final manuscript.

Funding

This study was funded by Amhara Regional State Health Bureau. However, the funder had no role in study design, data collection, analysis, preparation of the manuscript and decision to publish.

Competing interests

The authors declared that they have no any competing interests.

Author details

[1]Boru Meda District Hospital, South Wollo Zone, Amhara Region, Southeast, Ethiopia. [2]University of Gondar, College of Medicine and Health Science, School of Nursing, Gondar, Ethiopia.

References

1. World Health Organization. Responsible self-care and self-medication; a worldwide review of consumers' survey; the world self-medication industry. 2010.
2. Lam CLCM, Munro C, Lauder IJ. Self-medication among Hong Kong Chinese. Soc Sci Med. 1994;39(12):1641–7.
3. Sanghani SZH, Patel VJ. Self medication: prevalence and pattern in urban community. J Pharmacovigilance Drug Safety. 2008;5:95–8.
4. Phalke VDPD, Durgawale PM. Self-medication practices in rural Maharashtra. Indian J Commun Med. 2006;31(1):34–5.
5. Ayalew MB. Self-medication practice in Ethiopia: a systematic review. Patient preference and adherence. 2017;11:401.
6. WHO. Essential medicines in WHO regions. 2017.

7. Ganguly NKAN, Chandy SJ, Fairoze MN, Gill JP, Gupta U, Hossain S, Joglekar S, Joshi PC, Kakkar M, Kotwani A, Rattan A, Sudarshan H, Thomas K, Wattal C, Easton A, Laxminarayan R, Global Antibiotic Resistance Partnership (GARP) - India Working Group. Rationalizing antibiotic use to limit antibiotic resistance in India. Indian J Med Res. 2011;134:281–94.
8. Li LJWP. Self-medication with antibiotics: a possible cause of bacterial resistance. Med Hypotheses. 2005;65:1000–1.
9. WHO. WHO drug information. General Policy Issues. 2000;14(1):18–26. http://apps.who.int/medicinedocs/en/d/Jh1462e/.
10. Kumar R, Goyal A, Padhy BM, Gupta YK. Self-medication practice and factors influencing it among medical and paramedical students in India: a two-period comparative cross-sectional study. journal of natural science, biology and medicine. 2016;7(2):143–8.
11. Lukovic JA, Miletic V, Pekmezovic T, Trajkovic G, Ratkovic N, et al. SelfMedication Practices and Risk Factors for SelfMedication among Medical Students in Belgrade, Serbia. PLoS ONE. 2014;9(12):e114644. https://doi.org/10.1371/journal.pone.0114644.
12. Johnson D, Sekhar HS, Alex T, Kumaraswamy M, Chopra RS. Self medication practice among medical, pharmacy and nursing students. Int J Pharm Pharm Sci. 2016;8(7). ISSN-0975-1491.
13. Kumar N, Kanchan T, Unnikrishnan B, Rekha T, Mithra P, et al. Perceptions and Practices of Self-Medication among Medical Students in Coastal South India. PLoS ONE. 2013;8(8):e72247. https://doi.org/10.1371/journal.pone.0072247.
14. Zhu X, Pan H, Yang Z, Cui B, Zhang D, Ba-Thein W. Self-medication practices with antibiotics among Chinese university students: Elsevier Ltd; 2015.
15. Gama ASM, Secoli SR. Self-medication among nursing students in the state of Amazonas – Brazil. Rev Gaúcha Enferm. 2017;38(1):e65111. http://dx.doi.org/10.1590/1983-1447.2017.01.65111.
16. Banerjee TB I. Self-medication practice among undergraduate medical students in a tertiary care medical college. West Bengal J Postgrad Med. 2012;58(2):127–31.
17. Gutema GB, Gadisa DA, Kidanemariam ZA, Berhe DF, Berhe AH, Hadera MG, Hailu GS, Gebresamuel N, Abrha NG, Yarlagadda R, Dagne AW. Self-medication practices among health sciences students: the case of Mekelle university. Journal of Applied Pharmaceutical Science. 2011;01(10):183–9.
18. Ahmed NM. Self-medication practice among patients attending a sample of primary health care centers in Erbil City. Journal of Education and Practice. 2016;7(24):73–79.
19. Albalawi AH, Alanazi BD, Althmali KA, Alzhahrani OM, Aloqbi HS. A descriptive study of self-medication practices among patients in a public health care system in Tabuk City. International Journal of Academic Scientific Research. 2015;3(4):127–33.
20. KomalRaj MR, Bhat PK, Aruna CN. Self medication practices for ORAL health problems among DENTAL patients in Bangalore: a cross sectional study. IOSR Journal Of Pharmacy. 2015;5(10):68–75.
21. Kagashe GAB, BM. Self medication among patients seen at ophthalmology clinics at four hospitals in Dar Es Salaam Tanzania. IOSR Journal of Pharmacy. 2012;2(5):21–5.
22. Hossein Ansari SMH. Salehodin Boya, Fariba Zare, Mostafa, Peyvand ME. Prevalence of self-medication practices and drug use in patients with diabetes mellitus type 2: a cross sectional study in southeast of Iran. Pharm Lett. 2016;8(8):192–7.
23. Afolabi A. Self medication, drug dependency and self-managed health care-a review: INTECH open access Publisher; 2012.
24. Shaghaghi A, Asadi M, Allahverdipour H. Predictors of self-medication behavior: a systematic review. Iranian journal of public health. 2014; 43(2):136.
25. Yadav S, Rawal G. Self-medication practice in low income countries. Int J Pharmaceut Chem Anal. 2015;2(3):139–42.
26. Arrais PSD, Fernandes MEP, da Silva Dal Pizzol T, Ramos LR, Mengue SS, Luiza VL, et al. Prevalence of self-medication in Brazil and associated factors. Rev Saude Publica. 2016;50(suppl 2):13s.
27. Balamurugan E, Ganesh K. Prevalence and pattern of self medication use in coastal regions of South India. Br J Med Pract. 2011;4(3):a428.
28. Garofalo L, Di Giuseppe G, Angelillo IF. Self-medication practices among parents in Italy. Biomed Res Int. 2015;2015. https://doi.org/10.1155/2015/580650.
29. Ararsa A, Bekele A. Assessment of self-medication practice and drug storage on private pharmacy clients in Jimma town, Oromia, south West Ethiopia. Trends in Drug Delivery. 2014;1(3):17–29.
30. Marak A, Borah M, Bhattacharyya H, Talukdar K. A cross-sectional study on self-medication practices among the rural population of Meghalaya. International Journal of Medical Science and Public Health. 2016;5(6):1134–8.
31. Abrha S, Fantahun Molla WM. Self-medication practice: the case of Kolladiba town. North West Ethiopia: International Journal of Pharma Sciences and Research (IJPSR); 2014.
32. Luca Garofalo, Gabriella Di Giuseppe, and Italo F. Angelillo, "Self-Medication Practices among Parents in Italy," BioMed Research International. 2015;2015: 8. https://doi.org/10.1155/2015/580650.
33. Sado E, Gedif T. Drug utilization at household level in Nekemte town and surrounding rural areas, western Ethiopia: a cross-sectional study. Open Access Library Journal. 2014;1(03):1.
34. Divya M, Bharatesh S, Vasudeva G, Varalakshmi C. Self-Medication Among Adults in Urban Udupi Taluk, Southern India. International Journal of Medicine and Public Health. 2016;6(3):126–129.
35. Tena M. Self-medication practices with antibiotics among urban dwellers of Bahir Dar town. North West Ethiopia: AAU; 2014.
36. Jaleta A, Tesema S, Yimam B. Self-medication practice in sire town, West Ethiopia: a cross-sectional study. Cukurova Medical Journal. 2016;41(3):447–52.
37. Wabe NT, Ahmed D, Angamo MT. Self-medication with antibiotics and antimalarials in the community of Silte zone, South Ethiopia. TAF Preventive medicine Bulletin. 2012;11(5):529–36.
38. Aqeel T, Shabbir A, Basharat H, Bukhari M, Mobin S, Shahid H, et al. Prevalence of self-medication among urban and rural population of Islamabad, Pakistan. Trop J Pharm Res. 2014;13(4):627–33.
39. Wen Y, Lieber E, Wan D, Hong Y. A qualitative study about self-medication in the community among market vendors in Fuzhou, China. Health & social care in the community. 2011;19(5):504–13.
40. Abdulraheem I, Adegboye A, Fatiregun A. Self-medication with antibiotics: empirical evidence from a Nigerian rural population. BRITISH JOURNAL OF PHARMACEUTICAL RESEARCH. 2016;11(5):1–13. https://doi.org/10.9734/BJPR/2016/25268.
41. Befekadu A, Dhekama NH, Mohammed MA. Self-medication and contributing factors among pregnant women attending antenatal care in Ethiopia: the case of Jimma University specialized hospital. Medicine Science. 2014;3(1):969–81. https://doi.org/10.5455/medscience.2013.02.8098.
42. Ocan M, Bwanga F, Bbosa GS, Bagenda D, Waako P, Ogwal-Okeng J, et al. Patterns and predictors of self-medication in northern Uganda. PLoS One. 2014;9(3):e92323.
43. Mbarambara PM, Songa PB, Wansubi LM, Mututa PM, Minga BBK, Bisangamo CK. Self-medication practice among pregnant women attending antenatal care at health centers in Bukavu, eastern DR Congo. International Journal of Innovation and Applied Studies. 2016;16(1):38.
44. Helal R, Abou-Elwafa H. Self-medication in university students from the City of Mansoura, Egypt. J Environ Public Health. 2017;2017. https://doi.org/10.1155/2017/9145193.
45. Abebe B, Bizatu M. Self medication practices and associated factors among house holds in Dire Dawa town. Eastern Ethiopia: Harmaya University; 2016.
46. Borah H, Kakati R, Borah M, Deka C. Self-medication practices and its determinants among urban dwellers of Dibrugarh town, Assam. Scholars Journal of Applied Medical Sciences (SJAMS). 2016;4(8E):3100–3106. https://doi.org/10.21276/sjams.2016.4.8.71.
47. Jafari F, Khatony A, Rahmani E. Prevalence of self-medication among the elderly in Kermanshah-Iran. Global journal of health science. 2015;7(2):360.

15

Inflammation down-regulates CYP3A4-catalysed drug metabolism in hemodialysis patients

Hadi Molanaei[1], Abdul Rashid Qureshi[1], Olof Heimbürger[1], Bengt Lindholm[1], Ulf Diczfalusy[2], Björn Anderstam[1], Leif Bertilsson[3†] and Peter Stenvinkel[1*†]

Abstract

Background: Recent studies indicate that inflammation may also affect CYP3A4 activity. Associations of CYP3A4-mediated metabolism of quinine, with inflammatory biomarkers were investigated in patients undergoing maintenance hemodialysis (HD).

Methods: A single dose of 100 mg quinine was given to 44 HD patients and the plasma concentration of quinine and its metabolite 3-OH-quinine were measured 12 h after drug intake. The ratios of quinine/3-OH-quinine and 4β-OH-cholesterol/cholesterol were used as markers of CYP3A4 activity. Inflammatory biomarkers, high-sensitive CRP (hsCRP), pentraxin 3 (PTX3) and orosomucoid were followed during 4 weeks prior to quinine administration.

Results: The quinine/3-OH-quinine ratio correlated with median concentrations of hsCRP (Rho = 0.48; $p = 0.001$) and orosomucoid (Rho = 0.44; $p = 0.003$), and also with interleukin-6 at 12 h after drug intake (Rho = 0.43; $P = 0.004$) but not PTX3. In multivariate regression analysis, the correlation between CYP3A4 activity and median hsCRP remained borderline significant ($p = 0.05$). 4β-OH-cholesterol/cholesterol ratio correlated with quinine/3-OH-quinine ($p = 0.008$), but not with any of the inflammation markers.

Conclusions: The association between CYP3A4 activity and inflammatory biomarkers suggest that the activity of CYP3A4 is reduced by inflammation in HD patients. Further studies are needed to confirm this finding and to assess to what extent magnitude and duration of inflammation as well as the microbiota affect drug metabolism.

Keywords: Inflammation, CYP3A4, hemodialysis, Drug metabolism, quinine

Background

Chronic kidney disease (CKD) patients are at a high risk for drug side effects due to accumulation of drugs, which normally are excreted via the kidneys. It is believed that drugs that are metabolized by the liver are safe to prescribe in normal doses to end-stage renal disease (ESRD) patients. However, emerging data show that kidney failure itself can affect enzymes and drug transporters [1, 2]. Thus, the concentration of many drugs that normally are metabolized by the liver increases significantly in CKD patients. It is also possible that renal failure modifies drug interactions, including the affinity of some drugs to their receptor, the number of receptors, and the cell responses upon receptor activation. Taken together, all these factors contribute to a high risk of both under- and overdosing of drugs in this patient group.

A common feature of the uremic phenotype that may affect drug metabolism is persistent inflammation [3, 4]. Inflammation has been shown to reduce the activity of both drug metabolizing enzymes and transporters [5–8]. Pro-inflammatory cytokines are thought to be principal mediators of the impact of inflammation on these enzymes and transporters [6]. The mechanism of this inhibitory effect is not clear so far but the transcriptional suppression is thought to be a major factor in the down-regulation of many cytochrome P450s and there could

* Correspondence: peter.stenvinkel@ki.se
†Leif Bertilsson and Peter Stenvinkel contributed equally to this work.
[1]Division of Renal Medicine and Baxter Novum, Department of Clinical Science, Intervention and Technology, Karolinska Institutet, Karolinska University Hospital, SE-141 86 Stockholm, Sweden
Full list of author information is available at the end of the article

be multiple posttranscriptional effects involved as well [6]. Presence of the above mentioned factors increases the risk of side effect and drug interactions even more, especially in ESRD patients who on a daily basis take > 20 pills per day [9]. No doubt, such a large number of prescribed pills contributes to unintentional poor compliance in this patient group and adherence to drug prescriptions is in general much lower in dialysis patients than anticipated [10, 11].

By using alprazolam as a test drug we previously showed that a low degree of inflammation significantly reduced the activity of CYP3A4 [12], which is the most important hepatic drug-metabolizing enzyme accounting for the metabolism of almost 50% of all drugs currently used [13, 14]. Thus, any changes in its activity may alter drug metabolism of a number of drugs, leading potentially to serious consequences in terms of effects of drugs, risk of side effects and, ultimately, quality of life, safety and survival of the dialysis patient. Although the exact mechanism of enzyme inhibition by inflammation is not clear, previous studies have discussed the possible causative effect of inflammatory markers, such as C-reactive protein (CRP) on the activity of CYP3A4 [15, 16]. Moreover, the inflammatory marker orosomucoid has been shown to bind drugs and could thereby potentially raise their concentration in plasma [17]. Thus, this effect could be misinterpreted as a decreased activity of the drug-metabolizing enzyme.

The aim of this study was to investigate the effect of inflammation on the activity of CYP3A4. We investigated 44 prevalent hemodialysis (HD) patients using quinine (substrate of CYP3A4) as a test drug to investigate the effect of inflammation over four weeks on drug metabolism. Quinine is an anti-malaria drug with spasmolytic effects that commonly is prescribed in low doses (100–250 mg) to HD patients suffering leg cramps.

Table 1 Demography and laboratory parameters

Age, years	71 (61–77)
Female/male, n	11/33
Dialysis vintage, months	36 (20–72)
Body mass index, kg/m^2	25.0 (23.0–29.5)
Diabetes mellitus, n	23
Cardiovascular disease, n	30
Primary kidney disease, n	
Diabetes mellitus	12
Chronic glomerulonephritis	5
Nephrosclerosis	7
Polycystic kidney disease	4
Vasculitis	2
Other or unknown disease	14
Medications, n	
Beta-blockers	25
ACEi/ARBs	9
Statins	15

Data presented as number of patients (n), or as median and interquartile range (IQR). *Abbreviations: ACEi* angiotensin converting enzyme inhibitor, *ARBs* angiotensin receptor blockers

Methods

Patients

Fifty-four prevalent HD patients with no or minimal residual renal function agreed to participate in the study. Ten patients did not complete the study, see below. Baseline characteristics of the patients are shown in Table 1. All patients underwent three HD sessions per week (3.5–5.0 h/session) using high-flux polysulphone membrane dialyzers. All the patients were included in the study during between Nov. 2011 and March 2012. They were followed up during five weeks from the initiation of the study and until the study was completed.

Study design

Study design and time points for blood samples taken during the study are shown in Table 2. Four patients decided not to continue with the study. One patient was excluded due to a prolonged infectious episode. Two other patients were excluded from the study due to undetectable levels of both quinine and 3-OH-quinine in their plasma indicating that they did not take the test drug. Two patients died before the end of the study and another patient underwent kidney transplantation before completing the study. Each patient was given 100 mg quinine (Kinin®100 mg) orally in the evening before the day of a regular dialysis day. Samples of 10 ml peripheral blood were drawn into EDTA containing tubes at the beginning of the dialysis session. Plasma was separated and stored frozen at − 80 °C until analysis. The concentration of quinine and its metabolite 3-OH-quinine was measured in the blood sample collected 12 h after drug intake at the beginning of the dialysis. The ratio of quinine and 3-OH-quinine was used as a marker for CYP3A4 activity [18]. The levels of hsCRP, orosomucoid, and pentraxin 3 (PTX3) were measured weekly before dialysis sessions during the four weeks prior to the drug test (Table 2). Measurements were repeated in plasma samples collected 12 h after drug intake concomitantly with measurements of 4β-OH-cholesterol, cholesterol, hemoglobin, albumin, iron, N-terminal-pro-Natriuretic peptide (NT-pro-BNP), parathyroid hormone (PTH) and IL-6 (Table 2). No side effects of the drug were reported. None of the patients was treated with CYP3A4 inhibitors or inducers. Exclusion criteria were signs of local or systemic infection such as chill, fever, fatigue, increasing white blood counts or median hsCRP> 50 mg/L.

Table 2 Study design, patient flow and samples taken during the study

Week 1 $n = 54^a$	Week 2 $n = 50^b$	Week 3 $n = 49^c$	Week 4 $n = 47^d$	Week 5 (n:44)[e]	
				Day 1	Day 2
Inclusion hsCRP, PTX3, orosumucoid	hsCRP, PTX3, orosomucoid	hsCRP, PTX3, orosomucoid	hdCRP, PTX3, orosomucoid	Administration of 100 mg quinine	hdCRP, PTX3, IL-6 and orosomucoid Hb, P-Iron, P-albumin, NT-pro-BNB and PTH 4β-OH-Cholesterol and P-Cholesterol Concentrarion of quinine and 3-OH-quinine

[a]At screening, [b]Four patients decided to withdraw their consent and did not continue with the study, [c]One patient underwent kidney transplantation, [d]Two patients died before completing the study, [e]Three patients were excluded; one due to an infectious episode and two because of undetectable levels of quinine and 3-OH-quinine in plasma

Analyses

The concentrations of quinine and its metabolite 3-OH-quinine were determined by high-performance liquid chromatography with tandem mass spectrometric detection (UPLC-MS/MS) following sample separation by protein precipitation with acetonitrile containing internal standards [18]. A 100 μL volume of the sample was protein precipitated with 200 μL of the internal standard solution. The extract was injected into the UPLC-MS/MS system. Separation of the analytes was achieved on an Acquity UPLC BEH C18-column (2.1 × 50 mm 1.7 μm), using gradient run with mobile phase A (11 mM ammonium formate) and mobile phase B (0.1% formic acid in acetonitrile). The analytes were detected using a Micromass Quattro Primer XE mass spectrometer operating in positive electrospray ionization (ESI) mode utilizing selected reaction monitoring (SRM) for the transitions 325 → 160 m/z for quinine and 341 → 160 m/z for 3-OH-quinine. IL-6 was analyzed in serum by an immunometric assay on an Immulite 1000 Analyzer (Siemens Healthcare, Los Angeles, CA, USA) according to the instructions of the manufacturers. PTX3 was analyzed in EDTA plasma with sandwich ELISA from R&D systems (Abingdon, UK). Cholesterol was determined on a Roche/Hitachi Modular instrument using a commercial enzymatic method (Cholesterol CHOD-PAPP, Roche Diagnostics, GmbH, Mannheim, Germany). The between-day variation was 1.3% at 5 mmol/L. Orosomucoid, hemoglobin, iron, NT-pro-BNP, albumin, and hsCRP in plasma were measured by validated routine methods used by the accredited clinical chemistry laboratory at Karolinska University Hospital, Stockholm. Plasma 4β-OH-cholesterol was determined by isotope-dilution gas chromatography-mass spectrometry, using deuterium labeled 4β-OH-cholesterol as internal standard as described previously [19, 20]. The within-day variation was 4.5% and the between-day variation was 8.2%. The lower limit of quantification was 4.8 ng/mL and the method was linear up to 600 ng/mL. The ratio of 4β-OH-cholesterol/cholesterol was used as an additional marker of CYP3A4 activity [20].

Statistical methods

All variables are expressed as mean ± SD or as median (25th and 75th percentile), unless otherwise indicated. Statistical significance was set at the level of $p \leq 0.05$. Non-parametric Spearman's rank correlation analysis was used to determine associations between various variables. We used one way non-parametric ANOVA to study variation of CRP, PTX3 and orosomucoid. Determinants of ratio quinine/3-0H-quinine were explored using multivariate linear regression analysis. All statistical analyses were performed using statistical software SAS version 9.4 (SAS Campus Drive, Cary, NC, USA).

Results

Characteristics of the patients

Laboratory data in the 44 HD patients on the day of investigation, i.e., 12 h after intake of a single dose of 100 mg quinine ("Day 2" in Table 2), and median values for hs-CRP, orosomucoid and PTX3, calculated from five samples taken during 4 weeks prior to the study plus on Day 2, are shown in Table 3.

Correlations

Significant correlations were observed between plasma albumin and both preceding time on dialysis, dialysis vintage (Rho = 0.37; $p = 0.013$) and age (Rho = – 0.39; $p = 0.0085$). As expected, inflammatory markers correlated with each other: median orosomucoid vs. median hsCRP (Rho = 0.83; $p < 0.001$), median orosomucoid vs. IL-6 (Rho = 0.46; $p = 0.0016$) and IL-6 vs. median hsCRP (Rho = 0.45; $p = 0.0023$). A significant correlation was also observed between 4-beta-OH-cholesterol and cholesterol (Rho = 0.75; $p < 0.0001$) (Fig. 1). As 15 of the 44 patients were treated with statins, we investigated this correlation in patients with or without statins (Fig. 1). Significant correlations were observed both in patients on statins (Rho = 0.67; $p = 0.006$) and not on statins (Rho = 0.83; $p < 0.0001$) (Fig. 1). Significant correlations between CYP3A4 activity (expressed as ratio of quinine/ 3-OH-quinine) and median hsCRP (Rho = 0.48; $p = 0.001$), median orosomucoid (Rho = 0.44, $p = 0.003$) and

Table 3 Laboratory values in 44 HD patients on the final day of investigation (Week 5, Day 2; see Table 2); however, values for inflammatory markers, hsCRP, orosomucoid and PTX3, are shown as median values over 4 weeks plus the final day of investigation

Laboratory parameters	
hsCRP, mg/L [a]	4.5 (1.5–14.0)
Interleukin-6, pg/ml	6.0 (3.0–10.6)
Orosomucoid, g/L [a]	1.0 (0.8–1.3)
Pentraxin 3, ng/ml [a]	1.3 (1.1–2.0)
NT-pro-brain natriuretic peptide, ng/L	6330 (1285–21,830)
Parathyroid hormone, ng/L	322 (151–587)
Albumin, g/L	33 (32–36)
Iron, µg/L	10 (8–13)
4β-OH-Cholesterol, ng/ml	26 (14–26)
Cholesterol, mmol/L	3.9 (3.4–4.7)
Urea reduction rate, %	74 (70–78)
Hemoglobin, g/L	115 (106–121)

Data presented as median and interquartile range (IQR). [a] Median values for high sensitive (hs) CRP, orosomucoid and pentraxin-3 are calculated from the five samples taken during 4 weeks prior to the study plus the last day of the study. The rest of the parameters are sampled at day 2 of week 5

IL-6 at day 2 at the end of week 5 (Rho = 0.42; p = 0.004) were observed (Fig. 2a). Median values of hsCRP, PTX3 and orosomucoid were calculated from the measurements four weeks prior to the study plus the values taken at the last day of the study. We observed no statistically significant variations (non-parametric ANOVA) of CRP, PTX3 and orosomucoid during the study period (data not shown). Also the last value (samples taken at the same day as quinine) of hsCRP (Rho = 0.59; p < 0.001) and orosomucoid (Rho = 0.45; p = 0.002) correlated to the ratio of quinine/3-OH-quinine. We did not observe any correlation of the ratio of quinine/3-OH-quinine with NT-pro-BNP (Rho = 0.15; p = 0.332,) and plasma albumin (Rho = – 0.18; p = 0.237), respectively. A significant correlation (Rho = – 0.40; p = 0.008) was also found between ratio of quinine/3-OH-quinine and 4β-OH-cholesterol/cholesterol; a marker of CYP3A4 activity. No correlations were observed between the ratio of 4β-OH-cholesterol/cholesterol and median hsCRP (Rho = – 0.12; p = 0.44), median orosomucoid (Rho = – 0.09; p = 0.57) and IL-6 (Rho = – 0.14; p = 0.35) (Fig. 2b), respectively. We did not find any correlation between median PTX3 and CYP3A4 activity expressed as either quinine/3-OH-quinine (Rho = – 0.17; p = 0.26) or 4β-OH-cholesterol/cholesterol (Rho = – 0.21; p = 0.16). Sixteen participants in the study where treated with statins which is considered as an inhibitor of CYP3A4 but our results showed no significant difference between the participants with or without statin (P: 0.96).

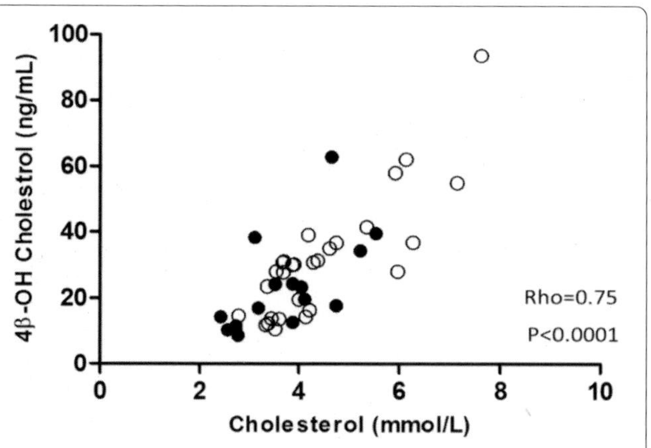

Fig. 1 Correlation between 4-beta-OH-cholesterol and cholesterol. Closed circles represent 15 patients treated with statins and open circles represent 29 patients without statin treatment

Multivariate analysis

The association between CYP3A4 activity expressed as quinine/3-OH-quinine and hsCRP showed a trend to be significant (β = 0.44; p = 0.05) in a multivariate analysis after full adjustment for age, gender, diabetes mellitus, dialysis vintage, PTH, orosomucoid and medication with angiotensin-converting enzyme inhibitors (ACEIs), angiotensin receptor blockers (ARBs), beta-blockers or statins (Table 4).

Discussion

In the present study, a single dose of 100 mg quinine was given to 44 ESRD patients undergoing maintenance HD and plasma quinine and its metabolite 3-OH-quinine were measured after 12 h immediately prior to the next HD session. Patients with signs of inflammation - according to weekly measurements of several biomarkers of inflammation over 4 weeks prior to the investigation – had a higher quinine/3-OH-quinine ratio, indicating decreased CYP3A4 activity, suggesting that the activity of CYP3A4 is reduced by inflammation in HD patients.

As kidney failure can alter the pharmacokinetics of many drugs at different levels [21, 22], drug dosing has always been a challenge in this vulnerable patient population [23]. The absorption of orally administered drugs in the gastrointestinal system may be affected by reduced gut motility, increased pH, increased paracellular transport across the intestinal epithelium [24] and reduced activity of drug metabolizing enzymes and transporters [1, 25]. This may result in increased rate of absorption and consequently increased bioavailability of drugs. The absorbed drugs need to be bound to albumin or other plasma proteins during the transport of drugs to the target organ or liver. However, as the concentrations of plasma proteins, including albumin, in general are decreased in ESRD patients, protein binding of drugs

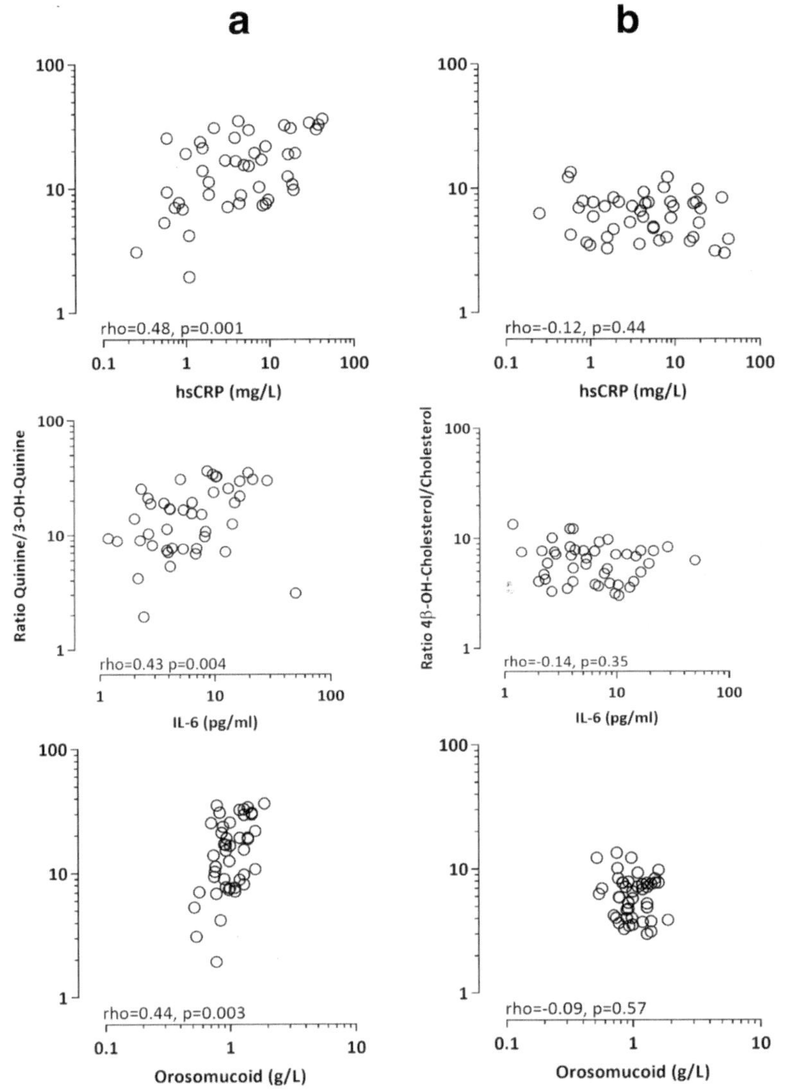

Fig. 2 Correlation between CYP3A4 activity, expressed as the ratio of quinine/3-OH-quinine (**a**) and 4β-OH-cholesterol/cholesterol (**b**), respectively, and median concentrations of hsCRP and orosomucoid as well as with a single measure of IL-6 (on Day 2 at week 5 of the study)

is reduced, and the free circulating concentration of the drug may therefore increase [26]. Furthermore, the uremic milieu per se could reduce the non-renal elimination of drugs by affecting the function of drug metabolizing enzymes and transporters leading to even larger risk of drug accumulation and drug intoxication [1].

As dialysis patients are often subjected to polypharmacy this increases the risk of drug-drug interactions [9, 27]. Furthermore, the concentration of circulating drugs is not only affected by the changes in drug metabolism and pharmacokinetics, but also by the dialysis treatment per se. The dialyzability of a drug depends on several factors, such as molecular weight, protein binding, volume of distribution, blood and dialysis flow rates during the dialysis treatment, and type of the dialysis membrane [22, 28]. Another important observation is that HD is reported to increases the metabolic activity of CYP3A4 suggesting that dialyzable uremic toxins may inhibit the activity of this enzyme [29, 30]. Thus, nephrologists need to consider a myriad of factors when a drug is prescribed to a dialysis patient. Further, as inflammation may alter the activity of drug metabolizing enzyme and transporters [7], this condition which is common in dialysis patients may add to the difficulties to prescribe drugs [28].

So far most studies on the impact of inflammation on drug metabolism have been conducted in animal models [7, 31]. In the current study, we studied pharmacokinetics of quinine, a substrate for CYP3A4, in a group of HD patients. Quinine is commonly used in dialysis wards against leg cramps in HD patients during the dialysis treatment and the risk of side effects is small for current doses prescribed to HD patients (100-250 mg). Our

Table 4 Multivariate linear regression models for determinants of the ratio quinine/3-OH-quinine in 44 prevalent hemodialysis patients. Data are expressed as adjusted r^2, beta (β) and significance

	Unadjusted (β, *P*) (r^2 = 0.23)	Model 1 (β, *P*) (r^2 = 0.27)	Model 2 (β, *P*) (r^2 = 0.27)	Model 3 (β, *P*) (r^2 = 0.21)
hsCRP (mg/L)	0.49 (**0.001**)	0.52 (**0.001**)	0.54 (**0.001**)	0.44 (**0.05**)
Age (years)		0.02 (0.90)	−0.002 (0.98)	− 0.03 (0.85)
Gender (female)		0.28 (**0.04**)	0.27 (0.07)	0.30 (0.07)
Diabetes mellitus		−0.13 (0.32)	−0.18 (0.22)	− 0.14 (0.44)
Vintage (months)		−0.11 (0.42)	−0.10 (0.50)	− 0.08 (0.62)
Betablockers			0.14 (0.38)	0.12 (0.46)
ACEi/ARBs			−0.21 (0.19)	−0.21 (0.21)
Statins			0.18 (0.31)	0.18 (0.31)
PTH (ng/L)				−0.01 (0.93)
Orosomucoid (g/L)				0.14 (0.56)

*Abbreviations***:** *hsCRP* High sensitivity C reactive protein, *ACEi* Angiotensin converting enzyme inhibitors, *ARBs* Angiotensin receptor blockers, *PTH* Parathyroid hormone
Bold text indicate significance levels

results show that CYP3A4 activity associate to biomarkers of inflammation. Since the already complicated drug metabolism in dialysis patients may be affected also by systemic inflammation, this adds novel challenges to correct drug dosing in this inflamed patient population [32]. Further, as Shah and Smith [33] reported that phenoconversion of drug metabolizing enzymes may be an important modifier of drug metabolism, the scenario may be even more complicated. Since inflammation may induce phenoconversion [34] this implies that genetically extensive metabolizers could be converted to a phenotypic poor metabolizer. Clearly, we need to individualize drug dosing to reduce the complications related to drug side effects and interactions. For this purpose we need to identify which factors in addition to traditionally known factors that affect pharmacokinetics and pharmacodynamics of drugs.

The results of the present study should be considered in light of the following strengths and caveats. The careful repeated monitoring of inflammation biomarkers during four weeks preceding the pharmacokinetic study of quinine strengthens the ascertainment of the inflammatory burden of the investigated patients. Some caveats deserve mentioning. As the sample size is rather small, the results need to be confirmed in larger cohorts. In a prior study, using alprazolam as a test drug, we demonstrated that inflammation associated to reduced activity of CYP3A4 in another cohort of HD patients [12]. Since orosomucoid can be considered as a confounder due to its ability to bind drugs [17], thereby raising the plasma concentration of quinine, this could lead to misinterpretation of reduced CYP3A4 activity. However, the correlation between quinine/3-OH-quinine and hsCRP showed a trend to being significant ($p = 0.05$) after multivariate regression analysis (Table 4) implying that inflammation per se affect the activity of CYP3A4. In the present study, no correlation between CYP3A4 activity and PTX3 was observed. However, it has been reported that PTX3 may primarily reflect endothelial dysfunction rather than systemic inflammation [35]. Another limitation is that the impact of accumulation of uremic toxins and its putative effects on drug functions and metabolism was not assessed.

Although we report a significant correlation between CYP3A4 activity expressed as quinine/3-OH-quinine and the ratio of 4β-OH-cholesterol/cholesterol; the latter being another marker for CYP3A4 activity [36], no correlation between the inflammatory biomarkers and the ratio of 4β-OH-cholesterol/cholesterol was observed. This finding is in accordance to our prior study using alprazolam as test drug [12]. Although 4β-hydroxycholesterol is considered to be a useful marker for CYP3A4 activity in healthy individuals, this marker may not be suitable for detecting CYP3A4 activity in HD patients. One reason could be that this cholesterol metabolite is very slowly eliminated after induction and therefore the relatively faster variation of the degree of inflammation may not be reflected by changes in metabolism of the slowly eliminated 4β-OH-cholesterol [12]. CYP3A accounts for 80% of total P450 content in intestines [37], and although the CYP3A content in intestine is only about 1% of the amount in the liver, its predominance in human intestine can lead to several fold more efficacy of the enzyme in intestine compared to liver [38, 39]. Indeed, the intestine is suggested to be of equal or even greater importance than liver for metabolism of drugs [40]. Furthermore, since the inflamed uremic milieu is associated with changes in gut microbiota [41], the discrepant findings with regard to the relation of quinine/3-OH-quinine and 4β-OH-cholesterol/cholesterol with inflammation could imply a role of uremic dysbiosis on the pharmacokinetic profile [42]. In a previous study in 440 healthy subjects representing three major populations in Africa, Asia and Europe, the coefficient of correlation between 4β-OH-cholesterol and cholesterol was low ($R = 0.30$), but significant ($p < 0.0001$); i.e. only 9% of the variation in 4β-OH-cholesterol concentration was due to the variation in cholesterol concentration [43]. Thus, a major determinant of the level of 4β-OH-cholesterol might be the CYP3A4 activity and not the concentration of the substrate i.e., cholesterol. In the present study, we found a much stronger correlation (rho = 0.75); fairly independent of statin treatment (Fig. 1). In our previous study using alprazolam as a marker of CYP3A4 activity, we also found a fairly high coefficient of correlation between 4β-OH-cholesterol and cholesterol (Rho = 0.58; $p = 0.0018$) (calculated from data of ref. [12]). In these two studies on HD patients the variation in 4β-OH-cholesterol concentration is determined to a pronounced extent by cholesterol (56% in the present study and 34% in [12]), which is higher than the 9% reported in healthy subjects [43]. We propose that 4β-OH-cholesterol/cholesterol is a better marker of CYP3A4 activity in healthy subjects while it is an inadequate marker in HD patients which could explain the absence of a relationship between CYP3A4 activity measured by 4β-OH-cholesterol and markers of inflammation in two independent groups of HD patients investigated by our group. Further Björkhem-Bergman et al. [44] have shown that whereas statin treatment had no effect on the hepatic CYP3A mRNA content, it significantly reduced 4β-OH-cholesterol, while there was no significant effect on the 4β-OH-cholesterol/cholesterol ratio [45]. An earlier in vitro study showed that the CYP3A4 enzyme is saturated at a cholesterol concentration of 100 μM [19]. Both 4β-OH-cholesterol and cholesterol are transported in lipoproteins in the circulation [19]. These data indicate that during statin treatment it is mainly the cholesterol-dependent lipoprotein binding capacity in the circulation that will determine the 4β-OH-cholesterol concentration in plasma, rather than a direct effect on the hepatic CYP3A4 enzyme. A disturbed cholesterol-dependent lipoprotein binding capacity in HD patients may also be operative [46]. Taken together, our results suggest that the ratio 4β-OH-cholesterol/cholesterol rather than 4β-OH-cholesterol alone, is the preferred measure of CYP3A4 activity.

Conclusion

In summary, a higher degree of inflammation associates with decreased activity of CYP3A4 in HD patients. Further studies are needed to find out if this consequence of inflammation will have a clinical significant impact on risk of drug interactions and side effects in dialysis patients.

Abbreviations

ACEi: Angiotensin converting enzyme inhibitor; ARBs: Angiotensin receptor blockers; CKD: Chronic kidney disease; CRP: C-reactive protein; CYP3A4: Cytochrome P450 3A4; ESRD: End stage renal disease; HD: Hemodialysis; hsCRP: High sensitive CRP; NT-pro-BNP: N-terminal pro-Brain Natriuretic peptide; PTX3: Pentraxin 3

Acknowledgements

We would like to thank the patients and personnel involved in this study. Also, we are indebted to our research staff at KBC (Annika Nilsson, Sofia Garpemo, Yvonne Eklöf and Ulrika Jensen) and to Department of Clinical Pharmacology at Karolinska University Hospital, Huddinge for the skilful analysis of drug concentrations. Part of the study was published as an abstract [47].

Funding

Peter Stenvinkel acknowledges grants from the Swedish Research Council, Medicine (K2014-65X-15320-10-3), Westmans Foundation and the Stockholm County Council (ALF). Baxter Novum is the result of a grant from Baxter Healthcare to Karolinska Institutet. The funding bodies did not take part in the design of the study, collection, analysis, and interpretation of data as well as in writing the manuscript.

Authors' contributions

HM, PS and LB designed the study. Recruitment of patients in the study and collection of all data was performed by HM. HM, PS, OH, BL and LB analyzed data and participated in the interpretations of the results. Statistical analyzes were performed by ARQ and HM. Analyses of 4β-OH-cholesterol/cholesterol were done by UD and analyses of other biomarkers were supervised and/or done by BA. All the authors participated in the revision of the manuscript and the paper was finally approved by all the authors.

Competing interests

Bengt Lindholm is employed by Baxter Healthcare Corporation. None of the other authors declare any conflict of interest.

Author details

[1]Division of Renal Medicine and Baxter Novum, Department of Clinical Science, Intervention and Technology, Karolinska Institutet, Karolinska University Hospital, SE-141 86 Stockholm, Sweden. [2]Division of Clinical Chemistry Department of Laboratory Medicine, Karolinska Institutet, Karolinska University Hospital, Stockholm, Sweden. [3]Division of Clinical Pharmacology, Department of Laboratory Medicine, |Karolinska Institutet, Karolinska University Hospital, Stockholm, Sweden.

References

1. Nolin TD, Naud J, Leblond FA, Pichette V. Emerging evidence of the impact of kidney disease on drug metabolism and transport. Clin Pharmacol Ther. 2008;83(6):898–903.
2. Yeung CK, Shen DD, Thummel KE, Himmelfarb J. Effects of chronic kidney disease and uremia on hepatic drug metabolism and transport. Kidney Int. 2014;85(3):522–8.
3. Stenvinkel P, Alvestrand A. Inflammation in end-stage renal disease: sources, consequences, and therapy. Semin Dial. 2002;15(5):329–37.
4. Kooman J, Dekker M, Usvyat LA, Kotanko P, van der Sande F, Schalkwijk CG, Shiels P, Stenvinkel P. Inflammation and premature aging in advanced chronic kidney disease. Am J Physiol Renal Physiol. 2017;313(4):F938–50.
5. Morgan ET. Regulation of cytochrome p450 by inflammatory mediators: why and how? Drug Metab Dispos. 2001;29(3):207–12.
6. Morgan ET. Impact of infectious and inflammatory disease on cytochrome P450-mediated drug metabolism and pharmacokinetics. Clin Pharmacol Ther. 2009;85(4):434–8.
7. Morgan ET, Goralski KB, Piquette-Miller M, Renton KW, Robertson GR, Chaluvadi MR, et al. Regulation of drug-metabolizing enzymes and

transporters in infection, inflammation, and cancer. Drug Metab Dispos. 2008;36(2):205–16.

8. Harvey RD, Morgan ET. Cancer, inflammation, and therapy: effects on cytochrome p450-mediated drug metabolism and implications for novel immunotherapeutic agents. Clin Pharmacol Ther. 2014;96(4):449–57.
9. Burnier M, Pruijm M, Wuerzner G, Santschi V. Drug adherence in chronic kidney diseases and dialysis. Nephrol Dial Transpl. 2015;30(1):39–44.
10. Weir MR, Fink JC. Safety of medical therapy in patients with chronic kidney disease and end-stage renal disease. Curr Opin Nephrol Hypertens. 2014; 23(3):306–13.
11. Ponticelli C, Sala G, Glassock RJ. Drug management in the elderly adult with chronic kidney disease: a review for the primary care physician. Mayo Clin Proc. 2015;90(5):633–45.
12. Molanaei H, Stenvinkel P, Qureshi AR, Carrero JJ, Heimburger O, Lindholm B, et al. Metabolism of alprazolam (a marker of CYP3A4) in hemodialysis patients with persistent inflammation. Eur J Clin Pharmacol. 2012;68(5):571–7.
13. Wrighton SA, Stevens JC. The human hepatic cytochromes P450 involved in drug metabolism. Crit Rev Toxicol. 1992;22(1):1–21.
14. Shimada T, Yamazaki H, Mimura M, Inui Y, Guengerich FP. Interindividual variations in human liver cytochrome P-450 enzymes involved in the oxidation of drugs, carcinogens and toxic chemicals: studies with liver microsomes of 30 Japanese and 30 Caucasians. J Pharmacol Exp Ther. 1994; 270(1):414–23.
15. Aitken AE, Morgan ET. Gene-specific effects of inflammatory cytokines on cytochrome P450 2C, 2B6 and 3A4 mRNA levels in human hepatocytes. Drug Metab Dispos. 2007;35(9):1687–93.
16. Charles KA, Rivory LP, Brown SL, Liddle C, Clarke SJ, Robertson GR. Transcriptional repression of hepatic cytochrome P450 3A4 gene in the presence of cancer. Clin Cancer Res. 2006;12(24):7492–7.
17. Piafsky KM, Borga O, Odar-Cederlof I, Johansson C, Sjoqvist F. Increased plasma protein binding of propranolol and chlorpromazine mediated by disease-induced elevations of plasma alpha1 acid glycoprotein. New Engl J Med. 1978;299(26):1435–9.
18. Björkhem-Bergman L, Backstrom T, Nylen H, Ronquist-Nii Y, Bredberg E, Andersson TB, et al. Quinine compared to 4beta-hydroxycholesterol and midazolam as markers for CYP3A induction by rifampicin. Drug Metab Pharmacokinet. 2014;29(4):352–5.
19. Bodin K, Bretillon L, Aden Y, Bertilsson L, Broome U, Einarsson C, et al. Antiepileptic drugs increase plasma levels of 4beta-hydroxycholesterol in humans: evidence for involvement of cytochrome p450 3A4. J Biol Chem. 2001;276(42):38685–9.
20. Diczfalusy U, Nylen H, Elander P, Bertilsson L. 4beta-hydroxycholesterol, an endogenous marker of CYP3A4/5 activity in humans. Br J Clin Pharmacol. 2011;71(2):183–9.
21. Naud J, Nolin TD, Leblond FA, Pichette V. Current understanding of drug disposition in kidney disease. J Clin Pharm. 2012;52(1 Suppl):10S–22S.
22. Velenosi TJ, Urquhart BL. Pharmacokinetic considerations in chronic kidney disease and patients requiring dialysis. Expert Opin Drug Metab Toxicol. 2014;10(8):1131–43.
23. Verbeeck RK, Musuamba FT. Pharmacokinetics and dosage adjustment in patients with renal dysfunction. Eur J Clin Pharmacol. 2009;65(8):757–73.
24. Magnusson M, Magnusson KE, Sundqvist T, Denneberg T. Impaired intestinal barrier function measured by differently sized polyethylene glycols in patients with chronic renal failure. Gut. 1991;32(7):754–9.
25. Dreisbach AW, Lertora JJ. The effect of chronic renal failure on drug metabolism and transport. Expert Opin Drug Metab Toxicol. 2008;4(8): 1065–74.
26. Steinman TI. Serum albumin: its significance in patients with ESRD. Semin Dial. 2000;13(6):404–8.
27. Chiu YW, Teitelbaum I, Misra M, de Leon EM, Adzize T, Mehrotra R. Pill burden, adherence, hyperphosphatemia, and quality of life in maintenance dialysis patients. Clin J Am Soc Nephrol. 2009;4(6):1089–96.
28. Baillie G, Mason N, editors. Dialysis of drugs: LLC, saline Michigan USA 2013.
29. Nolin TD, Appiah K, Kendrick SA, Le P, McMonagle E, Himmelfarb J. Hemodialysis acutely improves hepatic CYP3A4 metabolic activity. J Am Soc Nephrol. 2006;17(9):2363–7.
30. Michaud J, Nolin TD, Naud J, Dani M, Lafrance JP, Leblond FA, et al. Effect of hemodialysis on hepatic cytochrome P450 functional expression. J Pharm Sci. 2008;108(2):157–63.
31. Coutant DE, Kulanthaivel P, Turner PK, Bell RL, Baldwin J, Wijayawardana SR, et al. Understanding disease-drug interactions in Cancer patients: implications for dosing within the therapeutic window. Clin Pharmacol Ther. 2015;98(1):76–86.
32. Snaedal S, Heimburger O, Qureshi AR, Danielsson A, Wikstrom B, Fellstrom B, et al. Comorbidity and acute clinical events as determinants of C-reactive protein variation in hemodialysis patients: implications for patient survival. Am J Kid Dis. 2009;53(6):1024–33.
33. Shah RR, Smith RL. Addressing phenoconversion: the Achilles' heel of personalized medicine. Br J Clinical Pharm. 2015;79(2):222–40.
34. Shah RR, Smith RL. Inflammation-induced phenoconversion of polymorphic drug metabolizing enzymes: hypothesis with implications for personalized medicine. Drug Metab Dispos. 2015;43(3):400–10.
35. Witasp A, Ryden M, Carrero JJ, Qureshi AR, Nordfors L, Naslund E, et al. Elevated circulating levels and tissue expression of pentraxin 3 in uremia: a reflection of endothelial dysfunction. PLoS One. 2013;8(5):e63493.
36. Diczfalusy U, Kanebratt KP, Bredberg E, Andersson TB, Bottiger Y, Bertilsson L. 4beta-hydroxycholesterol as an endogenous marker for CYP3A4/5 activity. Stability and half-life of elimination after induction with rifampicin. Br J Clinical Pharm. 2009;67(1):38–43.
37. Paine MF, Hart HL, Ludington SS, Haining RL, Rettie AE, Zeldin DC. The human intestinal cytochrome P450 "pie". Drug Metab Dispos. 2006;34(5):880–6.
38. Yang J, Tucker GT, Rostami-Hodjegan A. Cytochrome P450 3A expression and activity in the human small intestine. Clin Pharmacol Ther. 2004;76(4):391.
39. Galetin A, Gertz M, Houston JB. Contribution of intestinal cytochrome p450-mediated metabolism to drug-drug inhibition and induction interactions. Drug Metab Pharmacokinet. 2010;25(1):28–47.
40. Basheer L, Kerem Z. Interactions between CYP3A4 and dietary polyphenols. Oxidative Med Cell Longev. 2015;2015:854015.
41. Ramezani A, Raj DS. The gut microbiome, kidney disease, and targeted interventions. J Am Soc Nephrol. 2014;25(4):657–70.
42. Bezirtzoglou EE. Intestinal cytochromes P450 regulating the intestinal microbiota and its probiotic profile. Microb Ecol Health Dis. 2012;23. https://doi.org/10.3402/mehd.v23i0.18370.
43. Diczfalusy U, Miura J, Roh HK, Mirghani RA, Sayi J, Larsson H, et al. 4Beta-hydroxycholesterol is a new endogenous CYP3A marker: relationship to CYP3A5 genotype, quinine 3-hydroxylation and sex in Koreans, Swedes and Tanzanians. Pharmacogenet Genomics. 2008;18(3):201–8.
44. Björkhem-Bergman L, Bergstrom H, Johansson M, Parini P, Eriksson M, Rane A, et al. Atorvastatin treatment induces uptake and efflux transporters in human liver. Drug Metab Dispos. 2013;41(9):1610–5.
45. Björkhem-Bergman L, Nylen H, Eriksson M, Parini P, Diczfalusy U. Effect of statin treatment on plasma 4beta-hydroxycholesterol concentrations. Basic Clin Pharmacol Toxicol. 2016;118(6):499–502.
46. Perez GO, Hsia SL, Christakis G, Burr J. Serum cholesterol binding reserve and high density lipoprotein cholesterol in patients on maintenance hemodialysis. Horm Metab Res. 1980;12(9):449–54.
47. Molanaei H, Qureshi AR, Heimbürger O, Lindholm L, Diczfalusy U, Anderstam B, et al. Inflammation down regulates cytochrome P450 mediated drug metabolism in hemodialysis patients. Nephrol Dial Transpl. 2016;i561:31.

16

Characterization of serious adverse drug reactions as cause of emergency department visit in children: a 5-years active pharmacovigilance study

Niccolò Lombardi[1*†], Giada Crescioli[1†], Alessandra Bettiol[1], Ettore Marconi[1], Antonio Vitiello[1], Roberto Bonaiuti[1], Anna Maria Calvani[2], Stefano Masi[3], Ersilia Lucenteforte[1], Alessandro Mugelli[1], Lisa Giovannelli[1] and Alfredo Vannacci[1]

Abstract

Background: To describe frequency, preventability and seriousness of adverse drug reactions (ADRs) in children as cause of emergency department (ED) admission and to evaluate the association between specific factors and the reporting of ADRs.

Methods: A retrospective analysis based on reports of suspected ADRs collected between January 1st, 2012 and December 31st, 2016 in the ED of Meyer Children's Hospital (Italy). Demographics, clinical status, suspected drugs, ADR description, and its degree of seriousness were collected. Logistic regression was used to estimate the reporting odds ratios (RORs) with 95% confidence intervals (CIs) of potential predictors of ADR seriousness.

Results: Within 5 years, we observed 834 ADRs (1100 drug-ADR pairs), of whom 239 were serious; of them, 224 led to hospitalization. Patients were mostly treated with one drug. Among patients treated with more than one drug, 78 ADRs presented a potential interaction. The most frequently reported ADRs involved gastrointestinal system. The most frequently reported medication class was antinfectives. Risk of serious ADR was significantly lower in children and infants compared to adolescents (ROR 0.41 [95% CI: 0.27–0.61] and 0.47 [0.32–0.71], respectively), and it was significantly increased in subjects exposed to more than one drug (ROR 1.87 [1.33–2.62] and 3.01 [2.07–4.37] for subjects exposed to 2 and 3 or more drugs, respectively). Gender, interactions and off-label drug use did not influence the risk of serious ADRs.

Conclusion: Active surveillance in pharmacovigilance might represent the best strategy to estimate and characterize the clinical burden of ADRs in children.

Keywords: Pediatrics, Adverse events, Safety, Observational study, Preventability, Drug interactions

Background

Adverse drug reactions (ADRs) are the most common cause of iatrogenic harm in health care and have recently received attention in national patient safety initiatives [1]. Moreover, ADRs are a significant cause of emergency department (ED) visits [2].

* Correspondence: niccolo.lombardi@unifi.it
†Equal contributors
[1]Department of Neurosciences, Psychology, Drug Research and Child Health, Section of Pharmacology and Toxicology, University of Florence, viale G. Pieraccini, 6, 50139 Florence, Italy
Full list of author information is available at the end of the article

Most studies on hospital admissions related to medication use focus on adult patients [3–8]. Fortunately, the burden of ADR-related ED admissions in children seems to be lower than observed in adults (5%–25% of all ED admissions) [3, 9], ranging from 0.4% to 10.3% of all children with a pooled estimate of 2.9% [10].

In this context, risk factors for ADRs in children are still poorly characterized. In fact, pharmacotherapy in children differs from adults, thus the spectrum of ADRs in children may differ as well [11], and certain subgroups are at higher risk, such as children exposed to cancer chemotherapy [12]. Furthermore, children are more often exposed to off-label medications, that potentially represent a greater risk for ADRs [13]. Because part of these medication-related events may be preventable [14], more knowledge on occurrence and content of ADRs in pediatric setting is necessary, with efforts focused on reducing medication errors and inappropriate prescribing [1].

EDs are an essential part of health care systems, serving as an interface between hospitals and communities, and could constitute the most important source of information about the frequency, seriousness, and economic burden of ADRs [15, 16].

Preventing ADRs and their related ED admissions in outpatients remains a public health and a patient safety challenge. Aims of this study are to describe frequency, preventability and seriousness of ADRs in children, and to evaluate the association between specific factors and the reporting of ADRs, by means of a 5-years long active pharmacovigilance study in ED.

Methods

This is a retrospective study performed on reports of suspected ADRs collected between January 1st, 2012 and December 31st, 2016 in the ED of Anna Meyer Children's University Hospital of Florence (Italy), as part of the study "Epidemiological Monitoring of Adverse Drug Reactions in Emergency Department" (MEREAFaPS), an on-going multicenter Italian active pharmacovigilance project. We analyzed all suspected ADRs reported from patients having at least one drug- or vaccine-related event.

All suspected ADRs leading to ED admission were identified from ED clinical charts and hospitalization data from the hospital discharge database. For each ADR report, we recorded demographic characteristics (age, gender, ethnic group), and patient clinical status on ED admission. Anatomical Therapeutic Chemical (ATC) classification system was used to code ongoing therapy (suspect and concomitant medications, administration route, therapy duration, and dosages). We also recorded all therapeutic indications of suspected drugs. The description of the ADR according to diagnosis and symptoms, was coded using the Medical Dictionary for Regulatory Activities (MedDRA) and organized by System Organ Class (SOC) [17]. ADR seriousness was classified according to the World Health Organization (WHO) criteria [17] as fatal, life-threatening, or requiring hospitalization of the patient, or causing serious/permanent disability.

The primary outcome was the frequency of total and serious ADRs leading to ED admission. The most frequently reported SOC and ATC classes were also evaluated. For each drug-ADR pair, causality and preventability (categorized as definitely or probably preventable, or not preventable) were assessed using the Naranjo [18] scale and Schumock and Thornton [19] algorithm, respectively. For the causality assessment of vaccine-related ADRs, the specific WHO [20, 21] algorithm was used. Data on medications were also analysed for drug-drug interactions (DDIs) by using the drug interaction software Micromedex Drug-REAX System (Thomson Reuters Healthcare Inc., Greenwood Village, Colorado, United States), available online with restricted access [22, 23].

The specific factors associated with the reporting of ADRs, such as age classes, sex, number of suspected drugs, DDIs and on-label vs off-label use were also analysed. The off-label use in children was defined as the use of a drug already covered by a Marketing Authorisation, in an unapproved way in terms of therapeutic indication, posology, formulation and route of administration [24].

Descriptive statistics was used to summarize data. Categorical data were reported as frequencies and percentages, whereas continuous data were reported as means with standard errors. Univariate and multivariate logistic regression were used to estimate the reporting odds ratios (RORs) with 95% confidence intervals (CIs) of potential predictors of ADR seriousness. ROR values for each variable were reported both as crude values and adjusted for all the other considered variables. All results were considered to be statistically significant at $p < 0.05$. Data management and statistical analysis were carried out using STATA 14.

Tuscany approved the present study with the Notification number 1225 - December 21, 2009. The local institutional ethics committee of the coordinating center (*Comitato Etico di Area Vasta Nord "CEAVNO" per la Sperimentazione Clinica, Azienda Ospedaliero-Universitaria Pisana*) approved the study according to the legal requirements concerning observational studies (*Study number 3055/2010, Protocol number 45288 - August 6, 2014*).

Results

During the 5-year study period, a total of 221,528 ED admissions was evaluated; of them, 492 were ADR-related, with an overall rate of 2.2 per 1000 ED admissions. Table 1 shows data of pediatric patients who experienced an ADR-related ED admission. We observed 834 ADRs, of whom 239 were serious (28.66%) and, of them, 224 led to hospitalization. No ADR led to death. Most of ADRs occurred in Caucasians (90.65%), with a mean patients' age (± standard error) of 62.53 ± 2.09 months. The male/female rate of ADRs was 1.17, i.e. comparable to the all-cause ED admission rate observed in Meyer Children's University Hospital. A total of 483 ADRs (57.91%) had an improvement and 48 (5.76%) had a complete resolution. For 285 ADRs (34.17%) data on the outcome were not available. Overall, patients were mostly treated with only one drug at time of ADR occurrence. Among patients treated with two or more drugs, 78 ADRs (20.21%) presented a potential DDI, which was

Table 1 Characteristics of pediatric patients admitted to ED for ADR

	Tot ADRs N (% out of 834)
N involved patients	492
N ADRs/patients	
1	256 (52.03)
2	155 (31.50)
3+	81 (16.46)
Age	
Mean ± standard error, months	62.53 ± 2.09
Age classes	
New-borns (< 1 month)	7 (0.84)
Infants (1–23 months)	332 (39.81)
Children (24–143 months)	368 (44.12)
Adolescents (144–192 months)	127 (15.23)
Sex	
Male	449 (53.48)
Female	385 (46.16)
Ethnic group	
Caucasian	756 (90.65)
Others	25 (3.00)
Not available	53 (6.35)
Tot number of drugs	
1	448 (53.72)
2	255 (30.58)
3+	131 (15.71)
Seriousness	
Hospitalization	224 (26.86)
Congenital abnormalities/ Deficit	1 (0.12)
Other clinically relevant conditions	14 (1.68)
Outcome	
Complete resolution	48 (5.76)
Improvement	483 (57.91)
Invariant situation/worsening	18 (2.16)
Not available	285 (34.17)
Drug-drug interactions[a]	
No	308 (79.79)
Yes	78 (20.21)
Mild	4 (1.04)
Moderate	17 (4.40)
Severe	57 (14.77)
	Tot drug ADR-pairs N (% out of 1100)
Drugs (vaccines excluded)	711 (64.64)
Causality	
In doubt	18
Possible	301
Probable	310
Certain	82
Vaccines	389 (35.36)
Causality	
Not associable	6
Undefined	50
Associable	333

[a]Percentage calculated on the total number of ADRs occurred in patients with more than one drug

severe in 57 cases (14.77%). The total number of drug-ADR pairs was 1100. Of them, 711 drug-ADR pairs were related to non-vaccines drugs; considering causality assessment, 82 were certain, 310 probable, 301 possible and 18 in doubt. On the other hand, 389 (35.36%) were related to vaccines; in particular, considering the evaluation of causality assessment, 333 were considered as associable, 50 as undefined and 6 were not associable.

Table 2 reported the distribution of ADRs according to SOC classification. The most frequently reported SOCs were: gastrointestinal disorders (27.34%), followed by general disorders and administration site conditions (21.46%), skin and subcutaneous tissue disorders (16. 19%), nervous system disorders (12.95%) and metabolism and nutrition disorders (3.60%). The majority of ADRs for each SOC were non-serious.

The drug-ADR pairs (stratified by ATC classes, level I) most commonly involved in ED admissions, overall and stratified according to ADRs seriousness, preventability and off-label use are listed in Table 3. Out of 1100 drug-ADR pairs, 711 were not related to vaccines; of them more than 30% were serious, 24% preventable and 8.7% related to off-label use. The most frequently reported ATC class was antinfectives for systemic use (ATC class J, excluded J07*) accounting for 288 drug-ADR pairs (40. 51%). Of them, 23.96% were serious, 24.19% were preventable and 0.69% were related to off-label use. The second most frequently reported ATC class was nervous system medication (ATC class N), accounting for 168 drug-ADR pairs (23.63%), of whom 48.21, 48.81 and 10. 71% were serious, preventable and related to off-label use, respectively. All other ATC classes accounted for 8. 30 to 0.56% of drug-ADR pairs.

The most frequent suspected active principles (APs) among antinfectives for systemic use agents and nervous system medications are reported in Additional file 1: Table S1.

Out of 1100 drug-ADR pairs, 389 were related to vaccines (35.36%); of them, 28% and 6.9% were serious and preventable, respectively (Table 3). The most

Table 2 Distribution of ADRs according to SOC classification

	Tot ADRs N (% out of 834)	Serious ADRs N (% out of corresponding SOC)
SOC		
Gastrointestinal disorders	228 (27.34)	*68 (29.82)*
General disorders and administration site conditions	179 (21.46)	*41 (23.56)*
Skin and subcutaneous tissue disorders	135 (16.19)	*17 (12.59)*
Nervous system disorders	108 (12.95)	*45 (41.67)*
Metabolism and nutrition disorders	30 (3.60)	*11 (36.67)*
Respiratory, thoracic and mediastinal disorders	27 (3.24)	*8 (29.63)*
Musculoskeletal and connective tissue disorders	27 (3.24)	*11(40.74)*
Psychiatric disorders	18 (2.16)	*7 (38.89)*
Eye disorders	13 (1.56)	*5 (38.46)*
Cardiac disorders	12 (1.44)	*5 (41.67)*
Ear and labyrinth disorders	10 (1.20)	*1 (10)*
Investigations	8 (0.96)	*3 (37.50)*
Infections and infestations	8 (0.96)	*1 (12.50)*
Vascular disorders	7 (0.84)	*2 (28.57)*
Injury, poisoning and procedural complications	7 (0.84)	*4 (57.14)*
Blood and lymphatic system disorders	5 (0.60)	*3 (60.00)*
Reproductive system and breast disorders	4 (0.48)	*0 (0.00)*
Renal and urinary disorders	4 (0.48)	*3 (75.00)*
Immune system disorders	3 (0.36)	*3 (100.00)*
Surgical and medical procedures	1(0.12)	*1 (100.00)*

Table 3 Distribution of drug-ADR pairs according to ATC classification (level I), overall and stratified according to seriousness, preventability and off-label use

	Tot drug-ADR pairs N (% out of 1100)	Seriousness N (% out of ATC level I)	Preventability N (% out of ATC level I)	Off-label use N (% out of ATC level I)
Related to Vaccines	389 (35.36)	*109 (28.02)*	*27 (6.94)*	–
Not related to Vaccines (ATC level I)	711 (64.64)	*226 (31.79)*	*172 (24.19)*	*62 (8.72)*
J - Antinfectives for systemic use (excluded vaccines - J07)	288 (40.51)	*69 (23.96)*	*15 (5.21)*	*2 (0.69)*
N - Nervous system	168 (23.63)	*81 (48.21)*	*82 (48.81)*	*18 (10.71)*
A - Alimentary tract and metabolism	59 (8.30)	*16 (27.12)*	*25 (42.37)*	*3 (5.08)*
M - Musculoskeletal system	53 (7.45)	*18 (33.96)*	*9 (16.98)*	*0 (0.00)*
C - Cardiovascular system	39 (5.49)	*17 (43.59)*	*22 (56.41)*	*18 (46.15)*
H - Systemic hormonal preparations	31 (4.36)	*7 (22.58)*	*6 (19.35)*	*5 (16.13)*
R - Respiratory system	27 (3.80)	*3 (11.11)*	*2 (7.41)*	*3 (11.11)*
L - Antineoplastic and immunomodulating agents	13 (1.83)	*4 (30.77)*	*2 (15.38)*	*2 (15.38)*
B- Blood and blood-forming organs	11 (1.55)	*6 (54.55)*	*3 (27.27)*	*5 (45.45)*
D - Dermatologicals	10 (1.41)	*3 (30.00)*	*1 (10.00)*	*0 (0.00)*
G - Genitourinary system and sex hormones	4 (0.56)	*2 (50.00)*	*4 (100.00)*	*4 (100.00)*
P - Antiparasitic products	4 (0.56)	*0 (0.00)*	*0 (0.00)*	*0 (0.00)*
S - Sensory organs	4 (0.56)	*0 (0.00)*	*1 (25.00)*	*2 (50.00)*

frequent suspected vaccines were Meningococcus B, multicomponent vaccine ($n = 67$, of whom 32.84% serious), Diphtheria-haemophilus influenzae B-pertussis-poliomyelitis-tetanus-hepatitis B ($n = 57$, of whom 45.61% serious), and Pneumococcus, purified polysaccharides antigen conjugated ($n = 55$, of whom 32.73% serious) (Additional file 2: Table S2).

Table 4 reports the distribution of serious and non-serious drug-ADR pairs and the potential associations between serious ADR risk and age, gender, total number of pharmacological treatments and presence of DDIs. On-label and off-label use and relative associations were also evaluated. Seriousness of ADRs significantly differed among age classes and according to the total number of drugs administered ($p < 0.001$). Risk of having an ADR reported as serious was significantly lower in children and infants compared to adolescents (adjusted ROR of 0.41 [95% CI: 0.27–0.61] and 0.47 [0.32–0.71], respectively). Risk of serious ADRs was significantly increased in subjects exposed to more than one drug (adjusted ROR of 1.87 [1.33–2.62] and 3.01 [2.07–4.37] for subjects exposed to 2 and 3 or more drugs, respectively) compared to subjects exposed to only one drug. On the other hand, the gender, the presence of DDIs and the on-label or off-label drug use did not influence the risk of having an ADR reported as serious.

Discussion

This study aimed to explore the frequency, preventability and seriousness of ADRs observed over a 5-year period in a single pediatric center in Italy, and to our knowledge it is the first study focused on serious ADRs with the aim of addressing the factors associated with the reporting of this kind of ADRs, in an Italian clinical pediatric setting.

In the present analysis, the rate of ADR-related ED admissions was 2.2 per 1000 admissions, notably lower than what is generally reported in literature (0.4% to 10.3% of all children, pooled estimate of 2.9%) [10]. In fact in a large systematic review [10], the rates of ADRs causing hospital admission ranged from 0.4% to 10.3% of all children (pooled estimate of 2.9% (2.6%, 3.1%)). This can be explained by the fact that we calculated the actual rate of ADRs on all ED admissions, including also those not related to drug utilization. These findings are in keeping with what was reported in another Italian study [25] that showed similar results in terms of ATC classes and SOCs most frequently associated with ADRs in children. According to Rosafio et al. (2017) [25], the medication classes most frequently implicated were anti-infective drugs for systemic use (28.9%) and central nervous system agents (22.3%). The three most common symptom manifestations were dermatologic conditions (46.1%), general

Table 4 Distribution of serious and non-serious drug-ADR pairs, and association between serious ADR risk and different factors, expressed as Reporting Odds Ratio (ROR)

	Non-serious drug-ADR pairs N (% out of 765)	Serious drug-ADRs pairs N (% out of 335)	*p*-value	Adjusted ROR of serious ADR [95% CI]	*p*-value
Age classes (FDA classification)					
Adolescents (144–192 months)	86 (11.24)	72 (21.49)	< 0.001	Ref	
Children (24–143 months)	335 (43.79)	123 (36.72)		0.41 [0.27–0.61]	< 0.001
Infants (1–23 months)	336 (43.92)	137 (40.90)		0.47 [0.32–0.71]	0.001
New-borns (< 1 month)	8 (1.05)	3 (0.90)		0.42 [0.10–1.70]	*0.224*
Sex					
Male	353 (46.14)	144 (42.99)	*0.333*	Ref.	
Female	412 (53.86)	191 (57.01)		0.77 [0.59–1.02]	*0.072*
Tot number of drugs					
1	347 (45.36)	101 (30.15)	< 0.001	Ref.	
2	276 (36.08)	128 (38.21)		1.87 [1.33–2.62]	< 0.001
3+	142 (18.56)	106 (31.64)		3.01 [2.07–4.37]	< 0.001
Drug-drug interactions					
No	268 (64.11)	165 (70.51)	*0.097*		
Yes	150 (35.89)	69 (29.49)		0.77 [0.54–1.11]	*0.166*
Off-label vs on-label use[a]					
On-Label	447 (92.36)	201 (88.94)	*0.133*	Ref.	
Off-label	37 (7.64)	25 (11.06)		1.56 [0.90–2.73]	*0.115*

Adjusted ROR values are shown along with the respective 95% Confidence Intervals
[a]Calculated only on non-vaccine medications

disorder and administration site conditions (29.7%) and gastrointestinal symptoms (16.0%).

Among the ADR reports collected in our study, "Antinfectives for systemic use" were the most common drugs, in agreement with a major national ADRs overview conducted in Italy in the last decade [16, 26]. In particular, amoxicillin and amoxicillin/clavulanate were the most frequently involved APs. This evidence could be attributable to the fact that in Tuscany amoxicillin and amoxicillin/clavulanate are generally the most prescribed antibiotics in the pediatric population (14.06 and 23.08 defined daily dose/1000 inhabitants per day, respectively) [27]. The most reported SOC in the present study was "Gastrointestinal disorders", whereas in literature "Skin and subcutaneous tissue disorders" is generally the first SOC to be reported in this population subset [28]. This discrepancy could be related to the fact that dermatological ADRs are generally less serious than gastrointestinal ones, and therefore could be mainly managed by out-of-hospital healthcare professionals rather that in EDs.

Regarding vaccine-related ED admission, this study showed a higher number of drug-ADR pairs for "Meningococcus B multicomponent vaccine" than reported by Rosafio et al. [25]. This data are not surprising given the peculiar Tuscan scenery of meningococcal B disease high incidence and the correlated high vaccination rate in children in the past few years [29]. Anyway, in our study the most common ADRs related to vaccines were fever, injection-site hypersensitivity and edema, and local vasodilatation (data not shown), that cannot be considered life-threatening, although they led to an ED admission. Thus, considering the high number of vaccine doses administered in Tuscany every year [30], the total number of vaccines-related ADRs detected in the present study is reasonably low and provides a general perception of safety of vaccination in children [31].

The rate of serious ADRs compared to non-serious ones, was lower than observed in other studies, performed in both general and pediatric populations [17, 28]. The lower rate of serious ADRs in this sample may indicate a better quality and safety of prescribing in the setting evaluated. Among the drug classes that deserve particular attention in terms of preventable ADRs, there are "Antinfectives for systemic use" (ATC class J) and "Nervous system medications" (ATC class N). The clinical evaluation of the collected ADR reports identified several cases of misuse and abuse due to accidental drug ingestion for class N. Unintentional exposure among children is an important public health problem [32]. One out of 180 two-year-old child visits an ED for a medication poisoning each year [33], and, during 2010–2011, an average of 1499 children/year aged less than 6 years were evaluated in ED in the United States for unintentional exposure to drugs, including agents of ATC class N [34]. In this context, our evidences underline the importance of careful drug management by parents and caregivers [35], with the final goal of improving the strategies to prevent these kind of adverse events [36].

This study also showed a correlation between the risk of serious ADR and age classes. Children and infants had a significantly lower risk of serious ADRs compared to adolescents, as reported in other studies [37, 38]. To the best of our knowledge, no other publications have previously reported age as a risk factor for serious ADR-related ED admission in children. In general, age-based analyses do not follow a clear pattern and are difficult to evaluate due to the variety of age classifications [10]. Healthcare professionals have to consider important factors related to age, such as pharmacokinetic and pharmacodynamic differences during children growth (i.e., immature tubular function and hypoalbuminemia in neonates, immaturity of blood brain barrier, reduced metabolism and liver function, etc.) [39].

Concerning risk factors associated with ADRs in children, polypharmacy was found as a potential predictor of adverse events. Multiple regression analysis showed a statistically significant correlation between polypharmacy (use of more than 3 drugs) and the risk of presenting to the ED for a serious ADR. Our results are consistent with several published investigations conducted in pediatric patients that also show polypharmacy to be an important factor that predisposes to ADRs [38]. Polypharmacy as a risk factor for ADRs is well characterized in adults and older subjects [40] and descriptive data are also available in children [41], but the risk of serious ADRs had not been addressed previously.

Off-label prescribing has been widely observed in children [42]. However, administration of a drug outside the conditions assessed during clinical trials may result in ADRs [43]. The present study shows no statistically significant difference between on-label and off-label use in terms of ADRs occurrence. Our evidence confirms the data already reported by Palmaro and colleagues on the safety of off-label drug utilization [44].

It is well known that the lack of reliable data on drug safety in the pediatric population is associated with specific issues, among which are the lack of dedicated clinical trials and the non-linear development of pharmacokinetic parameters [45]. Serious ADRs are generally not observed during pediatric clinical trials, especially in case of a latency period before onset [46], and in children as in adults it is not possible to fully investigate the spectrum of serious ADRs prior authorization of most medications [47]. Pharmacovigilance spontaneous reporting systems are subjected to under-reporting of ADRs, including serious ones [48]. Thus, an active pharmacovigilance study like the one presented here represents one of the best strategies to systematically collect, analyze and interpret data on ADRs [17], by means of protocols designed to actively detect ADRs on an ongoing basis within a defined group of people (i.e., children in ED).

The present study has several points of strength. First, we used a computerized monitoring programs and all participants were specifically trained healthcare professionals, who systematically analyzed each single ED clinical record. Furthermore, this is the first retrospective analysis evaluating serious ADRs as cause of ED admission in children over a long period of time in Italy. However, this study has also some limitations. The retrospective nature of our study may have led to an underestimation of the rate of ADR-related ED admissions as a result of missing documented clinical data. Indeed, not all pediatric ADRs were identified, since not all pediatric patients presenting an ADR, even if serious, attend ED. Therefore, the real prevalence of ADR is not known. Last, a control group with no ADRs was not available and this is also a limitation with regard to assessment of causality between ADRs and ED admission.

Conclusions

Serious ADRs are a relevant clinical event in children and a challenge for pediatricians and health care systems. The present research provided new insights on the factors that might increase the risk of serious pediatric ADRs. Future prospective, large-sample and multicenter studies should focus on other at-risk pediatric settings such as oncology, hematology, neurology, etc. to better understand the impact of ADRs and the effect of programmed preventive actions. In this context, we believe that active surveillance in pharmacovigilance might represent the best strategy to estimate and characterize the clinical burden of ADRs in children, with the final goal of improving the appropriateness of prescribing in the fragile population of pediatric patients.

Abbreviations

ADR: Adverse Drug Reaction; AP: Active Principles; ATC: Anatomical Therapeutic Chemical; CI: Confidence Interval; DDI: Drug-Drug Interactions; ED: Emergency Department; ROR: Reporting Odds Ratio; SOC: System Organ Class; WHO: World Health Organization

Funding

This study was funded by a research grant from the AIFA (the Italian Medicines Agency), Rome, Italy, Tuscan County resolution DGRT 790/2016 All. C. The funder of the study had no role in the collection, analysis and interpretation of data, nor in the writing of the report, nor in the decision to submit the article for publication.

Authors' contributions

NL, GC, AM, LG, AV (Vannacci) made substantial contributions to conception and design of the study. EM, AV (Vitiello), RB, AMC, SM made substantial contributions to acquisition of data. NL, GC, AB, RB, EL, AV (Vannacci) made substantial contributions to analysis and interpretation of data. NL, GC, AB were involved in drafting the manuscript. EL, AM, LG, AV (Vannacci) were involved in revising the manuscript critically for important intellectual content. All authors gave final approval of the version to be published. All authors agreed to be accountable for all aspects of the work in ensuring that questions related to the accuracy or integrity of any part of the work are appropriately investigated and resolved. All authors read and approved the final manuscript.

Competing interests

The authors declare that they have no competing interests.

Author details

[1]Department of Neurosciences, Psychology, Drug Research and Child Health, Section of Pharmacology and Toxicology, University of Florence, viale G. Pieraccini, 6, 50139 Florence, Italy. [2]Department of Pharmacy, Anna Meyer Children's University Hospital, viale G. Pieraccini, 24, 50139 Florence, Italy. [3]Department of Emergency Medicine, Anna Meyer Children's University Hospital, viale G. Pieraccini, 24, 50139 Florence, Italy.

References

1. Shehab N, Lovegrove MC, Geller AI, Rose KO, Weidle NJ, Budnitz DS. US emergency department visits for outpatient adverse drug events, 2013-2014. JAMA. 2016;316(20):2115–25.
2. Budnitz DS, Lovegrove MC, Shehab N, Richards CL. Emergency hospitalizations for adverse drug events in older Americans. N Engl J Med. 2011;365(21):2002–12.
3. Pirmohamed M, James S, Meakin S, Green C, Scott AK, Walley TJ, Farrar K, Park BK, Breckenridge AM. Adverse drug reactions as cause of admission to hospital: prospective analysis of 18 820 patients. BMJ. 2004;329(7456):15–9.
4. Marengoni A, Pasina L, Concoreggi C, Martini G, Brognoli F, Nobili A, Onder G, Bettoni D. Understanding adverse drug reactions in older adults through drug-drug interactions. Eur J Intern Med. 2014;25(9):843–6.
5. Davies EA, O'Mahony MS. Adverse drug reactions in special populations - the elderly. Br J Clin Pharmacol. 2015;80(4):796–807.
6. Alhawassi TM, Krass I, Bajorek BV, Pont LG. A systematic review of the prevalence and risk factors for adverse drug reactions in the elderly in the acute care setting. Clin Interv Aging. 2014;9:2079–86.
7. Salvi F, Marchetti A, D'Angelo F, Boemi M, Lattanzio F, Cherubini A. Adverse drug events as a cause of hospitalization in older adults. Drug Saf. 2012; 35(Suppl 1):29–45.
8. Dehours E, Bounes V, Bagheri H, Valle B, Ducasse JL, Montastruc JL. Adverse drug reactions in an emergency medical dispatching Centre. Eur J Clin Pharmacol. 2014;70(7):881–7.
9. Samoy LJ, Zed PJ, Wilbur K, Balen RM, Abu-Laban RB, Roberts M. Drug-related hospitalizations in a tertiary care internal medicine service of a Canadian hospital: a prospective study. Pharmacotherapy. 2006;26(11):1578–86.
10. Smyth RM, Gargon E, Kirkham J, Cresswell L, Golder S, Smyth R, Williamson P. Adverse drug reactions in children–a systematic review. PLoS One. 2012; 7(3):e24061.
11. Kearns GL, Abdel-Rahman SM, Alander SW, Blowey DL, Leeder JS, Kauffman RE. Developmental pharmacology–drug disposition, action, and therapy in infants and children. N Engl J Med. 2003;349(12):1157–67.
12. Mitchell AA, Lacouture PG, Sheehan JE, Kauffman RE, Shapiro S. Adverse drug reactions in children leading to hospital admission. Pediatrics. 1988; 82(1):24–9.
13. Turner S, Longworth A, Nunn AJ, Choonara I. Unlicensed and off label drug use in paediatric wards: prospective study. BMJ. 1998;316(7128):343–5.
14. Bates DW, Spell N, Cullen DJ, Burdick E, Laird N, Petersen LA, Small SD, Sweitzer BJ, Leape LL. The costs of adverse drug events in hospitalized patients. Adverse drug events prevention study group. JAMA. 1997;277(4): 307–11.

15. Zed PJ, Haughn C, Black KJ, Fitzpatrick EA, Ackroyd-Stolarz S, Murphy NG, MacKinnon NJ, Curran JA, Sinclair D. Medication-related emergency department visits and hospital admissions in pediatric patients: a qualitative systematic review. J Pediatr. 2013;163(2):477–83.
16. Carnovale C, Brusadelli T, Zuccotti G, Beretta S, Sullo MG, Capuano A, Rossi F, Moschini M, Mugelli A, Vannacci A, et al. The importance of monitoring adverse drug reactions in pediatric patients: the results of a national surveillance program in Italy. Expert Opin Drug Saf. 2014;13(Suppl 1):S1–8.
17. Perrone V, Conti V, Venegoni M, Scotto S, Degli Esposti L, Sangiorgi D, Prestini L, Radice S, Clementi E, Vighi G. Seriousness, preventability, and burden impact of reported adverse drug reactions in Lombardy emergency departments: a retrospective 2-year characterization. Clinicoecon Outcomes Res. 2014;6:505–14.
18. Naranjo CA, Busto U, Sellers EM, Sandor P, Ruiz I, Roberts EA, Janecek E, Domecq C, Greenblatt DJ. A method for estimating the probability of adverse drug reactions. Clin Pharmacol Ther. 1981;30(2):239–45.
19. Schumock GT, Thornton JP. Focusing on the preventability of adverse drug reactions. Hosp Pharm. 1992;27(6):538.
20. Causality assessment of adverse event following immunization (AEFI): user manual for the revised WHO. classification. Available at: **http://www.who.int/vaccine_safety/publications/aevi_manual.pdf** [Last Accessed 13 Oct 2017].
21. Tozzi AE, Asturias EJ, Balakrishnan MR, Halsey NA, Law B, Zuber PL. Assessment of causality of individual adverse events following immunization (AEFI): a WHO tool for global use. Vaccine. 2013;31(44):5041–6.
22. Micromedex® Medication, Disease and Toxicology Management. Available at: **http://www.micromedexsolutions.com/home/dispatch**.
23. Santos TRA, Silveira EA, Pereira LV, Provin MP, Lima DM, Amaral RG. Potential drug-drug interactions in older adults: a population-based study. Geriatr Gerontol Int. 2017;17(12):2336-46.
24. Neubert A, Wong IC, Bonifazi A, Catapano M, Felisi M, Baiardi P, Giaquinto C, Knibbe CA, Sturkenboom MC, Ghaleb MA, et al. Defining off-label and unlicensed use of medicines for children: results of a Delphi survey. Pharmacol Res. 2008;58(5–6):316–22.
25. Rosafio C, Paioli S, Del Giovane C, Cenciarelli V, Viani N, Bertolani P, Iughetti L. Medication-related visits in a pediatric emergency department: an 8-years retrospective analysis. Ital J Pediatr. 2017;43(1):55.
26. Ferrajolo C, Capuano A, Trifiro G, Moretti U, Rossi F, Santuccio C. Pediatric drug safety surveillance in Italian pharmacovigilance network: an overview of adverse drug reactions in the years 2001 - 2012. Expert Opin Drug Saf. 2014;13(Suppl 1):S9–20.
27. Lusini G, Lapi F, Sara B, Vannacci A, Mugelli A, Kragstrup J, Bjerrum L. Antibiotic prescribing in paediatric populations: a comparison between Viareggio, Italy and Funen, Denmark. Eur J Pub Health. 2009;19(4):434–8.
28. Priyadharsini R, Surendiran A, Adithan C, Sreenivasan S, Sahoo FK. A study of adverse drug reactions in pediatric patients. J Pharmacol Pharmacother. 2011;2(4):277–80.
29. Signorelli C, Chiesa V, Odone A. Meningococcal serogroup B vaccine in Italy: state-of-art, organizational aspects and perspectives. J Prev Med Hyg. 2015; 56(3):E125–32.
30. The Medicines Utilization Monitoring Centre. National Report on medicines use in Italy 2016. Rome: Italian Medicines Agency; 2017. **http://www.aifa.gov.it/sites/default/files/Rapporto_OsMed_2016_AIFA.pdf** [Last Accessed 13 Oct 2017
31. Staltari O, Cilurzo F, Caroleo B, Greco A, Corasaniti F, Genovesi MA, Gallelli L. Annual report on adverse events related with vaccines use in Calabria (Italy): 2012. J Pharmacol Pharmacother. 2013;4(Suppl 1):S61–5.
32. Lavonas EJ, Banner W, Bradt P, Bucher-Bartelson B, Brown KR, Rajan P, Murrelle L, Dart RC, Green JL. Root causes, clinical effects, and outcomes of unintentional exposures to buprenorphine by young children. J Pediatr. 2013;163(5):1377–83. e1371–1373
33. Schillie SF, Shehab N, Thomas KE, Budnitz DS. Medication overdoses leading to emergency department visits among children. Am J Prev Med. 2009; 37(3):181–7.
34. Franklin RL, Rodgers GB. Unintentional child poisonings treated in United States hospital emergency departments: national estimates of incident cases, population-based poisoning rates, and product involvement. Pediatrics. 2008;122(6):1244–51.
35. Wiley CC, Wiley JF 2nd. Pediatric benzodiazepine ingestion resulting in hospitalization. J Toxicol Clin Toxicol. 1998;36(3):227–31.
36. Kaushal R, Bates DW, Landrigan C, McKenna KJ, Clapp MD, Federico F, Goldmann DA. Medication errors and adverse drug events in pediatric inpatients. JAMA. 2001;285(16):2114–20.
37. Knopf H, Du Y. Perceived adverse drug reactions among non-institutionalized children and adolescents in Germany. Br J Clin Pharmacol. 2010;70(3):409–17.
38. Impicciatore P, Choonara I, Clarkson A, Provasi D, Pandolfini C, Bonati M. Incidence of adverse drug reactions in paediatric in/out-patients: a systematic review and meta-analysis of prospective studies. Br J Clin Pharmacol. 2001; 52(1):77–83.
39. Anderson GD, Lynn AM. Optimizing pediatric dosing: a developmental pharmacologic approach. Pharmacotherapy. 2009;29(6):680–90.
40. Nobili A, Licata G, Salerno F, Pasina L, Tettamanti M, Franchi C, De Vittorio L, Marengoni A, Corrao S, Iorio A, et al. Polypharmacy, length of hospital stay, and in-hospital mortality among elderly patients in internal medicine wards. The REPOSI study. Eur J Clin Pharmacol. 2011;67(5):507–19.
41. Morden NE, Goodman D. Pediatric polypharmacy: time to lock the medicine cabinet? Arch Pediatr Adolesc Med. 2012;166(1):91–2.
42. Lindell-Osuagwu L, Hakkarainen M, Sepponen K, Vainio K, Naaranlahti T, Kokki H. Prescribing for off-label use and unauthorized medicines in three paediatric wards in Finland, the status before and after the European Union Paediatric regulation. J Clin Pharm Ther. 2014;39(2):144–53.
43. Cuzzolin L, Atzei A, Fanos V. Off-label and unlicensed prescribing for newborns and children in different settings: a review of the literature and a consideration about drug safety. Expert Opin Drug Saf. 2006;5(5):703–18.
44. Palmaro A, Bissuel R, Renaud N, Durrieu G, Escourrou B, Oustric S, Montastruc JL, Lapeyre-Mestre M. Off-label prescribing in pediatric outpatients. Pediatrics. 2015;135(1):49–58.
45. Napoleone E. Children and ADRs (adverse drug reactions). Ital J Pediatr. 2010;36:4.
46. Clavenna A, Berti A, Gualandi L, Rossi E, De Rosa M, Bonati M. Drug utilisation profile in the Italian paediatric population. Eur J Pediatr. 2009; 168(2):173–80.
47. Clavenna A, Bonati M. Adverse drug reactions in childhood: a review of prospective studies and safety alerts. Arch Dis Child. 2009;94(9):724–8.
48. Langerova P, Vrtal J, Urbanek K. Adverse drug reactions causing hospital admissions in childhood: a prospective, observational, single-Centre study. Basic Clin Pharmacol Toxicol. 2014;115(6):560–4.

17

Comparison of topical tofacitinib and 0.1% hypochlorous acid in a murine atopic dermatitis model

Tomoki Fukuyama[1], Sarah Ehling[1,2], Jenny Wilzopolski[1,2] and Wolfgang Bäumer[1,2*]

Abstract

Background: Topical administration of PR022, 0.05% hypochlorous acid (HOCl) in gel has been demonstrated to be beneficial in a chronic murine atopic dermatitis model. In a follow up study we tested a higher concentration (0.1%) of PR022 HOCl gel in comparison to the Janus kinase inhibitor tofacitinib, both of which are currently in clinical phase studies for treatment of human atopic dermatitis.

Methods: The effect of topically administered HOCl (0.1%) in gel was compared to a topical formulation of tofacitinib (0.5%) in a therapeutic setting on atopic dermatitis-like lesions in NC/Nga mice as well as itch behaviour. NC/Nga mice were sensitized with house dust mite allergen. After reaching visible lesions, mice were treated either topically with HOCl or tofacitinib or gel vehicle for 17 days. After termination of the study, dorsal root ganglia were isolated for ex vivo stimulation and skin samples were taken for cytokine determination in inflamed skin.

Results: When administered onto lesional skin of NC/Nga mice, both HOCl and tofacitinib reduced lesions and scratching behaviour. The reduced inflammatory response by HOCl and tofacitinib treatment was demonstrated by diminished inflammatory cytokines in affected skin tissue from NC/Nga mice. Dorsal root ganglia neurons re-stimulated with a range of mediators of itch showed a reduced response compared to the vehicle control mice, when isolated from tofacitinib or HOCl treated mice.

Conclusions: These data indicate a similar beneficial potential of topical high dose PR022 HOCl (0.1%) in gel and tofacitinib, in a translational murine model of atopic dermatitis.

Keywords: Atopic dermatitis, Dorsal root ganglia, Hypochlorous acid, Tofacitinib, IgE, IL-4, IL-13, NC/Nga mice, Sensory neurons

Background

Although the incidence of atopic dermatitis (AD) is still increasing, topical pharmaceutical treatment options for AD are limited. Mostly traditional pharmaceutical treatments like topical calcineurin inhibitors or glucocorticoids are still used, but both have dose limiting side effects [1]. Currently there are some small clinical investigations on the use of hypochlorous acid (HOCl) for the topical treatment of AD [2]. It has been reported that HOCl has anti-itch and anti-inflammatory potential in human AD patients [2]. Thus, our group recently performed a detailed preventive and therapeutic intervention study of PR022, HOCl (0.05%) in gel in a chronic mouse model of AD, namely the NC/Nga mice sensitized to a human-relevant allergen (house dust mite allergen). We found a significant inhibition of lesion development and scratching behaviour in the preventive setting and a reduction of lesions and itch in a therapeutic setting accompanied by reduced immunoglobulin E (IgE) response, cytokine secretion in skin and responsiveness of sensory neurons. In vitro experiments with murine bone marrow derived dendritic cells and dorsal root ganglia neurons also revealed an inhibition of MAP kinase activity, inhibition of NFκB pathway and sensory response by pre-incubation of low concentrations of HOCl [3].

* Correspondence: Wolfgang.baeumer@fu-berlin.de
[1]Department of Molecular Biomedical Sciences, College of Veterinary Medicine, North Carolina State University, Raleigh, NC, USA
[2]Institute of Pharmacology and Toxicology, Faculty of Veterinary Medicine, Freie Universität Berlin, Koserstraße 20, 14195 Berlin, Germany

Therefore, the present study was performed to test a higher concentration (0.1%) of hypochlorous acid in the NC/Nga mice model in comparison to the Janus kinase (JAK) inhibitor tofacitinib, both of which are currently in clinical studies for treatment of human AD [4]. Apart from efficacy, a further target was to evaluate local tolerability of a higher HOCl concentration.

Methods

Materials and reagents

Hypochlorous acid (HOCl) was used as a gel formulation (0.1% AFC, pH 5.5 ± 0.5) and was supplied as "PR022" by Realm Therapeutics, Inc. (Malvern, PA, USA). PR022 is a proprietary formulation of stabilized hypochlorous acid in a gelling agent and an emollient in development for the treatment of atopic dermatitis. In the Phase 2 clinical study, 2 concentrations of PR022 are being evaluated, 0.05 and 0.1% (NCT03351777). For active sensitization, house dust mite allergen (*Dermatophagoides farina,* GREER, Lenoir, NC, USA) was used. Poly-L-lysine, laminin, capsaicin, allyl isothiocyanate (AITC), 2-mercaptoethanol and mineral oil were obtained from Sigma (St. Louis, MO, USA). Dispase was purchased from STEMCELL Technologies Inc. (Cambridge, MA, USA). Fura-2-acetoxymethyl ester (Fura-2 AM), phosphate buffered saline (PBS), collagenase, chloroquine, histamine, and SLIGRL-NH_2 were ordered from Thermo Fisher Scientific Inc. (Waltham, MA, USA). Fetal bovine serum (FBS), Dulbecco's modified eagle medium with L-glutamine (DMEM) and RPMI-1640 medium, Ca^{2+} and Mg^{2+}-free hank's balanced salt solution (HBSS), penicillin-streptomycin and fetal bovine serum (FBS) were from Mediatech Inc. (Manassas, VA, USA). MEM eagle (EMEM) medium was obtained from Lonza Group Ltd. (Allendale, NJ, USA). For determination of protein content DCs protein assay kit was used (BIO-RAD, Richmond, CA, USA). The murine IgE ELISA (OptEIA) set was ordered from Becton, Dickinson and Company (Franklin Lakes, NJ). Recombinant mouse interleukin (IL-)1β, IL-31, and tumor necrosis factor (TNF)α were purchased from Pepro Tech, Inc. (Rocky Hill, NJ, USA). Enzyme linked immunosorbent assay (ELISA) kits for IL-1β, IL-4, IL-13, thymic stromal lymphopoietin (TSLP), thymus and activation regulated chemokine (TARC), and TNFα were obtained from R&D systems (Minneapolis, MN, USA). Serotonin and tofacitinib were ordered from Tocris Bioscience (Bristol, UK).

Mice

NC/Nga (female) mice were ordered from Charles River Japan Laboratories (Tokyo, Japan). The mice arrived at 35 to 40 days of age and were kept in quarantine for at least 1 week. The facility offered a controlled environment (including individually ventilated cages and sentinel animals). The animals were housed at 22 °C with 50% humidity with a 12-h light cycle. The mice were fed with certified pellet diet and received water ad libitum. The study protocol was approved by the Animal Care and Use Committee of the North Carolina State University (IACUC Protocol No. 13–111-B).

Murine model of atopic dermatitis in NC/Nga mice

Prior to first sensitization, NC/Nga mice were clipped on their back. The following day, mice were sensitized with 30 μl of house dust mite allergen (HDM) suspended (10 mg/ml) in mineral oil and applied topically onto the back twice weekly. To accelerate sensitization, mild tape stripping ("Staples" office tape) was performed weekly just before the first HDM sensitization. Tape stripping was terminated as soon as visible lesions had developed. Treatment of HOCl (0.1% in gel, $n = 8$), tofacitinib (0.5% in lipoderm, $n = 8$) or vehicle (gel, $n = 8$) was started on day 15, where the mice showed a mean lesional score of 2.1. The mice were equally distributed according to their clinical score, that each treatment group represents the mean of 2.1. One group of mice ($n = 6$) was left untreated and served as a base control. The dose selection for tofacitinib was according to a former study in which 0.5% tofacitinib inhibited itch behaviour and inflammation in a mouse model of allergic contact dermatitis, higher doses (when given in acetone) led to irritation of mouse skin, thus it was decided to select a concentration of 0.5% [5].

During the experimental period, back skin thickness, body weight, clinical scores and scratching behavior were monitored once every week. The clinical score was determined as according to the following system: No symptoms, 0; mild, 1; moderate, 2; severe, 3 and extreme, 4. The mean was calculated from the score for erosions, edema, and erythema as well as skin dryness, as described previously [3]. To monitor scratching behaviour mice were video monitored for 30 min directly after sensitization with HDM once a week. Video monitoring was performed with mouse pairs (belonging to the same treatment group) at the same cage. Only repeated strokes with the hindlimb directed to the area of HDM sensitization were counted as scratching bout. Mice were sacrificed by CO_2 inhalation according to AVMA Guidelines for the Euthanasia of Animals and tissue was collected from each group on day 32.

The back skin, blood and dorsal root ganglia (DRG) were obtained from single mice 1 h after last HOCl or tofacitinib application (this means 24 h after last HDM challenge). Samples were processed (or stored) for IgE determination, histology, cytokine determination and functional measurement of intracellular Ca^{2+} in DRG neurons.

Histology

Tissue samples from rostral neck skin were excised, fixed in paraformaldehyde (4% solution), sectioned and stained with haematoxylin-eosin. Edema and cell influx were evaluated semiquantitatively (0, no influx, no edema; 1, mild; 2, moderate; and 3, severe influx, severe edema) in a blinded manner in skin sections of each mouse back skin ($n = 8$ for treatment groups, $n = 6$ for untreated control).

Cytokine determination of skin tissues

One part of the rostral neck skin tissue was snap-frozen in liquid nitrogen. Cytokine determination for skin tissues was performed as described previously [6]. IL-1β, – 4, – 13, TARC, TSLP and TNFα were measured by ELISA. Intra-assay variance was < 10%, inter-assay variance was not calculated as each ELISA (30 samples) was done in one setting (= one plate) for the present study.

Determination of total IgE in serum

Blood samples collected from single mice was centrifuged at 3000 g to isolate serum. We used an ELSA according to the manufacturer's protocol to determine total IgE level present in serum.

Isolation of DRG and calcium imaging on DRG cell culture

Preparation and cultivation of the DRG neurons from the NC/Nga mice was done as described previously [7]. Briefly, DRGs were dissected along the thoracic vertebral column. Single ganglia were digested by means of dispase and collagenase which was dissolved in HBSS for 30 min at 37 °C. A trituration of DRG using fire-polished Pasteur pipettes helped with dissociation. Single cells were centrifuged/washed in DMEM medium containing 10% FBS, resuspended in 50 μl medium and placed onto poly-D-lysine and laminin-coated coverslips. Cells were incubated at 37 °C for 2 h and then flooded with 1 ml of medium and further incubated at 37 °C. Calcium experiments were performed within 24 h of culture.

Changes in intracellular [Ca^{2+}] free concentration in single neurons were measured by digital microscopy connected to equipment for ratiometric recording of single cells as described elsewhere [8]. In brief, coverslips attached dorsal root ganglia cells were loaded with fura-2 (8 μmol/L) in DMEM media and incubated at 37 °C for 30 min. For ratiometric imaging, the cells were transferred to a tempered (37 °C) incubation chamber on the stage of the microscope and constantly perfused with Locke solution. Cells that incorporated fura2 were identified using fluorescence microscopy before starting the ratiometric experiment. Cells were marked with region of interest circles and monitored by sequential dual excitation, 340 and 380 nm. The frequency of image acquisition was 100 ms. DRG neurons were initially exposed to IL-1β (1 μg/ml), TNFα (1 μg/ml), histamine (1 mmol/l), followed by IL-31 (1 μg/ml), chloroquine (10 μmol/l), serotonin (1 mmol/l), AITC (100 μmol/l), capsaicin (1 μmol/l) and KCl (75 mmol/l). However, none of the cells were stimulated with more than 3–4 stimuli in the row and the order was switched randomly from slide to slide always ending with KCl. The cells were superfused with a steady Locke solution flux for at least 180 s. after each stimulus as a recovery for the cells prior to the next stimulus.

Statistical analysis

All data are displayed as mean (±SD). Statistical significance of the difference was estimated at the 5 and 1% levels of probability. If only the significance of differences between mean values of 2 groups were tested, Student t test was used. For comparisons of more than 2 groups we used a one-way ANOVA followed by Dunnett's multiple comparison test. Comparisons of proportions (study with dorsal root ganglia) were made by means of the Fisher exact test. The data analysis was performed with Prism 4 (GraphPad Software, San Diego, CA, USA).

Results

High dose of hypochlorous acid and tofacitinib reduce lesions and itch in the murine NC/Nga model of AD

To monitor the disease severity of the murine atopic like lesions we scored these according to the four major clinical symptoms of atopic dermatitis, namely excoriations, edema, and erythema and skin dryness. After starting HDM application, the lesional score gradually increased in the vehicle group starting from day 6. Topical administration of 0.1% HOCl and 0.5% tofacitinib resulted in reduction in skin lesions compared to the vehicle-only group. This difference became significant 10 days after initiation of HOCl treatment and 6 days after tofacitinib treatment initiation (Fig. 1a). In analogy to the lesion severity scratching bouts steadily increased throughout the study in the vehicle control group. This scratching behaviour was significantly reduced by topical administration of HOCl or tofacitinib compared to that of vehicle control group (Fig. 1b). A decrease of back skin thickness was observed in both treatment groups indicating a reduced lichenification (Fig. 1c). There was no difference in bodyweight in vehicle control, tofacitinib and hypochlorous acid gel indicating a lack of systemic effect of these two topical treatment options (data not shown).

The histological evaluation confirmed the in vivo findings: At day 32 vehicle treated mice had markedly increased edema formation and inflammatory cell influx. This was significantly reduced by topical treatment with HOCl and tofacitinib compared to vehicle treatment (Fig. 2a and b).

As a more objective measure of allergic inflammation in the skin and to corroborate histological findings,

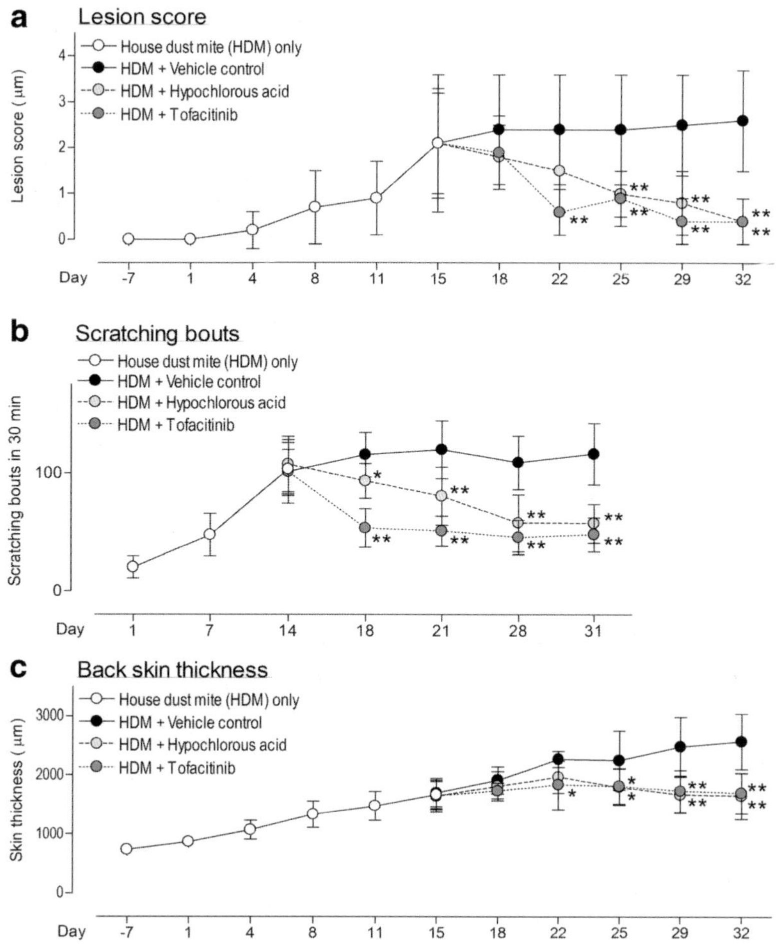

Fig. 1 Topical application of tofacitinib and hypochlorous acid, respectively, significantly reduced lesion formation, scratching behaviour and lichenification in NC/Nga mice. **a** Mice developed moderate lesions 15 days after HDM challenge. A therapeutic intervention with hypochlorous acid or tofacitinib significantly reduced the lesion score and hyperplasia at study day 32; **b** Scratching bouts steadily increase during repetitive challenge with house dust mite antigen within the first 14 days. Under therapeutic conditions, hypochlorous acid or tofacitinib significantly reduced scratching behaviour. **c** Back skin thickness was also significantly reduced by treatment with hypochlorous acid or tofacitinib indicating a positive impact on lichenification. $n = 8$ per group, $n = 6$ for untreated control), $^{*}p < 0.05$, $^{**}p < 0.01$ compared to vehicle treated mice

tissue cytokines were determined in back skin. In addition to an impact on pleiotropic pro-inflammatory cytokines like IL-1β, and TNFα, the level of classical Th2 cytokines like TARC, IL-4 and IL-13 was strongly diminished by treatment with hypochlorous acid gel or tofacitinib compared to the vehicle control treatment in back skin. In addition, the cytokine TSLP which has been described to be a direct pruritogen, was also significantly reduced (Table 1). By direct comparison of reduction of cytokines by tofacitinib and HOCl it seems that tofacitinib was more potent in reducing the cytokines (significantly for IL-4).

Total IgE was vastly increased compared to untreated age matched mice after chronic treatment with HDM. This increase was significantly reduced by topical administration of hypochlorous acid gel or tofacitinib compared to vehicle control treatment (Fig. 2c).

The ex-vivo-response of sensory neurons to different pruritus stimuli is diminished after HOCl or tofacitinib treatment

Both, HOCl and tofacitinib application had a significant effect on itch behavior. Thus, in a next step we assessed whether this response could also be retraced on dorsal root ganglia (DRG) ex vivo. For this, DRG were obtained from NC/Nga mice treated with vehicle, HOCl gel or tofacitinb and the ex vivo response of DRG neurons to histamine and non-histaminergic stimuli (serotonin, chloroquine, IL-31) were compared to DRG obtained from vehicle treated, house dust mite sensitized mice and a basal control (i.e. untreated, age matched NC/Nga mice). When DRG of hypochlorous acid gel or tofacitinib treated mice were monitored, histamine as well as non-histaminergic stimuli led to significant less

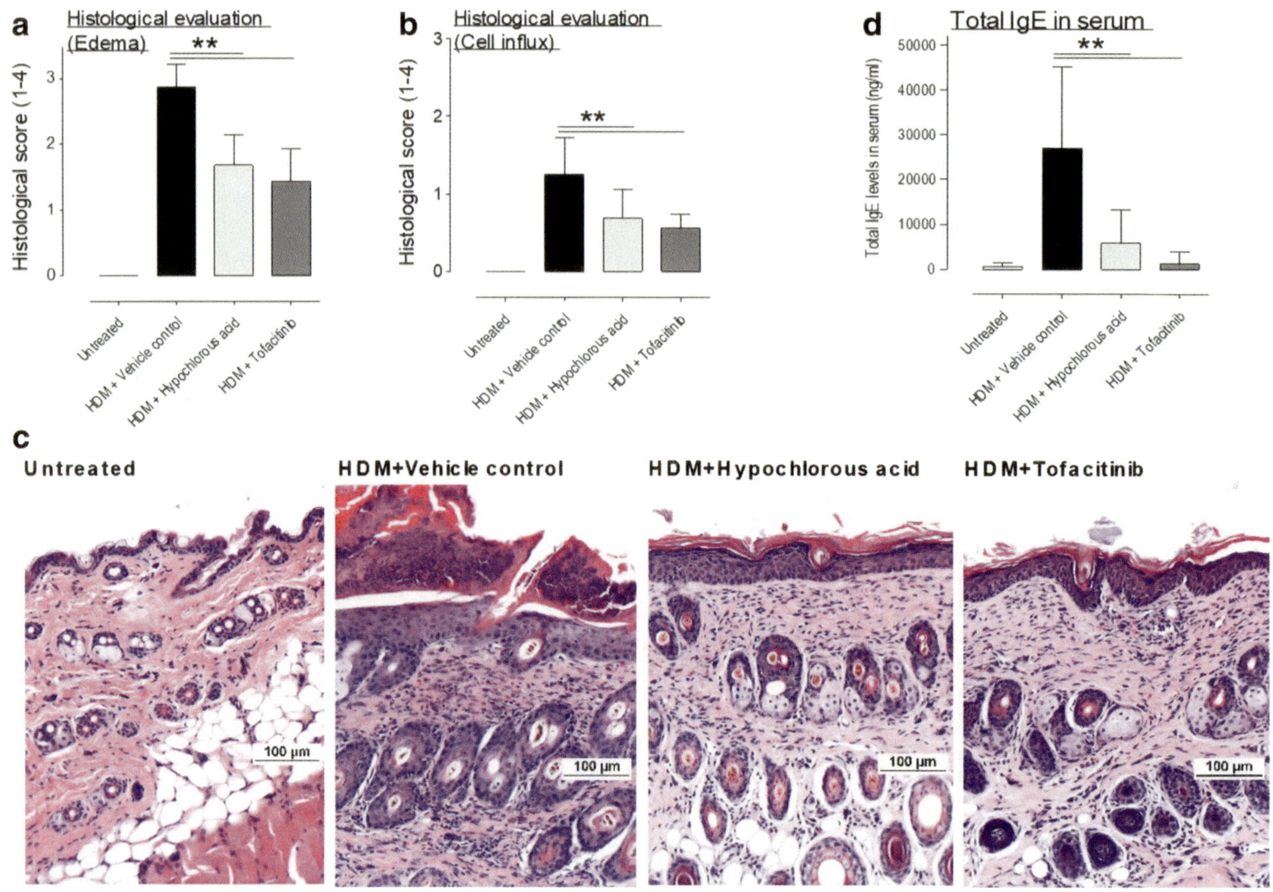

Fig. 2 Hypochlorous acid and tofacitinib significantly reduced edema and inflammatory cell influx as well as total IgE in serum. **a** NC/Nga mice were sacrificed on study day 32 and histological samples were taken for the detrermination of edema and inflammatory cell influx. Both treatment options led to significantly reduced edema (**a**, **c**) and inflammatory cell influx (**b**, **c**) compared to vehicle treated and HDM challenged mice. **d** Whereas a HDM challenge led to a vast increase of total IgE in vehicle treated mice, this concentration was significantly reduced by topical treatment with HOCl or tofacitinib., n = 8 per group, $n = 6$ for untreated control), *$p < 0.05$, **$p < 0.01$ compared to vehicle treated mice

sensory nerve activation compared to vehicle treated mice (Fig. 3a). In addition, we observed that an enhanced response to AITC (TRPA1 channel activator) as well as capsaicin (TRPV1 channel activator) was also reduced, which can be interpreted as a sign of reduced peripheral sensitization (Fig. 3b).

Discussion

Atopic dermatitis (AD), a multifactorial allergic-inflammatory disease with complex pathophysiology, remains incurable and affects 10 to 20% of children [9, 10]. The two major symptoms of AD are pruritus (itch) and inflammatory lesions. Topical treatment options

Table 1 Cytokine production in back skin of topical application of hypochlorous acid or tofacitinib in NC/Nga mice

Group	Untreated	HDM + Vehicle control	HDM + Hypochlorous acid	HDM + Tofacitinib
IL-1β (pg/mg)	84 ± 25	140 ± 60	83 ± 27 *	41 ± 17 **
IL-4 (pg/mg)	32 ± 18	157 ± 57	87 ± 28 **	36 ± 19 **†
IL-13 (pg/mg)	183 ± 101	739 ± 451	321 ± 68 *	162 ± 76 **
TARC (pg/mg)	32 ± 16	100 ± 49	53 ± 12 *	27 ± 10 **
TNFα (pg/mg)	98 ± 50	453 ± 230	207 ± 37 **	108 ± 40 **
TSLP (pg/mg)	69 ± 19	186 ± 96	115 ± 26 **	76 ± 25 **

Back skin tissue was collected 24 h after last HDM challenge and 1 h after last HOCl or tofacitinib application. Results are expressed as mean ± S.D. (pg/mg protein; $n = 8$ per group, $n = 6$ for untreated group)

*: $P < 0.05$ and **: $P < 0.01$ (Dunnett's multiple comparison test) vs. HDM + vehicle control group. †: $P < 0.05$ (Tukey's Multiple Comparison Test) HDM + Tofacitinib vs. HDM + Hypochlorous acid group

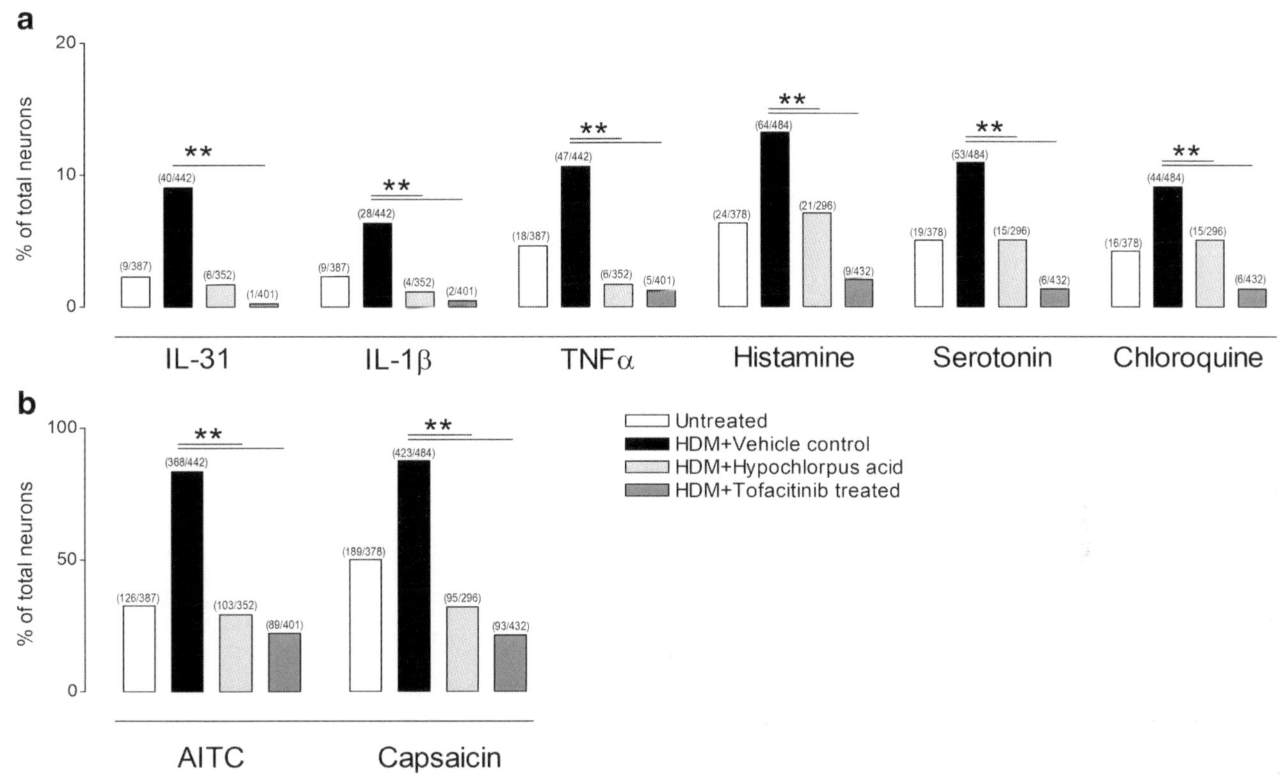

Fig. 3 Ex vivo response of sensory neurons stimulated with different pruritogens. **a** The ex vivo response of DRG neurons to IL-31 (1 μg/ml), IL-1β (1 μg/ml), TNFα (1 μg/ml), histamine (1 mmol/l), serotonin (1 mmol/l) and chloroquine (10 μmol/l) and (**b**) AITC (100 μmol/l) as well as capsaicin (1 μmol/l) were compared to DRG obtained from age matched vehicle treated and house dust mite antigen sensitized and challenged NC/Nga mice. The sensory nerve activation in dorsal root ganglia isolated from hypochlorous acid or tofacitinib treated mice were reduced in response to all stimuli compared to vehicle treated. Absolute number of neurons in brackets, $^{**}p < 0.01$ compared to vehicle treated mice

are limited and the frequently used glucocorticoids and calcineurin inhibitors have side effects, particularly with their long-term use [11].

In the present study employing the NC/Nga mouse model of AD, topical treatment with 0.1% hypochlorous acid showed a therapeutic effect in an established atopic dermatitis mouse model, significantly reducing both lesions and allergic itch throughout the experimental period. Results showed HOCl gel to have equivalent efficacy to the topical JAK inhibitor tofacitinib in reducing clinical manifestations of the disease (such as lesion score) as well as reducing the itch response. Although the reduction sets in faster in the tofacitinib group, the overall effect on day 31 were comparable. Tofacitinib was chosen as a comparator, as first results of a clinical phase II study revealed a great benefit of this topically administered JAK inhibitor. As a glucocorticoid was chosen as comparator in a former study, this offers the comparison with another topical therapeutic with a different mechanism of action.

In the present study we used a gel that is formulated at a pH range 6 (+/− 0.5). In this specific formulation available free chlorine is present in the form of hypochlorous acid at a concentration of ca. 0.1% (1000 ppm), a concentration which displayed no safety concerns in mice in this study. Although no side-by-side comparison has been performed, compared to the former study, the onset of reduction of itch and lesion score seems faster, when HOCl is formulated as 0.1% compared to 0.05% [3]. It took 17 treatment days to reduce the lesion score to > 50% compared to vehicle in the former study [3], whereas more than 50% reduction was already achieved after 10 treatment days in the current study.

During the study, a steady increase of scratching behavior was observed within the first 14 days of sensitization with house dust mite antigen (Fig. 1b). Comparable to the former study, we again observed a higher responsiveness to pruritic stimuli ex vivo in comparison to non-sensitized and age matched NC/Nga mice. The sensory neurons excised from vehicle treated and house dust mite antigen sensitized and challenged NC/Nga mice were generally more responsive to stimuli like IL-31, IL-1β, TNFα, histamine, chloroquine, serotonin, capsaicin and AITC. These results can be interpreted as a general state of peripheral sensitization often seen with stages of chronic itch [12]. Both therapeutic options (HOCl as well as tofacitinib) let to a significant reduction of this hyper responsiveness. These results can be interpreted as a reduction or normalization of sensory neurotransmission, which finds its in vivo correlation in the significant reduction of scratching behaviour. A limitation of this study is that the number of mice taken for each group do not allow a non-inferiority comparison between HOCl and tofacitinib (which was not the intention of this study).Thus, a comparison of the inhibitory effect can only be made descriptively. Nevertheless, compared to vehicle treated mice, both treatment options showed significant reduction of itch and lesions at the end of the study.

NC/Nga mice are frequently used for mechanistic studies as well as for testing new therapeutic options of AD [3, 13]. The advantage of this model is that lesions are induced with a relevant allergen (house dust mite antigen) and the phenotype is quite translational to the human counterpart (constant itch, Th2 cytokines, lichenification and enhanced IgE levels) [14]. Taken together, it seems that even a repeated/chronic administration of a hydrogel containing 0.1% available free chlorine hypochlorous acid is well tolerated and reveals significant anti-inflammatory and anti-itch properties, comparable to a JAK inhibitor (tofacitinib) which is currently in clinical phase III for the treatment of human AD. Reduced inflammation was confirmed histologically and by reduced concentrations of cytokines, which are frequently associated with atopic dermatitis (IL-4, IL-13, TARC [9]) and cytokines for which a major role in the mediation of itch has been described (TSLP [15]).

Conclusions

A repeated/chronic administration of a hydrogel containing 0.1% available free chlorine hypochlorous acid is well tolerated and reveals significant anti-inflammatory and anti-itch properties, comparable to a JAK inhibitor (tofacitinib) which is currently in clinical phase III for the treatment of human AD.

Abbreviations

AD: Atopic dermatitis; AITC: Allyl isothiocyanate; DRG: Dorsal root ganglia; ELISA: Enzyme linked immunosorbent assay; FBS: Fetal bovine serum; Fura-2 AM: Fura-2-acetoxymethyl ester; HBSS: Hank's balanced salt solution; HDM: House dust mite allergen; HOCl: Hypochlorous acid; IgE: Immunoglobulin E; IL: Interleukin; JAK: Janus kinase; KCl: Sodium chloride; ms: Millisecond; NFκB: Nuclear factor κB,; nm: Nanometer; PBS: Phosphate buffered saline; TARC: Thymus and activation regulated chemokine; TNFα: Tumor necrosis factor alpha; TSLP: Thymic stromal lymphopoietin

Acknowledgements

The authors would like to thank the College of Veterinary Medicine, NC State University for providing all facilities required to carry out the presented study.

Funding

The present study was supported by a grant from Realm Therapeutics Inc., PA, USA. Realm Therapeutics was not involved in collection, analysis, and interpretation of data or in writing the manuscript.

Authors' contributions

TF performed experiments, performed data analysis and wrote part of the manuscript, JW performed experiments and performed data analysis, SE performed experiments and performed data analysis, WB designed the study, performed data analysis and wrote most of the manuscript. All authors read and approved the manuscript.

Competing interests

The authors declare that they have no competing interests.

References

1. Akdis CA, Akdis M, Bieber T, Bindslev-Jensen C, Boguniewicz M, Eigenmann P, Hamid Q, Kapp A, Leung DY, Lipozencic J, et al. Diagnosis and treatment of atopic dermatitis in children and adults: European academy of Allergology and clinical immunology/American Academy of allergy, asthma and immunology/ PRACTALL consensus report. J Allergy Clin Immunol. 2006;118:152–69.
2. Draelos ZD. Antipruritic hydrogel for the treatment of atopic dermatitis: an open-label pilot study. Cutis. 2012;90:97–102.
3. Fukuyama T, Martel BC, Linder KE, Ehling S, Ganchingco JR, Baumer W. Hypochlorous acid is antipruritic and anti-inflammatory in a mouse model of atopic dermatitis. Clin Exp Allergy. 2018;48:78-88.
4. Bissonnette R, Papp KA, Poulin Y, Gooderham M, Raman M, Mallbris L, Wang C, Purohit V, Mamolo C, Papacharalambous J, Ports WC. Topical tofacitinib for atopic dermatitis: a phase IIa randomized trial. Br J Dermatol. 2016;175:902–11.
5. Fukuyama T, Ehling S, Cook E, Baumer W. Topically administered Janus-kinase inhibitors Tofacitinib and Oclacitinib display impressive antipruritic and anti-inflammatory responses in a model of allergic dermatitis. J Pharmacol Exp Ther. 2015;354:394–405.
6. Baumer W, Gorr G, Hoppmann J, Ehinger AM, Rundfeldt C, Kietzmann M. AWD 12-281, a highly selective phosphodiesterase 4 inhibitor, is effective in the prevention and treatment of inflammatory reactions in a model of allergic dermatitis. J Pharm Pharmacol. 2003;55:1107–14.
7. Fukuyama T, Ganchingco JR, Mishra SK, Olivry T, Rzagalinski I, Volmer DA, Baumer W. Janus kinase inhibitors display broad anti-itch properties: a possible link through the TRPV1 receptor. J Allergy Clin Immunol. 2017; 140:306–9. e303
8. Rossbach K, Nassenstein C, Gschwandtner M, Schnell D, Sander K, Seifert R, Stark H, Kietzmann M, Baumer W. Histamine H1, H3 and H4 receptors are involved in pruritus. Neuroscience. 2011;190:89–102.
9. Werfel T, Allam JP, Biedermann T, Eyerich K, Gilles S, Guttman-Yassky E, Hoetzenecker W, Knol E, Simon HU, Wollenberg A, et al. Cellular and molecular immunologic mechanisms in patients with atopic dermatitis. J Allergy Clin Immunol. 2016;138:336–49.
10. Leung DY, Bieber T. Atopic dermatitis. Lancet. 2003;361:151–60.
11. Schneider L, Tilles S, Lio P, Boguniewicz M, Beck L, LeBovidge J, Novak N, Bernstein D, Blessing-Moore J, Khan D, et al. Atopic dermatitis: a practice parameter update 2012. J Allergy Clin Immunol. 2013;131:295–9.
12. LaMotte RH, Dong X, Ringkamp M. Sensory neurons and circuits mediating itch. Nat Rev Neurosci. 2014;15:19–31.
13. Lim SJ, Kim M, Randy A, Nam EJ, Nho CW. Effects of Hovenia dulcis Thunb. Extract and methyl vanillate on atopic dermatitis-like skin lesions and TNF-alpha/IFN-gamma-induced chemokines production in HaCaT cells. J Pharm Pharmacol. 2016;68:1465–79.
14. Martel BC, Lovato P, Baumer W, Olivry T. Translational animal models of atopic dermatitis for preclinical studies. Yale J Biol Med. 2017;90:389–402.
15. Wilson SR, The L, Batia LM, Beattie K, Katibah GE, SP MC, Pellegrino M, Estandian DM, Bautista DM. The epithelial cell-derived atopic dermatitis cytokine TSLP activates neurons to induce itch. Cell. 2013;155:285–95.

Poisonings in Poland reported to the Polish National Health Fund in the years 2009–2011

Aleksandra Świderska[1], Marek Wiśniewski[2,3*], Marek Wiergowski[4], Anna Krakowiak[5] and Jacek Sein Anand [2,3]

Abstract

Background: Poisonings constitute a significant medical, social and economic problem worldwide. In Poland there is no nationwide registry of poisonings, which results in a lack of accurate epidemiological data. Few publications dealing with the problem are based on data obtained from toxicology units and therefore do not include information about cases treated at emergency departments and other non-toxicology units.

Methods: We analyzed all admissions due to poisonings reported to the Polish National Health Fund by all hospital units in Poland in the 2009–2011 period. Diagnoses were encoded according to the ICD-10 classification.

Results: A total of 254,425 admissions were reported, 85,398 in 2009, 85,230 in 2010 and 83,797 in 2011. The male to female ratios were 1.88, 1.75 and 1.80 respectively. The most frequent causes of admissions were poisonings with ethanol ($n = 121,874$; 47.9%), carbon monoxide ($n = 17,179$; 6.8%) and benzodiazepines ($n = 10,340$; 4.1%). Alcohols were the reason for 104,680 admissions in men (63.2%) and 22,612 admissions in women (25.5%; $p < 0.01$). Poisonings with pharmaceuticals and other drugs were reported in 34,616 men (20.9%) and 45,238 women (51%; $p < 0.01$). There were 1680 cases of fatal poisonings in the analyzed period. The hospital mortality due to poisonings increased from 1.1% in 2009 to 1.5% in 2011 ($p < 0.01$). The mortality in general Intensive Care Units increased from 14.4% in 2009 to 22.3% in 2011 ($p < 0.01$). The etiology of fatal poisonings was highly dependent on the type of hospital unit.

Conclusions: The overall number of admissions due to poisonings decreased slightly during the study period, but they remained a significant cause of morbidity and mortality. Alcohols were the main cause of admissions in the analyzed period. Alcohol intoxications were more frequent in men while poisonings with pharmaceuticals were more frequent in women. Carbon monoxide exposures were a significant cause of morbidity and mortality in the studied period in Poland. A national poison information and toxicovigilance system should be created in Poland, ideally allowing for near real-time monitoring of cases of poisonings.

Keywords: Poisoning, Epidemiology, Human toxicology, Poison control

Background

Poisonings constitute a significant medical, social and economic problem worldwide. Each case should be analyzed not only in the terms of associated morbidity and mortality, but also in the context of its influence on patient's family members, relatives and the whole community [1–5].

The epidemiology of poisonings can be studied from different perspectives. These include overall mortality, hospital admission rates and enquiries to Poisons Information Services. Analyzing epidemiology of poisonings presents challenges depending on the source of data and the parameters analyzed. Analysis based on poison information calls is often an indication of exposures (very common in small children where there is usually only a suspicion of poisoning) and the analysis of cases treated in specialized toxicology unit causes a significant selection bias because they usually admit the only the most severe cases. Epidemiology varies with the geographical

* Correspondence: emwu@gumed.edu.pl
[2]Department of Clinical Toxicology, Medical University of Gdansk, Kartuska 4/6, 80-104, Gdansk, Poland
[3]Pomeranian Center of Toxicology, Gdansk, Poland
Full list of author information is available at the end of the article

location. In developing countries poisoning by pesticides and herbicides is often common. In warmer countries people may be more often exposed to toxins from snakes or spiders. In most situations self-harm often involves agents that are available and may reflect local tradition. For example, in Sri Lanka pesticide and oleander poisoning are frequently encountered problems, in China herbicides and pesticides, and in the UK paracetamol are the most frequent poisons taken deliberately [6]. The epidemiology also changes with time, due to social trends, advances in medical care but also due to emerging new trends in substance abuse. The recent report from China shows decreasing mortality due to pesticide and alcohol poisonings [7]. Data from the United States shows increasing opioid mortality due to mostly abuse of heroin and synthetic opioids [8].

The system of poison control in Poland is based on Regional Centers of Clinical Toxicology (RCCTs) and was started in 1967. Currently, there are 11 RCCTs located in Gdansk, Poznan, Warsaw, Lodz, Lublin, Rzeszow, Tarnow, Wroclaw, Sosnowiec and Cracow (2 centers). All RCCTs in Poland are based on hospital units and include Intensive Care Units. The principal function of Polish RCCTs is the treatment of cases of poisonings which require specialist management (like antidote treatment or extracorporeal removal of poisons). The number of beds in the RCCTs is not big enough to treat all poisonings, so many less severe cases, which do not require intensive care, are treated at Emergency Departments (EDs) and other hospital units (mostly pediatric and internal medicine departments). Cases of severe poisonings which cannot be transferred to RCCTs are usually treated at general Intensive Care Units (ICUs). Since the creation of RCCTs there was no separate system of poison information. This service was provided by RCCTs without additional funding, usually by the physician on call at the RCCT. Until 2002 all Polish RCCTs sent annual reports of admissions to the RCCT in Lodz, which analyzed and published these data. The data on admissions to other units were never reported or analyzed. Until now there is no nationwide system of poison information or toxicovigilance in Poland. This situation results in a lack of accurate information on the morbidity and mortality of poisonings in Poland. Few published papers dealing with this problem are based or single-center experience or at best on the data obtained from all the RCCTs and do not include information about cases treated at EDs and other non-toxicology hospital units [4, 5, 9–13]. The most recent analysis of data from all the RCCTs in Poland covered years 1970–2002 and showed a decreasing overall mortality and an increasing number of admissions due to poisonings with alcohols [14]. The most recent analysis of mortality due to poisonings by Krakowiak et al. was based on data from only 5 of 11 active clinical toxicology centers in Poland [15]. Until now there has been no analysis of hospital admissions and mortality due to poisonings in Poland which included all types of hospital units.

The aim of this study was to analyze the epidemiology of poisonings based on the available data reported to the Polish National Health Fund (NHF) from 2009 to 2011.

Methods

The study was approved by the Independent Bioethics Committee at Medical University in Gdansk (approval NKBBN/508/2017).

The healthcare system in Poland is mostly publicly funded, but a large number of providers (especially in outpatient care) are private entities. The funds are managed by the NHF, which reimburses the hospitals and outpatient clinics for the services performed for the people covered by the public health insurance. In the studied period the NHF covered around 80% of the Polish population.

The NHF database was created in 2003. The database is not public, permission to use it for the purpose of this study was granted by the president of the National Health Fund. The database is in an electronic form and contains millions of datasets reported annually by the Polish healthcare providers. The database is used to reimburse providers for healthcare services and to monitor and plan expenses of the NHF. In the 2009–2011 period the dataset reported by providers included: identifiers of the provider, patient's personal identification number (contains age and sex information), time of admission and discharge, mode of admission and discharge, primary and secondary (optional) diagnoses (ICD-10), type of hospital unit and medical procedures performed (ICD-9). There was no regular quality control of the data reported by the healthcare providers to the NHF. The data used in this study were extracted from the NHF database. Data of all hospital admissions reported to the NHF in 2009–2011 were analyzed. We selected all cases in which primary diagnosis was within the T36-T65 range, according to the 10th revision of the International Statistical Classification of Diseases and Related Health Problems (ICD-10). The data on secondary diagnoses or intent of poisoning were not obligatorily reported to the NHF and because of it were only fragmentary (less than 20% of all reports) and were not used in this analysis. There were no other inclusion criteria, some incomplete records were excluded from the statistical analysis, as described in the results section.

Statistical analysis was performed using the Statistica 12 software (StatSoft, Inc., USA). Pearson's chi-squared test was used for categorical variables and Student's t-test was used for continuous data. All reported p values are two-sided, p values lower than the adopted level of significance ($\alpha = 0,05$) were considered significant.

Results

The number of hospitals (hospital units) which reported cases of poisonings to the NHF was 561 (2231) in 2009, 562 (1829) in 2010 and 553(2060) in 2011. The proportions of types of hospital units which reported cases of poisonings in the analyzed period are presented in Table 1.

A total of 254,425 admissions of 240,517 patients with the diagnosis of poisonings were reported in the 2009–2011 period. The total number of reported admissions was higher than the total number of admitted patients because some patients were admitted due to poisonings more than once a year. The annual number of admissions decreased slightly throughout the analyzed period. There were 85,398 admissions (82,306 patients) in 2009, 85,230 (80,238 patients) in 2010, and 83,797 (77,973 patients) in 2011. Most patients were men. Cases in which sex of the patient was not reported were excluded from the further analysis (7 cases in 2009, 7 cases in 2010 and 20 cases in 2011). All these admissions were treated solely at EDs.

Patient age

Distribution of patient age is shown in Fig. 1.

Patients 11–18 years of age ($n = 30{,}546$) were the largest group admitted between 2009 and 2011, followed by individuals aged 19–25 years ($n = 26{,}537$), 51–55 years ($n = 21{,}887$) and 46–50 years ($n = 20{,}500$). Cases where age was not reported were excluded from the age analysis.

Causes of poisonings

Most common diagnoses reported in the analyzed period are presented in Table 2.

The most common diagnoses were alcohols. Altogether, intoxications with ethanol (T51.0), partially coded alcohol (T51) or unspecified alcohol (T51.9) represented nearly half of all recorded admissions due to poisonings ($n = 121{,}874$; 47.9%). There was a slight increase in the number of admissions reported as T51.0 and a decrease of poisonings with unspecified (T51.9) or partially coded alcohol (T51). Summarily the proportion of admissions due to the T51, T51.0 and T51.9 codes decreased from 51.5% in 2009 to 48.2% in 2011 ($\chi2 = 187.64$; $p < 0.01$). There was an increase of admissions due to carbon monoxide poisonings in 2010 which amounted to 8.39% of all cases of poisonings, significantly higher than in 2009 and 2011 (5.93% and 5.92% respectively; $\chi2 = 546.26$; $p < 0.01$). There was a decline in number of poisonings with benzodiazepines, which constituted 4.3% of all admissions in 2009 and 3.72% in 2011 ($\chi2 = 36.82$; $p < 0.01$). There was a significant increase of admissions encoded as anticoagulants and antithrombotic drugs (T45.5) from 2.71% in 2009 to 3.84% in 2011 ($\chi2 = 170.83$; $p < 0.01$).

Table 1 Hospital units reporting cases of poisonings to the NHF in the 2009–2011 period

Type of hospital unit	2009	2010	2011
Regional Center of Clinical Toxicology	9	9	11
Intensive Care Unit	246	254	310
Internal Medicine Unit	493	487	483
Pediatric Unit	352	356	353
Emergency Department	528	544	546
other	603	179	357

The etiology of poisonings in the youngest groups of patients was different than in adults. The most common diagnoses in children and teenagers and the results of the statistical comparison between these groups are presented in Table 3.

Like in the whole group, carbon monoxide was a common diagnosis in the two youngest age groups. Other common diagnoses in the 0–10 group were typical for accidental poisonings (venom of arthropods, detergents, pesticides). The T51, T51.0 and T51.9 codes were the most common causes of admissions of teenagers ($n = 10{,}821$; 35,4%), but the proportion was much lower than in adults ($n = 110{,}286$; 54.5%; $\chi2 = 1349.94$; $p < 0.01$). Patients aged 11–18 were more often poisoned with non-steroidal anti-inflammatory drugs (NSAIDs) than adults (2,9% vs 0,7%; $\chi2 = 1158.18$; $p < 0.01$). Teenagers were less likely to overdose benzodiazepines than older patients (3% vs 4.4%; $\chi2 = 121.15$; $p < 0.01$). There were 938 (1.9%) admissions of patients ≤18 years old due to poisonings with antitussives in the analyzed period. The number of these cases rose by 35%, from 256 (1.52%) in 2009 to 345 (2.21%) in 2011. In the analyzed period there was also a higher proportion of admissions due to venom of other arthropods in the 0–18 group than in adults: 1569 (3.2%) and 1507 (0.7%) cases respectively ($\chi2 = 1875.14$; $p < 0.01$).

Etiology of poisonings differed significantly between the sexes. In the analyzed period there were 165,650 admissions of men and 88,741 admissions of women. Alcohols (all T51 codes) were the reason for 104,680 admissions in men (63.2%) and only 22,612 admissions in women (25.5%; $\chi2 = 32{,}873.6$; $p < 0.01$). Poisonings with pharmaceuticals and other drugs (all codes within the T36-T50 range) were reported in 34,616 men (20.9%) and 45,238 women (51%; $\chi2 = 24{,}277.5$; $p < 0.01$).

Treatment at ED vs. hospitalization

In the whole analyzed period the total number of poisoned patients who were treated solely at EDs (without

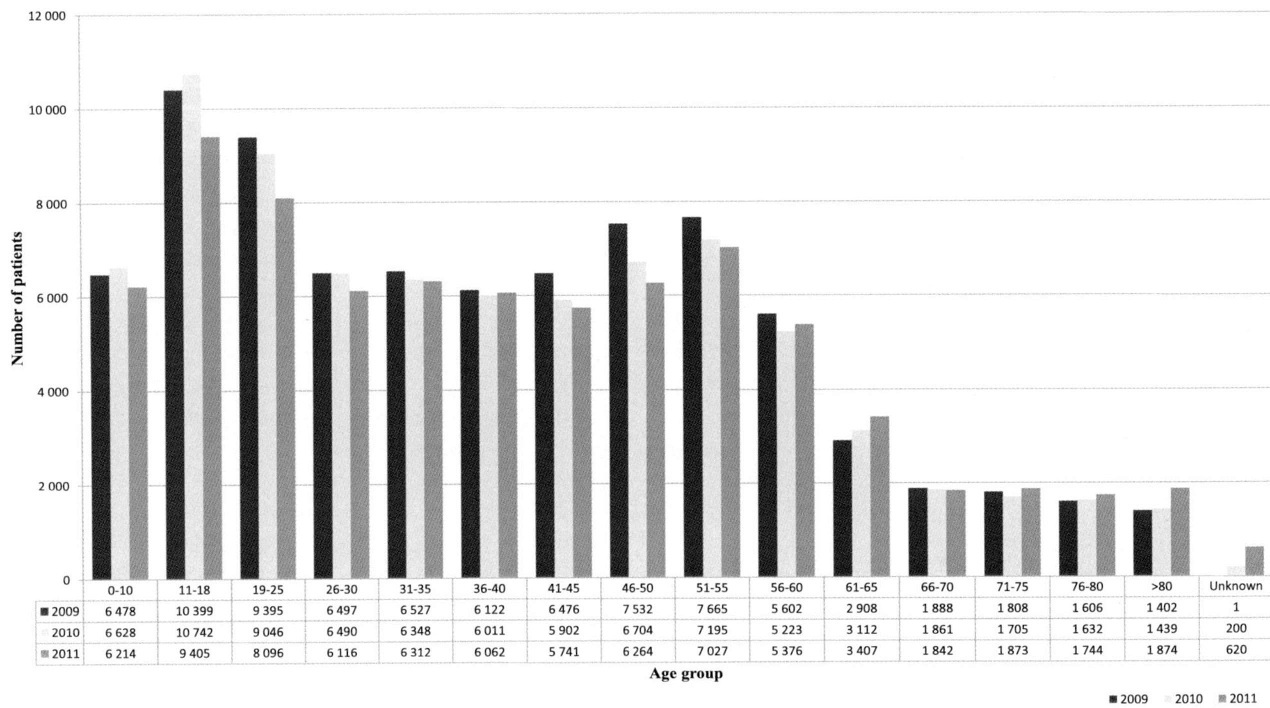

Fig. 1 Age structure of patients admitted due to poisonings in 2009–2011

further hospitalization) was 127,575 (50.1%). The proportion of patients treated solely at EDs and hospitalized and the sex distribution in these groups are shown in Table 4.

Women were generally more likely to be hospitalized and men were more frequently treated solely at EDs. The proportions of patients who were hospitalized in 2009, 2010 and 2011 were 66%, 66.4% and 63.5% for women and 42.8%, 42.8% and 39.1% for men ($\chi 2$ respectively 4146.56, 4337.91 and 4549.74; $p < 0.01$ for each analyzed year). The average age of patients treated solely at EDs was 40.3 ± 17.2 years and was significantly higher than the age of patients who were hospitalized (34.9 ± 22.3; $t = 68.4101$, $p < 0.01$). Alcohol poisonings (all T51 codes) constituted 70.8% of admissions which were treated solely at EDs compared with 25% of hospitalizations with this diagnosis in the 2009–2011 period ($\chi 2 = 49{,}989.3$; $p < 0.01$). Other common diagnoses for cases treated solely at EDs were carbon monoxide poisoning (5404 cases; 4.2%) and envenomation by arthropods (2106 cases; 1.7%). The most common diagnoses reported for hospitalized patients are presented in Table 5.

Table 2 Most common causes of admissions due to poisonings reported in the 2009–2011 period

ICD-10 code	Year			2009–2011 N (% of column)
	2009 N (% of column)	2010 N (% of column)	2011 N (% of column)	
T51.0 Ethanol	21,283 (24.9%)	19,471 (22.9%)	21,422 (25.6%)	62,176 (24.4%)
T51.9 Alcohol, unspecified or T51 partially coded	22,739 (26.6%)	17,975 (21.1%)	18,984 (22.7%)	59,698 (23.5%)
T58 Carbon monoxide	5064 (5.9%)	7151 (8.4%)	4964 (5.9%)	17,179 (6.8%)
T42.4 Benzodiazepines	3671 (4.3%)	3552 (4.2%)	3117 (3.7%)	10,340 (4.1%)
T45.5 Anticoagulants	2316 (2.7%)	2440 (2.9%)	3220 (3.8%)	7976 (3.1%)
T50.9 Other and unspecified drugs, medicaments and biological substances	1314 (1.5%)	1473 (1.7%)	1293 (1.5%)	4080 (1.6%)
T42.6 Other antiepileptic and sedative hypnotic drugs	1379 (1.6%)	1433 (1.7%)	1243 (1.5%)	4055 (1.6%)
T63.4 Venom of other arthropods	1023 (1.2%)	901 (1.1%)	1152 (1.4%)	3076 (1.2%)
T39.3 Other nonsteroidal anti-inflammatory drugs	966 (1.1%)	979 (1.2%)	982 (1.2%)	2927 (1.2%)
All admissions (T36-T65)	85,391 (100%)	85,223 (100%)	83,777 (100%)	254,391 (100%)

Table 3 Most common poisonings in children and teenagers in the 2009–2011 period

ICD-10 code	0–10 years old (% of column)	11–18 years old (% of column)	χ²(p) 0–10 vs. 11–18[a]	Total
T51.0 Ethanol	442 (2.3%)	7814 (25.6%)	4646.06 (< 0.01)	8256 (16.6%)
T51.9 Alcohol, unspecified or T51 (partially coded)	325 (1.7%)	3007 (9.8%)	1263.79 (< 0.01)	3332 (6.7%)
T58 Carbon monoxide	2807 (14.5%)	2782 (9.1%)	350.04 (< 0.01)	5589 (11.2%)
T50.9 Other and unspecified drugs, medicaments and biological substances	908 (4.7%)	1073 (3.5%)	43.82 (< 0.01)	1981 (3.9%)
T63.4 Venom of other arthropods	1091 (5.6%)	478 (1.6%)	647.53 (< 0.01)	1569 (3.2%)
T39.3 Other nonsteroidal anti-inflammatory drugs	526 (2.7%)	880 (2.9%)	1.07 (0.301)	1406 (2.8%)
T42.4 Benzodiazepines	463 (2.4%)	910 (3.0%)	14.96 (< 0.01)	1373 (2.8%)
T48.3 Antitussives	61 (0.3%)	877 (2.9%)	418.53 (< 0.01)	938 (1.9%)
T42.6 Other antiepileptic and sedative hypnotic drugs	204 (1.1%)	662 (2.2%)	85.57 (< 0.01)	867 (1.7%)
T55 Soaps, detergents	575 (3.0%)	48 (0.2%)	762.61 (< 0.01)	623 (1.2%)
T39.1 4-Aminophenol derivatives	75 (0.4%)	536 (1.8%)	182.51 (< 0.01)	611 (1.2%)
T60 Pesticides	513 (2.7%)	65 (0.2%)	616.5 (< 0.01)	578 (1.2%)
All admissions (T36-T65)	19,316 (100%)	30,550 (100%)	–	49,866 (100%)

[a]Pearson's chi-squared test

Hospital units

In the analyzed period 94,514 cases of poisonings were hospitalized in internal medicine and pediatric departments (74.5% of all hospitalizations). From 2009 to 2011 28,996 (22.9%) patients were treated at RCCTs, there was an increase from 21% in 2009 to 25% in 2011. Only 3206 cases (2.5%) were treated in general Intensive Care Units (ICUs). The proportion of hospitalizations at ICUs increased from 1.8% in 2009 to 3.1% in 2011.

Length of hospital stay

Mean duration of hospital stay due to poisonings remained constant throughout the analyzed period and amounted to 3 ± 11 days. We observed a slight decrease in the mean duration of hospital stays at RCCT: from 3.6 ± 5 days in 2009 to 3 ± 5 days in 2011.The proportion of hospitalizations longer than 10 days constituted less than 1% of the whole dataset.

Mode of discharge

The data on the mode of hospital discharge after admissions due to poisoning in the studied period are presented in Table 6 .

There was a decrease in the number of patients who were discharged against medical advice and concomitant increase in the number of individuals who self-willingly left the hospital without discharge.

Mortality

The proportion of hospitalizations during which the patients died increased throughout the analyzed period, amounting to 1.1%, 1.3% and 1.5% in 2009, 2010 and 2011, respectively ($\chi 2 = 196.89$; $p < 0.01$). The proportion of patients who died during hospitalization at RCCT (109, 96 and 109 cases respectively) remained at a relatively stable level (around 1%). The increase of mortality in ICUs, from 14.4% (114 cases) in 2009 to 22.3% (271 cases) in 2011, is worth emphasizing ($\chi 2 = 13.32$; $p < 0.01$). The proportion of patients who died during hospitalization in other units (usually internal medicine

Table 4 Number of admissions of acutely poisoned patients in the years 2009–2011, stratified by sex and place of treatment (Emergency Department vs. hospitalization)

Data category	Year									2009–2011		
	2009			2010			2011					
	M	F	Total	M	F	Total	M	F	Total	M	F	Total
All admissions	55,910	29,481	85,391	55,042	30,181	85,223	54,698	29,079	83,777	165,650	88,741	254,391
Cases treated solely in an Emergency Department (% of column)	31,969 (57.2%)	10,026 (34%)	41,995 (49.2%)	31,494 (57.2%)	10,152 (33.6%)	41,646 (48.9%)	33,326 (60,9%)	10,608 (36.5%)	43,934 (52.4%)	96,789 (58.4%)	30,786 (34.7%)	127,575 (50.1%)
Hospitalizations (% of column)	23,941 (42.8%)	19,455 (66%)	43,396 (50.8%)	23,548 (42.8%)	20,029 (66.4%)	43,577 (51.1%)	21,372 (39.1%)	18,471 (63.5%)	39,843 (47.6%)	68,861 (41.6%)	57,955 (65.3%)	126,816 (49.9%)

Table 5 Most common diagnoses of patients hospitalized due to poisonings in the 2009–2011 period

ICD-10 code	n (%)
T51.0 Ethanol	28,465 (22,4%)
T58 Carbon monoxide	12,333 (9.7%)
T42.4 Benzodiazepines	9497 (7.5%)
T45.5 Anticoagulants	7373 (5.8%)
T51.9 Alcohol, unspecified	3758 (3%)
T42.6 Other antiepileptic and sedative hypnotic drugs	3518 (2.8%)
T50.9 Other and unspecified drugs medicaments and biological substances	3004 (2.4%)
T39.3 Other nonsteroidal anti-inflammatory drugs	2693 (2.1%)
T43.0 Tricyclic and tetracyclic antidepressants	2134 (1.7%)
T43.2 Other and unspecified antidepressants	2063 (1.6%)
All hospitalizations (T36-T65)	126,816 (100%)

and pediatric departments) remained at a relatively constant level (268, 270 and 229 cases respectively; around 0.8% of all reported cases). The most common diagnoses of reported fatal poisonings are presented in Table 7.

Diagnoses associated with ethanol (T51.0, T51 and T51.9 codes) were recorded in 447 (26.6%) fatal poisonings reported in the analyzed period. Most of these cases (92.8%) were reported by departments other than RCCTs, 150 (33.6%) by ICUs and 265 (59.3%) by other departments. Surprisingly, anticoagulants (T45.5) were the second most common diagnosis of fatal poisonings overall. No such cases were reported by RCCTs, 9.5% of these fatalities were reported by ICUs and 90,5% by other departments. There were also 28 fatal cases reported as anticoagulant antagonist poisonings, none of these cases were reported by RCCTs. The most common causes of fatal poisonings reported by RCCTs were glycols, methanol, ethanol, carbon monoxide and benzodiazepines. Poisonings with pesticides (all T60 codes) were the cause of 24 fatal cases and mushroom ingestions caused 19 deaths. Most of these cases were reported by RCCTs (58.3% and 52.6%, respectively). The codes typically used for new psychoactive substances (T40.4, T40.6 and T40.9) were reported in 31 fatal cases in the analyzed period. Most of these cases (54.8%) were reported by ICUs. In the analyzed period only 9 fatal cases of opioid poisonings (T40.1, T40.2 and T40.3 codes) were reported to the NHF by all hospital units in Poland.

Discussion

Number of admissions

The total number of admissions due to poisonings recorded in the 2009–2011 period amounted to 254,425, which corresponded to 84,808 admissions per year on average. However, if adjusted for cases not reported to the NHF due to lack of health insurance, the true number of admissions due to poisonings would be approximately 300,000 in the analyzed period or 100,000 per year. Importantly, we observed a small decreasing tendency in the annual number of admissions due to poisonings. Irrespective of the analyzed year, the proportions of patients who were admitted solely to EDs and those who required longer hospitalization remained roughly similar (around 50% each).

Age and sex

The largest age group of patients who were admitted due to poisonings were teenagers, 11–18 years of age. Other authors reported similar age structure of poisoned patients [1, 2]. A relatively large proportion of middle-aged individuals (46–55 years of age) is worth emphasizing, as well as an increase in the number of poisoned subjects older than 80 years. The latter tendency most likely reflects the aging of Polish population and the changes in social and economic status of this age group [1–3, 16]. The increasing number of cases of poisonings in subjects older than 80 years is worrying, because of the increased mortality and longer hospital stay in this group [16].

Men constituted the vast majority of poisoned patients admitted during the analyzed period (average M/F ratio

Table 6 Mode of hospital discharge after poisonings in the 2009–2011 period

Mode of hospital discharge	Year			2009–2011 (% of column)
	2009 (% of column)	2010 (% of column)	2011 (% of column)	
Discharge without further referral	13,664 (31.5%)	13,458 (30.9%)	12,550 (31.5%)	39,672 (31.3%)
Referral to outpatient care	19,128 (44.1%)	19,165 (44%)	16,317 (41%)	54,610 (43.1%)
Referral to further hospitalization	4606 (10.6%)	5140 (11.8%)	5641 (14.2%)	15,387 (12.1%)
Discharge against medical advice	5506 (12.7%)	5137 (11.8%)	4452 (11.2%)	15,095 (12%)
Leaving hospital without discharge	0 (0%)	38 (0.1%)	250 (0.6%)	288 (0.2%)
Death	491 (1.1%)	580 (1.3%)	609 (1.5%)	1680 (1.3%)
Other/unspecified	1 (0.002%)	59 (0.1%)	24 (0.1%)	84 (0.1%)
Total number of hospitalizations	43,396 (100%)	43,577 (100%)	39,843 (100%)	126,816 (100%)

Table 7 Causes of fatal poisonings reported in the 2009–2011 period, stratified by the place of treatment

ICD-10 code	Number of fatal cases (% of column)			
	RCCTs	ICUs	other departments	all departments
T51.0 Ethanol	26 (8.3%)	79 (13.2%)	159 (20.7%)	264 (15.7%)
T45.5 Anticoagulants	0 (0%)	14 (2.3%)	134 (17.5%)	148 (8.8%)
T52.3 Glycols	56 (17.8%)	23 (3.8%)	32 (4.2%)	111 (6.6%)
T51.1 Methanol	34 (10.8%)	43 (7.2%)	23 (3.0%)	100 (6%)
T51.9 Alcohol, unspecified	5 (1.6%)	21 (3.5%)	69 (9%)	95 (5.7%)
T51 Alcohol, partially coded	1 (0.3%)	50 (8.3%)	37 (4.8%)	88 (5.2%)
T58 Carbon monoxide	18 (5,7%)	17 (2.8%)	22 (2.9%)	57 (3.4%)
T42.4 Benzodiazepines	16 (5.1%)	15 (2.5%)	25 (3.3%)	56 (3.3%)
T43.0 Tricyclic and tetracyclic antidepressants	12 (3.8%)	11 (1.8%)	9 (1.2%)	32 (1.9%)
T42.6 + T42.7 Other and unspecified antiepileptic and sedative-hypnotic drugs	6 (1.9%)	9 (1.5%)	16 (2.1%)	31 (1.8%)
T40.4 + T40.6 + T40.9 Other and unspecified narcotics and psychodysleptics (includes new psychoactive substances[a])	9 (2.9%)	17 (2.8%)	5 (0.7%)	31 (1.8%)
T43.3 Phenothiazine antipsychotics and neuroleptics	2 (0.6%)	20 (3.3%)	7 (0.9%)	29 (1.7%)
T51.8 Other alcohols	17 (5.4%)	13 (2.2%)	11 (1.4%)	28 (1.7%)
T47.5 Anticoagulant antagonists, vitamin K and other coagulants	0 (0%)	5 (0.8%)	23 (3.0%)	28 (1.7%)
T46.1 Calcium channel blockers	12 (3.8%)	7 (1.2%)	6 (0.8%)	25 (1.5%)
T60.0 + T60.3 + T60.9 Pesticides	14 (4.5%)	10 (1.7%)	0 (0%)	24 (1.4%)
T38.3 Insulin and oral hypoglycemic (antidiabetic) drugs	4 (1.3%)	10 (1.7%)	7 (0.9%)	21 (1.3%)
T62.0 Mushroom ingestion	10 (3.2%)	7 (1.2%)	2 (0.3%)	19 (1.1%)
T43.8 Other psychotropic drugs	1 (0.3%)	10 (1.7%)	5 (0,7%)	16 (1.0%)
T39.1 4-Aminophenol derivatives (includes acetaminophen[a])	7 (2.5%)	5 (0.8%)	3 (0.4%)	15 (0.9%)
T43.5 Other and unspecified antipsychotics and neuroleptics	1 (0.3%)	6 (1.0%)	8 (1.0%)	15 (0.9%)
T42.1 Iminostilbenes (includes carbamazepine[a])	8 (2.5%)	5 (0.8%)	0 (0%)	13 (0.8%)
T45.1 Antineoplastic and immunosuppressive drugs	0 (0%)	0 (0%)	13 (1.7%)	13
T43.2 Other and unspecified antidepressants	3 (1.0%)	5 (0.8%)	3 (0.4%)	11 (0.7%)
T46.9 Other and unspecified agents primarily affecting the cardiovascular system	1 (0.3%)	5 (0.8%)	5 (0.7%)	11 (0.7%)
T44.7 Beta-adrenoreceptor antagonists	1 (0,3%)	5 (0.8%)	4 (0.5%)	10 (0.6%)
Other	50 (15.9%)	187 (31.2%)	139 (18.1%)	389 (23.2%)
All fatal cases (T36-T65)	314 (100%)	599 (100%)	767 (100%)	1680 (100%)

[a]authors' comment

was 1.8). This observation is inconsistent with the data published by other authors according to which the majority of poisoned patients were women. This discrepancy can be explained by regional differences, e.g. status of health insurance or lack thereof and widely understood socioeconomic and cultural factors [2, 3, 17–19]. However we believe, that this difference is mostly due to two other factors. First, this study included not only cases treated in RCCTs, but also at EDs and men were much more frequently treated solely at EDs than women. Second, the main cause of poisonings in Poland in the reported period was ethanol and ethanol intoxication was much more common in men than in women (63.2% and 25.5% respectively). In our opinion these two factors were the main reason for the difference in sex distribution from other studies. Different sex distribution was seen for poisonings with pharmaceuticals and other drugs which were more frequent in women than in men (51% and 20.9% respectively).The available data were not sufficient to analyze the intent of poisoning (suicidal, accidental or recreational), but we believe, that the differences in diagnoses between men and women seen in our study are in line with previous findings that women were more likely to choose self-poisoning as a method of committing suicide than men [20].

Etiology of poisonings

Etiology of poisonings varies widely between countries, depending on many factors including availability of pharmaceuticals and other toxic substances and also cultural, social and economic differences. In our study irrespective of the analyzed year, the most common cause of admissions due to poisoning were alcohols, especially ethanol. The incidence of ethanol intoxications is known to vary considerably depending on social acceptance to alcohol consumption or religious background [1, 16, 19, 21–23]. Ethanol abuse and dependence are a long-time problem in Poland. According to the 2014 WHO global status report on alcohol and health, the average consumption of alcohol in Poland (12,5 l of 100% ethanol per year) was slightly higher than the mean value for the WHO European Region (10,9 l). However, because a significant part of the Polish population are lifetime abstainers (15.8% men and 37.8% women), the mean amount consumed by the drinkers was much higher (24,2 l per year) [24]. The results of our study showed that ethanol was a significant cause of morbidity and mortality in the Polish population, especially among men. Alcohols were the leading cause of both admissions and deaths due to poisonings in the analyzed period. Ethanol dependence and abuse are complex problems, and because of that many national, local and non-government organization entities in Poland are involved in long-time anti-alcohol interventions. Production and sale of alcoholic products is strictly regulated and the criminal law is severe for alcohol-related offences. Encouragingly, in the analyzed period there was a decreasing tendency of admissions due to alcohols.

Pharmaceutical agents and other drugs (all codes within the T36-T50 range) turned out to be the second most frequent cause of admissions and the leading cause of hospitalizations. The number of such cases remained relatively stable throughout the analyzed period. Noticeably, there was an increase in the number of admissions and deaths due to poisonings with anticoagulants recorded as a primary diagnosis. Interpreting this phenomenon, is difficult without access to all clinical data. It is likely that many of these cases were not really poisonings and that the T45.5 diagnosis was reported to the NHF in cases of adverse effects of antithrombotic therapy or even underdosing of these agents. It is worth noting that none of the fatal cases of anticoagulant overdose were reported by RCCTs. An additional analysis of all clinical data would be of most importance, especially for the fatal cases. The authors believe that anticoagulant overdose should rarely be fatal given the treatment options available in Poland. Full cooperation of the NHF and the involved hospitals would be necessary to perform such an analysis.

Carbon monoxide was still a significant cause of morbidity and mortality in the analyzed period. There was a significant increase of both admissions and fatalities due to CO exposure in 2010. This was probably due to the fact that the winter months of 2010 (winters of 2009/2010 and 2010/2011) were significantly colder than usual in Poland, which resulted in a higher risk of household exposure to CO due to heating with coal ovens [25].

The large number of admissions due to arthropod venom reported may have been due to insect bites, but also may have been caused by inaccurate encoding of ED interventions due to tick *(Ixodoidea)* bites.

There was a decreasing number of admissions due to benzodiazepine poisonings. This may be due to their declining use since safer and less addictive substances become more popular, but longer observation is necessary to fully support this conclusion.

There were significant differences in etiology of poisonings in the two youngest age groups. Most common causes of admissions were also alcohols and carbon monoxide. The most common diagnoses in the 0–10 group were in line with accidental poisonings (carbon monoxide, venoms, detergents) and in the 11–18 group they were more likely due to intentional overdoses or recreational substance use (alcohols, benzodiazepines, antitussives). The proportion of alcohol intoxications in the 11–18 age group was much lower than in adults, but higher than reported in other European countries [26]. The proportion of admissions due to poisonings with nonsteroidal anti-inflammatory drugs in this group was higher and poisonings with benzodiazepines were less frequent than in adults. This is most likely due to limited access to prescription medications in the younger group. Higher percentage of admissions due to arthropod venom in children and adolescents than in adults most likely reflects the differences in outdoor activity. In the analyzed period there was an increasing number of poisonings with antitussives, which was most likely due to recreational abuse of over-the-counter medications (mostly dextromethorphan) by Polish teenagers [27, 28]. In contrast to reports from other countries, the numbers of admissions and fatal cases due to poisonings with pesticides and opioids were relatively low in the analyzed period in Poland [23, 29, 30].

Hospitalizations

Mean duration of hospital stay of poisoned patients was relatively constant throughout the analyzed period. We observed a slight decrease in the mean duration of stays at RCCTs, which is consistent with the data reported by other authors according to whom the duration of relatively expensive hospitalization in specialized toxicology units was often shortened in favor of long-term treatment in other units, e.g. inpatient or outpatient psychiatric departments [4, 5]. The largest proportion of hospitalizations due to poisonings was reported by units other than RCCTs, such as internal medicine and pediatric departments. However, we observed an increase in the number of patients admitted to RCCTs, which implies that a growing number of poisoned patients were treated at specialized units. Another important finding of this study is a relatively high proportion of poisoned patients who had self-discharged home, against medical advice, as well as an increase in the number of patients who self-willingly left hospital without discharge. The largest proportion of patients who self-willingly left hospitals were treated at internal medicine and pediatric units, usually due to ethanol intoxications. Such patients are often reluctant to provide any health insurance data and their behavior markedly disorganizes functioning of a hospital unit and unnecessarily involves both their families and medical personnel [4, 5].

Mortality

A systematic increase in the proportion of patients who died during hospital stay is worth emphasizing. According to other authors, mortality rates of patients hospitalized due to poisoning vary from 0.4 to 3% depending on a country and etiology of poisoning [1, 3–5, 15, 17, 22, 29, 31–34]. Importantly, the mortality was lowest in the RCCTs, which implies that such specialized units are optimally prepared for management of even the most severe cases. We observed an increase in the mortality of patients hospitalized in general ICUs. This phenomenon can be only partially explained by the selection of patients admitted to the ICUs based on severity, because the similar selection applies to the RCCTs which have their own Intensive Care Units. The limited dataset available from the NHF made it impossible to properly compare the mortality between RCCTs and ICUs in this study, but previous research which included only poisonings with methanol and ethylene glycol showed more than 2 times higher mortality rate in ICUs than in RCCTs in this group of patients after adjusting for severity [35, 36]. The increase of mortality in ICUs is especially alarming because previous studies demonstrated that these units least often from all the departments referred their patients for further specialized treatment at RCCTs [4, 5].

The analysis of fatal cases revealed a striking difference in reported diagnoses between RCCTs and other departments. The most common diagnoses reported by RCCTs were associated with typically severe poisonings (methanol, ethylene glycol, carbon monoxide, pesticides, mushrooms, cardiovascular agents) while other departments reported codes which in the authors' opinion should not be associated with so high mortality (like anticoagulants and anticoagulant antagonists). This is very likely due to use of poisoning codes in cases of complications of therapeutic use of these agents or in cases where the real cause of death was the pathology for which the anticoagulants or anticoagulants were administered. The data available from the NHF did not allow us to explore this issue further.

Limitations of the study

Unlike previous studies, our analysis included not only the data of patients treated at RCCTs, but also those admitted to other hospital units, which has not been done before in Poland. Nevertheless, we are well aware of all potential limitations of the presented results, inherent to the fact that they are derived from the data gathered primarily for accounting purposes. In the NFH system the primary diagnosis is strictly associated with billing and as such may be a subject to bias. In order to maximize the reimbursement, hospitals may report secondary diagnoses (from medical perspective) as primary ones. We believe that in some cases ICD-10 classification was misinterpreted, including not only poisonings, but also adverse effects of treatment, which properly should be reported using other codes (eg. K29, D50-D76, T88.7). Another difficulty was due to the incomplete coding, which in many cases did not include the part of the ICD-10 code following the decimal mark, especially for cases treated solely at EDs. This was especially true for alcohol poisonings. Many such cases were coded as unspecified alcohol poisoning (T51.9) or only partially coded as T51 without specifying the type of alcohol (part of the code after the decimal mark). Almost all the admissions which were coded this way were treated solely at EDs. The T51 code includes ethanol (T51.0), methanol (T51.1), 2-propanol (T51.2), fusel oil (T51.3), other alcohols (T51.8) and unspecified alcohols (T51.9). In our opinion the diagnosis of ethanol poisoning was by far the most likely one for T51 and T51.9 codes. Similarly the part of the code identifying the intent of poisoning (X-Y codes), which would allow to distinguish suicidal overdoses from accidental and recreational ones was not required by the NHF for billing and this data was very fragmentary.

Another limitation is that the ICD-10 classification does not differentiate between acute and chronic exposures. We believe that a vast majority of analyzed cases were acute poisonings, because in Poland chronic exposures are usually treated in an outpatient setting, but the available data were not sufficient to confirm this.

The analyzed data did not include all admissions due to poisonings in the 2009–2011 period, because not all admissions were reported by the hospitals to the NHF. The reports for the NHF did not include the data of admissions of individuals who lacked the NHF health insurance, were imprisoned or were residents of countries outside the European Union. This can be a source of a significant bias, because it applied to up to 20% of all patients treated at RCCTs (personal communications during annual meetings of heads of Polish RCCTs). The proportion of patients without NHF health insurance treated in other hospital units might have been be similar or even higher (especially at ED's). We would like to be able to present more recent data, but so far we were not able to obtain the data for years 2012–2017 due to a change of NHF data sharing policy. Nevertheless, to the best of our knowledge, the hereby presented analysis is based on the largest of all datasets studied to date in Poland.

Conclusions

In conclusion, the overall number of admissions due to poisonings decreased slightly during the study period, but poisonings remained a significant cause of morbidity and mortality in Poland and caused around 100,000 admissions per year. Alcohols were the main cause of admissions due to poisonings, accounting for about 50% of all cases. Carbon monoxide exposures were a significant cause of morbidity and mortality in the studied period in Poland. The increasing number of poisonings with antitussives in adolescents is worth noting. Men were more likely to be admitted due to poisonings than women. Around half of the cases of poisonings were managed solely at Emergency Departments. Men were more likely to be treated solely at Emergency Departments and women were more likely to be hospitalized. The increasing number of patients older than 80 years may lead to increased treatment costs and mortality. There was an increase of hospital mortality due to poisonings, most evidently in general Intensive Care Units. We believe that a national poison information and toxicovigilance system should be created in Poland, ideally allowing for near real-time monitoring of cases of poisonings. This system could be based on Regional Centers of Clinical Toxicology, which should exist in all Polish regions.

Abbreviations

ED: Emergency Department; ICU: Intensive Care Unit; NHF: National Health Fund; RCCT: Regional Center of Clinical Toxicology

Acknowledgements

The authors want to thank dr Tadeusz Jędrzęjczyk, the president of the National Health Fund in Warsaw and dr Wojciech Waldman, the director of the Pomeranian Center of Toxicology in Gdansk for their support.

Funding

This research was funded by the Medical University of Gdańsk (grant 02–11/07/320).

Authors' contributions

AŚ main investigator, data gathering and quality control, writing of the manuscript. MW1 design and methodology of the study, statistical analysis, writing of the manuscript. MW2 review and writing of the manuscript. AK review and writing of the manuscript. JSA, coordination of the study and protocol, design of the study, review and writing of the manuscript. All authors read and approved the final manuscript.

Competing interests

The authors declare that they have no competing interests.

Author details

[1]National Health Fund Headquarters, Warsaw, Poland. [2]Department of Clinical Toxicology, Medical University of Gdansk, Kartuska 4/6, 80-104, Gdansk, Poland. [3]Pomeranian Center of Toxicology, Gdansk, Poland. [4]Department of Forensic Medicine, Medical University of Gdansk, Gdansk, Poland. [5]Toxicology Department, Nofer Institute of Occupational Medicine, Lodz, Poland.

References

1. Andiran N, Sarikayalar F. Pattern of acute poisonings in childhood in Ankara: what has changed in twenty years. Turk J of Pediatr. 2004;46:147–52.
2. Lipnik-Stangeli M. Hospitalizations due to poisonings in Slovenia – epidemiological aspects. Wien Klin Wochenschr. 2010;122:54–8.
3. Ramesha KN, Rao KB, Kumar GS. Pattern and outcome of acute poisoning cases in tertiary care hospital in Karnataka, India. Indian J Crit Care Med. 2009;13:152–5.
4. Sein Anand J, Świderska A. Selected data concerning acute intoxications with xenobiotics in Poland in the year 2009. Przegl Lek. 2010;67:559–65.
5. Świderska A, Sein AJ. Selected data concerning acute intoxications with xenobiotics in Poland in the year 2010. Przegl Lek. 2012;69:409–14.
6. Bateman DN. The epidemiology of poisoning. Medicine. 2012;40:42–5.
7. Wang L, Wu Y, Yin P, Cheng P, Liu Y, et al. Poisoning deaths in China, 2006-2016. Bull World Health Organ. 2018;96:314–326A. https://doi.org/10.2471/BLT.17.203943.
8. Gummin DD, Mowry JB, Spyker DA, et al. 2016 annual report of the American Association of Poison Control Centers' National Poison Data System (NPDS): 34th annual report. Clin Toxicol. 2017;55:1072–252. https://doi.org/10.1080/15563650.2017.1388087.
9. Czerczak S, Jaraczewska W. Acute poisonings in Poland. J Toxicol Clin Toxicol. 1995;33:669–75.
10. Jaraczewska W, Czerczak S. The pattern of acute poisonings in Poland. Vet Hum Toxicol. 1994;36:228.
11. Jaraczewska W, Czerczak S, Kotwica M. The National Poison Information Center in Poland. J Toxicol Clin Toxicol. 1996;34:669.
12. Kotwica M, Rogaczewska A. Acute poisonings in Poland during the period 1997-1999. An analysis of files from Krakow Poison Information Center. Przegl Lek. 2002;59:318.
13. Piekarska-Wijatkowska A, Czyzewska S, Kotwica M, Krakowiak A. Epidemiology of acute poisonings during 2002-2011 in toxicology unit; Department of Occupational Medicine and Toxicology, Nofer Institute of Occupational Medicine, Lodz, Poland. Przegl Lek. 2013;70(10):848–51.
14. Kotwica M, Czerczak S. Acute poisonings registered since 1970: trends and characteristics. Analysis of the files collected in the National Poison Information Centre, Łódź, Poland. Int J Occup Med Environ Health. 2007;20(1):38–43.
15. Krakowiak A, Piekarska-Wijatkowska A, Kobza-Sindlewska K, et al. Poisoning deaths in Poland: types and frequencies reported in Łódź, Kraków, Sosnowiec, Gdańsk, Wrocław and Poznań during 2009-2013. Int J Occup Med Environ Health. 2017;30:897–908.
16. Piekarska-Wijatkowska A, Kobza-Sindlewska K, Rogaczewska A, et al. Intentional poisoning among elderly people-residents of a large urban agglomeration in Poland. Hum Exp Toxicol. 2016;35:1328–36.
17. Ahmadi A, Pakravan N, Ghazizadeh Z. Pattern of acute food, drug, and chemical poisoning in Sari City, northern Iran. Hum Exp Toxicol. 2010;29:731–8.
18. Malangu N. Acute poisoning at two hospitals in Kampala-Uganda. J Forensic Legal Med. 2008;15:489–92.
19. Poplas-Susic T, Komericki-Grzinic M, Klemenc-Ketis Z, et al. Aetiological and demographical characteristics of acute poisoning in the Celje region, Slovenia. Eur J Emerg Med. 2009;16:127–30.
20. Schmidtke A, Bille-Brahe U, DeLeo D, et al. Attempted suicide in Europe: rates, trends and sociodemographic characteristics of suicide attempters during the period 1989-1992. Results of the WHO/EURO multicentre study on Parasuicide. Acta Psychiatr Scand. 1996;93:327–38.

21. Gude AB, Hoegberg LC, Pedersen M, et al. A study of 355 consecutive acute poisoning cases admitted to an emergency ward at Copenhagen University Hospital, Bispebjerg in 2001. Ugeskr Laeger. 2007;169:1793–7.
22. Hanssens Y, Deleu D, Tagi A. Etiologic and demographic characteristics of poisoning: a prospective hospital based study in Oman. J Toxicol Clin Toxicol. 2001;39:371–80.
23. Mowry JB, Spyker DA, Brooks DE, et al. 2015 annual Reportof the American Association of Poison Control Centers' National Poison Data System (NPDS): 33rd annual report. Clin Toxicol (Phila). 2016;54:924–1109.
24. World Health Organization. Global status report on alcohol and health. 2018. http://apps.who.int/iris/bitstream/10665/112736/1/9789240692763_eng.pdf?ua=1. Accessed 5 Oct 2018.
25. Wójcik R, Miętus M. Some features of long-term variability in air temperature in Poland (1951-2010). Prz Geogr. 2014;86:339–64.
26. Mintegi S, Azkunaga B, Prego J, et al. International epidemiological differences in acute poisonings in pediatric emergency departments. Pediatr Emerg Care. 2017. https://doi.org/10.1097/PEC.0000000000001031.
27. Zajac M, Andrzejczyk A, Kuich A, et al. Recreational usage of dextromethorphan-analysis based on internet users experiences. Przegl Lek. 2013;70:525–7.
28. Zając M, Schetz D, Sein AJ. Age and gender trends of inpatient recreational acute dextromethorphan intoxication hospitalized in Pomeranian Center of Toxicology between 2009-2011. Przegl Lek. 2014;71:488–90.
29. Lam SM, Lau AC, Yan WW. Over 8 year experience on severe acute poisoning requiring intensive care in Hong Kong, China. Hum Exp Toxicol. 2010;29:757–65.
30. Islambulchilar M, Islambulchilar Z, Kargar-Maher MH. Acute poisoning cases admitted to a university hospital in Tabriz. Iran Hum Exp Toxicol. 2009;28: 185–90.
31. Johansen SS, Jacobsen C, Muller IB, et al. Fatal cases of poisoning in eastern Denmark during a five-year period (1998-2002). Ugeskr Laeger. 2006;168: 3326–31.
32. Jonsson AK, Spigset O, Tiaderborn M, et al. Fatal drug poisonings in a Swedish general population. BMC Clin Pharmacol. 2009;27:7.
33. Lilleeng GH, Berg KJ, Giertsen F, Andrew E. Acute poisonings in Norway 1999-2004 – morbidity and mortality. Tidsskr Nor Laegeforen. 2007;127: 1023–7.
34. Ostapenko YN, Matveev SB, Gassimova ZM, Khonelidze RS. Epidemiology and medical aid at acute poisoning in Russia. Przegl Lek. 2001;58:293–6.
35. Sein Anand J, Świderska A, Pach J, Burda P. Selected data of acute intoxications with glycol and methanol in Poland in the year 2009. Przegl Lek. 2011;68:453–8.
36. Świderska A, Sein AJ. Selected data of acute poisonings with ethylene glycol and methanol in Poland in the year 2010. Przegl Lek. 2013;70:479–84.

19

Potentiating effect of imidacloprid on arsenic-induced testicular toxicity in Wistar rats

Lakshay Mahajan[1], Pawan Kumar Verma[2*], Rajinder Raina[3] and Shilpa Sood[4]

Abstract

Background: It is an established fact that humans and animals are exposed to more than one chemical concurrently from various sources such as food, air and water. In the past, much emphasis was laid on evaluating the toxic effects of a single chemical. Nowadays an increased attention is being paid to the interaction of xenobiotics with one another. Therefore, a study was aimed to evaluate the potentiating effect of imidacloprid (IMI) on arsenic-induced testicular toxicity in rats.

Methods: Adult male Wistar rats randomly divided into eight groups with six in each were subjected to daily oral administrations for 28 days. Group I served as control, group II received IMI at the dose rate of 16.9 mg/kg body weight, group III, IV and V received arsenic at the dose rate of 50, 100 and 150 ppb in drinking water whereas group VI, VII and VIII received both arsenic and IMI.

Results: Repeated oral administrations of IMI or arsenic (150 ppb) alone resulted in a significant ($P < 0.05$) elevation in the levels of malondialdehyde (MDA) and advanced oxidation protein product (AOPP) along with significant ($P < 0.05$) decline in total thiols and antioxidant enzymatic activities indicating reduced antioxidant defense in testicular tissue of exposed rats. These findings were further corroborated with histological alterations in testes like fluid accumulation in interstitial spaces in IMI administered rats. Similarly, rats provided access exclusively to arsenic-containing drinking water induced degenerative changes in seminiferous tubules in a concentration-dependent manner. Concurrent administration of IMI and arsenic produced more severe antioxidant and histopathological alterations of testes as compared to exposure to either toxicant.

Conclusions: Reduced antioxidant activities, increased MDA and AOPP levels with severe histopathological alterations in testes of rats on concurrent exposure indicated that IMI potentiated the arsenic-induced testicular toxicity in Wistar rats.

Keywords: Imidacloprid, Arsenic, Testes, Antioxidant, Oxidative damage

Background

The ability of the chemical pollutants to affect reproductive health has garnered significant attention in recent decades and is further compounded by the endocrine disruptive chemicals in the environment [1–3]. Chemicals that disrupt normal endocrine functions may interfere with the hormonal pathways responsible for the control of reproduction [4] triggering morphological and functional abnormalities in reproductive organs. Testicular toxicity of insecticides and other toxicants result in male infertility in mammals [5].

Various experimental studies have shown cellular and molecular aspects of gonadal damage in animals during spermatogenesis following chemical exposure including insecticides [5, 6]. Imidacloprid (IMI), a newer neonicotinoid has gained wide acceptance as an insecticide due to its extremely high insecticidal potency, broad insecticidal spectra, excellent systemic properties in pests and a low mammalian toxicity [7]. Agrochemicals along with heavy metals from emissions and groundwater are the main sources responsible for the environmental contamination [8]. Among heavy metals, Arsenic (As) is categorized as a

* Correspondence: drpawankv@yahoo.co.in
[2]Division of Veterinary Pharmacology and Toxicology, Faculty of Veterinary Science and Animal Husbandry, R S Pura, Jammu 181102, India
Full list of author information is available at the end of the article

ubiquitous trace element and is the 52nd most abundant element in the earth's crust. Arsenic finds a place in the priority list of hazardous substances published by the Agency for Toxic Substances and Disease Registry [9]. Studies revealed that arsenic interacts with sperm DNA which may contribute to the mechanisms for a trans-generational reproductive effect [9, 10].

The concurrent exposure of more than one environmental toxicant in mammals induce depletion in antioxidant defence system as indicated with reduced levels of total thiols (TTH) including reduced glutathione (GSH). Antioxidant defence system scavenges reactive oxygen/nitrogen species (ROS/RNS) generated in tissues and sub-cellular compartments during intoxication [11]. It has been reported that excessive generation of these free radicals in testicular tissue reduces antioxidant defence resulting in the disruption of the functional integrity of membrane structures of mitochondria and other cytoplasmic organelles through peroxidation of phospholipids, proteins and nucleotides [12, 13]. Hence, ROS plays an important role in the pathogenesis of male reproductive system due to the existence of high polyunsaturated fatty acid (PUFA) in the testes which makes it more sensitive to oxidative insults [14, 15]. Therefore, the present study was aimed to evaluate the potentiating effect of imidacloprid (IMI) on arsenic-induced testicular toxicity in male Wistar rats.

Methods

Experimental animals and chemicals used

The study was conducted on adult male Wistar rats (180–200 g, 12-14 weeks of age) procured from Indian Institute of Integrative Medicine (IIIM), Jammu. The animals were provided standard pelleted ration and tap water for drinking ad-libitum. All animals were maintained under standard managemental conditions (22 ± 3 °C, 50–60% relative humidity and 12 h light-dark cycles). Prior to the start of the experiment, Wistar rats were acclimatized in the laboratory conditions for a period of 15 days. All the experimental animals were kept under constant observation during the entire period of study. The experimental protocol was dully approved by Institutional Animal Ethics Committee (IAEC) vide letter no AU/ANN/13–14/IAEC/143–54, dated 24/05/2013. Imidacloprid (17.8% SL) used in the present study was commercially obtained from Mahindra and Mahindra Ltd. Agribusiness, Mumbai, India. Analytical grade Sodium Arsenate (Product no. 20237) procured from S.D. Fine-Chem. Limited, Mumbai was used as a source of arsenic. All other chemicals used in the study were of analytical grade and purchased from different standard firms.

Experimental protocol

The low observed adverse effect level (LOAEL) dose (16.9 mg/kg) of imidacloprid was used in the study to determine its effects alone and in conjunction with the different doses of arsenic in drinking water. As per the WHO guidelines, the maximum contaminant level (MCL) of arsenic in drinking water is 50 ppb [16] and in the present study, three dose levels viz. 50, 100 and 150 ppb in drinking water were used in the study [4.165 mg of Sodium arsenate used provided 1 mg arsenic].

Adult male Wistar rats were randomly allocated into eight groups with six rats each. Group I received distilled water (1 ml/day) and served as the control, whereas group II received IMI orally at the dose rate of 16.9 mg/kg body weight. Group III, IV and V were provided access exclusively to drinking water containing arsenic at the rate of 50, 100 and 150 ppb, respectively. The groups VI, VII and VIII received combined administration of IMI and arsenic at the dose rate of 16.9 mg/kg + 50 ppb, 16.9 mg/kg + 100 ppb and 16.9 mg/kg + 150 ppb, respectively. The animals received daily dosing of IMI between 9.00–10.00 AM daily for a period of 28 days. All animals were weighed weekly for modifying the total dose of IMI to be administered. The animals were observed for clinical signs if any, during the entire period of study.

Collection and processing of samples

After the end of 28 days of daily administrations of toxicants animals were sacrificed by cervical dislocation and testes 1 g each was collected in 10 ml ice-cold 0.5 M Phosphate buffer (pH 7.4) and formal saline (10%) for antioxidant parameters and histopathological studies, respectively. Tissue homogenate (10%) was prepared by homogenizing the testicular tissue using Teflon coated homogenizer at 1000 rpm for 5–7 min at 4 °C.

Determination of lipid peroxidation and protein oxidation product in testes

Levels of malondialdehyde (MDA) and advanced oxidation protein product (AOPP) were determined in the testicular tissue to determine the intensity of oxidation of membrane lipids and cellular proteins, respectively the following exposure to toxicant alone and in combination [17, 18].

Determination of antioxidant parameters in testes

Total thiols (TTH) level was determined in testes as per the standard method using reduced glutathione and was expressed in mM [19]. Various antioxidant enzymes in testicular tissue viz., catalase (CAT), superoxide dismutase (SOD), glutathione peroxidase (GPx), glutathione reductase (GR) and glutathione-s-transferase (GST) were determined spectrophotometrically (UV-1601, Shimadzu) to assess the alterations in antioxidant system following exposure to toxicant alone or in combination [20–24].

Histopathological studies

The histopathological studies were carried out according to standard methods. Formalin-fixed testes of the different group were embedded in paraffin, sectioned, stained with hematoxylin and eosin and examined under a light microscope for histopathological studies.

Statistical analysis

The biochemical and oxidative stress parameters were analyzed for analysis of variance at 5% level of significance using the Duncan Multiple Range test (SPSS 16.0).

Results

Antioxidant biomarkers in testicular tissue following repeated oral administration of IMI and arsenic alone and in combination in rats is presented in Table 1.

Glutathione-S-transferase (GST)

A significant ($P < 0.05$) decrease in GST activity was observed (34.5%) after repeated IMI administrations for 28 days considering the activity of the control group as 100%. Similarly, there was significant ($P < 0.05$) fall in GST activity within group III (14.2%), IV (29.7%) and V (48.3%) compared to the control. Similar significant ($P < 0.05$) decrease in the activities of GST were observed in group VI (58.9%), VII (65.0%) and VIII (75.3%).

Glutathione reductase (GR)

Significant ($P < 0.05$) decrease in GR activity was observed in IMI exposed animals (38.5%), as well as in groups III (15.6%), IV (24.5%) and V (35.4%) compared to control group. Such a significant fall in GR activity is also seen in combined exposed groups VI, VII and VIII (46.2–65.6%) as compared to the control group.

Glutathione peroxidase (GP_X)

GPx activity of testicular tissue had significantly ($P < 0.05$) declined in group II (35.8%), III (26.8%), IV(39.6%) and V (49.2%) as compared to following repeated oral exposure of toxicants. Similarly, GPx activity was profoundly declined in concurrent exposed groups (62.7–77.6%) compared to the control group.

Catalase (CAT)

CAT activity testes had significantly ($P < 0.05$) declined in all groups exposed to toxicants either alone (IMI or Arsenic) or in combination (IMI with arsenic) as to compared control group. The decline in CAT activity was observed to be concentration dependent with arsenic (25.8–39.8%). Such decline was more profound (56.0–67.8%) in combined exposed groups.

Superoxide dismutase (SOD)

A significant ($P < 0.05$) fall in SOD activity was observed in group II (30.7%), III (18.2%), IV (25.5%) and V (30.9%) as compared to control group. A similar decline in the activity of SOD was observed in different combined administered groups (34.5–57.2%).

Total thiols (TTH)

A significant ($P < 0.05$) decrease in mean TTH level was observed in IMI or arsenic alone administered groups - II (31.5%), III (16.8%), IV (26.1%) and V (32.1%) in comparison to control group. However decrease in TTH level a significant ($P < 0.05$) decrease in TTH level was observed in Group VI (39.5%), VII (42.2%) and VIII (49.6%) compared to control group.

Table 1 Activities of various antioxidant enzymes and total thiols (TTH) level in testes of Wistar rats following repeated oral administrations of IMI and arsenic alone and in combination

Groups	TTH	GST	GR	GPx	SOD	CAT
I. Control	$4.76^{c} \pm 0.540$	$59.03^{f} \pm 3.34$	$25.56^{f} \pm 1.88$	$26.89^{e} \pm 2.99$	$196.80^{d} \pm 13.12$	$1694.41^{e} \pm 62.69$
II. Imidacloprid (IMI) (16.9 mg/kg)	$3.26^{ab} \pm 0.105$	$38.65^{d} \pm 2.83$	$15.72^{bcd} \pm 1.73$	$17.26^{cd} \pm 1.30$	$136.44^{bc} \pm 14.02$	$1152.61^{d} \pm 42.63$
III. Arsenic (50 ppb)	$3.96^{bc} \pm 0.151$	$50.65^{e} \pm 3.64$	$21.58^{ef} \pm 1.44$	$19.68^{d} \pm 1.19$	$160.96^{cd} \pm 15.02$	$1256.72^{d} \pm 58.52$
IV. Arsenic (100 ppb)	$3.52^{ab} \pm 0.302$	$41.48^{d} \pm 1.90$	$19.30^{de} \pm 1.50$	$16.24^{cd} \pm 1.24$	$146.71^{bc} \pm 13.59$	$1189.93^{d} \pm 51.57$
V. Arsenic (150 ppb)	$3.23^{ab} \pm 0.341$	$30.50^{c} \pm 1.83$	$16.51^{cd} \pm 1.33$	$13.65^{bc} \pm 0.923$	$135.89^{bc} \pm 14.95$	$1020.15^{c} \pm 32.86$
VI. IMI + As (50 ppb)	$2.88^{ab} \pm 0.229$	$24.28^{bc} \pm 1.73$	$13.75^{bc} \pm 1.42$	$10.02^{ab} \pm 0.806$	$128.90^{bc} \pm 12.97$	$744.78^{b} \pm 36.45$
VII. IMI + As (100 ppb)	$2.75^{a} \pm 0.425$	$20.65^{ab} \pm 1.30$	$11.59^{ab} \pm 1.09$	$8.75^{a} \pm 0.899$	$117.26^{ab} \pm 12.86$	$687.69^{b} \pm 33.43$
VIII. IMI + As (150 ppb)	$2.40^{a} \pm 0.457$	$14.60^{a} \pm 0.350$	$8.50^{a} \pm 0.967$	$6.01^{a} \pm 0.753$	$84.25^{a} \pm 9.90$	$544.78^{a} \pm 34.73$

Values are given as mean ± SE of 6 animals unless otherwise stated
Values having different superscript (a,b,c,d,e,f) in a column are statistically different from one another at 5% level of significance
Values of TTH (total thiols) are expressed in μM
Values of GST (glutathione S transferase) are expressed in μmol of CDNB conjugate formed/ min/ g of tissue
Values of GR (glutathione reductase) are expressed nmol of NADPH/min
Values of GPx (glutathione peroxidase) are expressed in Unit/ g of tissue
Values of SOD (Superoxide dismutase) are expressed in Unit/ g of tissue
Values of CAT (Catalase) are expressed in μmol H_2O_2 decomposed/ min/ g of tissue

Testicular damage indicators

MDA and AOPP levels in testes of different groups of animals exposed IMI or arsenic alone and in combination are shown in Fig. 1a and b respectively.

Significant ($P < 0.05$) increase in lipid peroxidation (MDA levels) were observed in group II (120.4%), III (62.0%), IV (102.5%) and V (151%) after repeated administration of IMI or arsenic for 28 days. However such rise was significantly higher ($P < 0.05$) in combined administered groups viz. VI (206.3%), VII (251.4%) and VIII (278.4%) compared to the control group.

A significant ($P < 0.05$) increase in protein oxidation (AOPP) levels was observed in IMI exposed group (37.4%) as compared to the control group. Arsenic in different used concentrations was less effective in increasing the AOPP levels (15.6–23.8%). However, increased AOPP levels were higher in co-exposed groups (43.5–53.1%).

Histopathological alterations

The histopathological alterations in the testes following repeated oral administrations of IMI and arsenic alone or in combination in Wistar rats are shown in Fig. 2. In normal rats, histologically the testes had normal morphological features comprising of seminiferous tubules with central tubular lumen surrounded by a basement membrane and no microscopic lesion of pathological significance was observed. All stages of spermatogenesis could be appreciably seen and mature spermatozoa, interstitial tissue contained Leydig cells, macrophages were present in the lumen of control animal testes. In IMI exposed group, the testicular parenchyma did not show any significant histological alterations when compared to control, other than mild edematous fluid accumulation in the interstitial spaces. Testes in rats belonging to group III had appreciable but only mild

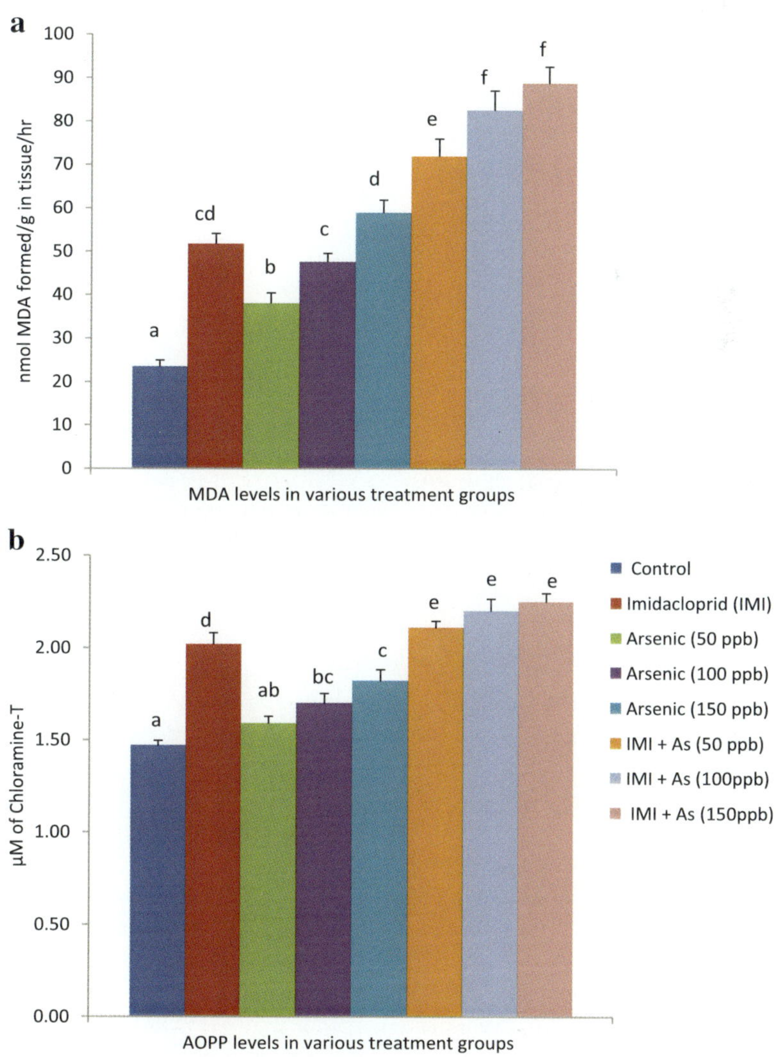

Fig. 1 Effect of repeated oral administrations of IMI and arsenic alone and in combination on (**a**) MDA and (**b**) AOPP levels in testes of Wistar rats. (Mean values having different superscripts (**a**, **b**, **c**) are statistically different from one another at 5% level of significance)

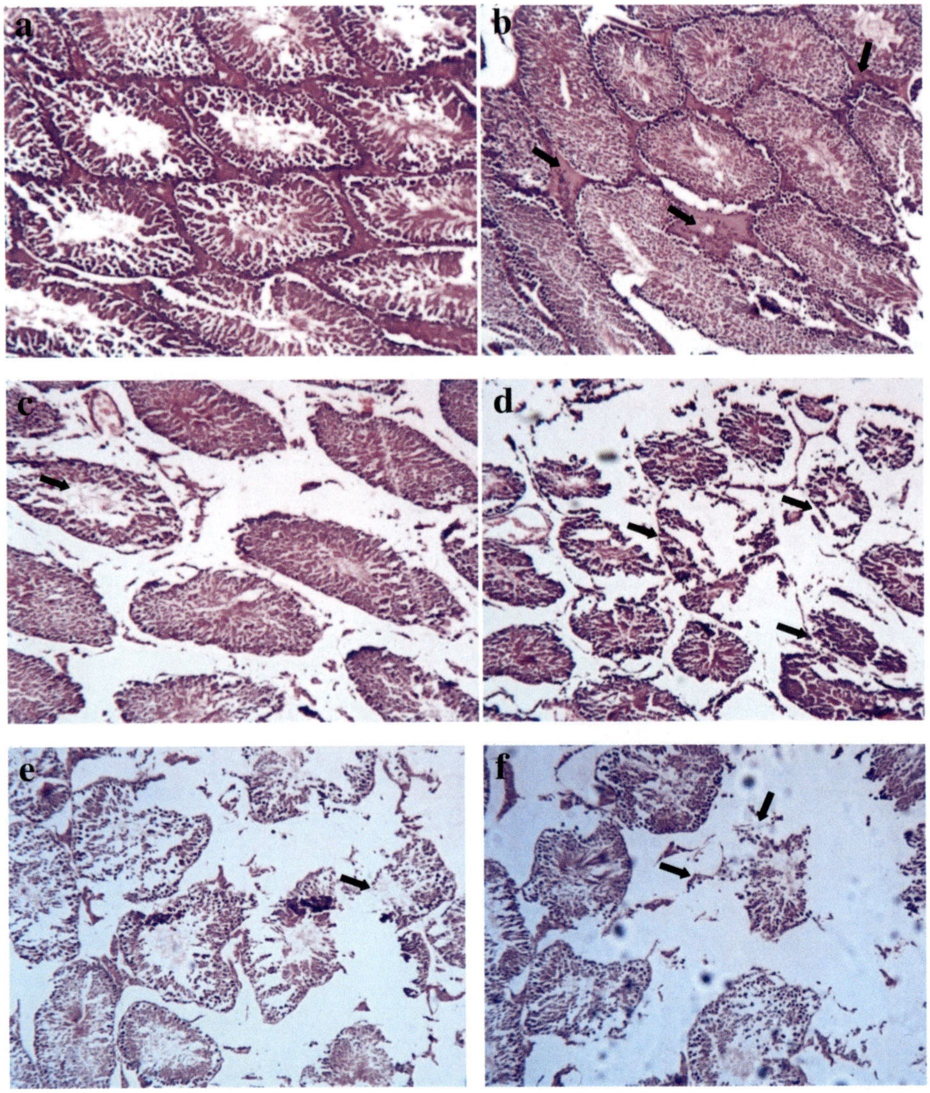

Fig. 2 Photomicrograph of H & E (10X) stained sections of formalin fixed testes (**a**) Control: normal testicular parenchyma with seminiferous tubules and interstitial tissue (**b**) IMI administered group: mild edema in the interstitial spaces (**c**) Arsenic group: mild degeneration and necrosis in germ cells (**d**) group VI disruption of seminiferous tubules and necrosis of germ cells (**e**) Group VII: Severely necrotic seminiferous tubules and (**f**) Group VIII: fibrillar debris representing the remnants of seminiferous tubules of testes in Wistar rats

degenerative changes in few seminiferous tubules. In rats belonging to group V appreciable degenerative and necrotic changes of germ cells were observed and such changes were not seen in rats administered lower concentration of arsenic.

In co-exposed rats (group VI) severe degenerative changes in seminiferous tubules with their number reduced along with degeneration and depletion of germ cells of all the lineages was observed. Increased concentrations of arsenic in drinking water and IMI induced more severe histopathological changes in the testes. Severe testicular necrosis was seen in group VII characterized by tubular shrinkage, decreased lumen diameter along with generalized necrosis and depletion of germ cells. More severe changes were appreciable in group VIII where tubules became severely necrotic with only remnants of fibrillar necrotic debris seen in testicular sections.

Discussion

Arsenic endemic areas groundwater is the major source of intoxication to mammals. Similarly, IMI is most commonly used neonicotinoid insecticide for pest and insects management in agricultural and animal practices. Therefore the coexistence of arsenic and IMI in the environment is reality and concurrent exposure to humans and animals could be potentially hazardous.

Effect of repeated oral administrations of arsenic alone and in-conjunction with IMI on antioxidant parameters in testicular tissue

Free radicals like hydroxyl (OH^-), superoxide ($O_2^{\cdot-}$), nitric oxide ($NO^{\cdot}$), hydrogen peroxide (H_2O_2) are commonly generated by auto-oxidation processes and/or enzymatic metabolic reactions are scavenged by cellular antioxidant system [25]. Repeated oral administrations of arsenic alone or in-conjunction with IMI increased cellular metabolic reactions leading to increased generation of free radicals. The inability of enzymatic antioxidant components like CAT, SOD and GPx to scavenge these excessively produced free radicals during metabolism of toxicants may induce testicular damage as indicated by increased levels of lipid peroxidation (MDA) and protein oxidation (AOPP) product after exposure with IMI and arsenic in Wistar rats. The increasing concentration levels of arsenic in drinking water proportionately increase the AOPP and MDA levels in testes of rats [26–28].

Protein and non-protein thiols (-SH group) play a significant role in scavenging free radicals including ROS. Thiols protect cellular components from oxidative insults either by direct scavenging of the free radicals and/or acts as the substrate for various antioxidant enzymes like SOD, GPx and GST [29]. In the present study, a significant reduction in the level of TTH in testicular tissue of rats exposed either to arsenic alone at 150 ppb or in concurrently exposed groups may be primary contributor of oxidative insults in testicular tissue. The replenishment of GSH during oxidative stress can be achieved by either increasing its biosynthesis or recycling by the activity of GR [30]. In the present study, reduction in the activity of GR may be responsible for the failure in replenishment resulting in the reduced level of GSH which decreases the direct and indirect scavenging of free radicals during intoxication [30]. The reduction in the activity of enzymes utilizing glutathione as a substrate (SOD, GPx and GST) may be due to the reduced level of thiols. The decreased antioxidant enzymes have been reported to induce oxidative damage of cellular membranes of spermatozoa due to generated free radicals which inhibit their number and increase their abnormality rate [31, 32]. Arsenic exposure along with IMI administration to Wistar rats produced a more profound decrease in antioxidant enzymatic activities than the administrations of either IMI or arsenic which is in consonance with reported findings [26].

The increased free radicals interact with the cellular proteins and lipids leading to the peroxidation as indicated by increased levels of MDA and AOPP in rats administered with arsenic (150 ppb) alone or in the combination of Arsenic at various concentrations with IMI administered group. These results are in accordance with the reported findings on interaction studies of insecticides and metals [33–35]. Administration of both IMI and arsenic induce significant fall in tissue levels TTH as compared to the sole administration of toxicants. Co-exposure of rats to IMI and arsenic may have generated excessive free radicals in testicular tissue and its sub-cellular compartments which may have resulted in depletion of antioxidants, as indicated with decreased TTH level in testes [36].

The significant increase in the lipid peroxidation and protein oxidation product was observed testicular tissue of the IMI administered group. These observations have also been in agreement with the finding reported in the male reproductive system following administrations of insecticides [33, 37]. The exposure of arsenic through drinking water also induces a significant rise in MDA and AOPP levels in the testes of Wistar rats. Various studies have also reported similar results on chemical induced oxidative damage in testes [28, 38, 39]. Concurrent exposure of both the toxicants produced a more significant increase in lipid and protein oxidation levels as compared to individual administration of either toxicant. The testes are rich in PUFA and prone to lipid peroxidation [40]. Peroxidation of membrane lipids can result in disruption of cell structural integrity [41] leading to cellular damage. Hence, the increase in MDA and AOPP levels caused by both the toxicants in the rat testes suggests peroxidation of PUFA in testicular cells, which can cause impairment of normal testicular and sperm abnormalities [41].

Histopathology alterations in testes

Microscopic examination of testes in rats of control group revealed normal mature seminiferous tubules with complete series of spermatogenesis and high spermatozoa concentration in the lumen. However, repeated oral administrations of IMI alone in rats showed progressive congestion in blood vessels and mild oedema in the interstitial space. IMI and arsenic in drinking water induced mild to severe degenerative changes of germ cells in testes of Wistar rats [34]. Increased concentration of arsenic along with IMI induced severe testicular necrosis characterized by tubular shrinkage, decreased lumen diameter along with generalized necrosis and depletion of germ cells. More severe changes were appreciable in animals co-exposed with arsenic at 150 ppb along with IMI made tubules severely necrotic with only remnants of fibrillar necrotic debris seen in testicular sections. The pronounced histopathological alterations are further corroborated by the increased levels of MDA, AOPP and reduced TTH and antioxidant defence increased the testicular tissue damage in Wistar rats. Similarly, another insecticide like acetamiprid administration produced vacuolization of the seminiferous tubules with a reduced number of spermaids and interstitial Leydig cells in the testes of Wistar rats [42]. These results were similar to the effects of β-cypermethrin in male mice [43]. However, α-cypermethrin has been reported to induce oedema between the seminiferous tubules and vacuolization of the tubules in male mice [44, 45].

Arsenic exposure has been reported to produce ruptured follicles and few follicles showed a reduction in the number of spermatozoa in the testes of male albino rats [46]. In present study arsenic along with IMI showed severe degenerative changes in seminiferous tubules, tubular shrinkage, decreased lumen diameter with generalized necrosis and depletion of germ cells which became more prominent with the increasing concentration of arsenic doses in the combination groups and such observed alterations are in agreement with reported findings [32, 33, 47].

Conclusion

The finding of the present study suggests that repeated oral administrations of arsenic or IMI alone produce testicular damage in male Wistar rats. Reduced antioxidant enzymatic activities, increased MDA, AOPP levels and severe histopathological alterations in testes observed following concurrent repeated exposure indicated that IMI potentiated the arsenic-induced testicular toxicity in Wistar rats.

Abbreviations

AOPP: Advanced oxidation protein product; CAT: Catalase; GPx: Glutathione peroxidase; GR: Glutathione reductase; GST: Glutathione-s-transferase; IMI : Imidacloprid; MDA: Malondialdehyde; SOD: Superoxide dismutase; TTH: Total thiols

Acknowledgements

Authors thank the Head, Division of Veterinary Pharmacology and Toxicology, Faculty of Veterinary Science and Animal Husbandry, R S Pura, Jammu for providing necessary facilities for conducting the research.

Funding

Part of Master's thesis and no additional funding was obtained for this study.

Authors' contributions

L. Mahajan – Planning and execution of research work. P. K. Verma – Experimental design and statistical analysis of research work. R. Raina – Supervision and interpretation. S. Sood – Histopathological study. All authors read and approved the final manuscript.

Competing interests

The authors declares that they have no competing interests.

Author details

[1]Division of Veterinary Pharmacology and Toxicology, Faculty of Veterinary Science and Animal Husbandry, R S Pura, Jammu 181102, India. [2]Division of Veterinary Pharmacology and Toxicology, Faculty of Veterinary Science and Animal Husbandry, R S Pura, Jammu 181102, India. [3]Division of Veterinary Pharmacology and Toxicology, Faculty of Veterinary Science and Animal Husbandry, R S Pura, Jammu 181102, India. [4]Division of Veterinary Pathology, Faculty of Veterinary Science and Animal Husbandry, R S Pura, Jammu 181102, India.

References

1. Kumar S. Occupational exposure associated with reproductive dysfunction. J Occup Health. 2004;46(1):1–19.
2. Yeung BH, Wan HT, Law AY, Wong CK. Endocrine disrupting chemicals: multiple effects on testicular signalling and spermatogenesis. Spermatogenesis. 2011;1(3):231–9.
3. Rana SV. Perspectives in endocrine toxicity of heavy metals--a review. Biol Trace Elem Res. 2014;160(1):1–14.
4. Diamanti-kandarakis E, Bourguignon JP, Giudice LC, et al. Endocrine-disrupting chemicals: an Endocrine Society scientific statement. Endocr Rev. 2009;30(4):293–342.
5. Mantovani A, Maranghi F. Risk assessment of chemicals potentially affecting male fertility. Contraception. 2005;72(4):308–13.
6. Mandal TK, Das NS. Testicular gametogenic and steroidogenic activities in chlorpyrifos insecticide-treated rats: a correlation study with testicular oxidative stress and role of antioxidant enzyme defence systems in Sprague-Dawley rats. Andrologia. 2012;44(2):102–15.
7. Solecki R. Pesticide residues in food. Toxicological evaluations- Imidacloprid. J med plants res. 2001:1–34.
8. Kacmar P, Pistl J, Mikula I. Immunotoxicology and veterinary medicine. Acta veterinaria. 1999;68:57–79.
9. ATSDR. CERCLA priority list of hazardous substances. Agency for Toxic substances and disease registry. Atlanta, GA: U.S. Department of Health and Human services; 2007.
10. Ali S, Chaspoul F, Anderson L, et al. Mapping fifteen trace elements in human seminal plasma and sperm DNA. Biol Trace Elem Res. 2017;175(2):244–53.
11. Naziroğlu M, Kutluhan S, Uğuz AC, Celik O, Bal R, Butterworth PJ. Topiramate and vitamin E modulate the electroencephalographic records, brain microsomal and blood antioxidant redox system in pentylentetrazol-induced seizure of rats. J Membr Biol. 2009;229(3):131–40.
12. Nagda G, Bhatt DK. Alleviation of lindane induced toxicity in testes of swiss mice (Mus musculus) by combined treatment with vitamin C, vitamin E and alpha-lipoic acid. Ind J Exper Biol. 2011;49(3):191–9.
13. Kovacic P, Somanathan R. Novel, unifying mechanism for mescaline in the central nervous system: electrochemistry, catechol redox metabolite, receptor, cell signaling and structure activity relationships. Oxidative Med Cell Longev. 2009;2(4):181–90.
14. Turner TT, Lysiak JJ. Oxidative stress: a common factor in testicular dysfunction. J Androl. 2008;29(5):488–98.
15. Mathur PP, D'cruz SC. The effect of environmental contaminants on testicular function. Asian J Androl. 2011;13(4):585–91.
16. Steinmaus CM, Yuan Y, Smith AH. The temporal stability of arsenic concentrations in well water in western Nevada. Environ Res. 2005;99(2):164–8.
17. Shafiq-ur-rehman. Lead-induced regional lipid peroxidation in brain. Toxicol Lett. 1984;21:333–7.
18. Witko-sarsat V, Friedlander M, Capeillère-blandin C, et al. Advanced oxidation protein products as a novel marker of oxidative stress in uremia. Kidney Int. 1996;49(5):1304–13.
19. Motchnik AP, Frei B, Ames NB (1994) Measurement of antioxidants in human blood plasma, protein thiols. In: packer L, eds. Oxygen radicals in biological systems, methods in enzymology. California, Academic Press 234(D):273–274.
20. Aebi HE. Catalase. In: Bergmeyer HU, editor. Methods of enzymatic analysis. New York: Academic Press; 1983. p. 276–86.
21. Marklund S, Marklund G. Involvement of superoxide anion radical in autoxidation of pyrogallol and a convenient assay for superoxide dismutase. Eur J Biochem. 1974;47:469–74.

22. Hafeman DG, Sunde RA, Hoekstra WG. Effect of dietary selenium on erythrocyte and liver glutathione peroxidase in the rat. J Nutr. 1974;104(5):580–7.
23. Habig WH, Pabst MJ, Jakoby WB. Glutathione S-transferases. The first enzymatic step in mercapturic acid formation. J Biol Chem. 1974; 249(22):7130–9.
24. Carlberg I, Mannervik B. Purification and characterization of the flavoenzyme glutathione reductase from rat liver. J Biol Chem. 1975;250(14):5475–4580.
25. Circu ML, Aw TY. Reactive oxygen species, cellular redox systems, and apoptosis. Free Radic Biol Med. 2010;48:749–62.
26. Aggarwal M, Naraharisetti SB, Sarkar SN, Rao GS, Degen GH, Malik JK. Effects of subchronic coexposure to arsenic and endosulfan on the erythrocytes of broiler chickens: a biochemical study. Arch Environ Contam Toxicol. 2009; 56(1):139–48.
27. Khan S, Telang AG, Malik JK. Arsenic-induced oxidative stress, apoptosis and alterations in testicular steroidogenesis and spermatogenesis in wistar rats: ameliorative effect of curcumin. Wudpecker J Pharmacy Pharmacol. 2013; 2(3):33–48.
28. Sumedha NC, Miltonprabhu S. Diallyl trisulfide (DATS) abrogates arsenic induced testicular oxidative stress in rats. Int J Pharmacol Toxicol. 2014; 2(2):30–7.
29. Lushchak VI. Glutathione homeostasis and functions: potential targets for medical interventions. J Amino Acids. 2012;736837
30. Johnson WM, Wilson-delfosse AL, Mieyal JJ. Dysregulation of glutathione homeostasis in neurodegenerative diseases. Nutrients. 2012;4(10):1399–440.
31. Mittal M, Flora SJ. Vitamin E supplementation protects oxidative stress during arsenic and fluoride antagonism in male mice. Drug Chem Toxicol. 2007;30(3):263–81.
32. Bal R, Türk G, Tuzcu M, et al. Assessment of imidacloprid toxicity on reproductive organ system of adult male rats. J Environ Sci Health B. 2012; 47(5):434–44.
33. Aggarwal M, Wangikar PB, Sarkar SN, et al. Effects of low-level arsenic exposure on the developmental toxicity of anilofos in rats. J Appl Toxicol. 2007;27(3):255–61.
34. Lonare M, Kumar M, Raut S, et al. Evaluation of ameliorative effect of curcumin on imidacloprid-induced male reproductive toxicity in wistar rats. Environ Toxicol. 2016;31(10):1250–63.
35. Olayinka ET, Ore A. Hepatotoxicity, nephrotoxicity and oxidative stress in rat testes following exposure to Haloxyfop-p-methyl ester, an arylphenoxypropionate herbicide. Toxics. 2015;3:373–89.
36. Tomizawa M, Casida JE. Selective toxicity of neonicotinoids attributable to the specificity of insect and mammalian nicotinic receptors. Annu Rev Entomol. 2003;48:339–64.
37. Taib IS, Budin SB, Ghazali AR, Jayusman PA, Louis SR, Mohamed J. Fenitrothion induced oxidative stress and morphological alterations of sperm and testes in male Sprague-Dawley rats. Clinics (Sao Paulo). 2013; 68(1):93–100.
38. Muthumani M, Miltonprabhu S. Silibinin ameliorates oxidative stress-mediated testicular damage by arsenic in rats. Asian Pacific J Tropical Biomed. 2012;1:1–7.
39. Kumar BA, Reddy AG, Kumar PR, Reddy YR, Rao TM, Haritha C. Protective role of N-acetyl L-cysteine against reproductive toxicity due to interaction of lead and cadmium in male wistar rats. J Nat Sci Biol Med. 2013;4(2):414–9.
40. Aitken RJ, Roman SD. Antioxidant systems and oxidative stress in the testes. Oxidative Med Cell Longev. 2008;1(1):15–24.
41. Bell M, Sikka S, Rajasekaran M, Hellstrom W. Time course of hydrogen peroxide induced changes in the lipid peroxidation of human sperm membranes. Adv Contracept Deliv Syst. 1992;8(1–2):144–1450.
42. Lenzi A, Gandini L, Picardo M, Tramer F, Sandri G, Panfili E. Lipoperoxidation damage of spermatozoa polyunsaturated fatty acids (PUFA): scavenger mechanisms and possible scavenger therapies. Front Biosci. 2000;5:E1–E15.
43. Zhang JJ, Wang Y, Xiang H, Li M, Li W, Ma K, Wang X, Zhang J. Oxidative stress: role in acetamiprid-induced impairment of the male ice reproductive system. Agri Sci China. 2011;10(5):786–96.
44. Wang XZ, Liu SS, Sun Y, Wu JY, Zhou YL, Zhang JH. Beta-cypermethrin impairs reproductive function in male mice by inducing oxidative stress. Theriogenology. 2009;72(5):599–611.
45. Manna S, Bhattacharyya D, Mandal TK, Das S. Repeated dose toxicity of alfa-cypermethrin in rats. J Vet Sci. 2004;5(3):241–5.
46. El-demerdash FM, Yousef MI, Radwan FM. Ameliorating effect of curcumin on sodium arsenite-induced oxidative damage and lipid peroxidation in different rat organs. Food Chem Toxicol. 2009;47(1):249–54.
47. Dopp E, Hartmann LM, Florea AM, et al. Uptake of inorganic and organic derivatives of arsenic associated with induced cytotoxic and genotoxic effects in Chinese hamster ovary (CHO) cells. Toxicol Appl Pharmacol. 2004; 201(2):156–65.

20

Effect of astragaloside IV on indoxyl sulfate-induced kidney injury in mice via attenuation of oxidative stress

Chunlan Ji[†], Yueming Luo[†], Chuan Zou, Lihua Huang, Ruimin Tian and Zhaoyu Lu[*]

Abstract

Background: *Astragalus membranaceus*, a traditional Chinese medicine (TCM), has been widely used in the treatment of chronic kidney disease (CKD) in China. Astragaloside IV is one of the major compounds of *Astragalus membranaceus*. Recent research has shown that astragaloside IV demonstrates pharmacological effects, such as anti-inflammatory, anti-fibrotic and anti-oxidative stress activities. Our aim was to investigate the effects of astragaloside IV on indoxyl sulfate (IS)-induced kidney injury in vivo, and to study the underlying mechanism.

Methods: Forty C57BL/6 mice with ½ nephrectomy were divided into four groups: control group ($n = 10$), IS group ($n = 10$), IS plus 10 mg/kg of astragaloside IV group ($n = 10$) and IS plus 20 mg/kg of astragaloside IV group ($n = 10$). IS intraperitoneal injection and astragaloside IV treatment were administered continuously for 1 month. Next, the blood urea nitrogen (BUN) level, serum IS level, tubulointerstitial injury, renal oxidative stress and inflammatory injury were assessed.

Results: The IS intraperitoneal injection mouse group showed increasing levels of serum IS, BUN, tubulointerstitial injury, renal oxidative stress and inflammatory injury. Astragaloside IV treatment couldn't reduce the serum IS level or renal nuclear factor-κB and interleukin-1β levels. However, 20 mg/kg astragaloside IV treatment reduced the BUN level and significantly attenuated IS-induced tubulointerstitial injury. Renal oxidative stress was decreased by the administration of astragaloside IV.

Conclusions: These results suggest that astragaloside IV prevents IS-induced tubulointerstitial injury by ameliorating oxidative stress and may be a promising agent for the treatment of uremia toxin-induced injury.

Keywords: Astragaloside IV, IS, Tubulointerstitial injury, Oxidative stress

Background

In chronic kidney disease (CKD), metabolic changes, disorders of gut microflora and impaired urinary excretion of metabolites lead to the accumulation of uremic toxins in the body [1]. Indoxyl sulfate (IS), one of the most extensively studied uremic toxins, has been increasingly recognized as an important contributor to kidney and heart dysfunction [2–4].

The pathophysiologic importance of protein-bound uremic toxins has been neglected for a long time [5, 6]. Dialysis is not powerful enough to remove protein-bound uremic toxins alone [7, 8]. Removing IS is very difficult in CKD patients. Consequently, identifying effective measures to reduce IS-induced injury is of significant value.

Indeed, the mechanism by which IS induces its toxic effects has now been clarified. Previous studies have demonstrated IS-induced tubulointerstitial injury in patients with CKD via the induction of oxidative stress and activation of the nuclear factor (NF)-κB pathway, producing various cytokines and inflammatory mediators, thereby promoting kidney damage [9–11].

Astragalus membranaceus, a traditional Chinese medicine (TCM), has been widely used for the treatment of CKD in China [12]. Astragaloside IV is one of the major compounds of *Astragalus membranaceus*. Astragaloside

* Correspondence: luzhaoyu111@163.com
[†]Chunlan Ji and Yueming Luo contributed equally to this work.
National Key Unit of Clinical Research of TCM on Chronic Kidney Diseases, Key Unit of Kidney Diseases, Guangdong Provincial Hospital of Chinese Medicine, The Second Clinical College of Guangzhou University of Chinese Medicine, 111th Dade Road, Guangzhou 510120, People's Republic of China

IV exerts considerable pharmacological effects, such as anti-inflammatory, anti-fibrotic and anti-oxidative stress activities [13, 14]. Although the wide use of *Astragalus* in CKD, and the antioxidant and anti-inflammatory properties of astragaloside IV, have been well demonstrated, studies regarding its efficacy in the prevention and attenuation of IS-induced tubulointerstitial injury have not been undertaken. Based on previous research, we hypothesize that astragaloside IV may affect IS-induced tubulointerstitial injury. Therefore, the aim of this study was to evaluate the effect of astragaloside IV on IS-induced tubulointerstitial injury in vivo, and to study its mechanism of action.

Methods

Animals, reagents and experimental drugs

Forty eight-week-old male C57BL/6 mice were used for this study. The C57BL/6 mice were purchased from Beijing Vital River Laboratory Animal Technology Company (Beijing, China). Each mouse was housed in our animal facility under pathogen-free conditions and was fed a standard laboratory diet, with free access to water.

Astragaloside IV (purity > 99%) was provided by Shanghai Winherb Medical Technology (Shanghai, China). IS potassium salt (purity 99.8%) and anti-β-actin antibody were obtained from Sigma (St. Louis, MO, USA). Anti-8-OHdG and anti-NF-κB were procured from Abcam (Cambridge, UK). Anti-cytochrome C was purchased from Santa Cruz Biotechnology (Santa Cruz, CA, USA). Fluorescein isothiocyanate (FITC)-conjugated anti-mouse immunoglobulin G (IgG), cy3-conjugated anti-rabbit IgG, horseradish peroxidase (HRP)-conjugated anti-mouse and rabbit IgG were purchased from Beyotime Biotechnology Company (Jiangsu, China).

Establishment of an animal model

The IS-induced tubulointerstitial injury model was carried out as described previously [15]. Forty C57BL/6 mice all underwent nephrectomy. All mice were anesthetized with an intraperitoneal injection of 2.0% pentobarbital sodium (30 mg/kg body weight). Next, the mice were randomly divided into four groups: control group ($n = 10$), IS group ($n = 10$), IS plus 10 mg/kg astragaloside IV group ($n = 10$), and IS plus 20 mg/kg astragaloside IV group ($n = 10$).

The experimental mice received an intraperitoneal injection of IS at a dosage of 100 mg/kg/day for 1 month. The control mice received daily phosphate-buffered saline (PBS) injection at the same volume. Astragaloside IV was suspended in 1% carboxymethyl cellulose (CMC) solution. Astragaloside IV group mice received astragaloside IV treatment by oral simultaneously at a dosage of 10 mg/kg or 20 mg/kg daily for 1 month. IS group mice received 1% CMC solution by oral at the same volume.

At the end of the study, all mice were anesthetized with an intraperitoneal injection of 2.0% pentobarbital sodium and then sacrificed. The sacrifice was implemented by the method of rapid decapitation and then collected the abdominal aorta blood and kidney sample. Blood were centrifugation at 3000 rpm for 15 min to take serum. The blood urea nitrogen (BUN) level, serum IS level, tubulointerstitial injury, renal oxidative stress and inflammatory injury were assessed.

The kidney was decapsulated and divided into several parts. One part was fixed in 10% formalin/PBS and processed for histopathological analysis, while another part was fixed in optimum cutting temperature (OCT) compound and stored at − 80 °C for immunofluorescence (IF) analysis. The remaining kidney tissue were isolate, quickly frozen in liquid nitrogen and stored at − 80 °C for Western-blot and ELISA detection The serum levels of BUN were measured using an auto-biochemical analyzer.

Indoxyl sulfate measurement

The serum IS concentration was detected by high-performance liquid chromatography (HPLC) tandem mass spectrometry, as described in our previous study [16].

The detection chemical included the standard IS potassium salt (purity 99.8%) and internal standard of hydrochlorothiazide (purity 99.5%), and was obtained from the Institute for Drug Control (Guangzhou, China).

Briefly, the serum samples were deproteinized by the addition of three parts of methanol to one part of serum for the determination of IS. All analyses were performed using an Acquity HPLC system (Agilent Technologies, Santa Clara, CA, USA) and an API3000 triple quadrupole mass spectrometer (Applied Biosystems, Foster City, CA, USA). Separation was performed using a reversed-phase HPLC ZORBAX Eclipse XDB-C18 column (Narrow-Bore 2.1 × 150 mm, 3.5-μm; Agilent). All data were assessed using Analyst14.1 software (Applied Biosystems). Standard curves were constructed using the linear regression formula $y = 0.0665 \times - 0.0294$, $R^2 = 0.9995$. The limit of quantification (LOQ) was defined as the lowest concentration for which acceptable precision and accuracy could be guaranteed (< 20%). The limit of detection (LOD) was 0.25 μg/ml.

Renal histopathological studies

Kidney slices were fixed in 10% formalin/PBS and embedded in paraffin. Sections of 2-μm thickness were prepared and stained with hematoxylin and eosin to evaluate the renal tubulointerstitial injury level. Renal histopathology studies were carried out under an Olympus BX61 microscope equipped with an Olympus DP72 digital camera.

Immunofluorescence staining

Sections were fixed in 4% paraformaldehyde for 15 min and washed with PBS twice for 10 min. Next, the sections were blocked in 10% casein/PBS (Vector, Burlingame, CA, USA) in PBS for 30 min. The sections were then incubated with primary antibodies overnight in a moisture chamber and washed sufficiently with PBST to remove unbound antibody. Next, the sections were incubated with secondary antibody, FITC-conjugated anti-mouse IgG or cy3-conjugated anti-rabbit IgG for 60 min at room temperature, and were washed as described for the primary antibody. Finally, the sections were stained with 4′,6-diamidino-2-phenylindole solution, washed for 5 min and then mounted on glass slides and analyzed under an Olympus BX61 fluorescence microscope equipped with an Olympus DP72 digital camera (Tokyo, Japan).

Western blot analysis

Kidney tissues were lysed in RIPA buffer. The lysates were clarified by centrifugation at 12,000 rpm for 30 min at 4 ° C, and the protein concentration in each lysate was determined using the BCA Protein Assay Kit (Pierce, Rockford, IL, USA). The protein samples were separated by sodium dodecyl sulfate–polyacrylamide gel electrophoresis and electroblotted onto nitrocellulose membranes. The membranes were blocked with 10% casein/PBS, incubated with a primary antibody at 4 °C overnight, and then incubated with HRP-conjugated secondary antibody. Immunoreactive bands were visualized using enhanced chemiluminescent reagent and exposure to the Bio-Rad ChemiDoc XRS + system (Hercules, CA, USA).

Enzyme-linked immunosorbent assay (ELISA) for interleukin (IL)-1β and IL-6

The concentrations of IL-1β and IL-6 in kidney tissues were determined using mouse IL-1β and IL-6 ELISA kits (R&D Systems, Minneapolis, MN, USA) according to the manufacturer's instructions.

Evaluation of 8-hydroxy-2′-deoxyguanosine (8-OHdG) expression and malondialdehyde (MDA) content, as well as superoxide dismutase (SOD) activity, in renal tissue

The expression of 8-OHdG, a marker of oxidative stress [17], in the kidney was examined by IF using anti-8-OHdG. The MDA level was assayed using the Lipid Peroxidation MDA Assay Kit (S0131; Beyotime, Nanjing, China). SOD activity was assayed using the Total Superoxide Dismutase Assay Kit (S0101; Beyotime) following the manufacturer's instructions.

Statistics

All data analyses were performed using SPSS software (ver. 13.0; SPSS, Inc., Chicago, IL, USA). The data are expressed as means ± standard error (SE). Comparisons among groups were conducted using analysis of variance. A value of $P < 0.05$ was deemed to indicate statistical significance.

Results

Astragaloside IV cannot reduce the serum levels of indoxyl sulfate in IS intraperitoneal injection mice

In our study, the IS intraperitoneal injection group mice showed a significantly increased serum level of IS compared with that in control group mice. The administration of astragaloside IV did not significantly decrease the serum levels of IS (Fig. 1).

Astragaloside IV inhibits tubulointerstitial injury in indoxyl sulfate intraperitoneal injection mice

The control group mice showed low levels of serum BUN and normal glomerular and tubulointerstitial morphology. The level of serum BUN was significantly increased in IS intraperitoneal injection group mice ($P <$ 0.001). In addition, IS intraperitoneal injection mice showed partial tubular epithelial cell degeneration, loss of the brush border, enlargement of the tubular lumen and interstitial expansion (Figs. 2 and 3).

The level of BUN of IS intraperitoneal injection mice was significantly decreased after 20 mg/kg of astragaloside IV treatment ($P = 0.048$). The administration of 20 mg/kg astragaloside IV attenuated the histopathological changes in IS intraperitoneal injection mice (Figs. 2 and 3). Astragaloside IV (10 mg/kg) did not exhibit any effect.

Astragaloside IV cannot ameliorate renal inflammatory injury in indoxyl sulfate intraperitoneal injection mice

Renal inflammatory injury was evaluated based on the expression of NF-κB, IL-1β, and IL-6. The expression of NF-κB was detected by western blotting and IF staining. The expression level of NF-κB was increased in both glomeruli and tubules in the IS group mice (Figs. 4 and 5). In addition, ELISA showed significantly increased levels of IL-1β expression in kidney homogenates (Fig. 6). The level of IL-6 expression was a bit increased in IS group mice (Fig. 6).

Astragaloside IV treatment could not attenuate the NF-κB expression in glomeruli and tubules. The expression of IL-1β and IL-6 in the astragaloside IV treatment group mice also showed no significant difference compared with that in IS group mice (Figs. 4, 5 and 6).

Astragaloside IV ameliorates renal oxidative stress in indoxyl sulfate intraperitoneal injection mice

Renal tissue oxidative stress was evaluated by 8-hydroxy-2′-deoxyguanosine (8-OHdG) IF staining, a

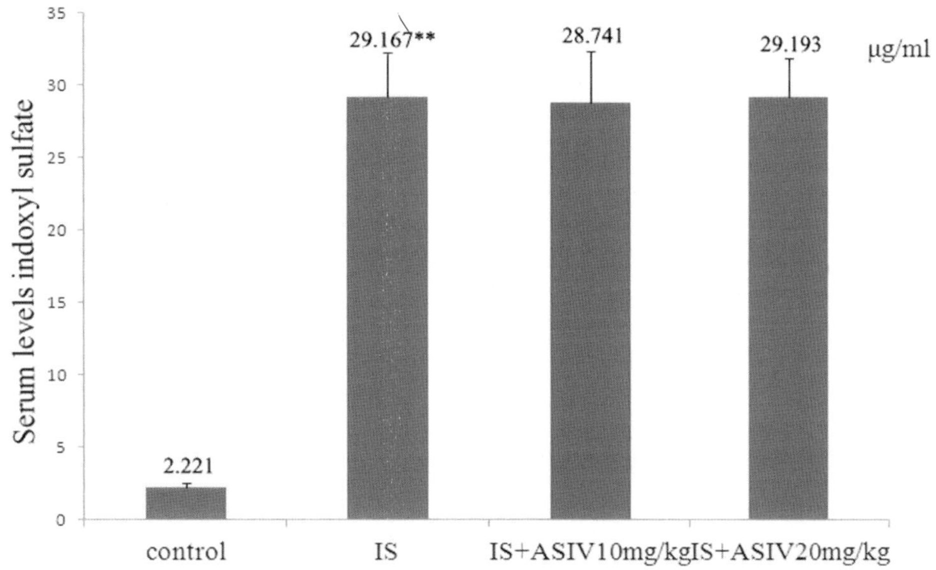

Fig. 1 Serum levels of indoxyl sulfate. The serum indoxyl sulfate concentration of mice was detected by high-performance liquid chromatography (HPLC) tandem mass spectrometry. Data were presented as means ± SE. **$P < 0.001$ vs. control group. IS: indoxyl sulfate. ASIV: astragaloside IV

critical biomarker of oxidative stress, measurement of the MDA level, and the SOD activity assay.

IS group mice showed increased 8-OHdG-positive areas in both glomeruli and tubules (Fig. 4). Increased 8-OHdG staining was associated with an increased MDA level and decreased SOD activity in the kidney (Fig. 7).

Astragaloside IV treatment can attenuate 8-OHdG expression in both glomeruli and tubules. In addition, 20 mg/kg of astragaloside IV decreased the MDA level and enhanced SOD activity (Figs. 4 and 7).

Cytochrome C is a marker linking mitochondrial oxidative stress and apoptosis [18]. In our study, the expression of cytochrome C was also increased in IS group mice. In addition, treatment with 20 mg/kg of astragaloside IV significantly attenuated cytochrome C expression (Fig. 5).

Discussion

In the present study, the protective effect of astragaloside IV against IS-induced tubulointerstitial injury was investigated. Our results showed that astragaloside IV

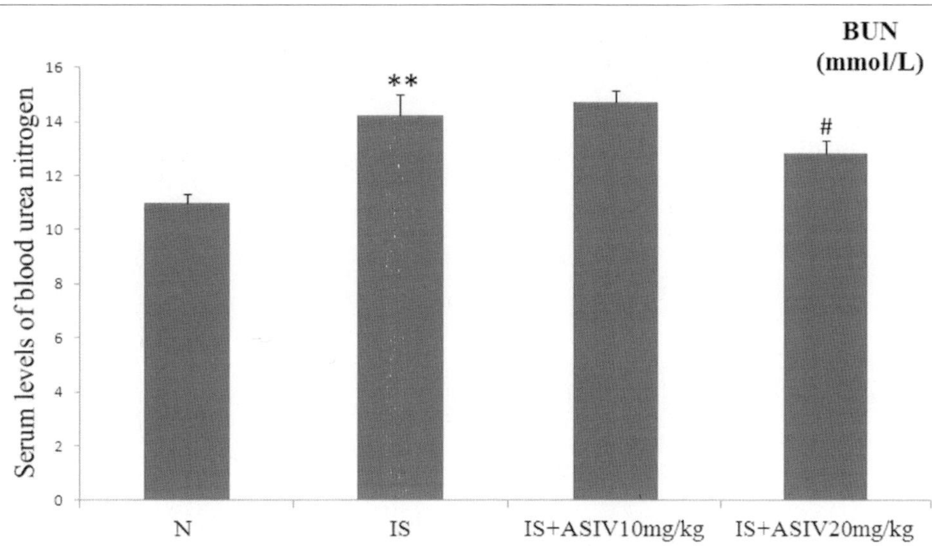

Fig. 2 Serum levels of blood urea nitrogen (BUN). IS: indoxyl sulfate. ASIV: astragaloside IV. **$P < 0.001$ vs. control group. $^{\#}P = 0.048$ vs. IS group

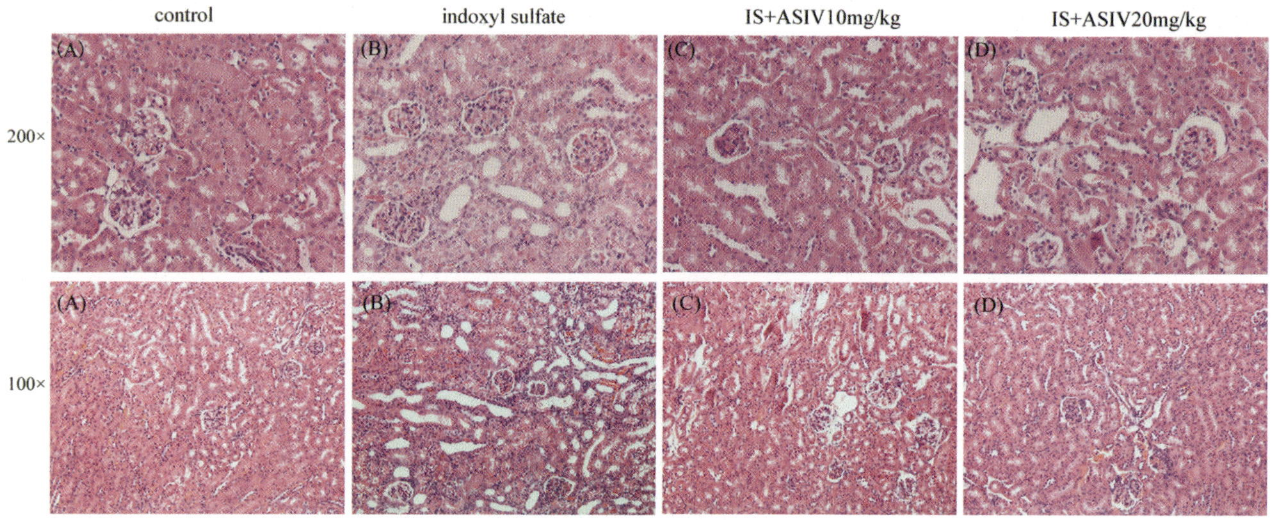

Fig. 3 Representative histopathology in IS intraperitoneal injection mice treated with or without astragaloside IV (HE staining). IS intraperitoneal injection mice showed partial tubular epithelial cell degeneration, loss of the brush border, enlargement of the tubular lumen and interstitial expansion. **a**: control group; **b**: IS group; **c**: IS plus 10 mg/kg astragaloside IV treatment group; **d**: IS plus 20 mg/kg astragaloside IV treatment group

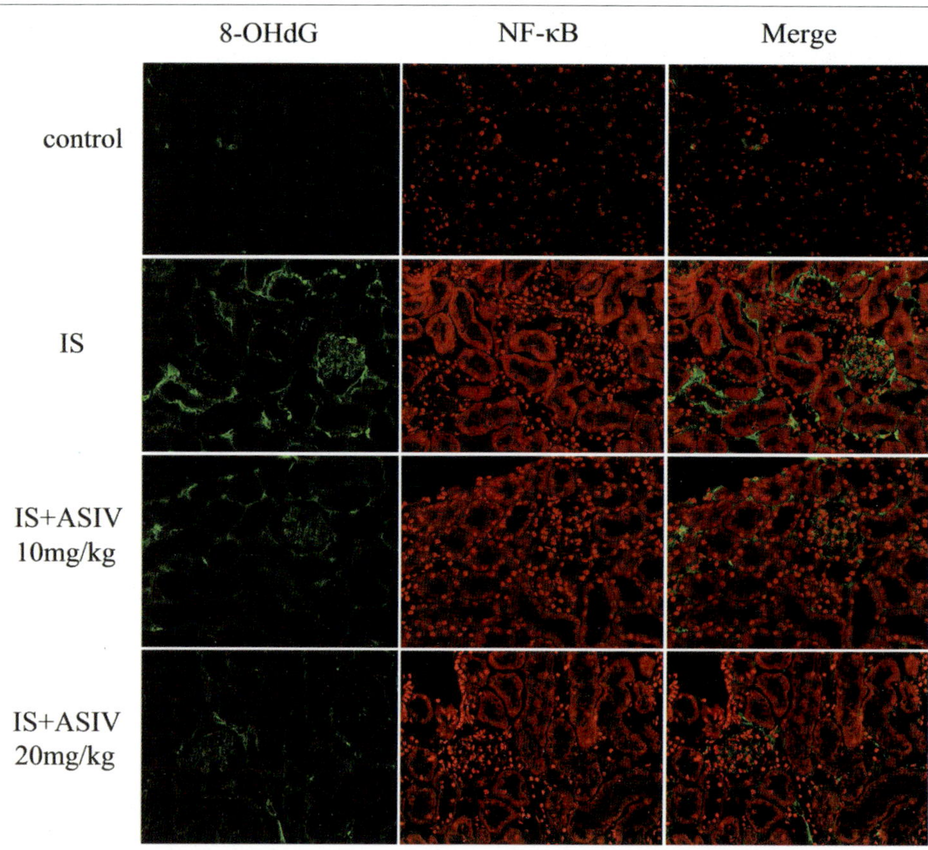

Fig. 4 Expression levels of 8-hydroxy-2′-deoxyguanosine (8-OHdG) and nuclear factor (NF)-κB in frozen sections of kidney. Localization of 8-OHdG and NF-κB in frozen sections was determined by immunofluorescence (IF) (× 200) with 8-OHdG antibody (green) and NF-κB ant (red)

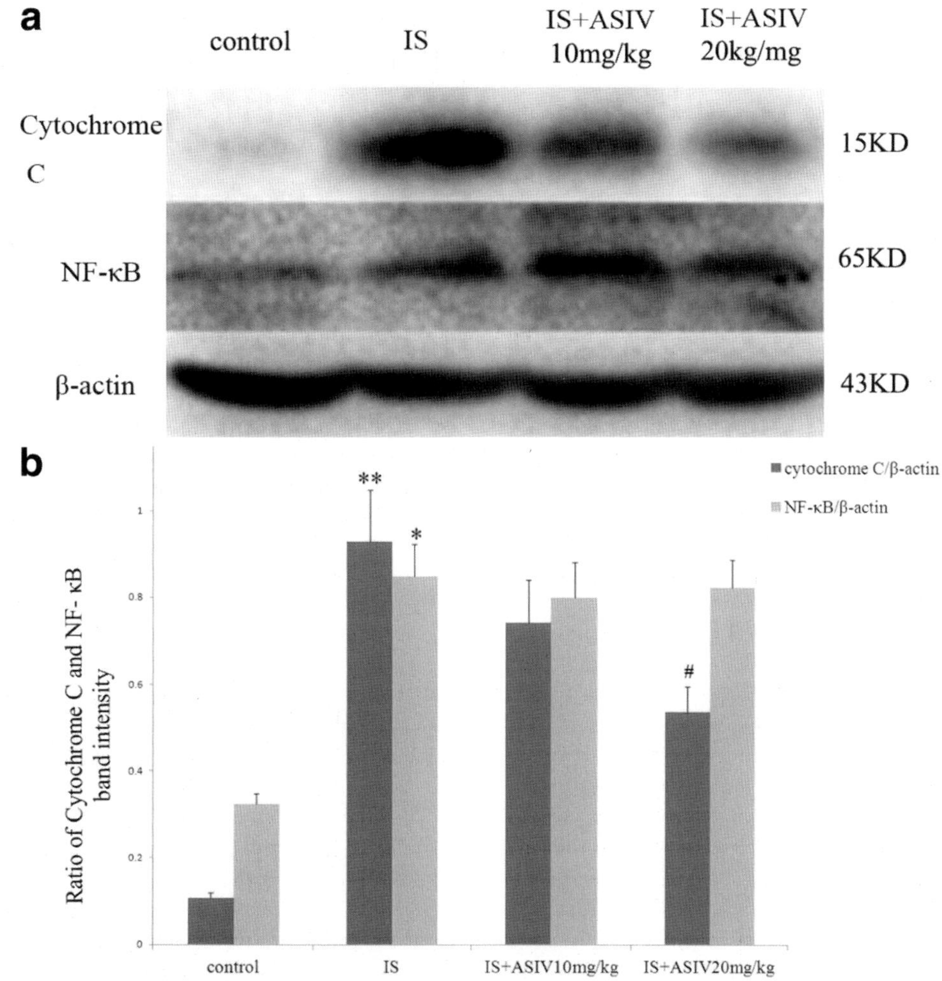

Fig. 5 Expression of NF-κB and cytochrome C in kidney tissue. Western blot analysis of the NF-κB and cytochrome C protein levels. **a** Representative western blot of NF-κB and cytochrome C in control and IS mice treated with or without astragaloside IV. **b** The data was shown as ratio of NF-κB or cytochrome C density to β-actin density. The values were expressed as mean ± SE and were compared by analysis of variance. *$P = 0.003$ vs. control group, **$P < 0.001$ vs. control group. $^{\#}P = 0.011$ vs. IS group

could reduce serum levels of BUN, inhibit renal tubulointerstitial injury and ameliorate renal oxidative stress in IS intraperitoneal injection mice. The evidence supported the effect of astragaloside IV on IS-induced tubulointerstitial injury.

CKD is recognized as a worldwide health problem, and the roles of individual cardiovascular risk factors in CKD are important [19].

Recent studies have found that the colon is an major organ in which uremic toxins are generated. In CKD patients, the imbalance mainly occurs in the colon, presenting as decreased levels of probiotics such as *Lactobacillus* and *Bifidobacteria* and increased pathogenic bacteria such as *Escherichia coli* and *Enterococcus* [20, 21]. Under these conditions, bacteria (mostly *E. coli*) produce numerous toxins from glycolysis of the retained proteins. For example, a fraction of tryptophan is metabolized into indole by *E. coli* in the colon, which is absorbed into blood through the intestinal wall and metabolized into IS in the liver [22].

Uremic toxins such as IS are protein-bound toxins with a molecular weight greater than 200 Da that are difficult to remove [23]. Dialysis is not powerful enough to remove protein-bound uremic toxins alone [7, 8]. Removing IS is very difficult in CKD patients; thus, finding effective measures to reduce IS-induced injury is of significant value.

Previous studies have demonstrated IS-induced tubulointerstitial injury in patients with CKD via the induction of oxidative stress and activation of the NF-κB pathway, producing various cytokines and inflammatory mediators and promoting kidney damage [9–11].

Astragaloside IV (3-O-β-D-xylopyranosyl-6-O-β-D--glucopyranosyl cycloastragenol) is a natural saponin

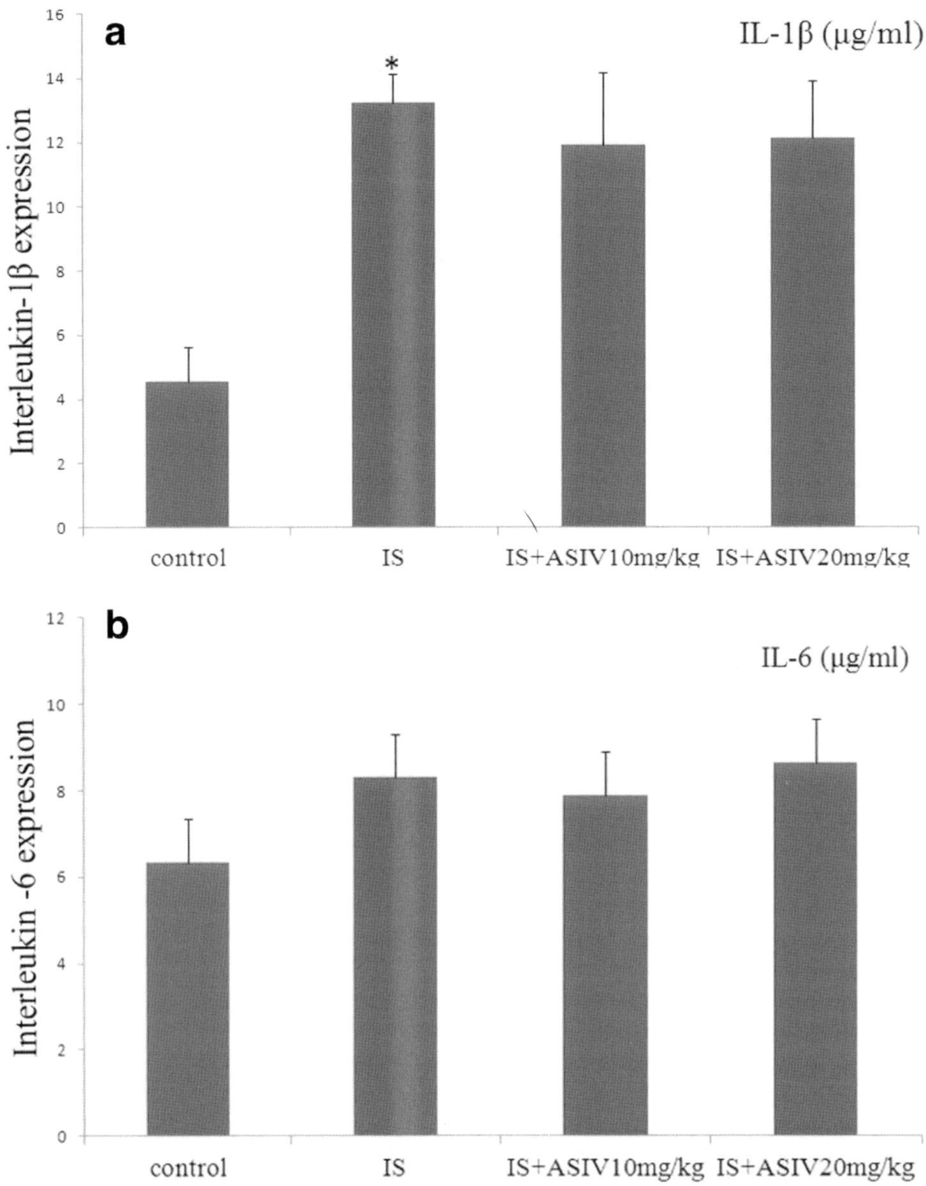

Fig. 6 Expression of IL-1β and IL-6 in kidney tissue. Expression of IL-1β and IL-6 protein in the kidney determined with Enzyme-linked immunosorbent assay (ELISA) in IS mice treated with or without astragaloside IV. **a** ELISA analysis of IL-1β in kidney tissues. **b** ELISA analysis of IL-6 in kidney tissues. *$P = 0.016$ vs. control group

purified from the roots of *Astragalus membranaceus* with antioxidant and anti-inflammatory effects [13, 14]. The anti-inflammatory effects of astragaloside IV have been demonstrated through the inhibition of NF-κB-mediated inflammatory gene expression [24]. Moreover, astragaloside IV exhibits antioxidant effects through the inhibition of reactive oxygen species (ROS) production, reduction of lipid peroxidation, and stimulation of antioxidant enzymes [25]. As mentioned previously, antioxidant treatment strategies are being developed to treat IS-induced tubulointerstitial injury. Oxidative stress is the most critical mechanism of kidney injury induced by indoxyl sulfate, and inflammatory injury is produced after the activation of inflammasome and NF-κB pathway [26]. We speculate that Astragaloside IV pre-intervents the most important oxidative stress step and has weaker pharmacological effects in inflammatory injury induced by indoxyl sulfate in this study.

These studies suggest that astragaloside IV may have a protective effect against IS-induced tubulointerstitial injury and its mechanisms of action may be associated with inhibiting oxidative stress Additional file 1.

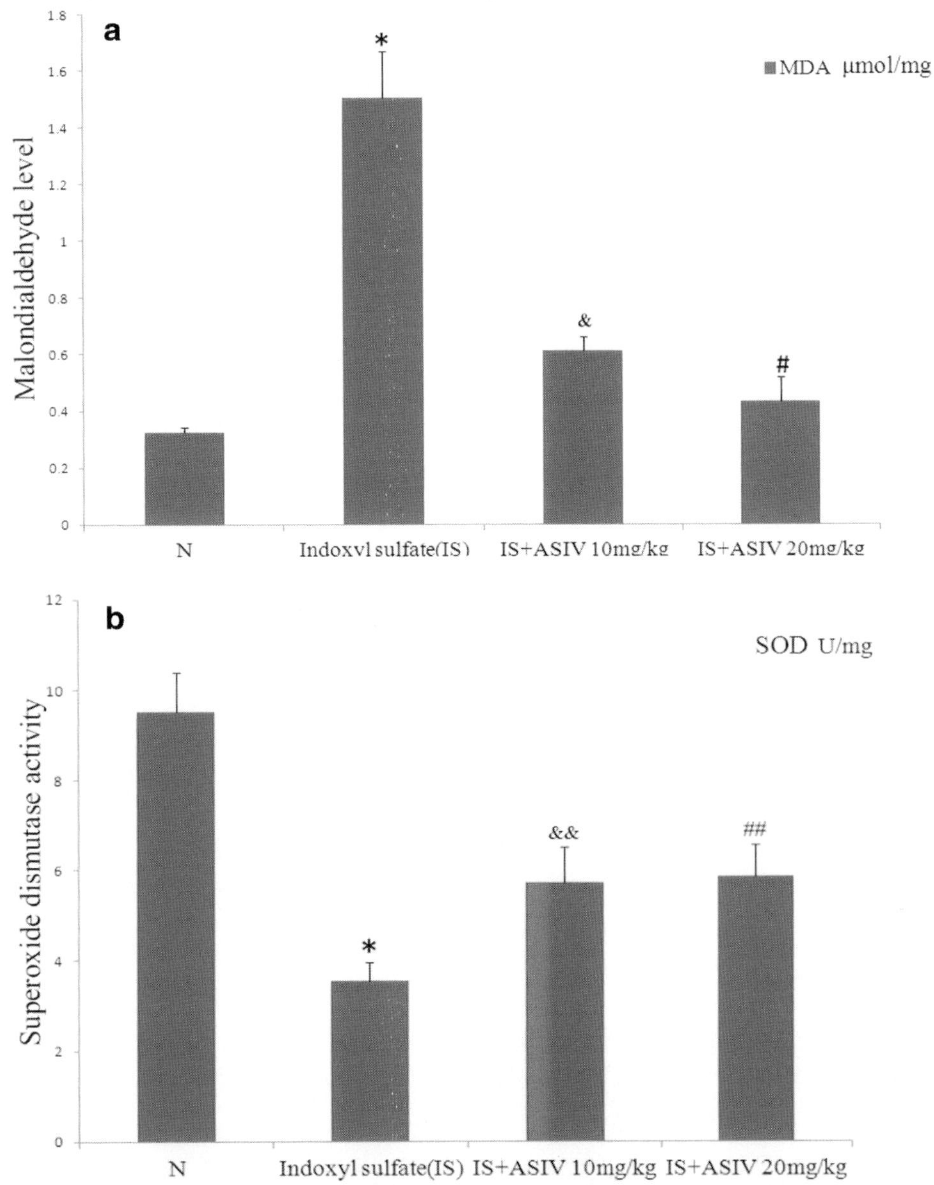

Fig. 7 Malondialdehyde (MDA) and superoxide dismutase (SOD) activity assays. Kidney oxidative stress was determined with MDA and SOD activity assays. **a** MDA levels of kidney tissues. **b** SOD activity of kidney tissues. IS group mice showed higher MDA and lower SOD values than control group mice. **P* < 0.001 vs. the control group. The MDA value was significantly lower, and SOD activity was significantly higher, after treatment with 20 mg/kg of astragaloside IV. $^{\#}P = 0.036$ vs IS group, $^{\&}P = 0.068$ vs IS group, $^{\&\&}P = 0.043$ vs IS group, $^{\#\#}P = 0.031$ vs IS group

Conclusions

Our study showed that astragaloside IV significantly prevented IS-induced tubulointerstitial injury. Astragaloside IV cannot suppress IS-induced elevation of NF-κB and IL-1β. Treatment with Astragaloside IV remarkably decreased the levels of MDA and 8-OHdG, and simultaneously increased the level of SOD. These results suggest that astragaloside IV could decrease IS-induced oxidative stress, which might constitute an important protective mechanism against tubulointerstitial injury induced by IS.

Abbreviations

As-IV: Astragaloside IV; BCA: Bicinchoninic acid; BUN: Blood urea nitrogen; CKD: Chronic kidney disease; DAPI: 4′,6-diamidino-2-phenylindole; ECL: Enhanced chemiluminescent; FITC: Fluoresceine isothiocyanate; HE: Hematoxylin eosin; HPLC: High Performance Liquid Chromatography; IL-1β: Interleukin-1β; IL-6: Interleukin-6; IS: Indoxyl sulfate; NF-κB: Nuclear factor-κB; RIPA: Radio-Immunoprecipitation Assay; SDS-PAGE: dodecyl sulfate, sodium salt-Polyacrylamide gel electrophoresis

Acknowledgements

The author thanks the nephrology Laboratory and Medical Foundation of the Guangdong Provincial Hospital of Chinese medicine for support.

Funding

This work was supported by grants from the Science and technology research project of Guangdong Provincial Hospital of Chinese medicine (NO.YN2016QJ16).

Authors' contributions

CJ, YL and ZL conceived the study. CJ, YL, LH and RT performed the experiments. CZ helped to design the study and participated in the statistical analysis; ZL made substantial contributions to conception and design of the study and agreed to be accountable for all aspects of the work. All authors read and approved the final manuscript. Each author contributed important intellectual content during manuscript drafting or revision.

Competing interests

The authors declare that they have no competing interests.

References

1. Vanholder R, Baurmeister U, Brunet P, Cohen G, Glorieux G, Jankowski J. European uremic toxin work group: a bench to bedside view of uremic toxins. J Am Soc Nephrol. 2008;19:863–70.
2. Watanabe H, Miyamoto Y, Otagiri M, Maruyama T. Update on the pharmacokinetics and redox properties of protein-bound uremic toxins. J Pharm Sci. 2011;100:3682–95.
3. Wu IW, Hsu KH, Lee CC, Sun CY, HsuHJ TCJ, et al. P-Cresyl sulphate and indoxyl sulphate predict progression of chronic kidney disease. Nephrol Dial Transplant. 2011;26:938–47.
4. Chiu CA, Lu LF, Yu TH, HungWC CFM, Tsai IT, et al. Increased levels of total P-Cresylsulphate and indoxyl sulphate are associated with coronary artery disease in patients with diabetic nephropathy. Rev Diabet Stud. 2010;7:275–84.
5. Vanholder R, Schepers E, Pletinck A, Neirynck N, Glorieux G. An update on protein-bound uremic retention solutes. J Ren Nutr. 2012;22:90–4.
6. Glorieux G, Vanholder R. New uremic toxins, which solutes should be removed? Contrib Nephrol. 2011;168:117–28.
7. Evenepoel P, Meijers BKI, Bammens BRM, Verbeke K. Uremic toxins originating from colonic microbial metabolism. Kidney Int. 2009;76:12–9.
8. Mei Jers BK, De Loor H, Bammens B, Verbeke K, Vanrenterghem Y, Evenepoel P. p-Cresyl sulfate and indoxyl sulfate in hemodialysis patients. Clin J Am Soc Nephrol. 2009;4:1932–8.
9. Palm F, Nangaku M, Fasching A, Tanaka T, Nordquist L, Hansell P, et al. Uremia induces abnormal oxygen consumption in tubules and aggravates chronic hypoxia of the kidney via oxidative stress. Am J Physiol Renal Physiol. 2010;299:380–6.
10. Tumur Z, Shimizu H, Enomoto A, Miyazaki H, Niwa T. Indoxyl sulfate Upregulates expression of ICAM-1 and MCP-1 by oxidative stress-induced NF-κB activation. Am J Nephrol. 2010;31:435–41.
11. Shimizu H, Bolati D, Adijiang A, Muteliefu G, Enomoto A, Nishijima F, et al. NF-κB plays an important role in indoxyl sulfate-induced cellular senescence, fibrotic gene expression, and inhibition of proliferation in proximal tubular cells. Am J Physiol Cell Physiol. 2011;301:C1201–12.
12. Zhong Y, Deng Y, Chen Y, Chuang PY, Cijiang HJ. Therapeutic use of traditional Chinese herbal medications for chronic kidney diseases. Kidney Int. 2013;84:1108–18.
13. Qiu LH, Xie XJ, Zhang BQ. Astragaloside IV improves homocysteine-induced acute phase endothelial dysfunction via antioxidation. Biol Pharm Bull. 2010; 33:641–6.
14. Xu C, Tang F, Lu M, Yang J, Han R, Mei M, et al. Pretreatment with Astragaloside IV protects human umbilical vein endothelial cells from hydrogen peroxide induced oxidative stress and cell dysfunction via inhibiting eNOS uncoupling and NADPH oxidase - ROS - NF-κB pathway. Can J Physiol Pharmacol. 2016;30:1–9.
15. Sun CY, Chang SC, Wu MS. Suppression of Klotho expression by protein-bound uremic toxins is associated with increased DNA methyltransferase expression and DNA hypermethylation. Kidney Int. 2012;81:640–50.
16. Lu Z, Zeng Y, Lu F, Liu X, Zou C. Rhubarb Enema attenuates renal Tubulointerstitial fibrosis in 5/6 Nephrectomized rats by alleviating Indoxyl sulfate overload. PLoS One. 2015;10:e0144726.
17. Torres-Gonzalez M, Gawlowski T, Kocalis H, Scott BT, Dillmann WH. Mitochondrial 8-oxoguanine glycosylase decreases mitochondrial fragmentation and improves mitochondrial function in H9C2 cells under oxidative stress conditions. Am J Physiol Cell Physiol. 2014;306:221–9.
18. Kroemer G, Galluzzi L, Brenner C. Mitochondrial membrane permeabilization in cell death. Physiol Rev. 2007;87:99–163.
19. Go AS, Chertow GM, Fan D, McCulloch CE, Hsu CY. Chronic kidney disease and the risks of death, cardiovascular events, and hospitalization. N Engl J Med. 2004;351:1296–305.
20. Tumur Z, Niwa T. Indoxyl sulfate inhibits nitric oxide production and cell viability by inducing oxidative stress in vascular endothelial cells. Am J Nephrol. 2009;29:551–7.
21. Friedman EA. Can the bowel substitute for the kidney in advanced renal failure? Curr Med Res Opin. 2009;25:1913–8.
22. Meijers BK, Evenepoel P. The gut-kidney axis: indoxyl sulfate, p-cresyl sulfate and CKD progression. Nephrol Dial Transplant. 2011;26:759–61.
23. Evenepoel P, Meijers BK, Bammens BR, Verbeke K. Uremic toxins originating from colonic microbial metabolism. Kidney Int Suppl. 2009;114:S12–9.
24. Gui D, Huang J, Guo Y, Chen J, Chen Y, Xiao W, Liu X, Wang N. Astragaloside IV ameliorates renal injury in streptozotocin-induced diabetic rats throughinhibiting NF-κB-mediated inflammatory genes expression. Cytokine. 2013;61:970–7.
25. Ko JK, Lam FY, Cheung AP. Amelioration of experimental colitis by Astragalus membranaceus through anti-oxidation and inhibition of adhesion molecule synthesis. World J Gastroenterol. 2005;11:5787–94.
26. Chao CT, Chiang CK. Uremic toxins, oxidative stress, and renal fibrosis: an interwined complex. J Ren Nutr. 2015;25:155–9.

21

Using superparamagnetic iron oxide nanoparticles to enhance bioavailability of quercetin in the intact rat brain

Rezvan Enteshari Najafabadi[1], Nasrin Kazemipour[1], Abolghasem Esmaeili[2*], Siamak Beheshti[2] and Saeed Nazifi[3]

Abstract

Background: Quercetin (QT) as a bioactive flavonoid has a potential therapeutic activity for numerous neuronal injuries and neurodegenerative diseases. However, the low absorption rate of QT, especially through the blood-brain barrier, restricts its bioactivity in the body. The current research took the advantage of superparamagnetic iron oxide nanoparticles (SPIONs) to enhance the bioavailability of quercetin.

Methods: Quercetin conjugated with SPIONs was prepared by means of nanoprecipitation method and was characterized by X-ray diffractometer, scanning electron microscope, and Fourier transformed infrared spectrometer analyses. Wistar male rats were orally fed by gavage with QT and QT-SPION at 50 and 100 mg/kg daily doses for 7 days. Using high-performance liquid chromatography (HPLC) method, biodistribution of QT was evaluated in plasma and brain tissue.

Results: The outcomes of this research revealed a higher concentration in the plasma and brain of the rats fed with QT-SPION in comparison to free QT.

Conclusion: The results of this study confirm that SPION as a targeted drug delivery system enhances the bioavailability of quercetin in the brain about ten folds higher than free quercetin and could be used for the treatment of neurodegenerative disorders.

Keywords: Oral drug delivery, HPLC, Nanoparticles, Quercetin, SPION

Background

Nanoparticles (NPs) are demarcated as particles up to 1000 nm especially less than 200 nm in diameter. NPs as capable vehicles have been applied to deliver some drugs and reagents into the numerous tissues and organs including the central nervous system (CNS). Superparamagnetic iron oxide nanoparticles (SPIONs, Fe_3O_4 NPs) is one of the most interesting NPs. These nanoparticles have magnetic properties and, therefore, using an external magnet, SPION could be used as a targeted drug delivery system. Also, SPIONs are considered for cell tracking, bioseparation, magnetic resonance imaging (MRI), and magnetic hyperthermia [1, 2].

Iron ions may release after utilization of iron oxide nanoparticles and accumulate in the body tissue [3]. This depends on the size, concentration, surface charge, and the type of coating and side-groups of iron oxide nanoparticle. Iron ions through oxidative stress may lead to macromolecule damage [3]. Accordingly, the application of iron oxide nanoparticles in the central nervous system needs serious care [4].

Several neurodegenerative disorders, such as Alzheimer's disease, affect the structure and function of the CNS. In spite of the gradually growing of drugs for the treatment of CNS disorders, there are few potential novel drugs available [5–7]. This is because of poor bioavailability and also the failure of many therapeutic molecules to cross the blood-brain barrier (BBB) [8]. Instead, any drug entry into the brain via parenteral administration is severely controlled by the BBB. A report suggests that over 98 % of small molecules and almost all the large molecules cannot penetrate to the brain [9].

* Correspondence: aesmaeili@sci.ui.ac.ir
[2]Cell, Molecular Biology and Biochemistry Division, Department of Biology, Faculty of Sciences, University of Isfahan, P.O. Box: 8174673441, Isfahan, Iran
Full list of author information is available at the end of the article

It has been attempted to increase the bioavailability of the therapeutic molecules. One approach is increasing the concentration of drug in blood circulation by nanoparticles. Another approach is increasing the permeability of the BBB. Strategies used to increase BBB permeability are categorized as invasive and non-invasive. The first strategy includes the momentary enhancement of the BBB permeability [10], agent intracerebral grafting [11], or direct infusion of the drug via intraventricular or intracerebral routes [12]. The invasive methods are expensive and are associated with problems, such as brain infections or edema [13]. The non-invasive strategies comprise an alteration of the drug molecules by means of chemical [14] or biochemical methods [15], accompanied by means of the olfactory route [16]. After modification, they may have certain disadvantages such as losing drug activity. As mentioned above the utilization of nanoparticles especially SPIONs could overcome these limitations.

Quercetin (3,3′,4′,5,7-pentahydroxyflavone, (QT)) is an active biological flavonoid found in large quantities in edible fruits, vegetables and medicinal plants such as onions, cabbage, and apples [17–19]. Quercetin has antiinflammatory [20], antioxidant [21], anti-cancer [22], antiviral [23], and anti-ischemic effects [24, 25]. Also, quercetin may alter glucose homeostasis in the brain [26]. Neuronal protection of QT has been reported in both in vitro and in vivo investigations [27–31]. Therefore, QT has a potential therapeutic for various neuronal injuries and neurodegenerative diseases [19]. However, the solubility of QT in water is low and it has a short biological half-life. Also, it has poor oral and CNS bioavailability. Accordingly, these limitations may overcome by means of the SPIONs [32–34]. Consequently, Kumar et al. and Akal et al. [35, 36] conjugated quercetin with SPIONs. Both studies used an in vitro method to evaluate the effect of quercetin conjugated with SPIONs on cells. None of them did investigate the bioavailability of quercetin-SPIONs in vivo.

Therefore, in the current study, the quercetin conjugated dextran coated Fe_3O_4 nanoparticles (QT- Fe_3O_4 NPs) were prepared by chemical precipitation method and the quercetin bioavailability enhancement in an experimental rat model was investigated.

In this requirement, Wistar rats were used because they are of the same purebred species. In addition, rats are used as models in medical testing due to their genetic, biological and behaviour characteristics closely resemble those of humans, and many symptoms of human conditions can be replicated in rats.

Methods

No additional purification was performed on reagents used in this study. The chemicals were bought from Fluka, Merck, and Sigma–Aldrich chemical companies.

Synthesis of quercetin conjugated iron oxide nanoparticles (QT-SPION).

Quercetin conjugated Fe_3O_4 nanoparticles were prepared as Kumar et al. described in 2014 with some modifications [35]. First, chemical coprecipitation method was used to synthesize dextran coated Fe_3O_4 nanoparticles. Briefly, 1.135 g $FeCl_3$ anhydrous, 0.695 g $FeCl_2$ and 0.45 g dextran were mixed and dissolved in 200 ml deionized (DI) water. The chemical reaction is as follow: Fe (II) + 2Fe (III) + 8OH $\rightarrow$ Fe3O4 + 4H2O. The mixture was then placed into a three-neck flask equipped with a mechanical stirrer. After complete mixing, ammonia solution was dropped into the mixture under argon protection with vigorous stirring. This operation was continued until the solution reached a pH of 9. Then the solution was kept at 90 °C for 2 h with constant moving. A strong magnet was applied to collect the subsequent precipitate. Then using DI water and ethanol the supernatant was washed several times. To dry out the supernatant, it was placed into an oven at 70 °C overnight.

QT-SPION nanoparticles were prepared by addition of QT to dextran-coated Fe_3O_4 nanoparticles. For this purpose, the pre-determined amount of 1-ethyl-3[3-dimethylaminopropyl] carbodiimide hydrochloride (EDC) and N-hydroxysuccinimide (NHS) was added to the dextran-coated Fe_3O_4 nanoparticles under ultrasonication according to related protocols. Then, under ultrasonication, a required amount of quercetin in dimethyl sulfoxide (DMSO) solution was added to the mixture and was stirred for 24 h at room temperature. To eliminate any free drug or any other biological scums, the precipitate was washed with DMSO and acetone. Then, the precipitate was collected using a strong external magnet and was dried out by means of a freeze drier.

Characterization techniques

Fourier transformed infrared (FTIR) spectroscopy was recorded on a Jasco 6300 spectrophotometer in the range of 400 and 4000 cm^{-1} by KBr pellet method. X-ray diffractometer (XRD) patterns of magnetite nanoparticles were carried out in a PANalytical X'PERT PRO powder X-ray diffractometer with Cu $K\alpha_1$ ($k =$ 1.54056 Å) radiation at room temperature. Hitachi S–4700 field emission–scanning electron microscope (FE–SEM), equipped with an energy-dispersive X-ray analysis (EDX) detector was used to obtain the morphological features of nanoparticles.

Drug release study and loading

To measure the in vitro release rate of QT from QT-SPIONs in phosphate buffer saline (PBS) medium a dialysis bag method was used. Briefly, by means of cellulose dialysis tube bags, 1 mg of QT (QT-SPIONs) was suspended in 1.5 mL of PBS (pH 7.4). The dialysis with a magnetic stirrer was performed at 37 °C. Two ml of the sample was picked up at regular time intervals for 20 h. To measure the amount of QT in the medium spectrophotometer at 374 nm wavelength was used.

Cumulative percentage quercetin release from QT-SPIONs, into PBS with pH values of 7.4 was calculated using the below equation,

$$\text{Cumulative percentage drug release } (\%) = \text{Volume of sample withdrawn (ml)/bath volume (v)} \times \text{P (t} - 1) + \text{Pt}$$

Where Pt is % release at time t and P (t − 1) is % release prior to 't'. The results were shown as mean ± SEM of triplicate experiments.

To measure quercetin loading in quercetin conjugate with iron oxide nanoparticles, the amount of quercetin was measured using a spectrophotometer at 260 nm and then, according to the amount of quercetin consumed, loading was calculated.

Animals

Adult male Wistar rats ($n = 42$), weighing between 180 and 200 g, were bought from Royan Institute (Isfahan, Iran). All experiments were carried out in accord with the guide for the care and use of laboratory animals (USA National Institute of Health publication No. 80–23, revised 1996). Also, all procedures were approved by the graduate studies committees of the University of Isfahan and Shiraz University. Rats were randomly divided into groups of 6 rats and were housed 3/cage in a room with a temperature of 25 °C ± 2 °C and a 12 h light/dark cycle (lights on at 07:00 a.m.). All animals had free access to tap water and diet for one week before the experiment. Not any problem was detected during the experimental procedures. Sample sizes were based on Mead's resource equation. Based on this formula the optimum size of an experiment usually has between 10 and 20 error degrees of freedom (E). In calculating the number of rats needed, the probable casualties were also considered.

Dosing and sampling

All of the treatments (QT, SPION, and QT-SPION) were dissolved in deionized water (DI) and gavaged (08:00–10:00 am) in separate groups of rats. Rats in treatment groups received 50 or 100 mg/kg of body weight QT, SPION, or QT-SPION.

Short-term feeding: Quercetin conjugated Fe_3O_4 nanoparticles (QT-SPIONs) were freshly prepared for ingesting administration via gavage. Group one was treated with a dose of free QT solution (100 mg/kg). Group two was administered with a dose of 100 mg/kg of QT-SPIONs. Then 3, 6, 9, 12, and 24 h later, blood samples (almost 1 ml) were collected from the tail vein and poured into centrifuge tubes containing heparin. Then, plasma was obtained via centrifugation at 4 °C (3000×g, 10 min) and kept at − 70 °C till use.

Long-term feeding: Rats in this test were divided into five groups. Group one and two were administered with 50 mg/kg and 100 mg/kg free QT solution, respectively. Group three received 50 mg/kg QT-SPIONs and group four treated with 100 mg/kg QT-SPIONs. All constructions were administered orally at a daily dose for a period of 7 days. Group five served as control and received neither QT nor QT-SPIONs. Twenty-four hours after of the last feeding each rat was anesthetized by intraperitoneal injection of sodium pentobarbital. Then the blood (1 ml for each rat) was taken from the heart and was put into tubes containing heparin. Plasma was collected as described above and stored at − 70 °C until use. To determine the distribution of the quercetin in the brain, rats were sacrificed after administration of a mixture of ketamine (100 mg/kg, i.p) and xylazine (10 mg/kg, i.p) anaesthesia. Samples of the brains were rapidly removed and kept at − 70 °C before the examination.

Preparation of plasma and brain samples

A 100 μl of plasma was supplemented with one ml of methanol, and the combination was vortexed for five minutes and then centrifuged (10,000 rpm, Eppendorf, 5417R, USA) for 10 min at 4 °C. The collected clear supernatant was filtered using 0.20 μm syringe filters. To measure QT in plasma, 20 μl of the sample was injected into the HPLC system. Approximately 100 mg of brain tissue was homogenized in 500 μl in 1× PBS (pH 7.4). Then, the homogenates were centrifuged at 10,000 rpm for 10 min at 4 °C. Then, 300 μl of methanol with 200 μl aliquots of the clear tissue homogenates were added and the scattering was vortexed for two minutes. Then the samples were centrifuged at 10,000 rpm for 10 min at 4 °C. The supernatant was filtered using 0.20 μm syringe filters and 20 μl of the brain sample was injected into the HPLC system to measure QT.

HPLC analysis of quercetin

HPLC was performed as previously described [19]. Briefly, quercetin was evaluated by HPLC equipped with a reverse-phase C18 column (150 mm × 4.6 mm, pore size 5 μm, ProntoSIL), a UV detector and a vacuum degasser run by Smartline-2600 software. Methanol and water (70:30 *v*/*v*) (pH adjusted to 3.64 with glacial acetic acid) was used as the mobile phase. To separate QT, an isocratic condition with column temperature of 25 °C, a constant flow rate of 1.0 ml/min, 20 μl injection volume and a detection wavelength of 374 nm, was performed. To evaluate the linear relationship between the peak areas and the concentrations of quercetin the calibration curves were generated. The coefficient of determination (r^2), slope, and intercept were calculated as regression parameters by weighted linear regression.

Iron determination

Plasma and brain samples were prepared as described above. The iron concentrations of plasma (at the time point of 3, 6, 9, 12, and 24) and brain tissue (24 h after oral administration of QT-SPIONs) were measured by ICP-OES (inductively coupled plasma-optical emission spectroscopy). To assay iron concentration, one gram of the sample was mixed with 1 ml sulphuric acid (98%) in a tube and heated at 100 °C for 5 min. Every ten minutes 3 ml of perchloric acid was added to the tube and heated for 40 min. After digestion, the solution was diluted to with 10 ml of distilled water for ICP-OES tests.

Liver histology

At the end of the study to investigate histopathologic alterations, animals were killed by ketamine anesthesia. Liver samples of control rats and animals treated with 100 mg/kg of free QT, SPION and QT-SPION were removed and fixed instantaneously in 10% formalin in order to routine paraffin embedding. Paraffin blocks with 3 mm thickness were prepared and stained with haematoxylin–eosin (H–E) method. Finally, sections were examined under Leitz microscope at 400_ magnification.

Statistical analysis

The results were reported as mean ± SEM (standard error mean) for the six independent experiments. One-way ANOVA followed by a multiple comparisons Tukey's test or Student's t-test was used to estimate the difference as multiple comparison tests. For these procedures, *GraphPad Prism* software version 6 was used. For all analyses, P values of less than of 0.05 were considered statistically significant.

Results

Physicochemical characterization of QT-SPIONs

The FTIR spectrum of dextran-coated Fe_3O_4 nanoparticles, quercetin, and quercetin conjugated magnetite nanoparticles (QT-SPIONs) are shown in Fig. 1A (a–c). The spectrum of dextran-coated Fe_3O_4 nanoparticle (Fig. 1A (a)) displayed a durable absorption band at 573 cm^{-1} that was allocated to the Fe–O vibration frequency of magnetite spinel structure and the broad peaks at 3377 cm^{-1} represent the OH stretching vibration of the hydroxyl groups. FTIR of quercetin (Fig. 1A (b)) showed characteristic bands corresponding to OH groups at 3388 cm^{-1}, to C=O absorption at 1656 cm^{-1} and a region corresponding to C-O stretching at 1150–1070 cm^{-1}. Also, the peak 931 cm^{-1} represents the C-H bending vibration of aromatic groups. The spectrum of the synthesized QT-SPIONs (Fig. 1A (c)) showed broad absorption bands at 3386 cm^{-1}, which were assigned to the stretching vibrations of hydroxyl groups and other characteristic bands that confirmed the successful conjugation of quercetin on the Fe_3O_4 nanoparticles.

The crystalline structure and phase analysis of magnetite nanoparticles were examined by XRD analysis. The pattern of powder XRD for the synthesized magnetic nanoparticles was close to that of crystalline magnetite Fe_3O_4 (Fig. 1B). In addition, the characteristic peaks of Fe_3O_4 NPs at 30.1°, 35.4°, 43.9°, 53.4°, 57.0° and 62.6° were detected for dextran coated and quercetin conjugated Fe_3O_4 NPs approving the existence of the crystalline structure of the magnetite.

The surface morphology and size of the quercetin conjugated Fe_3O_4 nanoparticles obtained were directly visualized by FE-SEM (Fig. 2a). As can be seen, the nanoparticles are spherical and have diameters in the

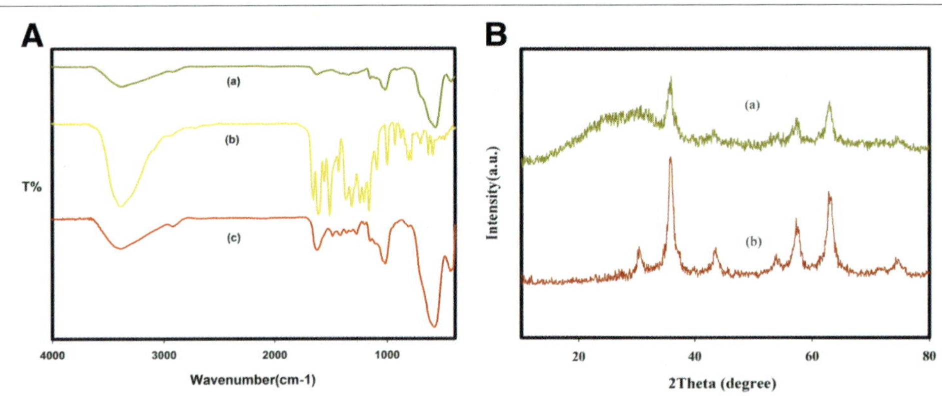

Fig. 1 FTIR and XRD profiles. **a** Comparison of FTIR spectra of dextran coated iron oxide nanoparticle, pure quercetin and quercetin conjugated Fe_3O_4 nanoparticles. The samples fro top to bottom are (a) dextran coated SPIONs and (b) pure quercetin and (c) quercetin conjugated Fe_3O_4 nanoparticles. **b** XRD pattern for the (a) dextran coated and (b) quercetin conjugated Fe_3O_4 nanoparticles

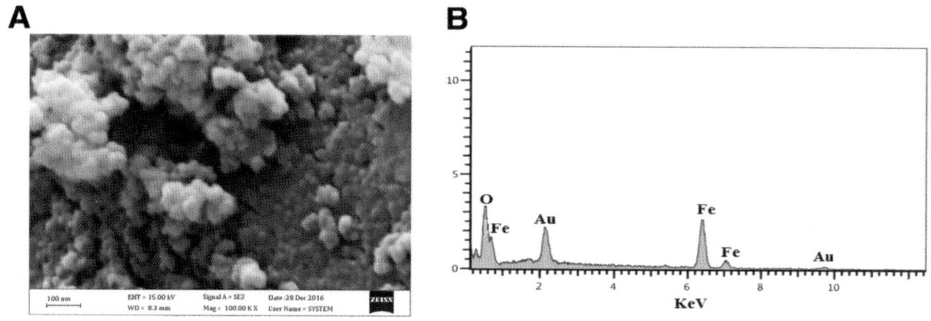

Fig. 2 a SEM image of quercetin conjugated Fe_3O_4 nanoparticles. **b** SEM-EDX spectrum of quercetin conjugated Fe_3O_4 nanoparticles

range of 30 to 50 nm. The presence of the iron and oxygen was also confirmed by the EDX detector coupled to the SEM (Fig. 2b).

The release rate of quercetin from either solution containing free quercetin or solution inclosing QT-SPION was primarily rapid and then it was slower as time continued. In the beginning, 71.8 ± 2.5% and 23.5 ± 1.8% of the drug was released in 4 h from free quercetin and QT-SPION respectively. This was progressively amplified and turn out to be a maximum value of 61.6 ± 0.8% in 8 h for quercetin released from QT-SPION. The release rate of QT from NPs was slower and more constant at the rate of around 60% over the period of 20 h (Fig. 3). These results showed that conjugation of quercetin with SPION decreased the release of QT from the NPs compared to that free from of QT.

To calculate quercetin loading, the difference in quercetin concentration used in the preparation of quercetin conjugate and the concentration of quercetin in the subfiltration solution was calculated and the quercetin concentration was used. The percentage of quercetin loading was 42%.

Detection of quercetin in plasma

There are numerous analytical techniques suitable for bioavailability study and measuring of QT in organic fluids. HPLC–UV, HPLC-FD (fluorometric detection), HPLC–ED (electrochemical detection) and GC–MS method have been used so far [37–40]. In this study, we used HPLC–UV which is adequate specificity and simplicity for quantifying of QT in plasma and brain tissue. The standard curve for quercetin was linear in the range of 0.05–0.6 μg/ml, which could be described by the regression equation: $Y = 95215X + 118$ ($r = 0.9976$) for quercetin where Y was the peak area of the analyte, and X was the concentration in μg/ml (Fig. 4). Figure 4

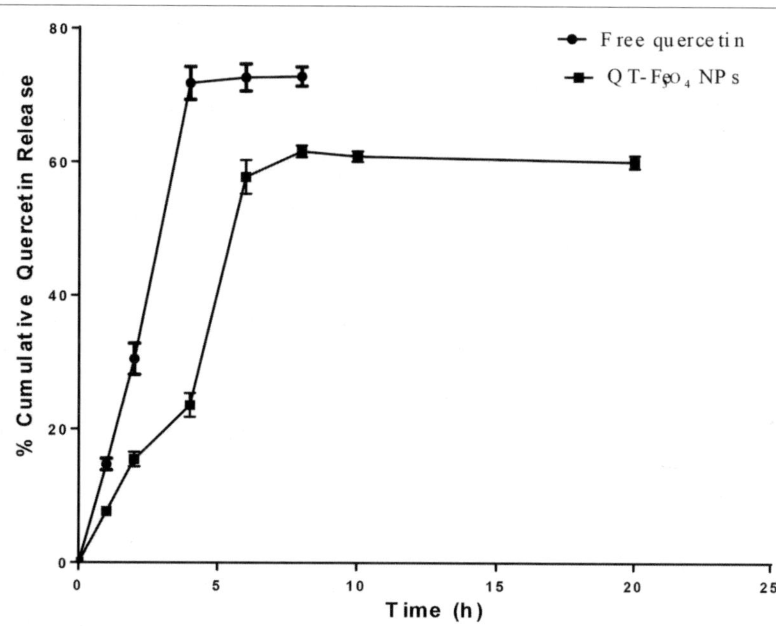

Fig. 3 In vitro cumulative percent drug release versus time profile of quercetin. Plot showing percent cumulative release of QT from QT-Fe_3O_4 NPs in comparison with the free QT in pH 7.4 phosphate-buffered saline (PBS). Results are presented as mean ± SEM ($n = 3$). h, hours

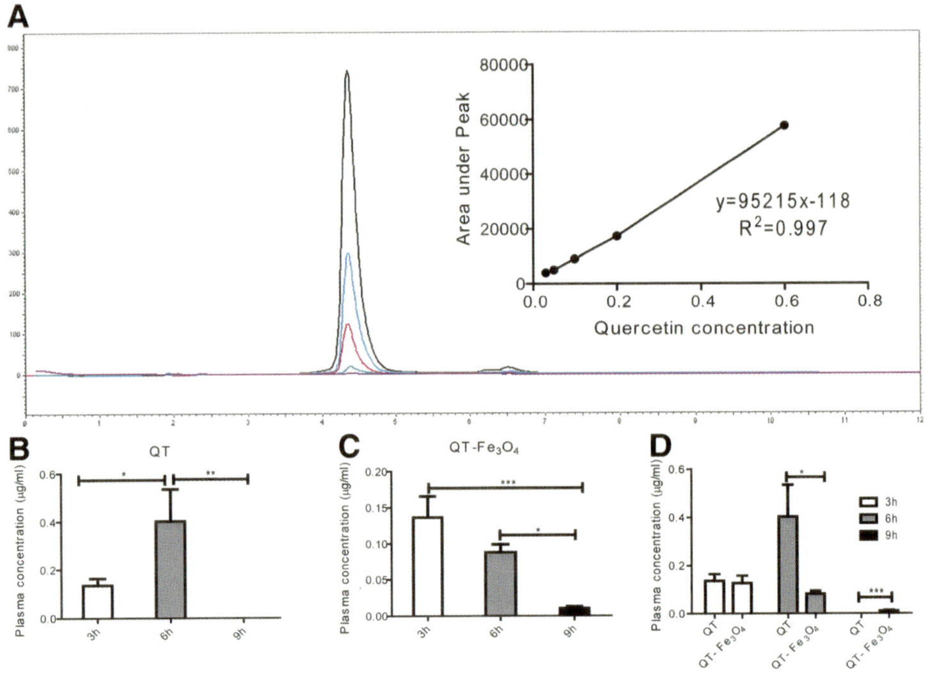

Fig. 4 HPLC analyses for the identification of quercetin in rat plasma after oral administration of quercetin and quercetin conjugated Fe3O4 nanoparticles in Wistar rats. **a** Quercetin standards. Different serial dilutions are shown: 0.6 µg/ml (black), 0.2 µg/ml (blue), 0.1 µg/ml (red), and 0.05 µg/ml (green). The inset shows the calibration curve (Peak area vs. Concentration). **b** free QT, and **c** QT-SPIONs, and **d** comparison of the concentration of free QT with QT-SPIONs. All values reported are mean ± SEM (*n* = 6). [* for p < 0.05, ** for p < 0.01 and *** for p < 0.001]. QT, quercetin; h, hours

shows the concentration-time profiles of an individual dosage of 100 mg/kg of free QT and QT-SPIONs in the plasma. The maximum plasma concentration of free QT solution (100 mg/kg) within 6 h after oral administration was 0.402 ± 0.133 µg/ml (Fig. 4b). This for 100 mg/kg in 3 h after oral administration of QT-SPIONs was 0.137 ± 0.029 µg/ml (Fig. 4c). The maximum plasma concentration of free QT was significantly higher ($p < 0.05$) in comparison to QT-SPIONs. While free QT disappears from plasma 6 h after administration, QT-SPIONs remains in plasma for 9 h (Fig. 4d). No quercetin was detected in control samples. Quercetin conjugated with SPIONs exhibited prolonged blood circulation compared to free ones.

Detection of quercetin in brain

HPLC was used to detect quercetin concentration in brain tissues. Figure 5 shows the quercetin concentration in brain tissue after treatment of animals with free QT, and QT-SPIONs over a time period of 7 days. The concentrations of QT in the brain for 50 mg/kg, and 100 mg/kg were 0.019 ± 0.003 and 0.053 ± 0.018 µg/ml, respectively. Nevertheless, the concentration of quercetin in the brain of rats treated with 50 mg/kg and 100 mg/kg of QT- Fe_3O_4 nanoparticles was 0.13 ± 0.04 and 0.52 ± 0.08 respectively. Brains of the rats were fed with QT-SPIONs shows higher concentrations of QT when compared with those that were fed with free QT.

Detection of iron in plasma and brain

The iron accumulations in the plasma at 0, 3, 6, 9, and 24 h after oral treatment of 100 mg/kg of QT-SPIONs were quantified by ICP-OES. For the brain tissue, this

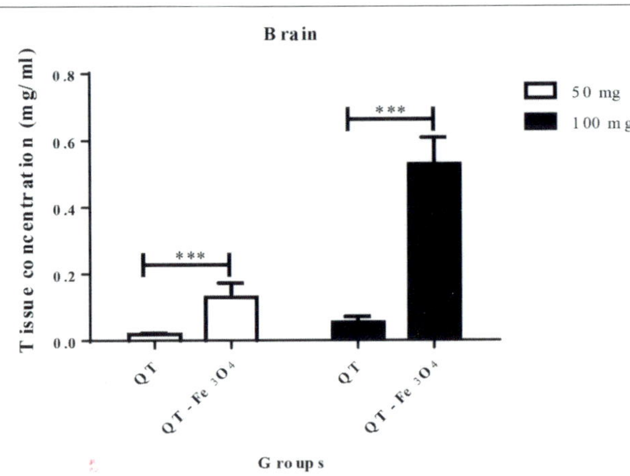

Fig. 5 HPLC analyses for the biodistribution of quercetin in rat brain after oral administration of quercetin and quercetin conjugated Fe_3O_4 nanoparticles. QT, quercetin. All values reported are mean ± SEM (n = 6). [* for *p* < 0.05, ** for *p* < 0.01 and *** for *p* < 0.001]. QT, quercetin

was down after 24 h of administration of QT-SPION. In control rats, the iron content of the plasma was 52.4 ± 1.8 μg/dL. Plasma iron concentrations in rats after 3, 6, 9, and 24 h were 83.3 ± 2.02, 96.6 ± 4.9, 63.3 ± 2.9, and 54.3 ± 1.7 μg/dL respectively. A time course showed that total serum iron levels were low at hour 3, increased significantly at hour 6, and decreased at hour 9 (Fig. 6a). Brain iron contents were 5.3 ± 0.3 μg/g tissue in control rats and 6.2 ± 0.1 μg/g tissue in rats 24 h after superparamagnetic iron oxide nanoparticles administration, which is less than the iron content in the plasma (Fig. 6b). There is no significant difference in brain iron contents in control and treated rats.

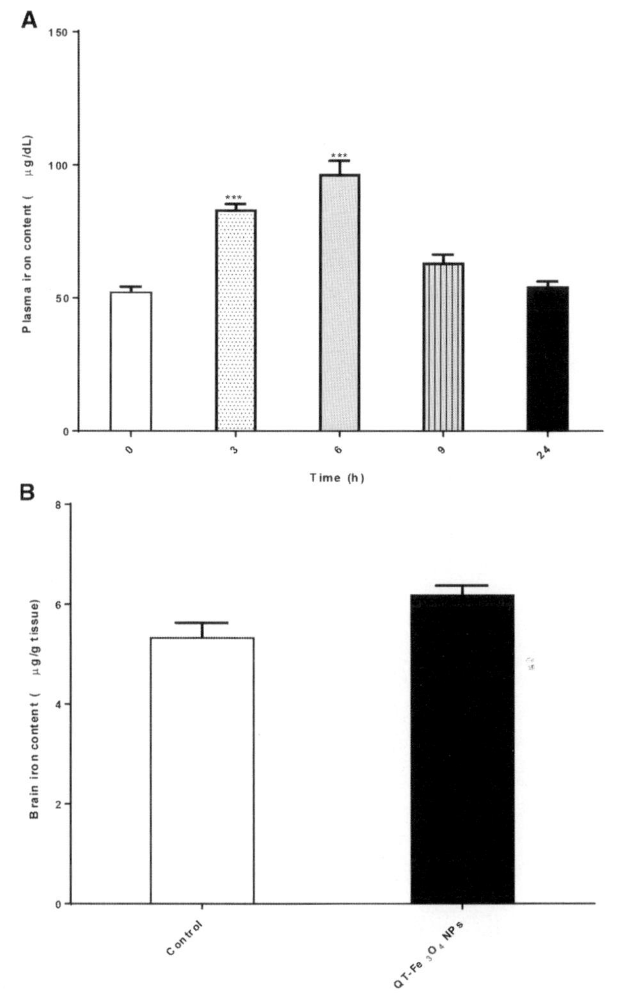

Fig. 6 Total iron concentration in plasma and brain. **a** analyses for the identification of total iron in rat plasma after oral administration of quercetin conjugated Fe_3O_4 nanoparticles (100 mg/kg) in Wistar rats. **b** analyses for the determination of iron content in rat brain after oral administration of quercetin conjugated Fe_3O_4 nanoparticles (100 mg/kg.) All values reported are mean ± SEM (n = 3). QT, quercetin; h, hours. [*** for $p < 0.001$]. QT, quercetin

Histopathologic alterations

Histology of liver tissues is shown in Fig. 7. Hepatic sections of control rats showed a regular lobular pattern with a central vein, slit-like sinusoids, and prominent nuclei. No histological alterations were detected in the liver tissue of treated rats.

Discussion

Quercetin has high antioxidant potential in comparison with a number of flavonoids and could be used to treat or prevent the development and progression of neurodegenerative diseases [28]. Quercetin in combination with ascorbic acid decreases glutathione (GSH) levels in the neural cells. These results were interpreted as a confirmation of the effect of quercetin on oxidative stress [41]. Oyama and colleagues as the first group of investigators who explored the effect of quercetin contained *Ginkgo biloba* extract on the neurons suffered from oxidative stress caused by hydrogen peroxide found that quercetin reduces the oxidative metabolism in a dose dependent way [42]. Naidu et al., studied the effect of quercetin on the lipid peroxidation and found that Superoxide Dismutase (SOD), and catalase enzymes levels decreased after the administration of quercetin. Hence they suggested that probable action mechanism of quercetin in order to inhibit activities of oxidases, and Nitric Oxide Synthase (NOS) enzymes include scavenging of free radicals and chelating the metal ions such as iron and copper [43]. Studying the effect of quercetin and its glycoside metabolite on the apoptosis rate of glioma cell line revealed that quercetin treatment inhibits cell death induced by oxidative stress [44]. Since the antioxidant effect of quercetin was verified in a number of studies, a new step initiated through studying the effect of this compound on the neurodegenerative diseases. Investigation of the neuroprotective effect of quercetin on the cognitive impairment induced by D-galactose was also in consistent with the previous studies. Therefore, the activity of SOD increased and the concentration of Ca^{2+} was controlled in the brain tissue that all indicate a more complexed action mechanism for quercetin [45]. The main limitation of quercetin is low solubility and bioavailability.

The current study describes a simple precipitation method to prepare the quercetin conjugated with superparamagnetic nanoparticles and investigates the bioavailability of quercetin using this approach in the intact rat brain. Recent studies designated successful loading of quercetin onto magnetic nanoparticles [35, 36, 46]. The novel QT-Fe_3O_4 nanoparticles described in this work have the desired characteristics to be used as a carrier system. The results of the physicochemical characterization of QT-SPIONs are in line with a previous report by Kumar et al. [35]. Results of this study

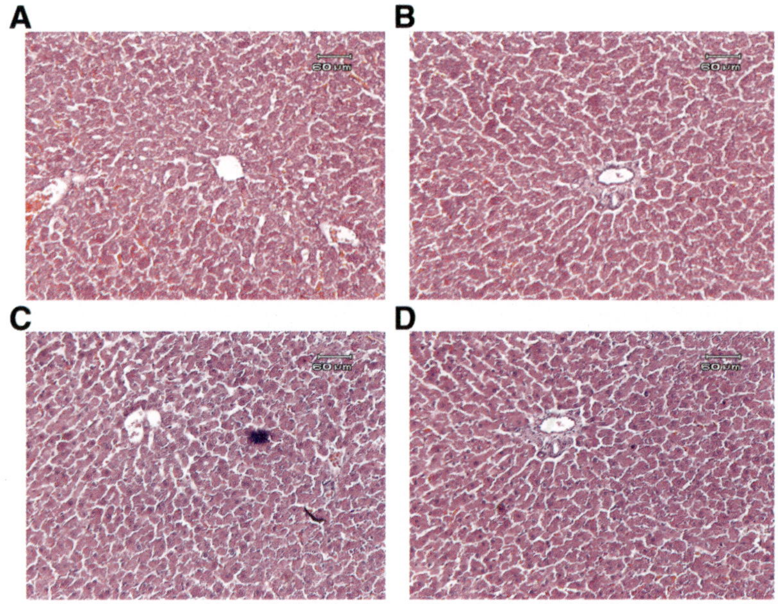

Fig. 7 Liver histology of the control and experimental rats. The figure shows the effect of Fe_3O_4NP, QT, QT-SPIONs (at a dose of 100 mg/kg, and 7 days) on histology of liver of rats. **a** control; **b** free quercetin (QT); **c** SPIONs; **d** QT-SPIONs. The histology shows the normal liver architecture for all treatments (H & E staining)

showed that the quercetin was effectively conjugated to the dextran coated superparamagnetic iron oxide nanoparticles (Fig. 1). In vivo study showed that Fe_3O_4 nanoparticles are relatively safe because they leave the body quickly and therefore, in vital organs no accumulation of nanoparticles occur [1, 47]. In our study, no mortalities were detected in rats fed with Fe_3O_4 NPs and QT-SPIONs. In a study [48], the toxicity of Fe_3O_4 ferrofluid (6 mg/rat) in rats were evaluated. No changes in mortality were detected in this study. Histopathological results showed at least during the period the rats were treated with NPs, QT-SPIONs and free QT no toxic effect was observed. As we previously reported rats fed with NPs showed a significant weight loss whereas those that fed QT-SPION didn't [49].

By entering nanoparticles into the gastrointestinal tract through the oral route, the NPs can be absorbed through the epithelium and enter the blood circulation. This route for NPs administration is the most useful one especially in the case of chronic diseases. Nanoparticles help to overcome limitations such as varied-range pH, enzymes degradation and poor solubility, penetrability, and dissolution in the gastrointestinal system. The small particle size of NPs increases the contact with the epithelial surfaces and leads in more uptake of the particles [50]. Nevertheless, several factors such as particle size, nanoparticle stability, surface charge, the intestinal contents, and the residence time of nanoparticles at the absorption site affect the absorption and bioavailability of the nanoparticles [51].

The size, composition and surface hydrophilicity of a drug affect its distribution in the body. The major site of metabolism of particles is the liver, where most of the metabolizing enzymes are found. The metabolism process involves adding or modifying a functional group on the surface of the drug or involves conjugation of the drug with endogenous groups. Metabolism of nanoparticles is a bit more complicated because of the difference in its structure. In the liver, the ligands associated with nanoparticles are metabolized along with them. Nevertheless, the precise pathway of NPs metabolism is unknown yet. The optimum demand for nanoparticles is readily clearance from the body without causing any toxic effects. The particle material, size, shape, surface chemistry, and charge of NPs determine their modifications. In summary, the size, shape, structure, and coating [52] have a significant effect on the cellular uptake, cytotoxicity, distribution and clearance of INOPs.

The drug release behavior of quercetin conjugated to the dextran-coated SPIONs was investigated using a dialysis membrane in basic medium. Our results showed that almost 60% of the drug released within 8 h of dialysis (Fig. 3). However, the quercetin release from SPIONs was slow and controlled in the basic release medium. It is clear that an efficient drug delivery system such as SPIONs, need to have the capability to release their drug cargo at an optimum amount. Nevertheless, it has been reported that a large part of the drug cargo is rapidly released from the in vivo administration of SPIONs. This phenomenon is called as a burst effect. Therefore, minor quantities of the drug reach the specific site after drug treatment. Different strategies such as using different coating [53], mesoporous structure [54] have been used to reduce the burst effect. Finally, the results of drug release in the current study are in line with findings of quercetin biodistribution in plasma.

In the next step, rats were fed with free quercetin and quercetin conjugated Fe_3O_4 nanoparticles to compare the bioavailability of the QT and QT in conjugated with Fe_3O_4 NPs in the plasma and the brain of healthy rats using HPLC assay. The plasma concentrations of the QT and QT-SPIONs deteriorated quickly after 6 h. The clearance rate of QT from the blood was significantly higher for the free QT than QT in conjugated with Fe_3O_4 NPs. This phenomenon could be due to quick distribution and metabolization of the free QT. Alongside with this study, Manach et al. reported rapid metabolization of the quercetin by the intestinal enzymes [55]. The plasma concentration of QT-SPIONs displayed an enhancement in oral bioavailability. This reveals more constant release of QT from NPs in comparison to free QT. Alternatively, the small size of QT-SPIONs causes a high quantity of quercetin in plasma. Additionally, dextran coating of Fe_3O_4 NPs may aid in holding the QT in the blood circulation for a long period [56, 57]. Jain and colleagues in 2013 reported that using self-emulsifying drug delivery systems could increase the plasma concentration of the quercetin in comparison with free QT solution [58]. Also, it has been reported that the encapsulation of the quercetin in polymeric nanoparticles increased the oral bioavailability of QT when compared with free QT [59]. Other research groups have reported coupling NPs with QT improved oral bioavailability of the quercetin [60–64].

It should be reminded that in our study the loading of the QT in QT-SPIONs is 42% which means QT significantly is lower than that of free QT because only a part of QT- Fe_3O_4 is quercetin. Furthermore, the concentration of QT in the brain of rats fed with 50 mg /kg QT-Fe_3O_4 NPs and 100 mg /kg QT- Fe_3O_4 NPs were significantly higher (*P*, 0.05) than rats treated with free QT (Fig. 5).

The concentration of quercetin in the brain delivered by Fe_3O_4 nanoparticles at the concentration of 50 and 100 mg/kg were about 7 and 10-folds higher respectively in comparison with the free quercetin. It designates that Fe_3O_4 nanoparticles increased the bioavailability of quercetin. From this observation, QT-SPIONs enhance the biodistribution of quercetin into the brain. Thus, because of the Fe_3O_4 nanoparticles, the levels of QT are significantly higher than the free quercetin in the plasma and the brain.

One advantage of nanoparticle drug delivery systems in comparison to the free drugs is mostly due to elongated blood circulation. In our study, the concentration of quercetin in the blood increased significantly. Prolonged quercetin circulation in the blood may enhance drug capability to interact with particular carriers or receptors localized inside of the blood-brain barrier endothelial cells and, accordingly, to passage the blood-brain barrier. It has been shown that receptor-mediated transport is the most effective carrying mechanism that occurs on the luminal side of the brain capillary endothelium.

It may be questioned whether quercetin enhancement of the brain tissues is because of the blood circulation in the brain due to lack of blood perfusion. As shown quercetin was almost disappeared completely from the blood circulation after nine hours of treatment. QT was determined in the brain after 24 h of the QT administration on day 7 of treatment. Therefore, the amount of quercetin in the brain couldn't be due to the existence of the QT in the blood vessels.

The blood-brain barrier (BBB) is contained of a contiguous layer of endothelial cells connected by tight junctions. These tight junctions are almost 100 times tighter than junctions of other capillary endothelium [65]. Therefore, the barrier allowing lipid-soluble molecules transport across the membrane while hydrophilic solutes exhibit insignificant permeation [66]. To overcome the barrier one approach is altering barrier integrity or characteristics, and another approach is changing the characteristics of the drug. Since there are risks related to changing the permeability of the BBB, efforts have been made to modify drugs to more readily cross the barrier.

To cross the BBB, the size and weight of nanoparticles should be in a certain range [67]. So that 20 to 100 nm is the optimum size in order to pass through BBB [68] and consequently smaller size of nanoparticles is associated with more efficient drug delivery. Nanoparticles by passive diffusion and receptor-mediated endocytosis can cross the BBB.

To verify whether SPIONs could cross the BBB, we measured the amount of iron contents of the plasma and brain. The results showed that superparamagnetic iron oxide nanoparticles penetrated from the digestive system to the blood circulation. Considering time points iron returned to the normal levels 9 h after SPIONs treatment. The profile of plasma iron contents is very similar to the profile of the plasma quercetin concentration. However, the iron contents of the brain were not significantly higher in the brain of treated rats than control rats. In line with the reported study [9], the results of the current research revealed that SPIONs couldn't cross the BBB [69]. This might be due to the existence of various proteins, for instance, multidrug resistance protein and P-glycoprotein on the BBB cells function as efflux proteins [70]. Some of these proteins such as multidrug resistance proteins are ATP-dependent and drive numerous external nanoparticles out of cells. However, magnetic nanoparticles could increase penetration of the BBB. The sensitivity of brain cells to these nanoparticles is higher than other organs cells [71, 72].

SPIONs can carry the loaded drug to the desired target area using an external magnetic field and at the same time tracking the biodistribution of the particles [73]. This approach as a modern technology is known as theragnositc (therapeutic and diagnostic). This method could reduce the side effects and the required dosage of the drugs [74–77]. Use of the exterior magnetic field facilitates uptake of Fe_3O_4 NPs by brain cells [78]. Therefore, nanoparticles-based drug carriers are promising to improve the special brain drug delivery system. However, the external magnetic field may increase NPs aggregation [79].

Although the research has reached to its aims, due to time, pricing and ethical concerns, there were some unavoidable limitations. First, because of the time limit, this study was conducted only for one week. Therefore, to generalize the results, the research should be done in a longer time. Second, due to the unavailability of funds, the current study has not investigated the lower or higher dosage of the treatment or has not included sex of the rats, cellular study and so on. Finally, measurement of quercetin and histological assessment have been done only for plasma and the brain, it is ideal to do these for other tissues of the body. To avoid the complexity of the subject it is necessary to study these limitations in separate studies.

Conclusions

In the current study, the capability of SPIONs covered with dextran was investigated for bioavailability improvement of the quercetin, in the brain of a healthy rat model. Neither QT nor QT-SPIONs remain in plasma more than of 9 h. The plasma concentrations of QT in rats treated with QT- SPIONs were higher than those of free quercetin. Therefore, it can be concluded that SPIONs coated with dextran enhance delivery of the poorly water soluble quercetin to the brain. Accordingly, this delivery system may be a promising feature in the clinical application. Also, these results propose a potential effective strategy for regulating the biodistribution of QT-SPIONs in the brain by means of an external magnetic field. In future nanoparticle carrier systems may have a significant role in the treatment of the neurological disorders.

Abbreviations

BBB: Blood–brain barrier; CNS: Central nervous system; FTIR: Fourier transformed infrared spectrometer; HPLC: high-performance liquid chromatography; NPs: Nanoparticles; QT: Quercetin; SEM: Scanning electron microscope; SPIONs: Superparamagnetic iron oxide nanoparticles; XRD: X-ray diffractometer

Acknowledgments

This work was supported by the grant from the University of Shiraz and help of the University of Isfahan. The authors thank Dr. Zari Pahlevanneshan of the University of Isfahan for her assistance with nanoparticle preparation.

Funding

The University of Isfahan supported this work.

Authors' contributions

AE and NK designed the study and drafted the manuscript. AE, NK, SB and SN analyzed and interpreted the data came from this study. REN performed the experiments and was a major contributor in writing the manuscript. All authors read and approved the final manuscript.

Competing interests

The authors declare that they have no competing interests.

Author details

[1]Department of Basic Sciences, School of Veterinary Medicine, Shiraz University, Shiraz, Iran. [2]Cell, Molecular Biology and Biochemistry Division, Department of Biology, Faculty of Sciences, University of Isfahan, P.O. Box: 8174673441, Isfahan, Iran. [3]Department of Clinical Science, School of Veterinary Medicine, Shiraz University, Shiraz, Iran.

References

1. Barreto A, Santiago V, Mazzetto S, Denardin JC, Lavín R, Mele G, et al. Magnetic nanoparticles for a new drug delivery system to control quercetin releasing for cancer chemotherapy. J Nanopart Res. 2011;13(12):6545–53.
2. Chowdhury P, Nagesh PK, Kumar S, Jaggi M, Chauhan SC, Yallapu MM. Pluronic nanotechnology for overcoming drug resistance. In: Bioactivity of Engineered Nanoparticles: Springer; 2017. p. 207–37.
3. Valdiglesias V, Kiliç G, Costa C, Fernández-Bertólez N, Pásaro E, Teixeira JP, et al. Effects of iron oxide nanoparticles: cytotoxicity, genotoxicity, developmental toxicity, and neurotoxicity. Environ Mol Mutagen. 2015;56(2): 125–48.
4. Vinzant N, Scholl JL, Wu C-M, Kindle T, Koodali R, Forster GL. Iron oxide nanoparticle delivery of peptides to the brain: reversal of anxiety during drug withdrawal. Front Neurosci. 2017;11:608.
5. Pardridge WM. Why is the global CNS pharmaceutical market so under-penetrated? Drug Discov Today. 2002;7(1):5–7.
6. Zheng M, Tao W, Zou Y, Farokhzad OC, Shi B. Nanotechnology-based strategies for siRNA brain delivery for disease therapy. In: Trends in biotechnology; 2018.
7. Durães F, Pinto M, Sousa E. Old drugs as new treatments for neurodegenerative diseases. Pharmaceuticals. 2018;11(2):44.

8. Neuwelt E, Abbott NJ, Abrey L, Banks WA, Blakley B, Davis T, et al. Strategies to advance translational research into brain barriers. Lancet Neurol. 2008; 7(1):84–96.
9. Huang Y, Zhang B, Xie S, Yang B, Xu Q, Tan J. Superparamagnetic Iron oxide nanoparticles modified with tween 80 pass through the intact blood–brain barrier in rats under magnetic field. ACS Appl Mater Interfaces. 2016;8(18): 11336–41.
10. Kiviniemi V, Korhonen V, Kortelainen J, Rytky S, Keinänen T, Tuovinen T, et al. Real-time monitoring of human blood-brain barrier disruption. PLoS One. 2017;12(3):e0174072.
11. Chauhan NB. Trafficking of intracerebroventricularly injected antisense oligonucleotides in the mouse brain. Antisense Nucleic Acid Drug Dev. 2002;12(5):353–7.
12. Westphal M, Ram Z, Riddle V, Hilt D, Bortey E, Group ECotGS. Gliadel® wafer in initial surgery for malignant glioma: long-term follow-up of a multicenter controlled trial. Acta Neurochir. 2006;148(3):269–75.
13. Abbott NJ, Romero IA. Transporting therapeutics across the blood-brain barrier. Mol Med Today. 1996;2(3):106–13.
14. Oldendorf WH. Measurement of brain uptake of radiolabeled substances using a tritiated water internal standard. Brain Res. 1970;24(2):372–6.
15. Wu D, Pardridge WM. Pharmacokinetics and blood-brain barrier transport of an anti-transferrin receptor monoclonal antibody (OX26) in rats after chronic treatment with the antibody. Drug Metab Dispos. 1998;26(9):937–9.
16. Illum L. Nasal drug delivery—possibilities, problems and solutions. J Control Release. 2003;87(1):187–98.
17. Kumari A, Yadav SK, Pakade YB, Singh B, Yadav SC. Development of biodegradable nanoparticles for delivery of quercetin. Colloids Surf B: Biointerfaces. 2010;80(2):184–92.
18. Wu T-H, Yen F-L, Lin L-T, Tsai T-R, Lin C-C, Cham T-M. Preparation, physicochemical characterization, and antioxidant effects of quercetin nanoparticles. Int J Pharm. 2008;346(1):160–8.
19. Bagad M, Khan ZA. Poly (n-butylcyanoacrylate) nanoparticles for oral delivery of quercetin: preparation, characterization, and pharmacokinetics and biodistribution studies in Wistar rats. Int J Nanomedicine. 2015;10:3921.
20. Stewart LK, Soileau JL, Ribnicky D, Wang ZQ, Raskin I, Poulev A, et al. Quercetin transiently increases energy expenditure but persistently decreases circulating markers of inflammation in C57BL/6J mice fed a high-fat diet. Metabolism. 2008;57(Supplement 1):S39–46.
21. Ramos FA, Takaishi Y, Shirotori M, Kawaguchi Y, Tsuchiya K, Shibata H, et al. Antibacterial and antioxidant activities of quercetin oxidation products from yellow onion (Allium cepa) skin. J Agric Food Chem. 2006;54(10):3551–7.
22. Chakraborty S, Stalin S, Das N, Choudhury ST, Ghosh S, Swarnakar S. The use of nano-quercetin to arrest mitochondrial damage and MMP-9 upregulation during prevention of gastric inflammation induced by ethanol in rat. Biomaterials. 2012;33(10):2991–3001.
23. Choi H-J, Kim J-H, Lee C-H, Ahn Y-J, Song J-H, Baek S-H, et al. Antiviral activity of quercetin 7-rhamnoside against porcine epidemic diarrhea virus. Antivir Res. 2009;81(1):77–81.
24. Duarte J, Pérez-Vizcaíno F, Zarzuelo A, Jiménez J, Tamargo J. Vasodilator effects of quercetin in isolated rat vascular smooth muscle. Eur J Pharmacol. 1993;239(1):1–7.
25. Davis JM, Murphy EA, Carmichael MD, Davis B. Quercetin increases brain and muscle mitochondrial biogenesis and exercise tolerance. Am J Phys Regul Integr Comp Phys. 2009;296(4):R1071–R7.
26. Sandeep M, Nandini C. Influence of quercetin, naringenin and berberine on glucose transporters and insulin signalling molecules in brain of streptozotocin-induced diabetic rats. Biomed Pharmacother. 2017;94:605–11.
27. Ossola B, Kääriäinen TM, Männistö PT. The multiple faces of quercetin in neuroprotection. Expert Opin Drug Saf. 2009;8(4):397–409.
28. Dajas F. Life or death: neuroprotective and anticancer effects of quercetin. J Ethnopharmacol. 2012;143(2):383–96.
29. Dajas F, Juan Andres A-C, Florencia A, Carolina E, Felicia R-M. Neuroprotective actions of flavones and flavonols: mechanisms and relationship to flavonoid structural features. Cent Nerv Syst Agents Med Chem. 2013;13(1):30–5.
30. Nichols M, Zhang J, Polster B, Elustondo P, Thirumaran A, Pavlov E, et al. Synergistic neuroprotection by epicatechin and quercetin: activation of convergent mitochondrial signaling pathways. Neuroscience. 2015;308: 75–94.
31. Lee YJ, Bernstock JD, Nagaraja N, Ko B, Hallenbeck JM. Global SUMO ylation facilitates the multimodal neuroprotection afforded by quercetin against the deleterious effects of oxygen/glucose deprivation and the restoration of oxygen/glucose. J Neurochem. 2016;138(1):101–16.
32. Rivera F, Urbanavicius J, Gervaz E, Morquio A, Dajas F. Some aspects of thein vivo neuroprotective capacity of flavonoids: bioavailability and structure-activity relationship. Neurotox Res. 2004;6(7–8):543–53.
33. Blasina F, Vaamonde L, Silvera F, Tedesco AC, Dajas F. Intravenous nanosomes of quercetin improve brain function and hemodynamic instability after severe hypoxia in newborn piglets. Neurochem Int. 2015;89:149–56.
34. Galho A, Cordeiro M, Ribeiro S, Marques M, Antunes M, Luz D, et al. Protective role of free and quercetin-loaded nanoemulsion against damage induced by intracerebral haemorrhage in rats. Nanotechnology. 2016;27(17):175101.
35. Kumar SR, Priyatharshni S, Babu V, Mangalaraj D, Viswanathan C, Kannan S, et al. Quercetin conjugated superparamagnetic magnetite nanoparticles for in-vitro analysis of breast cancer cell lines for chemotherapy applications. J Colloid Interface Sci. 2014;436:234–42.
36. Akal Z, Alpsoy L, Baykal A. Superparamagnetic iron oxide conjugated with folic acid and carboxylated quercetin for chemotherapy applications. Ceram Int. 2016;42(7):9065–72.
37. Bongartz D, Hesse A. Selective extraction of quercetrin in vegetable drugs and urine by off-line coupling of boronic acid affinity chromatography and high-performance liquid chromatography. J Chromatogr B Biomed Sci Appl. 1995;673(2):223–30.
38. Erlund I, Alfthan G, Siren H, Ariniemi K, Aro A. Validated method for the quantitation of quercetin from human plasma using high-performance liquid chromatography with electrochemical detection. J Chromatogr B Biomed Sci Appl. 1999;727(1):179–89.
39. Yochum L, Kushi LH, Meyer K, Folsom AR. Dietary flavonoid intake and risk of cardiovascular disease in postmenopausal women. Am J Epidemiol. 1999; 149(10):943–9.
40. Soleas G, Yan J, Goldberg D. Ultrasensitive assay for three polyphenols (catechin, quercetin and resveratrol) and their conjugates in biological fluids utilizing gas chromatography with mass selective detection. J Chromatogr B Biomed Sci Appl. 2001;757(1):161–72.
41. Skaper SD, Fabris M, Ferrari V, Dalle Carbonare M, Leon A. Quercetin protects cutaneous tissue-associated cell types including sensory neurons from oxidative stress induced by glutathione depletion: cooperative effects of ascorbic acid. Free Radic Biol Med. 1997;22(4):669–78.
42. Oyama Y, Fuchs PA, Katayama N, Noda K. Myricetin and quercetin, the flavonoid constituents ofGinkgo biloba extract, greatly reduce oxidative metabolism in both resting and Ca2+–loaded brain neurons. Brain Res. 1994;635(1–2):125–9.
43. Naidu PS, Singh A, Kulkarni SK. Quercetin, a bioflavonoid, attenuates haloperidol-induced orofacial dyskinesia. Neuropharmacology. 2003;44(8):1100–6.
44. Le Nest G, Caille O, Woudstra M, Roche S, Guerlesquin F, Lexa D. Zn–polyphenol chelation: complexes with quercetin,(+)-catechin, and derivatives: I optical and NMR studies. Inorg Chim Acta. 2004;357(3):775–84.
45. Lu J, Zheng YL, Luo L, Wu D-M, Sun D-X, Feng Y-J. Quercetin reverses D-galactose induced neurotoxicity in mouse brain. Behav Brain Res 2006; 171(2):251–260.
46. Malekzadeh AM, Ramazani A, Rezaei SJT, Niknejad H. Design and construction of multifunctional hyperbranched polymers coated magnetite nanoparticles for both targeting magnetic resonance imaging and cancer therapy. J. Colloid Interface Sci. 2017;490:64–73.
47. Boyer C, Whittaker MR, Bulmus V, Liu J, Davis TP. The design and utility of polymer-stabilized iron-oxide nanoparticles for nanomedicine applications. NPG Asia Mat. 2010;2(1):23–30.
48. Hong R, Feng B, Chen L, Liu G, Li H, Zheng Y, et al. Synthesis, characterization and MRI application of dextran-coated Fe 3 O 4 magnetic nanoparticles. Biochem Eng J. 2008;42(3):290–300.
49. Najafabadi RE, Kazemipour N, Esmaeili A, Beheshti S, Nazifi S. Quercetin prevents body weight loss due to the using of superparamagnetic Iron oxide nanoparticles in rat. Adv Biomed Res. 2018;7.
50. Pridgen EM, Alexis F, Farokhzad OC. Polymeric nanoparticle drug delivery technologies for oral delivery applications. Expert Opin Drug Deliv. 2015; 12(9):1459–73.
51. Alai M, Lin WJ. Application of nanoparticles for oral delivery of acid-labile lansoprazole in the treatment of gastric ulcer: in vitro and in vivo evaluations. Int J Nanomedicine. 2015;10:4029.
52. Feng Q, Liu Y, Huang J, Chen K, Huang J, Xiao K. Uptake, distribution, clearance, and toxicity of iron oxide nanoparticles with different sizes and coatings. Sci Rep. 2018;8(1):2082.

53. Mahmoudi M, Sant S, Wang B, Laurent S, Sen T. Superparamagnetic iron oxide nanoparticles (SPIONs): development, surface modification and applications in chemotherapy. Adv Drug Deliv Rev. 2011;63(1):24–46.
54. Guo S, Li D, Zhang L, Li J, Wang E. Monodisperse mesoporous superparamagnetic single-crystal magnetite nanoparticles for drug delivery. Biomaterials. 2009;30(10):1881–9.
55. Manach C, Texier O, Morand C, Crespy V, Régérat F, Demigné C, et al. Comparison of the bioavailability of quercetin and catechin in rats. Free Radic Biol Med. 1999;27(11):1259–66.
56. Sun M, Gao Y, Guo C, Cao F, Song Z, Xi Y, et al. Enhancement of transport of curcumin to brain in mice by poly (n-butylcyanoacrylate) nanoparticle. J Nanopart Res. 2010;12(8):3111–22.
57. Gulyaev AE, Gelperina SE, Skidan IN, Antropov AS, Kivman GY, Kreuter J. Significant transport of doxorubicin into the brain with polysorbate 80-coated nanoparticles. Pharm Res. 1999;16(10):1564–9.
58. Jain S, Jain AK, Pohekar M, Thanki K. Novel self-emulsifying formulation of quercetin for improved in vivo antioxidant potential: implications for drug-induced cardiotoxicity and nephrotoxicity. Free Radic Biol Med. 2013;65: 117–30.
59. Jain AK, Thanki K, Jain S. Co-encapsulation of tamoxifen and quercetin in polymeric nanoparticles: implications on oral bioavailability, antitumor efficacy, and drug-induced toxicity. Mol Pharm. 2013;10(9):3459–74.
60. Dhawan S, Kapil R, Singh B. Formulation development and systematic optimization of solid lipid nanoparticles of quercetin for improved brain delivery. J Pharm Pharmacol. 2011;63(3):342–51.
61. Zhao L, Liu A, Sun M, Gu J, Wang H, Wang S, et al. Enhancement of oral bioavailability of puerarin by polybutylcyanoacrylate nanoparticles. J Nanomater. 2011;2011:6.
62. Yordanov G. Influence of the preparation method on the physicochemical properties of econazole-loaded poly (butyl cyanoacrylate) colloidal nanoparticles. Colloids Surf A Physicochem Eng Asp. 2012;413:260–5.
63. Tian X-h, Lin X-N, Wei F, Feng W, Huang Z-C, Wang P, et al. Enhanced brain targeting of temozolomide in polysorbate-80 coated polybutylcyanoacrylate nanoparticles. Int J Nanomedicine. 2011;6:445–52.
64. Ghosh A, Mandal AK, Sarkar S, Panda S, Das N. Nanoencapsulation of quercetin enhances its dietary efficacy in combating arsenic-induced oxidative damage in liver and brain of rats. Life Sci. 2009;84(3):75–80.
65. Butt AM, Jones HC, Abbott NJ. Electrical resistance across the blood-brain barrier in anaesthetized rats: a developmental study. J Physiol. 1990; 429(1):47–62.
66. McConnell H. Ferumoxytol Iron oxide nanoparticles as a magnetic resonance contrast agent in central nervous system lesions. 2018.
67. Talegaonkar S, Mishra P. Intranasal delivery: an approach to bypass the blood brain barrier. Indian J Pharmacol. 2004;36(3):140.
68. Jo DH, Kim JH, Lee TG, Kim JH. Size, surface charge, and shape determine therapeutic effects of nanoparticles on brain and retinal diseases. Nanomedicine. 2015;11(7):1603–11.
69. Rousseau V, Denizot B, Pouliquen D, Jallet P, Le Jeune J. Investigation of blood-brain barrier permeability to magnetite-dextran nanoparticles (MD3) after osmotic disruption in rats. MAGMA. 1997;5(3):213–22.
70. Taccola C, Cartot-Cotton S, Valente D, Barneoud P, Aubert C, Boutet V, et al. High brain distribution of a new central nervous system drug candidate despite its P-glycoprotein-mediated efflux at the mouse blood-brain barrier. Eur J Pharm Sci. 2018;117:68–79.
71. Laurent S, Burtea C, Thirifays C, Häfeli UO, Mahmoudi M. Crucial ignored parameters on nanotoxicology: the importance of toxicity assay modifications and "cell vision". PLoS One. 2012;7(1):e29997.
72. Mahmoudi M, Laurent S, Shokrgozar MA, Hosseinkhani M. Toxicity evaluations of superparamagnetic iron oxide nanoparticles: cell "vision" versus physicochemical properties of nanoparticles. ACS Nano. 2011;5(9): 7263–76.
73. Shubayev VI, Pisanic TR II, Jin S. Magnetic nanoparticles for theragnostics. Adv Drug Deliv Rev. 2009;61(6):467–77.
74. Neuberger T, Schöpf B, Hofmann H, Hofmann M, Von Rechenberg B. Superparamagnetic nanoparticles for biomedical applications: possibilities and limitations of a new drug delivery system. J Magn Magn Mater 2005; 293(1):483–496.
75. Lübbe AS, Alexiou C, Bergemann C. Clinical applications of magnetic drug targeting. J Surg Res. 2001;95(2):200–6.
76. Rudge S, Peterson C, Vessely C, Koda J, Stevens S, Catterall L. Adsorption and desorption of chemotherapeutic drugs from a magnetically targeted carrier (MTC). J Control Release. 2001;74(1–3):335–40.
77. Zanganeh S, Ho J, Aieneravaie M, Erfanzadeh M, Pauliah M, Spitler R. Drug Delivery. Iron Oxide Nanoparticles for Biomedical Applications: Elsevier; 2018. p. 247–71.
78. Thomsen LB, Linemann T, Pondman KM, Lichota J, Kim KS, Pieters RJ, et al. Uptake and transport of superparamagnetic iron oxide nanoparticles through human brain capillary endothelial cells. ACS Chem Neurosci. 2013; 4(10):1352–60.
79. Hamley I. Nanotechnology with soft materials. Angew Chem Int Ed. 2003; 42(15):1692–712.

22

Gender-differences of in vitro colonic motility after chemo- and radiotherapy in humans

Maria Antonietta Maselli[1*], Antonia Ignazzi[1], Francesco Pezzolla[2], Annunziata Scirocco[1], Dionigi Lorusso[2], Fabrizio De Ponti[3] and Carola Severi[4]

Abstract

Background: The aim of the present in vitro study was to investigate, in different genders, motor responses in surgical colonic specimens from patients with rectal cancer undergoing and not undergoing chemotherapy with capecitabine and radiotherapy.

Methods: This in vitro study was conducted from October 2015 to August 2017 at the Experimental Pharmacology Laboratory at the National Institute "S. de Bellis" after collecting samples at the Department of Surgery. Segments of sigmoid colon were obtained from 15 patients (Male (M)/Female (F) = 8/7; control group, CG) operated on for elective colorectal resection for rectal cancer without obstruction and 14 patients (M/F = 7/7; study group, SG) operated on for elective colorectal resection for rectal cancer who also received chemotherapy, based on capecitabine twice daily, and radiotherapy. Isometric tension was measured on colonic circular muscle strips exposed to increasing carbachol or histamine concentrations to obtain concentration-response curves. The motor responses to electrically evoked stimulation were also investigated.

Results: In males, carbachol and histamine caused concentration-dependent contractions in the CG and SG. An increased sensitivity and a higher response to carbachol and histamine were observed in SG than CG ($P < 0.01$). On the contrary, in females, the response to carbachol was not significantly different in CG from the SG and the maximal responses to carbachol were greater in CG than in SG ($P < 0.001$). The same applied to histamine for half-maximal effective concentrations and maximal response in that they were not significantly different in CG from the SG. Electrically evoked contractions were significantly more pronounced in males, especially in the SG ($P < 0.05$).

Conclusions: This preliminary in vitro study has shown gender differences in motor responses of colonic circular muscle strips in patients who had received chemotherapy with capecitabine and radiotherapy.

Keywords: Chemotherapy, Radiotherapy, Capecitabine, Carbachol, Histamine, Nitrergic pathways, Motility, Human colon, Gender

Background

The clinical manifestations associated with exposure to chemotherapy and radiotherapy include diarrhea, abdominal cramps and associated pain and, most frequently, nausea and vomiting [1, 2]. Diarrhea involves the interaction of motor activity and epithelial transport. Mucositis is a key factor to be taken into account after chemo- and radiotherapy [3].

Some authors have shown hypercontractility in gastric fundic and duodenal muscle in rats after exposure to Fluorouracil (5-FU) [4] while others have found increased sensitivity to cholinergic stimulation in the duodenum and colon after whole-body irradiation in guinea pigs [4, 5]. This increased responsiveness after irradiation may be associated with colonic motor alterations consisting in giant contractions in dogs and intestinal migrating motor complexes disruption in rats [2, 6].

* Correspondence: antonella.maselli@irccsdebellis.it
[1]Experimental Pharmacology Laboratory, National Institute of Gastroenterology "S. de Bellis", Research Hospital - Castellana Grotte (BA), 70013 Castellana Grotte, Italy
Full list of author information is available at the end of the article

The use of chemo- and radiotherapy disrupts the mucosal barrier and represents a clinically significant risk factor for local infections and sepsis [7]. Some studies demonstrated significant enhancement in gastrointestinal muscle contractility in response to carbachol during infections and chronic inflammation [8, 9] and increased sensitivity to histamine in inflammatory conditions related to the release of leukotrienes that increase histamine receptor numbers [10]. Furthermore, the increase in gastrointestinal transit occurring during infection is mediated by endogenous tachykinins, modulated by the activation of nitric oxide (NO) biosynthesis [11]. This tachykinergic component is most probably expressed in elderly male patients per a gender-related difference in receptor density of human colon [12].

Nevertheless, this increased in sensitivity to contractile agonists is not universally observed. For instance, Sung et al. showed a significant reduction in contractility to carbachol in human stomach induced by cisplatin-based chemotherapy [13]. Besides, the response to histamine did not change in colitis in rats [14].

In 5-FU-induced oral mucositis, NO is also involved. In fact, previous reports showed that proinflammatory cytokines stimulate inducible NO synthase (iNOS)-derived NO production [7]. The NO increase is in agreement with studies reporting increased plasma nitric oxide after oral administration of anticancer drugs in rats and in disagreement with other studies reporting reduced expression of the inducible form of NOS in rats receiving cisplatin and no change in neural NO synthase (nNOS) expression in patients receiving chemotherapy [13, 15, 16].

These discrepancies in contractile response to agonists, carbachol and histamine, and NO production might be related to differences in species, intestinal tracts, duration of chemotherapy and radiotherapy or length of time after chemo-and radiotherapy as well as to gender.

Possible gender differences in the colonic response to chemotherapy and radiotherapy have not been well characterized. Therefore, the aim of the present in vitro study was to investigate, in different genders, the response to contracting agents (carbachol or histamine) and electrical stimulation in surgical colonic specimens from patients who had undergone standard chemotherapy with capecitabine and radiotherapy, compared to patients who had not undergone chemo- and radiotherapy.

Methods

This in vitro study was conducted at the Experimental Pharmacology Laboratory of The National Institute of Gastroenterology "S. de Bellis" Castellana Grotte (BA) after collecting samples at the Department of Surgery of the same institute. The in vitro experiments were carried out from October 2015 to August 2017. Segments of sigmoid colon obtained from 15 patients (M/F = 8/7) operated on for elective colorectal resection for rectal cancer served as a control group (CG) and 14 patients (M/F = 7/7) operated on for elective colorectal resection of rectal cancer who had received neoadjuvant therapy, based on capecitabine (Xeloda®, 825 mg/m^2, Welwyn Garden City, United Kingdom), twice daily and one dose of radiotherapy (50.4 Gy in 28 fractions of 180 cGy/die) before surgery served as a study group (SG). Patients were 15 men (8 CG, average age 73.4 ± 1.1 years; range 73–76 years and 7 SG, average age 73.3 ± 1.7 years; range 72–77 years) and 14 women (7 CG, average age 74.3 ± 1.6 years; range 72–76 years and 7 SG, average age 73.6 ± 1.3 years; range 72–78 years).

In all patients, preanaesthetic medication was intramuscular atropine (1 mg) and midazolam (5 mg). Anaesthesia was induced by propofol (2.5 mg/kg) intravenously (i.v.) and maintained with nitrous oxide/oxygen (N_2O/O_2) (1/2) and sevoflurane (0.5–2%). Patients received norcuronium (8 mg) i.v. during induction of anaesthesia.

Colonic strips were taken from a carcinoma-free area, 1–4 cm along the longitudinal axis.

Motility study in vitro

We used the same methods reported before [17]. In brief, tissues were gently deprived of the mucosa and the muscle segments were cut into strips (1.0 cm × 0.3 cm) transversely (circular) to the axis of bowel. Circular muscle strips were mounted in an organ bath (10 ml) containing oxygenated Krebs solution, maintained at a temperature of 37 °C and gassed with 5% carbon dioxide (CO_2) in O_2. The composition of the Krebs solution was as follows: sodium chloride (NaCl) 115.5 mM; potassium chloride (KCl) 4.6 mM; calcium chloride ($CaCl_2$) 2.5 mM; magnesium chloride ($MgCl_2$) 2.1 mM; sodium bicarbonate ($NaHCO_3$) 21.9 mM; monosodium phosphate ($NaHPO_4$) 1.2 mM; and glucose 15.5 mM. Tissues were stored overnight at 4 °C prior to use. Strips were tied with a silk ligature to an isometric transducer (Force 100, N. S/N 77648, 77645, 77631, ADInstruments Ltd., Unit B, Bishops Mews, Transport Way, Oxford OX4 6HD, UNITED KINGDOM), and contractions were recorded on a PowerLab/800 (Model ML119 Serial 2265, ADInstruments Ltd., Unit B, Bishops Mews, Transport Way, Oxford OX4 6HD, UNITED KINGDOM) acquisition program. The muscle length was measured directly in the bath by using a caliper. After gentle, repeated washings following by 1-h stabilization, tissues were placed under a tension of 20–24 mN (in preliminary tests it was shown that this baseline tension produces the maximal response to 1×10^{-6}M carbachol). After equilibration, at least two comparable responses to carbachol were recorded before tissues were exposed to increasing concentrations of carbachol, histamine or electrical field stimulation (EFS). The motor response to carbachol and histamine were investigated on circular strips obtained from male and female patients of both groups. Strips were exposed to increasing concentrations of carbachol (1×10^{-8}M-1×10^{-6}M, cumulatively) and histamine (1×10^{-8}M-1×10^{-6}M, cumulatively) in order to obtain concentration-response curves. The curves were repeated after 60 min and some washing steps.

The motor responses to EFS were investigated on circular strips obtained from male and female patients of both groups. EFS was performed with an electrical stimulator type 215/T (Hugo Sachs Elektronik, March/Freiburg, Germany) using two platinum wire electrodes (15 mm in length and 5 mm in width) placed parallel to the longitudinal axis of the strips. Electrodes were placed 4.5 mm from the strip. The duration of the train of electrical pulses was always 10 s, and stimulation was performed every 2 min (0.1–10 Hz, pulse duration 0.3 ms, supramaximal strength: 20 V) [18, 19]. The current applied across the bath was monitored and the compliance of voltage was also measured. The time interval between each train of electrical pulses was always 60 min, because preliminary experiments indicated that this allows to evoke reproducible control responses, apart from the first response, which was always discarded. Electrically evoked contractions were evaluated in the presence of atropine (2×10^{-6}M), guanethidine (5×10^{-6}M) and L-nitro arginine methyl ester (L-NAME 2×10^{-4}M), an inhibitor of NO synthase. The contact time was 30 min for atropine and guanethidine and 45 min for L-NAME. The concentration of atropine was chosen on the basis of previous experiments showing that they fully blocked the contraction produced by 1×10^{-4}M carbachol. The concentration of guanethidine was chosen on the basis of literature data [20, 21]. At the end of each experiment, strips were removed, blotted, and weighed.

Chemicals

Carbachol chloride, histamine dihydrochloride, atropine sulphate, guanethidine sulphate, and L-nitro arginine methyl ester (L-NAME) were purchased from Sigma Chemical Co. (St Louis, Missouri, United States). Other chemicals were of the highest quality and were obtained from commercial sources.

Statistical analysis

The results are given as means ± standard error (SE) (n indicates the number of patients). Carbachol- and histamine-induced contractions were measured as increases over baseline activity and were calculated as mN per cross sectional area (expressed in cm^2) [18, 19, 22, 23]. We then expressed concentration-response data as a percentage of the maximal response to carbachol or histamine and calculated half-maximal effective concentration (EC_{50}) values with 95% confidence intervals (CIs) from log concentration-response curves using non-linear regression analysis. Stress induced by electrical stimulation was expressed as mN per cross sectional area [18, 19, 22, 23]. We compared data sets with a paired Wilcoxon test (responses before and after treatment), unpaired Mann-Whitney U test (differences between groups), and unpaired Student's t test, as appropriate. We used a commercial statistical package (GraphPad Prism, version 5 for Windows, GraphPad Software, San Diego, California, United States) and considered statistical significance achieved when $P < 0.05$.

Results

Response to carbachol and histamine

In male patients, carbachol (1×10^{-8}M-1×10^{-6}M) and histamine (1×10^{-8}M-1×10^{-6}M) caused concentration-dependent contractions in circular muscle strips in the CG and SG (Fig. 1). EC_{50} values to carbachol were 8.54×10^{-6}M (95% CI $4.54–16.0 \times 10^{-6}$M) and 1.58×10^{-6}M (95% CI $0.68–3.70 \times 10^{-6}$M) in CG and SG respectively (Fig. 1). This response was greater in SG than in CG ($P < 0.01$). Moreover, the maximal responses to carbachol (expressed in mN/cm^2) were significantly higher in SG male patients (4623.0 ± 894.4 mN/cm^2 in SG vs 1621.0 ± 204.5 mN/cm^2 in CG; P < 0.01).

The same was true when we analyzed histamine-induced responses: EC_{50} values were 3.77×10^{-6}M (95% CI $1.79–7.94 \times 10^{-6}$M) and 0.37×10^{-6}M (95% CI $0.09–1.42 \times 10^{-6}$M) in CG and SG, respectively. This response was greater in SG than in CG ($P < 0.001$) (Fig. 2). Again, the maximal responses to histamine were significantly higher in

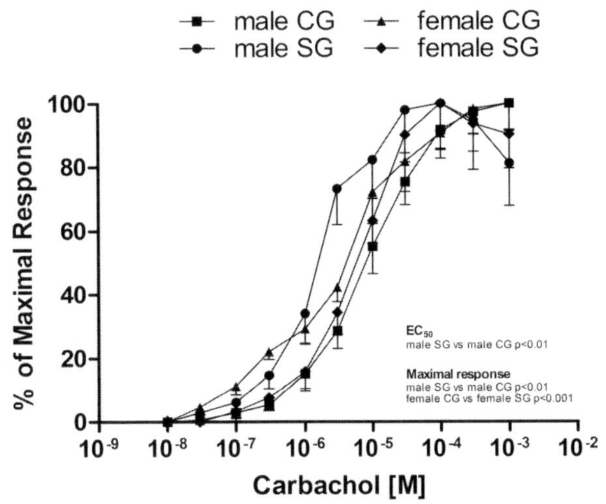

Fig. 1 Log concentration-response curves for carbachol in male and female patients [control group (CG), study group (SG)]. All responses are expressed as a percentage of the control maximal response to carbachol. Results are means ± standard error (SE) ($n = 15$ male patients and $n = 14$ female patients). $P < 0.01$, half-maximal effective concentration (EC_{50}) value in SG male patients vs CG male patients; P < 0.01, maximal response in SG male patients vs CG male patients; $P < 0.001$, maximal response in CG female patients vs SG female patients

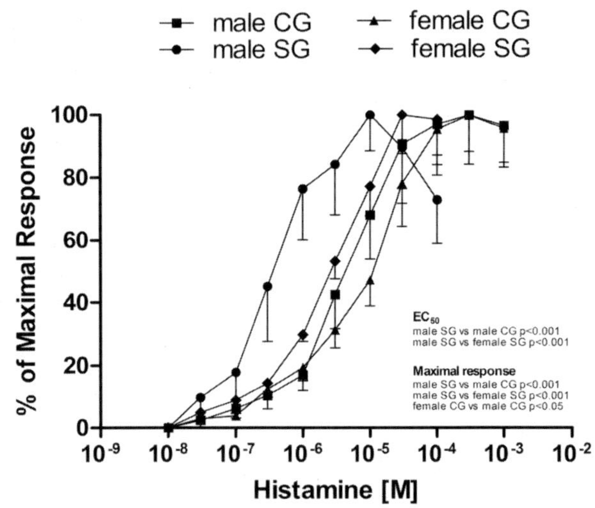

Fig. 2 Log concentration-response curves for histamine in male and female patients [control group (CG), study group (SG)]. All responses are expressed as a percentage of the control maximal response to histamine. Results are means ± standard error (SE) (n = 15 male patients and n = 14 female patients). P < 0.001, half-maximal effective concentration (EC_{50}) value in SG male patients vs CG male patients; P < 0.001, EC_{50} value in SG male patients vs SG female patients; P < 0.001, maximal response in SG male patients vs CG male patients; P < 0.001, maximal response in SG male patients vs SG female patients; *P* < 0.05, maximal response in CG female patients vs CG male patients

SG male patients (2895.0 ± 220.0 mN/cm^2 in SG vs 847.8 ± 123.9 mN/cm^2 in CG; P < 0.001).

Conversely, in female patients, the response to carbachol (1×10^{-8}M-1×10^{-6}M) was not significantly different in the two groups, with a trend towards a reduced response in SG: EC_{50} values for carbachol were 3.84×10^{-6}M (95% CI 1.85–7.96×10^{-6}M) and 6.84×10^{-6}M (95% CI 3.70–12.63×10^{-6}M) in CG and SG, respectively (Fig. 1). The maximal responses to carbachol were significantly higher in CG female patients (2247.0 ± 186.9 mN/cm^2 in CG vs 1354.0 ± 109.9 mN/cm^2 in SG; *P* < 0.001).

The response to histamine was not significantly different in the two groups, with a trend towards a reduced response in CG: EC_{50} values for histamine were 7.99×10^{-6}M (95% CI 4.27–14.97×10^{-6}M) and 3.85×10^{-6}M (95% CI 2.07–7.14×10^{-6}M) in CG and SG, respectively (Fig. 2) and the maximal responses to histamine were not significantly different in the two groups (1384 ± 154.6 mN/cm^2 in CG, 1292.0 ± 148.7 mN/cm^2 in SG).

Moreover, analyzing groups of different gender, in SG maximal responses to carbachol and histamine were significantly more pronounced in male vs female patients (P < 0.001) and EC_{50} values to histamine were significantly different in male vs female patients (P < 0.001). In CG, the maximal response to histamine was significantly more pronounced in female vs male patients (*P* < 0.05).

Electrically evoked contractions

In both patient groups, electrically evoked contractions in circular muscle strips were linearly related to stimulation frequency in the 0.1–10 Hz range: analyzing groups of different gender, electrically evoked contractions were significantly more pronounced in male than in female patients both in CG that in SG at all frequencies.

The contractions in male patients were much more marked in SG than in CG in the 0.3–10 Hz frequency range (Fig. 3). The same trend was observed in female patients, where electrically evoked contractions were more marked in SG than in CG at frequency 0.1 Hz, 1–10 Hz (Fig. 3).

Analyzing groups of different gender, electrically evoked contractions were significantly more pronounced in male than in female patients both in CG that in SG at all frequencies. In male patients, atropine and guanethidine per se inhibited electrically evoked contractions depending on stimulation frequency. The inhibition was significant in CG at all frequencies and in SG only at 3–10 Hz. The addition of L-NAME reversed atropine and guanethidine inhibition, increasing electrically evoked responses at all frequency in CG and in SG only at 1–3 Hz (Fig. 4a-b).

In females, also atropine and guanetidine inhibited electrically evoked contractions in CG at all frequency while in SG at the frequency 0.3–10 Hz. As in male patients, the addition of L-NAME reversed atropine and guanetidine inhibition increasing electrically evoked responses in CG

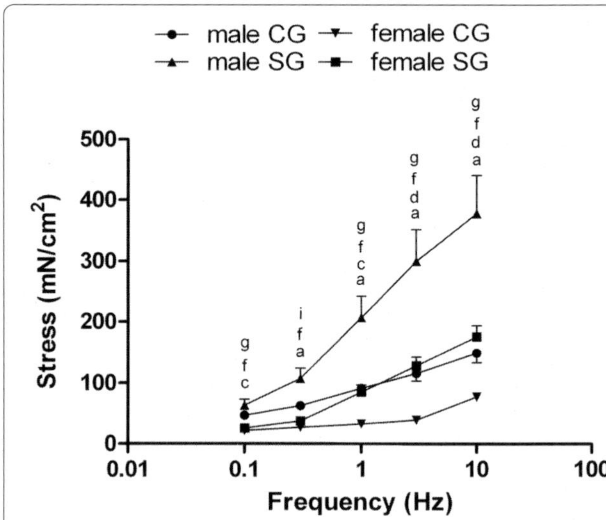

Fig. 3 Electrically evoked contractions related to stimulation frequency (range: 0.1–10 Hz) in male and female patients [control group (CG), study group (SG)]. Results are means ± standard error (SE) (*n* = 8 male CG, *n* = 7 male SG, n = 7 female CG, n = 7 female SG). [a]P < 0.05 and [b]P < 0.01, CG male patients vs SG male patients; [c]P < 0.05 and [d]P < 0.01, CG female patients vs SG female patients; [e]P < 0.01 and [f]P < 0.001, CG male patients vs CG female patients; [g]P < 0.05, [h]P < 0.01 and [i]P < 0.001, SG male patients vs SG female patients

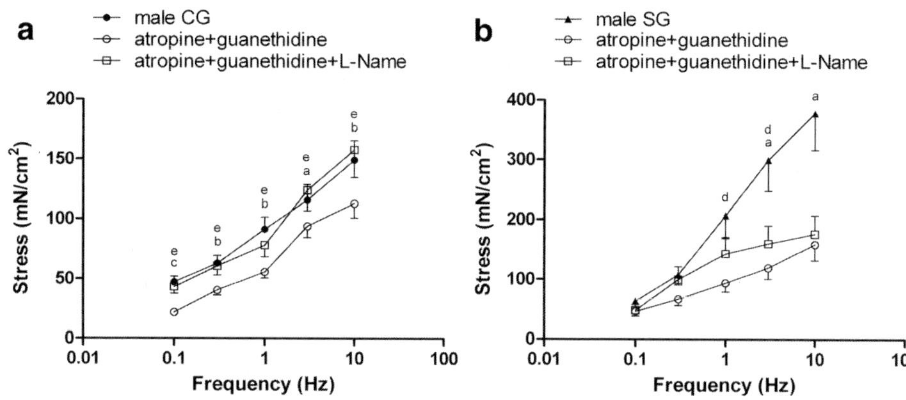

Fig. 4 Electrically evoked contractions in control group (CG) (**a**) and study group (SG) (**b**) male patients. CG and SG experiments in the presence of atropine and guanethidine or atropine, guanethidine, and L-nitro arginine methyl ester (L-NAME). Results are means ± standard error (SE); **a**, n = 8 patients; **b**, n = 7 patients. [a]$P < 0.05$, [b]$P < 0.01$ and [c]$P < 0.001$, atropine and guanethidine vs controls; [d]$P < 0.05$ and [e]$P < 0.01$, atropine and guanethidine vs atropine, guanethidine, and L-NAME

and in SG, but this was significant at all frequencies only in CG (Fig. 5a-b).

Notably, the effect of L-NAME was most marked in CG males and less pronounced in SG males, CG and SG females.

Discussion

In this study, in vitro colonic motor responses to carbachol, histamine or electrical stimulation after chemo- and radiotherapy were quite different in male and female patients. Some of the observed gender differences were so remarkable that in our opinion they deserve a preliminary report here, since they are also in line with circumstantial evidence already available in the literature. However, we must acknowledge important intrinsic limitations of our study: we could analyse only a limited number of surgical specimens, which did not allow us to further investigate mechanisms underlying the gender differences. Furthermore, we cannot completely rule out the possibility that at least some of the observed differences might be due to heterogeneity of the clinical condition in individual patients.

Colonic circular muscle strips after chemo- and radiotherapy in SG were more sensitive to carbachol and histamine with respect to controls in males. Sensitivity to carbachol in these patients is in line with previous findings showing hypercontractility in gastric fundic and duodenal muscle, in both inflammatory and post-inflammatory phases of 5-FU induced intestinal mucositis in rats [4]. Other authors showed increased sensitivity to cholinergic stimulation in the duodenum and colon after whole-body irradiation in guinea pigs [5]. This increased responsiveness may be associated with colonic motor alterations consisting in giant contractions in dogs and intestinal migrating motor complexes disruption in rats [2, 6]. The increased incidence of giant contractions has been

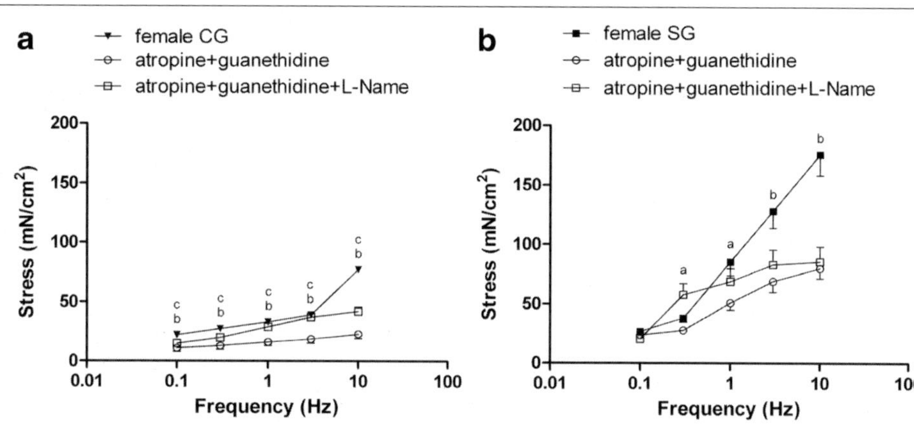

Fig. 5 Electrically evoked contractions in control group (CG) (**a**) and study group (SG) (**b**) female patients. CG and SG experiments in the presence of atropine and guanethidine or atropine, guanethidine, and L-NAME. Results are means ± standard error (SE); **a**, n = 7 patients, **b**, n = 7 patients. [a]$P < 0.05$ and [b]$P < 0.01$, atropine and guanethidine vs controls; [c]$P < 0.05$, atropine and guanethidine vs atropine, guanethidine, and L-NAME

suggested to be responsible for the iatrogenic side effects such as diarrhea, abdominal cramping and vomiting [2, 6, 24]. Furthermore, other studies have demonstrated significant enhancement in gastrointestinal muscle contractility in response to carbachol during chronic inflammation and infections [8, 9]. When the mucosal barrier is damaged, the use of chemo- and radiotherapy represents a risk factor for local infections and sepsis [7].

Increased sensitivity to histamine has also been reported in inflammatory conditions related to the release of leukotrienes enhancing histamine receptor numbers [10]. Nevertheless, this increased sensitivity to contractile agonists is somewhat controversial. Sung et al. showed significantly reduced contractility to carbachol in human stomach after cisplatin-based chemotherapy [13]. Besides, the response to histamine did not change in colitis in rats [14]. These discrepancies might be related to differences in species, intestinal tracts, duration of chemotherapy or length of time after chemotherapy as well as to gender.

In the present study, the sensitivity and the maximum response to carbachol or histamine were greater in male than in female SG patients. Even considering the mean age of our patients, this different response might at least in part be ascribed to female hormones, although we cannot rule out other factors. Indeed, Kaur et al. [25] showed increased estrogen levels after surgery even in postmenopausal women. This may be an indicator than under stress (as after chemo- and radiotherapy) estrogen levels can be higher even in postmenopausal women. Therefore the different responses that we observed might be relative to an effect of female hormones still released under stress. An alternative explanation is that gender differences might be ascribed to the fact that in postmenopausal women tissues, in any case, have been exposed to estrogens in previous years, so that, even when oestrogen levels decrease, tissue responses may still differ. Interestingly, ovariectomy in adult female rabbits caused altered receptor sensitivity and increased intrinsic smooth muscle sensitivity to histamine in vascular smooth muscle. This would further explain the gender-dependent difference that we observed in females compared to males [26].

In the CG, we confirm the data previously published in our recent study on elderly female and male patients, where females were more sensitive and showed higher maximal response to carbachol [17]. These observations are in line with previous findings, one showing increased response to carbachol in animals, while the other suggested that aging induces an increase in Calcium ions (Ca^{2+}) store with consequent Ca^{2+} overload, although these data do not specifically refer to gender differences [27, 28].

Also electrically evoked contractions were more marked in SG than in CG in both genders and this may be due to the formation of peroxynitrite. During severe inflammation, as observed after 5-FU treatment, a generation of reactive oxygen species (ROS) occurs. ROS directly damage cells, tissues, blood vessels and stimulate transcriptions factors, such as nuclear transcription factor-kB (NF-kB), which in turn causes up-regulation of pro-inflammatory cytokines, such as interleukin-1(IL-1), interleukin-6 (IL-6) and tumor necrosis factor alpha (TNF-alfa). Previous reports show that 5-FU induces oral mucositis causing proinflammatory cytokines that stimulate iNOS-derived NO production [7]. The reaction between NO and ROS produces peroxynitrite, a toxic compound that causes lipid peroxidation, oxidation of protein sulfhydryl groups, with tissue injury and local increase of inflammation [7, 29, 30].The increased electrically evoked contraction could also be attributed to tachykininergic components. The increase in gastrointestinal transit occurring during infection is mediated by endogenous tachykinins, which are modulated by the activation of NO biosynthesis [11]. This tachykininergic component is most probably expressed in elderly male patients. In fact, Burcher et al. showed a gender-related difference in receptor density of human colon, with binding capacity (B_{max}) lower in females than in males [12]. An increase in NO is in agreement with reports of an increased plasma nitric oxide after oral administration of anticancer drugs in rats and in disagreement with other reports of a reduced expression of the inducible form of NOS in rats receiving cisplatin and of no change in neural NO synthase (nNOS) expression in patients receiving chemotherapy [13, 15, 16].

It is difficult to explain why the electrically evoked contractile response were greater in males than in females after chemo- and radiotherapy. However, even in the control group, the response to electrical stimulation is greater in males than in females, as we have already shown in previous work [17]. Besides, the response to EFS and L-NAME was lower in females than in males both in CG and in SG, possibly because elderly females are not under the influence of female hormones unlike adult females, as suggested in our previous study [17].

One study hypothesized that advanced age is associated with decreased expression of neuronal NO synthase (nNOS) and concomitant reduction in synthesis of NO in rat colon [31]. That may contribute to explain our findings in females. Other studies showed that estrogens increase endothelial NO synthase (eNOS) [32, 33], but inhibit iNOS [32]. During inflammatory reactions, NO levels, produced by iNOS, increase and this may contribute to local tissue damage [34–37]. This may explain the lack of difference in response to L-NAME group SG in both genders.

In order to explain the increased sensitivity to carbachol and decreased response to EFS and L-NAME in CG female patients we hypothesize a decreased expression of nNOS with concomitant reduction in synthesis of NO [31].

Conclusions

This preliminary in vitro study indicates gender differences in the motor responses of colonic circular muscle strips exposed to cholinergic, histaminergic and electrical stimulation in patients who have received chemotherapy with capecitabine and radiotherapy. Further studies to elucidate the underlying mechanisms are warranted.

Abbrevations

5-FU: Fluorouracil; EFS: Electrically evoked stimulation; eNOS: Endothelial nitric oxide synthase; IL-1: interleukin-1; IL-6: interleukin-6; iNOS: inducible nitric oxide synthase; L-NAME: L-nitro arginine methyl ester; NF-kB: nuclear transcription factor-kB; nNOS: neuronal nitric oxide synthase; NO: nitric oxide; ROS: reactive oxygen species; TNF-alfa: tumor necrosis factor alpha; M: Male; F: Female; SE: standard error; N_2O/O_2: nitrous oxide/oxygen; B_{max}: binding capacity; CI: confidence interval; Ca^{2+}: Calcium ions; i.v.: intravenous

Acknowledgements

We wish to thank Dr. Maria Lucia Caruso for her collaboration as a pathologist.

Author contributions

All authors have reviewed the manuscript for its scientific content and approved its final version. MAM designed the study and drafted the manuscript; AI performed the experiments on muscle strips and analyzed the data; DL contributed to patients' selection, provided surgical specimens and contributed to data collection; FP contributed to patients' selection, provided surgical specimens and contributed to data collection; AS contributed to data analysis; FDP contributed to data analysis and interpretation and reviewed the draft of the manuscript; CS designed the study and drafted the manuscript.

Funding

The project was funded by the Italian Ministry of Health through Grant RO 06.17. The Italian Ministry of Health had no role in the design of the study, collection, analysis, and interpretation of data or in writing the manuscript.

Competing interests

The authors declare that they have no competing interests.

Author details

[1]Experimental Pharmacology Laboratory, National Institute of Gastroenterology "S. de Bellis", Research Hospital - Castellana Grotte (BA), 70013 Castellana Grotte, Italy. [2]Department of Surgery, National Institute of Gastroenterology "S. de Bellis", Research Hospital - Castellana Grotte (BA), 70013 Castellana Grotte, Italy. [3]Department of Medical and Surgical Sciences, University of Bologna, 40126 Bologna, Italy. [4]Department of Internal Medicine and Medical Specialities, University Sapienza, 00161 Rome, Italy.

References

1. Riezzo G, Clemente C, Leo S, Russo F. The role of electrogastrography and gastrointestinal hormones in chemotherapy-related dyspeptic symptoms. J Gastroenterol. 2005;40(12):1107–15.
2. Picard C, Wysocki J, Fioramonti J, Griffiths NM. Intestinal and colonic motor alterations associated with irradiation-induced diarrhoea in rats. Neurogastroenterol Mot. 2001;13(1):19–26.
3. Lockhart PB, Sonis ST. Alterations in the oral mucosa caused by chemotherapeutic agents. A histologic study. J Dermatol Surg Oncol. 1981; 7(12):1019–25.
4. Soares PM, Mota JM, Gomes AS, Oliveira RB, Assreuy AM, Brito GA, Santos AA, Ribeiro RA, Souza MH. Gastrointestinal dysmotility in 5-fluorouracil-induced intestinal mucositis outlasts inflammatory process resolution. Cancer Chemother Pharmacol. 2008;63(1):91–8.
5. Krantis A, Rana K, Harding RK. The effects of γ-radiation on intestinal motor activity and faecal pellet expulsion in the Guinea pig. Dig Dis Sci. 1996; 41(12):2307–16.
6. Summers RW, Hayek B. Changes in colonic motility following abdominal irradiation in dogs. Am J Phys. 1993;264(6 Pt 1):G1024–30.
7. Leitão RF, Ribeiro RA, Bellaguarda EA, Macedo FD, Silva LR, Oriá RB, Vale ML, Cunha FQ, Brito GA. Role of nitric oxide on pathogenesis of 5-fluorouracil induced experimental oral mucositis in hamster. Cancer Chemother Pharmacol. 2007;59(5):603–12.
8. Moreels TG, De Man JG, Bogers JJ, De Winter BY, Vrolix G, Herman AG, Van Marck EA, Pelckmans PA. Effect of Schistosoma mansoni-induced granulomatous inflammation on murine gastrointestinal motility. Am J Physiol Gastrointest Liver Physiol. 2001;280(5):G1030–42.
9. Vermillion DL, Collins SM. Increased responsiveness of jejunal longitudinal muscle in Trichinella-infected rats. Am J Phys. 1988;254(1 Pt 1):G124–9.
10. Pynaert G, Grooten J, van Deventer SJ, Peppelenbosch MP. Cysteinyl leukotrienes mediate histamine hypersensitivity ex vivo by increasing histamine receptor numbers. Mol Med. 1999;5(10):685–92.
11. Martínez-Cuesta MA, Barrachina MD, Beltrán B, Calatayud S, Esplugues J. Nitric oxide modulates the acute increase of gastrointestinal transit induced by endotoxin in rats: a possible role for tachykinins. J Pharm Pharmacol. 1997;49(10):988–90.
12. Burcher E, Shang F, Warner FJ, Du Q, Lubowski DZ, King DW, Liu L. Tachykinin NK2 receptor and functional mechanisms in human colon: changes with indomethacin and in diverticular disease and ulcerative colitis. J Pharmacol Exp Ther. 2008;324(1):170–8.
13. Sung EZ, Arasaradnam RP, Jarvie EM, James S, Goodyear SJ, Borman RA, Snead D, Sanger GJ, Nwokolo CU. Effects of neo-adjuvant chemotherapy for oesophago-gastric cancer on neuro-muscular gastric function. Mol Biol Rep. 2012;39(12):9989–94.
14. Wells RW, Blennerhassett MG. Persistent and selective effects of inflammation on smooth muscle cell contractility in rat colitis. Pflugers Arch. 2004;448(5):515–24.
15. Nagahama S, Korenaga D, Honda M, Inutsuka S, Sugimachi K. Assessment of the intestinal permeability after a gastrectomy and the oral administration or anticancer drugs in rats: nitric oxide release in response to gut injury. Surgery. 2002;131(1 Suppl):S92–7.
16. Wang Y, Aggarwal SK. Effects of cisplatin and taxol on inducible nitric oxide synthase, gastrin and somatostatin in gastrointestinal toxicity. Anti-Cancer Drugs. 1997;8(9):853–8.
17. Maselli MA, Trisolini P, Demma I, Pezzolla F, De Ponti F. Gender- and age-related differences in muscular and nerve-mediated responses in human colon. Dig Dis Sci. 2011;56(2):352–8.
18. Snape WJ Jr, Williams R, Hyman PE. Defect colonic smooth muscle contraction in patients with ulcerative colitis. Am J Phys. 1991;261(6 Pt 1):G987–91.
19. Snape WJ Jr, Kim BH, Willenbucher R, Koelbel CB, Mayer EA Jr, Walsh JH. Differences in the response of proximal and distal rabbit colonic muscle after electrical field stimulation. Gastroenterology. 1989;96(2 Pt 1):321–6.
20. Takeuchi T, Niioka S, Yamaji M, Okishio Y, Ishii T, Nishio H, Takatsuji K, Hata F. Decrease in participation of nitric oxide in nonadrenergic, noncholinergic relaxation of rat intestine with age. Jpn J Pharmacol. 1998;78(3):293–302.
21. Mitolo-Chieppa D, Mansi G, Rinaldi R, Montagnani M, Potenza MA, Genualdo M, Serio M, Mitolo CI, Rinaldi M, Altomare DF, Memeo V.

Cholinergic stimulation and nonadrenergic, noncholinergic relaxation of human colonic circular muscle in idiopathic chronic constipation. Dig Dis Sci. 1998;43(12):2719–26.

22. Snape WJ Jr, Mayer EA, Koelbel CB, Hyman PE, Williams R, Root D. Response of smooth muscle from proximal and distal human colon. Neurogastroenterol Motil. 1989;1:29–34.
23. Maselli MA, Piepoli AL, Guerra V, Caruso ML, Pezzolla F, Lorusso D, Demma I, De Ponti F. Colonic smooth muscle responses in patients with diverticular disease of the colon: effect of the NK2 receptor antagonist SR48968. Dig Liver Dis. 2004;36(5):348–54.
24. Otterson MF, Sarna SK, Moulder JE. Effects of fractionated doses of ionizing radiation on small intestinal motor activity. Gastroenterology. 1998;95(5): 1249–57.
25. Kaur G, Mishra S, Kaur A, Sehgal A, Nageswari KS, Prasad R. Retention of ovaries and oxidative stress of surgery. Int J Gynaecol Obstet. 2007;97(1):40–3.
26. Ma L, Yu Z, Xiao S, Thadani U, Robinson CP, Patterson E. Supersensitivity to serotonin- and histamine-induced arterial contraction following ovariectomy. Eur J Pharmacol. 1998 Oct 23;359(2–3):191–200.
27. Zhang L. Muscarinic receptors in developing rat colon. Eur J Pharmacol. 1996;304(1–3):211–9.
28. Lopes GS, Ferreira AT, Oshiro ME, Vladimirova I, Jurkiewicz NH, Jurkiewicz A, Smaili SS. Aging-related changes of intracellular Ca^{2+} stores and contractile response of intestinal smooth muscle. Exp Gerontol. 2006;41(1):55–62.
29. Rubbo H, Radi R, Trujillo M, Telleri R, Kalyanaraman B, Barnes S, Kirk M, Freeman BA. Nitric oxide regulation of superoxide and peroxynitrite-dependent lipid peroxidation. Formation of novel nitrogen-containing oxidized lipid derivatives. J Biol Chem. 1994;269(42):26066–75.
30. Radi R, Beckman JS, Bush KM, Freeman BA. Peroxynitrite oxidation of sulfhydryls. The cytotoxic potential of superoxide and nitric oxide. J Biol Chem. 1991;266(7):4244–50.
31. Takahashi T, Qoubaitary A, Owyang C, Wiley JW. Decreased expression of nitric oxide synthase in the colonic myenteric plexus of age rats. Brain Res. 2000;883(1):15–21.
32. Orshal JM, Khalil RA. Gender, sex hormones, and vascular tone. Am J Physiol Regul Integr Comp Physiol. 2004;286(2):R233–49.
33. Tostes RC, Nigro D, Fortes ZB, Carvalho MH. Effects of estrogen on the vascular system. Braz J Med Biol Res. 2003;36(9):1143–58.
34. Ajuebor MN, Virág L, Flower RJ, Perretti M, Szabó C. Role of inducible nitric oxide synthase in the regulation of neutrophil migration in zymosan-induced inflammation. Immunology. 1998;95(4):625–30.
35. Brenner T, Brocke S, Szafer F, Sobel RA, Parkinson JF, Perez DH, Steinman L. Inhibition of nitric oxide synthase for treatment of experimental autoimmune encephalomyelitis. J Immunol. 1997;158(6):2940–6.
36. Hierholzer C, Harbrecht B, Menezes JM, Kane J, MacMicking J, Nathan CF, Peitzman AB, Billiar TR, Tweardy DJ. Essential role of induced nitric oxide in the initiation of the inflammatory response after hemorrhagic shock. J Exp Med. 1998;187(6):917–28.
37. Lohinai Z, Benedek P, Fehér E, Györfi A, Rosivall L, Fazekas A, Salzman AL, Szabó C. Protective effects of mercaptoethylguanidine, a selective inhibitor of inducible nitric oxide synthase, in ligature-induced periodontitis in the rat. Br J Pharmacol. 1998;123(3):353–60.

23

Fractal properties and morphological investigation of Nano hydrochlorothiazide is used to treat hypertension

Amir Kazemi Korayem, Shahriar Ghamami* and Zahra Bahrami

Abstract

Purpose: High blood pressure (hypertension) is a relatively common condition that increases blood pressure in the arteries abnormally, causing problems such as heart disease and stroke. Blood pressure is a force that is felt through the walls of the blood vessels and has a direct relationship to the power of pumping the heart and vascular resistance to the blood flow. One of the lowing of blood pressure medications is hydrochlorothiazide (Hctz) which is used to treat high blood pressure and swelling from heart failure, liver damage, and other minor actions.

Procedures: This study explains the effectiveness of Hctz with the help of "fractal dimension". To perfect investigate the fractal dimension, we used the Hctz drug nanoparticle form then using MATLAB software, homogeneity levels or heterogeneity of Nano Hctz using SEM images were computed.

Results: We calculated histogram plot with SEM image by MATLAB software which that its standard deviation was eclose to zero and it can explain that the scattering of data is low and their amount is in one suffering. Fractal dimensions obtained from Matlab and SPSS software for normal distribution, correlation, standard deviation, mean, cumulative frequency and variance analysis were analyzed.

Conclusions: In this research, the association between Hctz treatment effects with the point of view of the fractal dimension of the drug was demonstrated to prove the properties of the drug in the body. in the near future, drug fractal studies can improve the development of new drugs and treatments with minimal cost than clinical approaches by linking chemistry, mathematical sciences and pharmaceutical sciences.

Keywords: Fractal, Cardiac, Hypertension, Hydrochlorothiazide, MATLAB, Drug delivery

Introduction

High blood pressure or blood pressure is one of the most important causes of heart disease and stroke worldwide [1–3]. According to available statistics, about 20% of the adult suffer from high blood pressure [4]. Blood pressure in men is twice that of women [5, 6]. The number of people with high blood pressure is expected to rise to 1.56 billion people worldwide by 2025 [6, 7]. Among the illnesses, blood pressure is known as a silent killer because it has no warning signs, and many people are not aware of it [8–10]. The increasing prevalence of the disease is attributable to lifestyle and dietary factors such as physical inactivity, acute stress, intensive exercise, alcohol and smoking, and a high sodium diet (usually from Processed and fatty foods) is shown in Fig. 1 [11–16]. Blood pressure increase in the morning. When blood pressure is measured in the morning, high blood pressure is associated with an increased risk of stroke and heart disease [17]. Drugs are generally started as monotherapy (just one drug) and at a low-dose [18]. Side-effects associated with antihypertensive drugs are usually minor [19–21]. Hctz is one of the drugs used to treat high blood pressure [4, 22].

Geometric shapes (circle, triangle, square, straight line, polygon, etc.) are quite familiar with Euclidean geometry, which actually help us to better classify our surroundings. However, the truth is that the visible nature does not have an Euclidean geometry, in other words, the real world shapes are not Euclidean! In fact, the

* Correspondence: shghammamy@yahoo.com
Department of Chemistry, Faculty of Science, Imam Khomeini International University, Qazvin 34148-96818, Iran

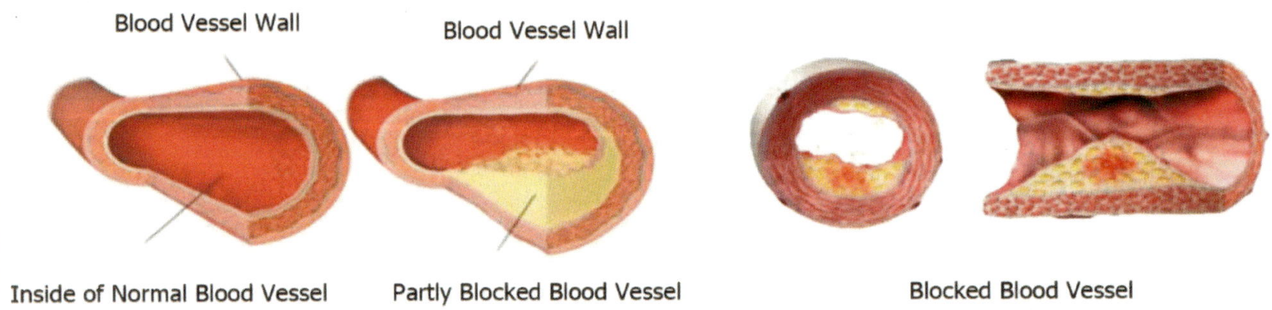

Fig. 1 Hypertension happens when the force on the walls of blood vessels from the blood within them is more than normal

geometry that can describe our world is called fractal geometry [23]. In fact, fractals have three characteristics from a geometric point of view:

1. Self-similar.
2. On a small scale, they are complex.
3. Dimension is not an integer (for example, 1.51).

But fractal calculations:

Contrarily, fractals do not have correct dimensions. When the dimension of a fractal it is said to be 1.2, it means that it is more complex than a line, and simpler than a page. Calculation of this dimension is obtained after a series of logarithmic formulas [24]. If the dimension along a line is equal to one, then the dimension of a page is equal to two, and the space dimension is three. An example of the fractal is presented herein using math intuition.

The Koch Snowflake!

Consider the equilateral triangle. Step by step:

- Draw an equilateral triangle.
- Divide each side into three equal parts.
- Draw an equilateral triangle on each middle part.
- Divide each outer side into thirds.
- Draw an equilateral triangle on each middle part.
- Repeat until you're satisfied with the number of iterations.

Decorate your snowflake how you like it. Regularly, it is performed repeatedly to have fractal shapes (Fig. 2).

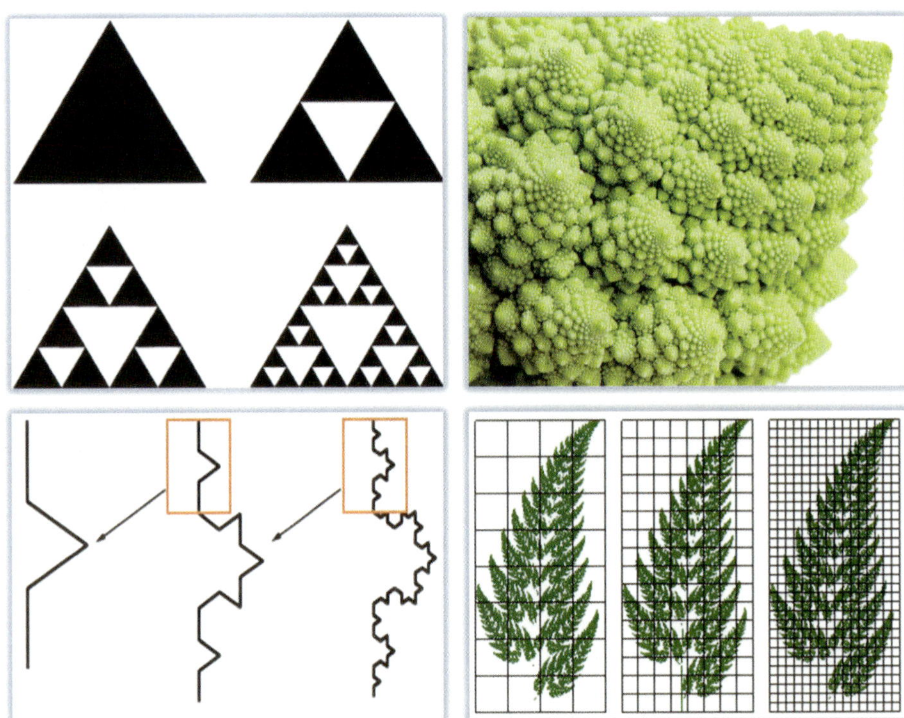

Fig. 2 Example of branching fractals, Selfsame Fractal Zoom-Zones, showing the structural elements, or elementary geometrical units

In nanoscale, many self-assembly processes create fractal patterns. Fractals are shapes that are repeated in many magnifications and are common throughout nature and appear in the natural environment, biological systems, and human physiology. As a biological example, the dendritic structure of the human neuron is a nanoscale nerve structure and uses this Fractal geometry connectivity to generate advanced information processing [25, 26]. The same connection can also be used with the use of artificial fractal electrical circuits for future commercial computers. By combining nano and fractal, many of the surrounding events can be justified. Regarding nanotechnology, drugs can with improved physical and chemical properties, such as high reactivity and the ability to select a cell membrane from pathogenic bacteria, can be produced [27]. Many fields are exciting at the start of this journey to improve the basic quality of human life. Fractal Property is a physical characteristic that is expressed at the supermolecular level, on a microscopic scale and on a macroscopic scale. To calculate fractal dimensions, image processing is performed in divided windows using MATLAB. This software can display a binary image with the characteristics of fractal nanoparticles. Fractal Geometry has recently been recognized as an analytical tool suitable for describing nanostructures. Also, fractals are infinitely complex models that are self-similar across different scales [28, 29]. The fractal dimension parameter is determined by calculating the predicted perimeter length by taking steps of a known length along the border and including the number of scales [30, 31].

One of the good applications of the fractal can be the development of anticancer drugs and this drug discovery. Cancer tumor cells exhibit irregular, heterogeneous, and very distinct structures, and therefore we have difficulty in making effective anticancer drugs [32, 33]. Fractal models can be used in nonhomogeneous systems and non-Fickian processes in pharmacokinetic models, such as cancer drugs [34].

Experimental

Materials and methods

Starting materials were obtained from Merck (Berlin, Germany) and used without further purification. The surface morphology of the product was characterized by a field emission scanning electron microscope (FESEM) (Hitachi S 4160, Japan) with an accelerating voltage of 20 kV. The size of selected samples was estimated using the Scherer method. For identification, FESEM samples were coated with gold. This is essentially a function in MATLAB (MathWorks, Natick, Massachusetts, USA) as a powerful software application widely used for data design and analysis e, programming and execution of engineering and research calculations. Thus, MATLAB data were analyzed with statistical packages to discuss statistical aspects and provide comparable results from this study (SPSS, IBM, Armonk, NewYork, USA). To obtain quantitative and qualitative information related to each image in addition to RGB, Histogram MATLAB scales were determined for the images, which shows the symmetry and/or asymmetry as well as the uniformity/non-uniformity between points on the image. The graphs determine differences between different parts of an image.

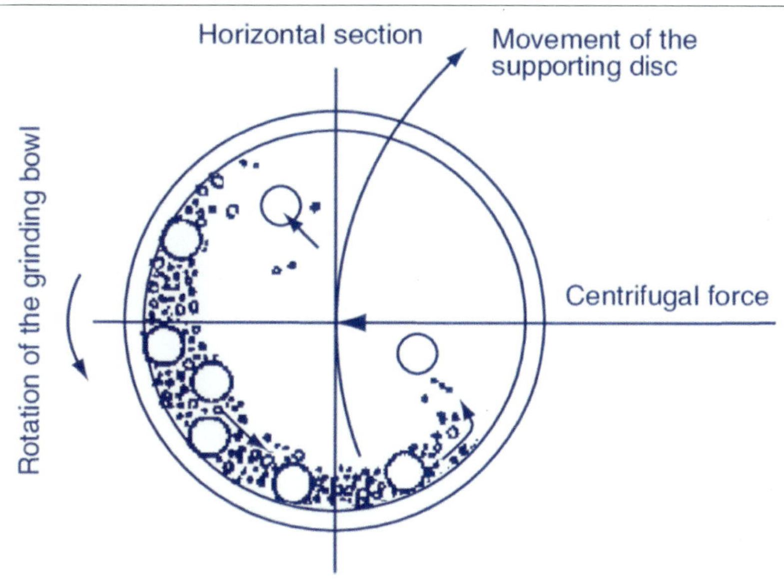

Fig. 3 Planetary ball mill process

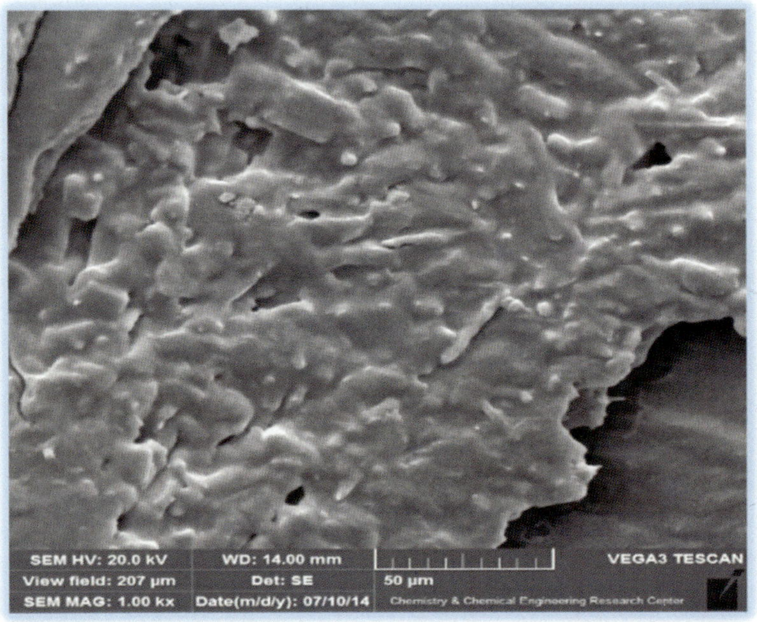

Fig. 4 SEM images of hydrochlorothiazide

Synthesis of Nano Hctz ($C_7H_8ClN_3O_4S_2$) is used to treat hypertension

Nanoscale particles were produced using the "top-down" method in this study. In this method, the particles are miniaturized by grinding to a nanometer size. The appropriate tool for this method is a ball mill process (Fig. 3). In order to make a nanoparticle in a ball mill, the grinding jar and balls should be made of an abrasion-resistant material such as ZrO_2 to minimize contamination of the sample material by abrasion. In this device, the rotation of the chamber and a plate around a single axis creates a force from the center that can reach 20 times the acceleration of gravity [35]. The drug was first placed in an oven at 70 °C for 1 h. Then, the dry drug was poured into a mill cup containing 15 different-sized metal-polymeric balls. It took around 5 hrs to become a nanoscale [36, 37].

Computational method

Twenty-five sections of SEM images were selected and their fractal dimensions calculated using MATLAB software. Then, fractal computations were transferred to SPSS software to analyze normal distribution, correlation, standard deviation, mean, cumulative frequency and variance [38]. Given the resulting numbers, we drew a logarithmic diagram in which the vertical and horizontal axes were log $(1/r)$ and log Nr, respectively, and Coefficient of the size as the box was 1.3. We used a program written in MATLAB to calculate the fractal dimension [39]. There are several methods for calculating the fractal definition, including (1) the self similarly definition [40], (2) the mass fractal dimension, (3) the spare-sphere fractal dimension, (4) the Euclid dimension, (5) the grid style, (6) an analytical approach for fractal diminishing, and (7) the box-counting fractal dimension. In this study, the self-similar method was used to determine the fractal dimension of FESEM images, which was analyzed using the box-counting method [41–43]. A variety of methods are used to estimate fractal dimensions. Due to the ease of mathematical calculation and empirical estimation, boxthe -counting dimension is one of the most widely used dimension assessment to determine the fractal dimension of different phenomena. The characteristics of this method include ample algorithm, a high precision with a relatively smaller grid selection, and usability in higher

Table 1 Chart analysis of fractal dimension boxes Hydrochlorothiazide

Log(res)	Log (boxnum)
0	9.93
0.6931	8.898
1.386	8.021
2.079	6.978
2.773	6.112
3.466	5.157
5.545	2.293
6.238	1.339

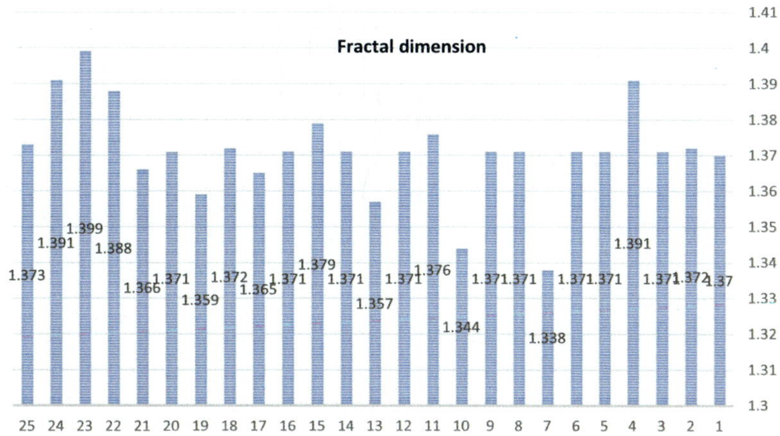

Fig. 5 Statistical values of the selected Hydrochlorothiazide nanoparticles

pixels. The fractal dimension was calculated theoretically by applying the following formula:

$$D = \lim_{r \to 0} \frac{\log Nr}{\log(1/r)} \quad (1)$$

Where D is the fractal dimension and $N\,r$ is the number of squares including a part of the considered fractal dimensions [44]. For the box-counting fractal dimension, we assumed that F is a nonempty and bounded subset of Rn and we supposed that (F) is the fewest number of collections witha maximum dimension of (r) that can cover (F). The box-counting dimensions under and above (F): if they are equal we say they are equal to the box-counting dimension or the F box dimension; then we define:

$$\dim_{B} F = \lim_{r \to 0} \frac{\log Nr(F)}{-\log(r)} \quad (2)$$

The circle of cubes in r coordinates from Rn implies cubes in the following form:

If $[m1r,(m1+1)r] \times \cdots \times [mnr,(mn+1)r]$, then $mn,\ldots,m1$ are integers.

Finally, $Nr\sqrt{(F)} \leq Nr'(F)$.

If $r\sqrt{n} < 1$,

Then

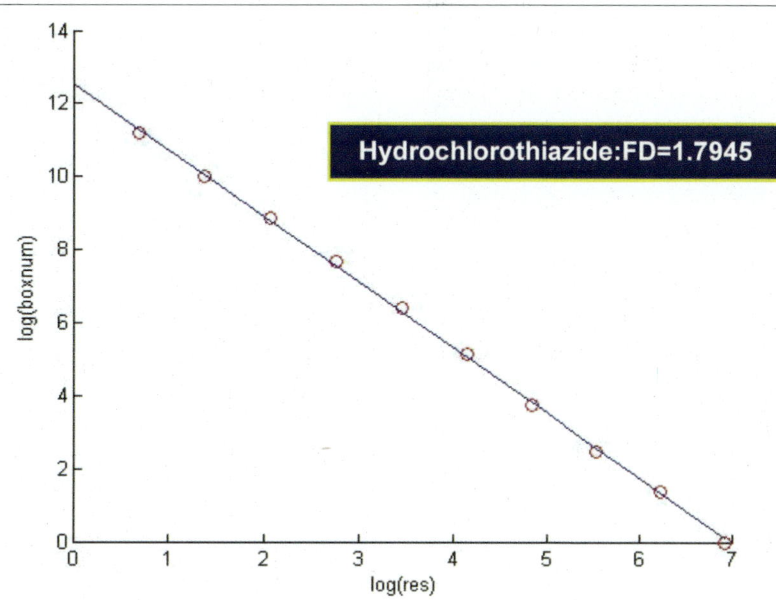

Fig. 6 Chart analysis of fractal dimension boxes hydrochlorothiazide

$$\frac{\log Nr\sqrt{(F)}}{\log (r\sqrt{n})} \leq \frac{\log Nr'(F)}{(-\log\sqrt{n} - \log r)} \quad (3)$$

If we limit $\dim_B F = \frac{\lim}{r \to 0} \frac{\log Nr'(F)}{-\log r.}$

Then

$$\dim_B F \leq \lim_{r \to 0} \frac{\log Nr'(F)}{-\log r} \quad (4)$$

Finally: $N_r'(F) \leq 3^n N_r(F)$.

Results

Analysis of the effective factors for creating the Nanodrug

It should be noted that the ball milling technique (as one of the high-to-low methods) was used to make nano Hctz [45]. which was confirmed through the analysis of SEM images taken from the sample. The SEM image (Fig. 4) shows that the particles are less than 100 nm confirming the formation of nano Hctz. Then, fractal dimensions were calculated 20 randomly selected SEM images using MATLAB software. For this fractal dimension, the standard image, average, maximum and minimum range histogram, asymmetry and also harmonics were obtained using SPSS software [46, 47].

Morphological properties

The images are taken from the outer structure and the morphological structure of the sample show that the nanopowder is made of very dense, porous and cavity holes, and its spherical particles are below 100 nm; The larger particles observed in the images, in fact, are the accumulation of smaller particles that appear in an irregular spherical shape [48]. The SEM images of the Nano Hctz are shown in Fig. 4. cumulative percentages are a simple way to compare different sets of data.

Analysis using MATLAB and SPSS data

The statistical and numerical interpretation of fractal dimensions is given in Table 1. According to FESEM images, fractal dimensions separated from the image are calculated. With the point of view, sometimes when the same value appears more than once, it is repeated as the frequency of a known number. The cumulative frequency was used to determine the number of explanations below or above a specific value. The total frequency of all modules calculated below the upper-class class is the cumulative frequency of that class, which adds a class interval to the frequency and frequencies of the first distances to the distance of that class. This is a different method for expressing frequency distribution. Figure 5 shows mean (1.919), median, maximum (1.399), minimum (1.338), range (0.94), variance (0.000174), standard deviation (0.013209), and skewness obtained for fractal dimension data using SPSS software.

Table 2 Correlation coefficient calculated between the points on the graph nano hydrochlorothiazide

Correlations*	LOGres	LOGboxnum
LOGres		
Pearson Correlation	1	−1.000
Sig. (2-tailed)		.000
N	8	8
LOGboxnum		
Pearson Correlation	−1.000	1
Sig. (2-tailed)	.000	
N	8	8

*Correlation is significant at the 0.01 level (2-tailed)

Discussion

There is a large deviation from the normal distribution in the assumptions of normal errors, all of which are shown by statistical calculations and calculated intervals for regression, and its value can have understandable effects on the accuracy of the results. A simple method for controlling error assumptions will normally be distributed if the likelihood of a probability fraction (PP) is correctly recognized by the software, also if it is accepted that the line is based on a normal assumption. The numerical value of RGB is calculated in the same amount of porous holes in dark and bright images. In the images of all images, dark areas with numbers less than 0.5 and 0.5 points are clearly displayed with more. Figure 6 shows the calculated dimension of nano box Hctz.

The distribution of pp. was obtained using a statistical statistic of the data. According to the results, the data on a line indicates that the population is normal. Nano-fractal dimensions of the drug were calculated as 1.371. The location was found anywhere in the chart using the MATLAB software (Table 1). Input (res) or X

Table 3 Regression coefficient nano hydrochlorothiazide

Coefficients [a] Model		Unstandardized Coefficients		Standardized Coefficients	t	Sig.
		B	Std. Error	Beta		
1	(Constant)	9.892	.023		432.537	.000
	LOGres	−1.371	.007	−1.000	−207.737	.000

[a] Dependent Variable: LOGboxnum

Table 4 Calculate the number of maximum, minimum, average and uncertainty of data related to nano hydrochlorothiazide

Residuals Statistics [a]	Minimum	Maximum	Mean	Std. Deviation	N
Predicted Value	1.34056	9.89152	6.09100	3.047221	8
Residual	−.063656	.038483	.000000	.035931	8
Std. Predicted Value	−1.559	1.247	.000	1.000	8
Std. Residual	−1.640	.992	.000	.926	8

[a] Dependent Variable: LOGboxnum

is an independent variable in this graph. This factor represents 1 / r, the size of the box image. Login (box num) is an associated variable or Y, which indicates the number of boxes (box-counting method) to obtain the position of these points. Obviously, the difference for each image in the log (box num) will produce a fractal pattern in each selected image. Regardless of the unrestrained and orderly images, a special order or pattern is carefully obtained in the figures.

The correlation coefficient between the points' data (Table 1) in our software SPSS was obtained using Pearson's correlation coefficient.

After obtaining the correlation coefficient, data were used for linear regression analysis of the charges (Table 2). The line slope was calculated narrowly as 1.371 with MATLAB and then computed by the software. Charts intercept was 9.892. Table 3 represents the obtained maximum and minimum values as well as uncertainty data.

The linear equation was obtained for the nano-medicine using Table 4.

$$\text{Log (box num)} = -1.371\ \text{Log(res)} + 9.892$$

As you can see, placing data on a straight line indicates that this is a normal population.

In RGB images, the brightness of each part of the image was processed and matched with MATLAB software. According to RG tables and images, none of them larger than half are not characteristic of the bright points of the image, while none of the half RG of the image is displayed in the image. RG Distribution of different points of the image, shown in Fig. 7.

Conclusion

The primary purpose of this study is to prove the fractal behavior of Nano drugs Pharmacy and Medicine Knowledge. In this research, after nano-making of a Hctz drug, the fractal dimensions of the nanoparticle were calculated and the results were entered into the SPSS software for statistical analysis. Subsequently, using MATLAB software, homogeneity levels or heterogeneity of Nano Hctz using SEM images were investigated. After calculation, it was found that the produced particles are not homogeneous and their size and morphology are different. The results show that the differences in magnification and reduction of SEM images cause distinctions in fractal dimensions. The nano Htze fractal indicates that its standard deviation is close to zero, and if the standard deviation of the data is close to zero or exactly zero, then it can be argued that the scattering of data is

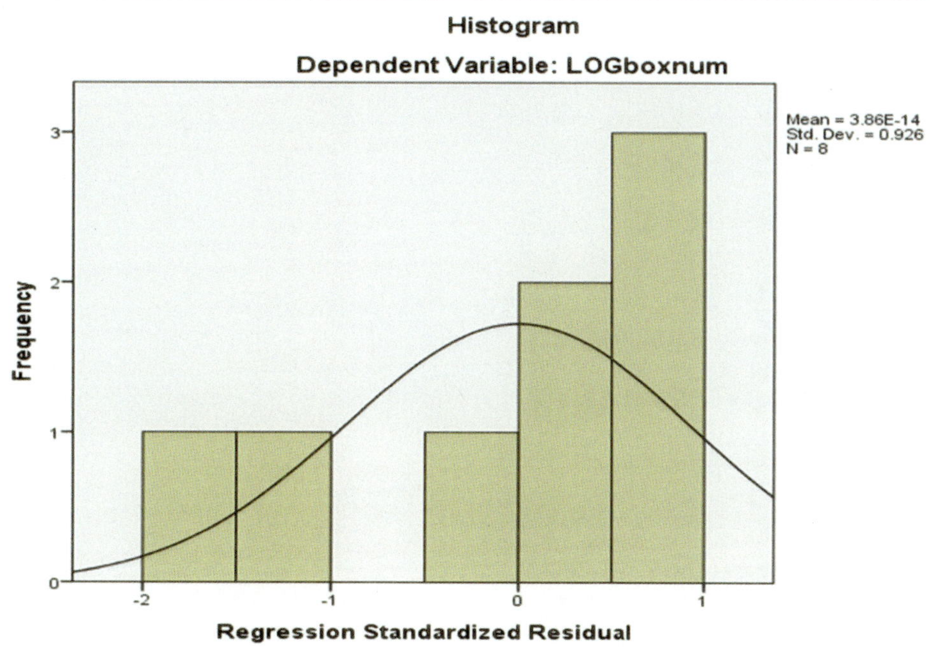

Fig. 7 Histograms of the nano hydrochlorothiazide

low and their amount is in one suffering. In scientific studies, data with a difference of more than two standard deviations from the mean value are usually considered as offset data and removed from the analysis. Some of the properties of Hctz, such as the beneficial effects of therapy, drug delivery, and medication degrees in the body, can be proven by studying and calculating fractal behavior, A research from this perspective, which was done for the first time, can be extensible for other drugs in medicine. We believe that in the not too distant future, fractal studies will be an effective tool for classifying drugs, diseases and tumors and will create a new horizon for disease prevention and treatment. Obviously, this type of study is much Cheaper and less risky than clinical studies.

Abbreviations

Hctz: Hydrochlorothiazide; SEM: Scanning electron microscope

Acknowledgments

The authors gratefully acknowledge the financial support of the Research Council of the International University Imam Khomeini.

Funding

Not applicable.

Authors' contributions

AK synthesized Nano medication and analyzed and interpreted fractal dimension with Nano hydrochlorothiazide (Hctz) which is used to treat high blood pressure, also explained the effectiveness of Hctz with the help of fractal dimension and was a major contributor in writing the manuscript. SG importing and processing the SPSS and MATLAB software information with SEM image and analyzed the relationship between fractal dimension, extracted images and software outputs. ZB conducted studies on heart disease and blood pressure in different people, especially elderly and athletes and also made numerical calculations of the fractal dimension in this manuscript. All authors read and approved the final manuscript.

Competing interests

The authors declare that they have no competing interests.

References

1. Christe V, Waeber G, Vollenweider P, Marques-vidal P. Antihypertensive drug treatment changes in the general population: the CoLaus study. BMC Pharmacol Toxicol. 2014;15:20.
2. Keil U. Coronary artery disease: the role of lipids, hypertension and smoking. Basic Res Cardiol. 2000;95:I52–8.
3. Kendall M. Hypertension in the elderly. Basic Res Cardiol. 1998;93:s043.
4. Chobanian AV, Bakris GL, Black HR, Cushman WC, Green LA, Izzo JL, Jones DW, Materson BJ, Oparil S, Wright JT. Seventh report of the joint national committee on prevention, detection, evaluation, and treatment of high blood pressure. hypertension. 2003;42:1206–52.
5. Rivas M, Garay RP, Escanero JF, Cia P, Alda JO. Soy milk lowers blood pressure in men and women with mild to moderate essential hypertension. J Nutr. 2002;132:1900–2.
6. Haapanen N, Miilunpalo S, Vuori I, Oja P, Pasanen M. Association of leisure time physical activity with the risk of coronary heart disease, hypertension and diabetes in middle-aged men and women. Int J Epidemiol. 1997;26: 739–47.
7. Bakris GL, Ritz E. The message for world kidney day 2009: hypertension and kidney disease: a marriage that should be prevented. J Clin Hypert. 2009;11: 144–7.
8. Moore J. Hypertension: catching the silent killer. Nurse Pract. 2005;30:16–35.
9. Sawicka K, Szczyrek M, Jastrzebska I, Prasal M, Zwolak A, Daniluk J. Hypertension–the silent killer. J Pre-Clin Clin Res. 2011;5.
10. Kawasoe S, Maruguchi Y, Kajiya S, Uenomachi H, Miyata M, Kawasoe M, Kubozono T, Ohishi M. Mechanism of the blood pressure-lowering effect of sodium-glucose cotransporter 2 inhibitors in obese patients with type 2 diabetes. BMC Pharmacol Toxicol. 2017;18:23.
11. Iestra J, Kromhout D, Van der Schouw Y, Grobbee D, Boshuizen H, Van Staveren W. Effect size estimates of lifestyle and dietary changes in all-cause mortality in coronary artery disease patients. Circulation. 2005;112:924–34.
12. Gupta R, Joshi P, Mohan V, Reddy K, Yusuf S. Epidemiology and causation of coronary heart disease and stroke in India. Heart. 2008;94:16–26.
13. Kaplan NM. Kaplan's clinical hypertension. Lippincott Williams & Wilkins; 2010.
14. Boden-Albala B, Sacco RL. Lifestyle factors and stroke risk: exercise, alcohol, diet, obesity, smoking, drug use, and stress. Curr Atheroscler Rep. 2000;2: 160–6.
15. Stampfer MJ, Hu FB, Manson JE, Rimm EB, Willett WC. Primary prevention of coronary heart disease in women through diet and lifestyle. N Engl J Med. 2000;343:16–22.
16. Kaplan GA, Keil JE. Socioeconomic factors and cardiovascular disease: a review of the literature. Circulation. 1993;88:1973–98.
17. Nayak UY, Shavi GV, Nayak Y, Averinen RK, Mutalik S, Reddy SM, Gupta PD, Udupa N. Chronotherapeutic drug delivery for early morning surge in blood pressure: a programmable delivery system. J Control Release. 2009;136:125–31.
18. Benz J, Black H, Graff A, Reed A, Fitzsimmons S, Shi Y. Valsartan and hydrochlorothiazide in patients with essential hypertension. A multiple dose, double-blind, placebo controlled trial comparing combination therapy with monotherapy. J Hum Hypertens. 1998;12.
19. Soffer BA, Wright JT, Pratt JH, Wiens B, Goldberg AI, Sweet CS. Effects of losartan on a background of hydrochlorothiazide in patients with hypertension. Hypertension. 1995;26:112–7.
20. Koch-Weser J. Vasodilator drugs in the treatment of hypertension. Arch Intern Med. 1974;133:1017–27.
21. Collins R, Peto R, MacMahon S, Godwin J, Qizilbash N, Hebert P, Eberlein K, Taylor J, Hennekens C, Fiebach N. Blood pressure, stroke, and coronary heart disease: part 2, short-term reductions in blood pressure: an overview of randomised drug trials in their epidemiological context. Lancet. 1990;335: 827–38.
22. Messerli FH, Makani H, Benjo A, Romero J, Alviar C, Bangalore S. Antihypertensive efficacy of hydrochlorothiazide as evaluated by ambulatory blood pressure monitoring: a meta-analysis of randomized trials. J Am Coll Cardiol. 2011;57:590–600.
23. Kazemi Korayem A, Ghamami S, Bahrami Z. Fractal properties and morphological investigation of nano-amiodarone using image processing. SIViP. 2018.
24. Theiler J. Estimating fractal dimension. JOSA A. 1990;7:1055–73.
25. Khire TS, Kundu J, Kundu SC, Yadavalli VK. The fractal self-assembly of the silk protein sericin. Soft Matter. 2010;6:2066–71.
26. Rothemund PW, Papadakis N, Winfree E. Algorithmic self-assembly of DNA Sierpinski triangles. PLoS Biol. 2004;2:e424.
27. Bueno J. Antimicrobial models in nanotechnology: from the selection to application in the control and treatment of infectious diseases. In: Nanotechnology in diagnosis, treatment and prophylaxis of infectious diseases. 2015. p. 19–38.
28. Leland WE, Taqqu MS, Willinger W, Wilson DV. On the self-similar nature of Ethernet traffic (extended version). IEEE/ACM Trans Networking. 1994;2:1–15.

29. Demetzos C, Pippa N. Fractal geometry as a new approach for proving nanosimilarity: a reflection note. Int J Pharm. 2015;483:1–5.
30. Russ JC. Fractal surfaces: Springer Science & Business Media; 2013.
31. Klinkenberg B. A review of methods used to determine the fractal dimension of linear features. Math Geol. 1994;26:23–46.
32. Jean-Quartier C, Jeanquartier F, Jurisica I, Holzinger A. In silico cancer research towards 3R. BMC Cancer. 2018;18:408.
33. Pereira LM. Fractal pharmacokinetics. Comput Math methods Med. 2010;11: 161–84.
34. Pang KS, Weiss M, Macheras P. Advanced pharmacokinetic models based on organ clearance, circulatory, and fractal concepts. AAPS J. 2007;9:E268–83.
35. EGe A, Senna M, Kosova N. Soft mechanochemical synthesis: a basis for new chemical technologies. In: Springer Science & Business Media; 2001.
36. Vickers G, Quan K. Ball-mills versus end-mills for curved surface machining. J Eng Ind. 1989;111:22–6.
37. Mishra B, Rajamani RK. The discrete element method for the simulation of ball mills. Appl Math Model. 1992;16:598–604.
38. Mathews JH, Fink KD. Numerical methods using MATLAB. London: Pearson; 2004.
39. Lynch S. Dynamical systems with applications using MATLAB: Boston: Birkhäuser; 2004.
40. Neimark AV. Calculating surface fractal dimensions of adsorbents. Adsorpt Sci Technol. 1990;7:210–9.
41. Yang R, He S, Yi J, Hu Q. Nano-scale pore structure and fractal dimension of organic-rich Wufeng-Longmaxi shale from Jiaoshiba area, Sichuan Basin: investigations using FE-SEM, gas adsorption and helium pycnometry. Mar Pet Geol. 2016;70:27–45.
42. Rodrigues Costa CA, Paula Leite CA, Fátima de Souza E, Galembeck F. Size effects on the microchemistry and plasticity of Stöber silica particles: a study using EFTEM, FESEM, and AFM-SEPM microscopies. Langmuir. 2001;17:189–94.
43. Jiao K, Yao S, Liu C, Gao Y, Wu H, Li M, Tang Z. The characterization and quantitative analysis of nanopores in unconventional gas reservoirs utilizing FESEM–FIB and image processing: an example from the lower Silurian Longmaxi shale, upper Yangtze region, China. Int J Coal Geol. 2014;128:1–11.
44. Packard NH, Crutchfield JP, Farmer JD, Shaw RS. Geometry from a time series. Phys Rev Lett. 1980;45:712.
45. Czekai DA, Seaman LP. Method of grinding pharmaceutical substances. In: Book Method of grinding pharmaceutical substances (editor ed.^eds.). City: Google Patents; 1999.
46. Coakes SJ, Steed L. SPSS: Analysis without anguish using SPSS version 14.0 for Windows. Wiley; 2009.
47. Verma J. Data analysis in management with SPSS software. Springer Science & Business Media; 2012.
48. Van Den Boomgaard R, Smeulders A. The morphological structure of images: the differential equations of morphological scale-space. IEEE Trans Pattern Anal Mach Intell. 1994;16:1101–13.

24

Anesthetic-sensitive ion channel modulation is associated with a molar water solubility cut-off

Robert J. Brosnan* and Trung L. Pham

Abstract

Background: NMDA receptor modulation by hydrocarbons is associated with a molar water solubility cut-off. Low-affinity phenolic modulation of $GABA_A$ receptors is also associated with a cut-off, but at much lower molar solubility values. We hypothesized that other anesthetic-sensitive ion channels exhibit distinct cut-off effects associated with hydrocarbon molar water solubility, and that cut-off values are comparatively similar between related receptors than phylogenetically distant ones.

Methods: Glycine or $GABA_A$ receptors or TREK-1, TRESK, $Na_v1.2$, or $Na_v1.4$ channels were expressed separately in frog oocytes. Two electrode voltage clamp techniques were used to study current responses in the presence and absence of hydrocarbon series from eight functional groups with progressively increasing size at saturated aqueous concentrations. Null response (cut-off) was defined by current measurements that were statistically indistinguishable between baseline and hydrocarbon exposure.

Results: Ion channels exhibited cut-off effects associated with hydrocarbon molar water solubility in the following order of decreasing solubility: $Na_v1.2 \approx Na_v1.4 \gtrsim$ TRESK $\approx$ TREK-1 > $GABA_A$ >> glycine. Previously measured solubility cut-off values for NMDA receptors were intermediate between those for $Na_v1.4$ and TRESK.

Conclusions: Water solubility cut-off responses were present for all anesthetic-sensitive ion channels; distinct cut-off effects may exist for all cell surface receptors that are sensitive to volatile anesthetics. Suggested is the presence of amphipathic receptor sites normally occupied by water molecules that have dissociation constants inversely related to the cut-off solubility value. Poorly soluble hydrocarbons unable to reach concentrations sufficient to out-compete water for binding site access fail to modulate the receptor.

Keywords: Anesthesia, Mechanism, Ion channel, Electrophysiology, Aliphatic

Background

Protein-ligand interactions are commonly described using a "lock-and-key" model in which the protein and ligand have to fit together to have a chemical effect [1]. Although inhaled anesthetics are presumed to exert their effects through ion channels and cell surface receptor proteins, the diverse nature of both anesthetic ligands and the proteins they modulate challenge assumptions of a conserved complementary structure [2, 3]. Current and historical inhaled anesthetics include single atoms, triatomic molecules, various alkanes (with and without halogens), various ethers (with and without halogens), and various alkenes (with and without halogens); experimental inhaled anesthetics demonstrate even greater structural variety. Hence, these drugs act as structurally diverse keys that each can open the same lock. Moreover, a single inhaled anesthetic can allosterically modulate function of a large number of structurally diverse and phylogenetically unrelated ion channels—including many different ligand-gated ion channels, voltage-gated ion channels, and leak channels—and cell surface receptors—including many different channel-linked receptors, enzyme-linked receptors, and G protein-coupled receptors. Hence, these agents also act like a key that can open many different locks.

* Correspondence: rjbrosnan@ucdavis.edu
Department of Surgical and Radiological Sciences, School of Veterinary Medicine, University of California, One Shields Avenue, Davis, CA 95616, USA

Inhaled anesthetics typically have high median effective concentrations consistent with low-affinity target interactions [4], and these agents can bind multiple amphipathic sites on a protein of which at least some may be associated with water molecules [5]. Anesthetic modulation of protein function firstly depends upon the presence of an agent in sufficient concentration to desolvate, displace weakly-bound water molecules within an allosteric binding site, and only then bind to the allosteric site. We postulate that drugs with insufficient water solubility to competitively displace water from this amphipathic allosteric site would be unable to bind and modulate the protein—a cut-off effect—even at a saturated aqueous phase drug concentration. These low-affinity amphipathic drug-receptor interactions could be associated with different hydrocarbon solubility cut-off values for different proteins since the water dissociation constants within critical allosteric sites could also be different for different proteins. In support, N-methyl-d-aspartate (NMDA) receptor whole-cell currents are unchanged by saturated concentrations of organic compounds once the hydrocarbon ω-end or ring size is increased such that the predicted molar water solubility is less than approximately 1.1 mM; yet these same hydrocarbons still are able to allosterically modulate γ-aminobutyric acid receptor type A ($GABA_A$) currents [6]. However, $GABA_A$ receptors may have their own hydrocarbon cut-off, as $GABA_A$ receptor whole-cell currents are unchanged by a series of substituted phenol and benzene rings once the predicted molar water solubility of these compounds is less than 0.1 mM [7].

We hypothesize that cut-off effects associated with molar water solubility is a generalizable feature of inhaled anesthetic-sensitive ion channels and receptors. As a test, we evaluated responses of anesthetic-sensitive channels and receptors to eight different functional groups of organic compounds, differing only by carbon additions to the ω-end of a chain or to a ring, so that we could study compounds of different molecular volumes and carbon atoms but similar molar water solubility values (and vice versa) and therefore distinguish between effects caused by drug size versus solubility. Although inhaled anesthetics bind many different proteins, we studied six channels and receptors reported to contribute to immobilizing effects in vivo: voltage-gated sodium channels type II and type IV ($Na_v1.2$ and $Na_v1.4$), [8] TWIK-related spinal cord channel (TRESK) [9], TWIK-related potassium channel type I (TREK-1) [10], $GABA_A$ receptors [11], and glycine receptors [12].

Methods

Oocyte collection

Adult female *Xenopus laevis* vivarium-maintained frogs (Xenopus Express, Brooksville, FL) were anesthetized with chilled 0.2% buffered tricaine, surgically ovariectomized, and were either administered morphine analgesia and recovered from anesthesia (first ovariectomy) or euthanized (second ovariectomy) by decapitation and double pithing while anesthetized. The theca externa and mesovarium of the removed ovary were disrupted manually, and oocytes were defolliculated enzymatically by use of 0.2% collagenase. Oocytes were stored in a modified Barth's electrolyte solution until ready for use. This protocol was approved by the Institutional Animal Care and Use Committee at the University of California, Davis.

Receptor expression

Each anesthetic-sensitive receptor type was separately expressed in different oocytes by injecting plasmids containing sequences for receptor subunits which were provided as gifts from the laboratory of R. Adron Harris (University of Texas, Austin). All plasmids were sequenced and their identity confirmed by comparison to National Center for Biotechnology Information databases. Human voltage-gated Type II sodium channels ($Na_v1.2$) were expressed by intracytoplasmic injection of 5 ng RNA per oocyte containing the SCN2A gene; human voltage gated Type IV sodium channels ($Na_v1.4$) were similarly expressed using RNA encoding the SCN4A gene. The human TRESK channel ($K_{2P}18.1$) was expressed by intracytoplasmic injection of 5 ng RNA per oocyte containing the KCNK18 gene; the human TREK-1 channel ($K_{2P}2.1$), was similarly expressed using RNA encoding the KCNK2 gene. Heterotrimeric $GABA_A$ receptors were expressed by a 1 ng oocyte intranuclear co-injection of three different plasmids containing cytomegalovirus promoters and coding DNA for one of thee subunits—human α_1 (GABRA1), rat β_2 (GABRB2), or rat γ_{2s} (GABRG2 short)—in a 1:1:10 ratio to ensure incorporation of the γ-subunit; this was confirmed by demonstrating receptor potentiation to 10 μM chlordiazepoxide during co-application with GABA. Glycine receptors were expressed by intracytoplasmic injection of 5 ng RNA per oocyte containing the gene for the human glycine α_1 subunit (GLRA1). Nuclease-free water-injected oocytes served as negative controls for all experiments.

Electrophysiology studies

Oocytes were incubated at 18 °C for 1–4 days in fresh and filtered modified Barth's solution composed of 88 mM NaCl, 1 mM KCl, 2.4 mM NaHCO3, 20 mM HEPES, 0.82 mM $MgSO_4$, 0.33 mM $Ca(NO_3)_2$, 0.41 mM $CaCl_2$, 5 mM sodium pyruvate, gentamycin, penicillin, streptomycin, and corrected to pH = 7.4. All salts and antibiotics were A.C.S. grade (Fisher Scientific, Pittsburgh, PA). Oocytes were studied in a 250 μL linear-flow chamber perfused with frog Ringer's (FR) solution composed of 115 mM NaCl, 2.5 mM KCl, 1.8 mM $CaCl_2$, and 10 mM HEPES prepared in 18.2 MΩ H2O and filtered and adjusted to pH = 7.4. All solutions were delivered to the perfusion chamber via a syringe pump with gastight glass syringes and foil-wrapped Teflon tubing.at a rate of 1.5 ml/min. Oocytes were impaled by two 3 M KCl-filled 0.2–1 MΩ borosilicate glass electrodes (KG-33, King Precision Glass, Claremont, CA) connected to separate headstages (Axon Instruments HS2A, Molecular Devices, San Jose, CA) through which voltage was measured and current was passed by use of a computer-controlled amplifier (Axon Instruments GeneClamp 500B, Molecular Devices, San Jose, CA) [6].

For oocytes expressing Na_v channels, the cell transmembrane potential was clamped at -80 mV with a 200 ms step increase to 0 mV applied approximately every minute. The Na_v channel response was calculated as the difference between the current required to maintain the holding potential and the largest negative current deflection produced by the voltage step. For oocytes expressing K_{2P} channels, the transmembrane potential was clamped at −60 mV, and voltage was stepped to + 60 mV each minute. The K_{2P} channel response was calculated as the difference between holding potential current and voltage step plateau current. For both channel types, baseline responses were measured during oocyte perfusion with FR for a minimum of three times to demonstrate response variability <10%. The perfusate was then switched to the hydrocarbon test drug dissolved at a saturated aqueous phase concentration in FR for 2 min after which the current response to the step voltage was measured. The hydrocarbon drug was then washed out for 5–10 min, and the current response was again measured to demonstrate that it was within 10% of the initial baseline response.

For two-electrode voltage clamp studies in oocytes expressing $GABA_A$ receptors or glycine receptors, the transmembrane potential was clamped at −80 mV while being perfused with FR. Approximately every 5 min, the perfusate was switched for 30 s to FR + EC_{10} agonist—20 μM 4-aminobutanoic acid for $GABA_A$ receptors or 40 μM aminoethanoic acid for glycine receptors—and then the perfusate was switched back to FR for agonist washout. The current response for each ligand-gated ion channel was calculated as the difference between the peak current measured in the presence of agonist and the whole-cell current measured immediately prior to agonist exposure. Baseline responses were measured in triplicate to confirm <10% variability of current responses in the absence of drug exposure. Next, the perfusate was switched to the hydrocarbon test drug dissolved at a saturated aqueous phase concentration for 2 min followed by a 30s exposure the same concentration of hydrocarbon dissolved in FR + agonist. The hydrocarbon drug was then washed out, and oocytes were exposed to FR + agonist 5 and 10 min later to verify return of the current response to within 10% of pre-drug baseline levels.

Drug solution preparation

Using predicted density values published in SciFinder (Chemical Abstracts Service, American Chemical Society, Columbus OH), drug solutions were prepared by anaerobic addition of a hydrocarbon volume to gastight glass syringes containing either FR or FR + agonist to create a concentration equal to its calculated molar water solubility (Table 1). After vigorous agitation, an immiscible hydrocarbon microbubble could be found in the syringe, confirming that a saturated solution had been achieved. However, butane is a gas a room temperature and pressure, and a saturated aqueous phase cannot be achieved because butane vapor pressure exceeds atmospheric pressure. Instead, using FR or FR + agonist containing 1 atm O_2 partial pressure in gastight glass syringes, butane drug solutions were prepared by repeated syringe headspace exchanges to yield solutions with gas partial pressures that were 90% butane and 10% O_2.

Data analysis

Drug responses were calculated as a percent change from the control (baseline) current responses as follows: $\%change = \frac{I_D - I_B}{I_B}$, where I_D and I_B are the current responses measured during perfusions with drug and without drug (baseline), respectively. Average current responses for each drug and channel were described by mean ± SEM. A positive current change indicated drug-induced positive allosteric modulation of the channel, whereas a negative current change indicated negative allosteric modulation (inhibition) of channel function. A drug-receptor cut-off response was defined as an absolute value change in current <10% from baseline that was statistically indistinguishable from zero using a two-tailed Student t-test. The log_{10} of the calculated solubility ($log_{10}S$) for compounds immediately below and above the cut-off for each hydrocarbon functional group were used to determine the receptor cut-off. For each hydrocarbon, there was a "grey area" of indeterminate solubility effect between sequentially increasing hydrocarbon chain lengths. Mean solubility cut-offs were calculated as the average $log_{10}S$ for the least soluble compound that modulated receptor function and the most soluble neighboring compound for which no effect was observed. From this result, a 95% confidence interval for $log_{10}S$ was calculated for receptor solubility cut-offs.

Results

Sample channel recordings are shown in Fig. 1, and hydrocarbon effects on each anesthetic-sensitive ion channel are summarized in Table 2. With increasing carbon additions to the ω-end or ring, all anesthetic-sensitive channels exhibited a cut-off effect, defined by <10% channel modulation, the smallest effect size that is reliably resolved

Table 1 Source, purity and physical properties of study compounds

Compound	CAS#	MW (amu)	P_{vap} (mmHg)	Solubility (M)	Carbon (#)	Volume (Å^3)	Source	Purity (%)
Alcohols								
1-octanol	111-87-5	130.23	1.14×10^{-1}	9.0×10^{-3}	8	262	Alfa Aesar	>99
1-nonanol	143-08-8	144.25	4.07×10^{-2}	2.7×10^{-3}	9	290	Alfa Aesar	>99
1-decanol	112-30-1	158.28	1.48×10^{-2}	6.5×10^{-4}	10	317	Aldrich	>99
1-undecanol	112-42-5	172.31	5.10×10^{-3}	1.7×10^{-4}	11	344	Acros	98
1-dodecanol	112-53-8	186.33	2.09×10^{-3}	4.1×10^{-5}	12	372	TCI	99
1-tridecanol	112-70-9	200.36	8.07×10^{-4}	1.2×10^{-5}	13	400	Aldrich	97
1-tetradecanol	112-72-1	214.39	1.47×10^{-4}	2.1×10^{-6}	14	427	Fluka	>99
1-pentadecanol	629-76-5	228.41	1.27×10^{-4}	4.7×10^{-7}	15	454	Aldrich	99
Aldehydes								
nonanal	124-19-6	142.24	5.32×10^{-1}	2.3×10^{-3}	9	289	Aldrich	95
decanal	112-31-2	156.27	2.07×10^{-1}	9.8×10^{-4}	10	316	Aldrich	98
undecanal	112-44-7	170.29	8.32×10^{-2}	4.2×10^{-4}	11	344	Aldrich	97
dodecanal	112-54-9	184.32	3.44×10^{-2}	1.8×10^{-4}	12	372	TCI	98
tridecanal	10486-19-8	198.34	1.46×10^{-2}	8.2×10^{-5}	13	399	TCI	98
tetradecanal	124-25-4	212.37	6.39×10^{-3}	3.7×10^{-5}	14	427	TCI	98
heptadecanal	629-90-3	254.45	6.22×10^{-4}	3.5×10^{-6}	17	509	TCI	>97
octadecanal	638-66-4	268.48	3.00×10^{-4}	1.7×10^{-6}	18	536	TCI	>95
docosanal	57402-36-5	324.58	2.02×10^{-5}	9.1×10^{-8}	20	646	Alfa Aesar	98
Alkanes								
butane	106-97-8	58.12	1.92×10^{3}	1.4×10^{-3}	4	156	Matheson	99.99
pentane	109-66-0	72.15	5.27×10^{2}	4.3×10^{-4}	5	184	Aldrich	>99
hexane	110-54-3	86.18	1.51×10^{2}	1.2×10^{-4}	6	211	Acros	>99
heptane	142-82-5	100.20	4.52×10^{1}	3.1×10^{-5}	7	239	Acros	>99
octane	111-65-9	114.23	1.42×10^{1}	6.9×10^{-6}	8	267	Acros	>99
nonane	111-84-2	128.26	4.63×10^{0}	1.4×10^{-6}	9	294	Acros	99
decane	124-18-5	142.28	1.58×10^{0}	2.6×10^{-7}	10	321	Acros	>99
undecane	1120-21-4	156.31	5.64×10^{-1}	4.2×10^{-8}	11	349	Acros	99
tetradecane	629-59-4	198.39	2.85×10^{-2}	6.1×10^{-9}	14	431	Aldrich	>99
eicosane	112-95-8	282.55	1.40×10^{-4}	2.9×10^{-9}	20	596	Aldrich	99
Alkenes								
1-pentene	109-67-1	70.13	6.37×10^{2}	1.4×10^{-3}	5	176	Aldrich	99
1-hexene	592-41-6	84.16	1.88×10^{2}	4.2×10^{-4}	6	203	Aldrich	>99
1-octene	111-66-0	112.21	1.79×10^{1}	2.6×10^{-5}	8	258	Aldrich	98
1-nonene	124-11-8	126.24	5.77×10^{0}	7.4×10^{-6}	9	286	Aldrich	96
1-decene	872-05-9	140.27	1.92×10^{0}	1.5×10^{-6}	10	313	Aldrich	>97
1-undecene	821-95-4	154.29	6.61×10^{-1}	2.6×10^{-7}	11	341	Aldrich	97
1-dodecene	112-41-4	168.32	2.34×10^{-1}	4.1×10^{-8}	12	368	Aldrich	>99
1-tridecene	2437-56-1	182.35	$8.56\ 10^{-2}$	5.8×10^{-9}	13	396	Aldrich	96
Alkynes								
1-hexyne	693-02-7	82.14	1.35×10^{2}	2.9×10^{-3}	6	184	Aldrich	97
1-heptyne	628-71-7	96.17	4.35×10^{1}	6.6×10^{-4}	7	212	Acros	99
1-octyne	629-05-0	110.2	1.44×10^{1}	1.9×10^{-4}	8	239	Acros	99
1-nonyne	3452-09-3	124.22	4.87×10^{0}	3.9×10^{-5}	9	267	Aldrich	99

Table 1 Source, purity and physical properties of study compounds *(Continued)*

Compound	CAS#	MW (amu)	P_{vap} (mmHg)	Solubility (M)	Carbon (#)	Volume (Å^3)	Source	Purity (%)
1-decyne	764-93-2	138.25	1.69×10^{0}	7.9×10^{-6}	10	294	Aldrich	98
1-undecyne	2243-98-3	152.28	6.05×10^{-1}	1.4×10^{-6}	11	322	TCI	98
1-dodecyne	765-03-7	166.30	2.22×10^{-1}	2.4×10^{-7}	12	349	TCI	98
Amines								
1-octadecanamine	124-30-1	269.51	4.88×10^{-5}	1.3×10^{-3}	18	546	TCI	97
1-eicosanamine	10525-37-8	297.56	8.96×10^{-6}	2.7×10^{-4}	20	601	Rambus	95
1-hexacosanamine	14130-10-0	381.72	8.91×10^{-8}	2.3×10^{-5}	26	766	ACC	98
1-octacosanamine	14130-12-2	409.77	2.21×10^{-8}	6.3×10^{-6}	28	821	ACC	98
1-triacontanamine	66214-00-4	437.83	5.85×10^{-9}	1.8×10^{-6}	30	876	ACC	98
Cycloalkanes								
cyclopentane	287-92-3	70.13	3.14×10^{2}	3.3×10^{-3}	5	147	Aldrich	>99
cyclohexane	110-82-7	84.16	9.37×10^{1}	1.0×10^{-3}	6	176	Aldrich	>99.7
cycloheptane	291-64-5	98.19	1.99×10^{1}	2.9×10^{-4}	7	206	Aldrich	96
cyclooctane	292-64-8	112.21	4.56×10^{0}	7.2×10^{-5}	8	236	Aldrich	>99
cyclodecane	293-96-9	140.27	4.47×10^{-1}	3.2×10^{-6}	10	295	Aldrich	95
cycloundecane	294-41-7	154.29	1.85×10^{-1}	5.7×10^{-7}	11	324	Aldrich	95
cyclododecane	294-62-2	168.32	4.13×10^{-2}	9.2×10^{-8}	12	353	TCI	>99
Ethers								
dibutyl ether	142-96-1	130.23	7.10×10^{0}	1.6×10^{-2}	8	277	Aldrich	99.3
dipentyl ether	693-65-2	158.28	1.00×10^{0}	3.0×10^{-3}	10	331	Fluka	>98.5
dihexyl ether	112-58-3	186.33	1.48×10^{-1}	5.8×10^{-4}	12	386	Aldrich	97
diheptyl ether	629-64-1	214.39	2.23×10^{-2}	1.2×10^{-4}	14	442	TCI	98
dioctyl ether	629-82-3	242.44	4.53×10^{-3}	2.4×10^{-5}	16	497	TCI	98
didecyl ether	2456-28-2	298.55	8.08×10^{-5}	1.2×10^{-6}	20	606	TCI	98
diundecyl ether	43146-97-0	326.60	1.24×10^{-5}	2.3×10^{-7}	22	661	TCI	98

CAS# Chemical Abstracts Service number, *MW* molecular weight, P_{vap} vapor pressure at 25 °C, molar solubility in pure water at pH = 7, and molecular volume are calculated estimates (rather than measured values) referenced by SciFinder Scholar

given the given baseline variability allowed in these studies. All current modulation above this value was statistically different from baseline.

The mean hydrocarbon molar water solubility cut-off value and 95% confidence interval range for each ion channel is as follows (Fig. 2): $Na_v1.2 = 1.4$ mM (0.81 mM–2.4 mM); $Na_v1.4 = 1.2$ mM (0.62 mM–2.3 mM); TRESK = 0.59 mM (0.26 mM–1.3 mM); TREK-1 = 0.51 mM (0.24 mM–1.1 mM); $GABA_A = 120$ μM (60 μM–250 μM); Glycine = 0.63 μM (0.24 μM–1.7 μM). Loss of ion channel modulation generally occurred in this same order for all organic compounds, with some clustering of cut-offs for the Na_v and K_{2P} at similar molar water solubility values.

For each ion channel, the calculated molar water solubility was the only physical-chemical property examined that was associated with similar cut-off values between different hydrocarbon functional groups. An example of this is shown in Fig. 3 in which the grey indeterminate bars that separate known regions of positive and absent modulation are clustered around a relatively narrow molar water solubility cut-off range. Other channels, when similarly graphed as a function of hydrocarbon molar water solubility, show qualitatively similar results but with clustering around each channel's own distinct molar water solubility cut-off value. In contrast, $GABA_A$ receptor cut-off effects are not associated with the number of molecular carbon atoms or molecular volume of the hydrocarbon (Fig. 4), and these results mirror those of the other anesthetic-sensitive ion channels studied here.

Both Na_v channels were inhibited by all of the hydrocarbons tested above their respective cut-off values, whereas both of the ligand-gated ion channels ($GABA_A$ and glycine receptors) were potentiated by all compounds above their respective cut-off values (Table 2). However, the K_{2P} channels were differently affected by compounds with different organic functional groups. Both were positively modulated by alkanes, alkenes, alkynes, cycloalkanes, and ethers, and both were negatively modulated by aldehydes and primary amines. However, whereas primary

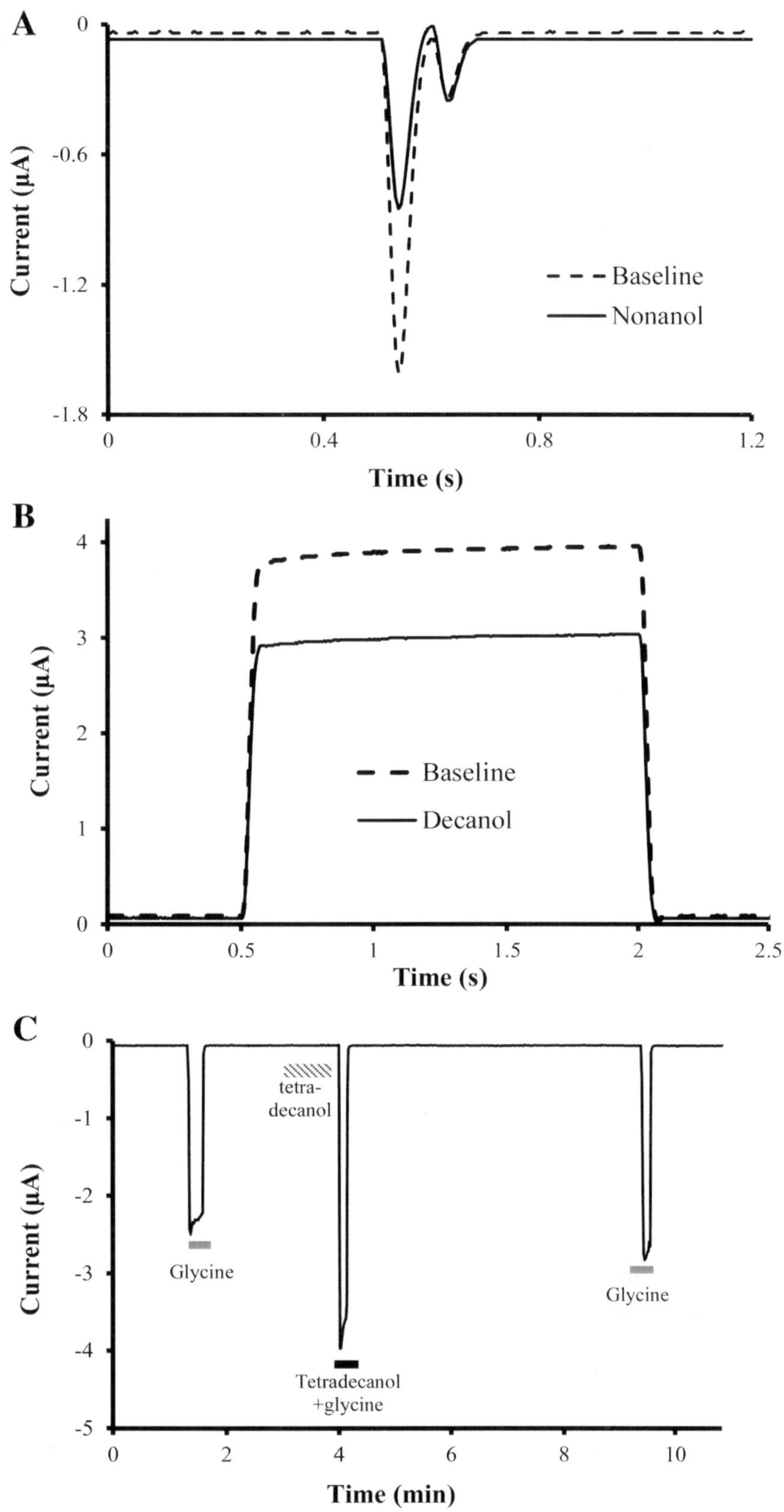

Fig. 1 Sample tracings for (**a**) $Na_V1.2$ channels, (**b**) TREK-1 channels, and (**c**) glycine receptors before and after alcohol exposure at saturated aqueous phase concentrations (Table 1). Whole cell current responses were qualitatively similar between both Na_v channels and between both K_{2P} channels. Electrophysiologic responses of $GABA_A$ receptors during similar hydrocarbon exposure studies have been published elsewhere [6, 7]

Table 2 Percent change ±SEM of whole-cell currents measured during two-electrode voltage clamp studies in response to administration of saturated concentration of each hydrocarbon (or 90% atm for butane)

Compound	$Na_v1.2$	$Na_v1.4$	TRESK	TREK-1	$GABA_A$	Glycine
Alcohols						
1-octanol			74 ± 5 (5)*			
1-nonanol	−62 ± 7 (5)*	−48 ± 4 (6)*	41 ± 4 (5)*	−36 ± 2 (6)*		
1-decanol	−4 ± 1 (5)	− 35 ± 6 (6)*	2 ± 1 (6)	−28 ± 4 (6)*	322 ± 29 (5)*	
1-undecanol	−2 ± 1 (5)	− 4 ± 1 (5)		0 ± 2 (5)	81 ± 13 (5)*	
1-dodecanol					39 ± 6 (7)*	
1-tridecanol					2 ± 1 (6)	
1-tetradecanol				5 ± 3 (5)	4 ± 2 (5)	38 ± 6 (6)*
1-pentadecanol						−7 ± 2 (5)
Aldehydes						
nonanal	−51 ± 1 (6)*		−22 ± 6 (5)*		119 ± 29 (7)*	
decanal	−24 ± 3 (5)*	−31 ± 3 (6)*	−4 ± 2 (5)	−45 ± 3 (5)*		
undecanal	−6 ± 1(5)	−2 ± 1 (5)		−20 ± 2 (6)*		
dodecanal				− 5 ± 1 (5)		
tridecanal					20 ± 3 (7)*	
tetradecanal					5 ± 2 (9)	
heptadecanal						31 ± 2 (5)*
octadecanal						20 ± 3 (5)*
docosanal						1 ± 2 (7)
Alkanes						
butane	−20 ± 2 (7)*	−22 ± 2 (5)*	25 ± 5 (6)*	61 ± 9 (5)*	523 ± 68 (5)*	
pentane	−1 ± 1 (5)	− 2 ± 1 (5)	7 ± 1 (5)	−3 ± 2 (5)	221 ± 10 (7)*	
hexane		− 1 ± 0 (2)		4 ± 3 (4)	29 ± 5 (6)*	61 ± 5 (5)*
heptane		0 ± 1 (5)			−3 ± 1 (5)	
octane					− 1 ± 4 (2)	206 ± 21 (5)*
nonane						62 ± 18 (5)*
decane					5 ± 2 (2)	20 ± 3 (6)*
undecane						8 ± 2 (5)
tetradecane						5 ± 1 (5)
eicosane						9 ± 4 (2)
Alkenes						
1-pentene	−28 ± 2 (5)*	−45 ± 4 (5)*			351 ± 38 (6)*	
1-hexene	1 ± 1 (5)	0 ± 0 (6)	37 ± 7 (5)*	157 ± 13 (5)*	83 ± 8 (6)*	
1-octene			2 ± 1 (5)	1 ± 1 (5)	7 ± 3 (5)	
1-nonene					7 ± 4 (6)	
1-decene						
1-undecene						54 ± 7 (5)*
1-dodecene						−3 ± 3 (5)*
1-tridecene						1 ± 1 (5)
Alkynes						
1-hexyne	−44 ± 2 (5)*	−34 ± 2 (5)*	44 ± 5 (5)*		313 ± 23 (6)*	
1-heptyne	−2 ± 4 (5)	−4 ± 2 (6)	29 ± 5 (7)*	55 ± 5 (4)*	78 ± 5 (7)*	
1-octyne		2 ± 1 (5)	5 ± 2 (5)	−1 ± 2 (9)	− 3 ± 1 (6)	

Table 2 Percent change ±SEM of whole-cell currents measured during two-electrode voltage clamp studies in response to administration of saturated concentration of each hydrocarbon (or 90% atm for butane) *(Continued)*

Compound	$Na_v1.2$	$Na_v1.4$	TRESK	TREK-1	$GABA_A$	Glycine
1-nonyne					6 ± 1 (4)	
1-decyne					7 ± 1 (6)	55 ± 14 (5)*
1-undecyne						223 ± 20 (6)*
1-dodecyne						3 ± 2 (5)
Amines						
1-octadecanamine	−15 ± 1 (6)*	−11 ± 1 (6)*	−23 ± 2 (6)*	−16 ± 1 (5)*	46 ± 5 (8)*	
1-eicosanamine	0 ± 0 (6)	− 2 ± 2 (5)	−1 ± 1 (7)	−2 ± 3 (5)	67 ± 7 (6)*	
1-hexacosanamine			0 ± 2 (6)	−1 ± 3 (6)	1 ± 2 (6)	
1-octacosanamine						26 ± 3 (7)*
1-triacontanamine						2 ± 1 (6)
Cycloalkanes						
cyclopentane	−45 ± 4 (5)*	−11 ± 1 (6)*	63 ± 9 (5)*	68 ± 13 (5)*	93 ± 8 (7)*	
cyclohexane	−1 ± 1 (5)	−2 ± 2 (5)	1 ± 1 (6)	63 ± 6 (6)*	321 ± 17 (5)*	
cycloheptane	0 ± 1 (6)		0 ± 1 (5)	−4 ± 2 (6)	6 ± 3 (5)	
cyclooctane						
cyclodecane						22 ± 3 (5)*
cycloundecane						3 ± 2 (5)
cyclododecane						0 ± 1 (5)
Ethers						
dibutyl ether	−33 ± 3 (5)*	−44 ± 5 (5)*		50 ± 9 (6)*	234 ± 24 (5)*	
dipentyl ether	1 ± 1 (5)	1 ± 0 (5)	20 ± 2 (8)*	65 ± 6 (6)*	111 ± 9 (7)*	
dihexyl ether		0 ± 1 (5)	2 ± 1 (6)	3 ± 2 (6)	13 ± 1 (5)*	143 ± 10 (5)*
diheptyl ether		−1 ± 2 (2)			−1 ± 4 (5)	74 ± 8 (6)*
dioctyl ether					1 ± 3 (5)	95 ± 8 (5)*
didecyl ether						28 ± 4 (6)*
diundecyl ether						2 ± 2 (7)

Positive changes indicate drug potentiation of channel function, and negative changes indicate drug inhibition of channel function. Drug-induced changes ≥10% in magnitude in either direction that are significantly greater than zero (**not** a cut-off response) are indicated by an asterisk. The number of oocytes studied for each channel and drug combination is shown in parentheses

alcohols potentiated TRESK currents, they inhibited TREK-1 currents.

As increasing hydrocarbon chain length decreased molar water solubility to values close to a channel cut-off value, there was commonly a decrease in the magnitude of current potentiation or inhibition (Table 2). Notable exceptions to this pattern are cyclohexane with $GABA_A$ receptors and undecyne with glycine receptors. Otherwise, there appeared no obvious relationship between hydrocarbon molar water solubility and either the magnitude or direction of receptor modulation.

Discussion

As shown previously for NMDA receptors, all of the anesthetic-sensitive ligand-gated, voltage-gated and leak channels examined in this study exhibited cut-off effects for each class of organic compounds, and these cut-offs were associated with the calculated molar water solubility of the hydrocarbon. The cut-offs occurred in a predictable order, with Na_v channels K_{2P} channels, and $GABA_A$ receptors cut-offs all clustered within roughly one order magnitude of saturated drug concentrations. In contrast, the glycine receptor cut-off was associated with drug molar water solubility values over two orders of magnitude lower. If previously determined NMDA receptor results are included [6], cut-off responses proceed in order of decreasing hydrocarbon solubility as follows: $Na_v1.2 \approx Na_v1.4 \gtrsim$ NMDA $\gtrsim$ TRESK $\approx$ TREK-1 $>$ $GABA_A$ $>>$ glycine (Fig. 2).

Hydrocarbon cut-off responses in the present study, defined by <10% effect, confirm data available in published literature. Horishita and Harris [13] found that the ability of primary alcohols to modulate $Na_v1.2$ channels was lost between 1-octanol and 1-decanol, and is consistent with

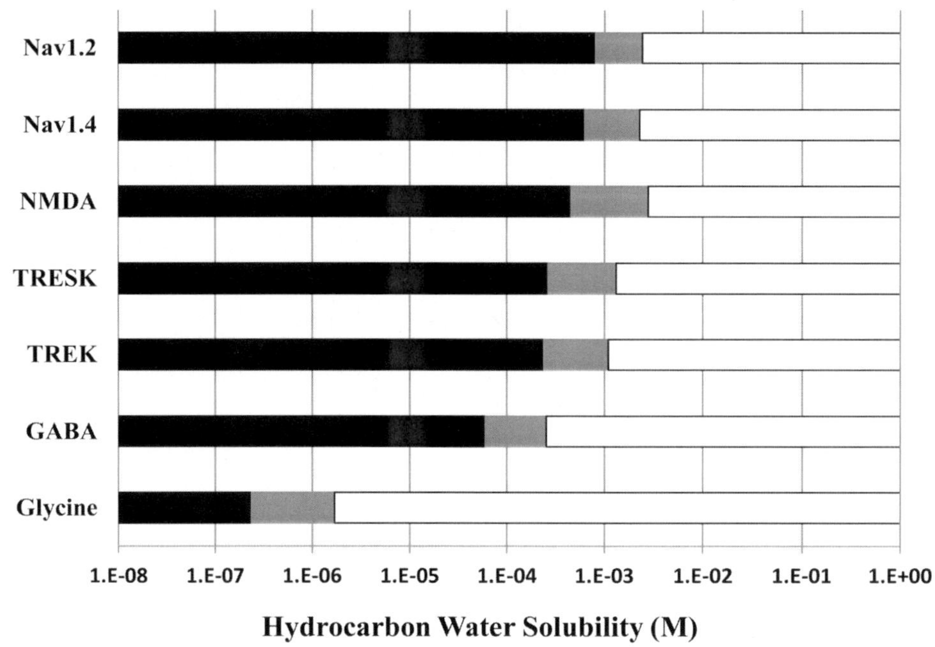

Fig. 2 Summary of ion channel response as a function of hydrocarbon molar water solubility. Hydrocarbons that modulate ion channel function are indicated by a white bar. Hydrocarbons that did not affect whole cell currents for an ion channel are indicated by a black bar. The grey bar represents the 95% confidence interval around the mean hydrocarbon molar water solubility cut-off value for each ion channel

our finding of a cut-off between 1-nonanol and 1-decanol for this channel. Likewise, Peoples and Weight [14] observed $GABA_A$ receptor potentiation with primary alcohol chains up to 1-dodecanol and a cut-off effect at 1-tridecanol and beyond, exactly where this cut-off was observed in the present study. The confidence interval for the $GABA_A$ receptor molar water solubility cut-off from this study also encompasses the calculated solubility cut-off values for substituted benzene and phenolic compounds [7].

Discrete water solubility-associated cut-off effects may be a common feature of all inhaled anesthetic-sensitive

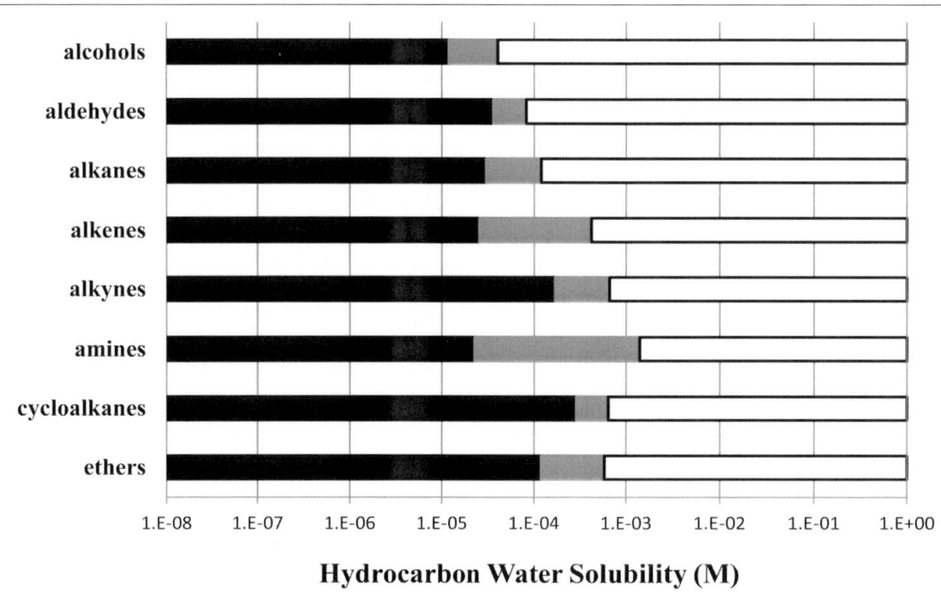

Fig. 3 $GABA_A$ receptor current potentiation (white bars) and absent whole cell current effects for eight different organic classes graphed as a function of the calculated hydrocarbon molar water solubility. The grey bars represent hydrocarbon solubility ranges within each organic class for which $GABA_A$ receptor modulation was not evaluated. Cut-off values are clustered between 6.0×10^{-5} and 2.5×10^{-4} M

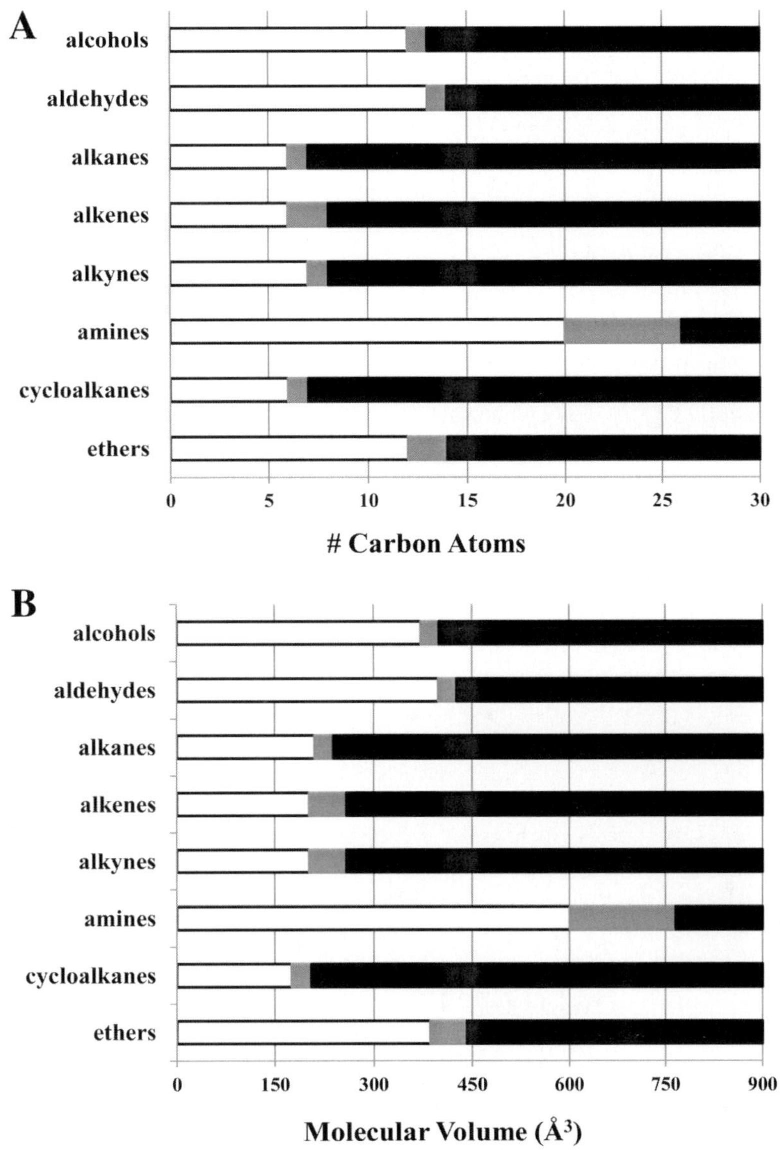

Fig. 4 Graph of $GABA_A$ receptor modulation as a function of the number of carbon atoms in a molecule (Panel **a**) and as a function of hydrocarbon molecular volume (Panel **b**). White and black bars indicate carbon numbers (Panel **a**) and molecular volumes (Panel **b**) associated with receptor potentiation and absent receptor modulation, respectively. Grey bars indicate regions for which hydrocarbon response data is not available. No pattern of consistent cut-off values associated with hydrocarbon chain length or molecular volume is evident

ion channels. Conventional volatile and gas anesthetics immobilize individuals at high aqueous phase concentrations [15] suggesting that they engage in low-affinity binding with target receptors. We postulate that these conventional anesthetic-receptor interactions mirror experimental hydrocarbon-receptor interactions, and we propose a molar water solubility hypothesis to describe non-specific drug binding to low-affinity and amphipathic allosteric sites on proteins. Before a ligand can alter protein function, it must first bind at a site capable of inducing a change in protein function. In order to bind, water molecules must be removed from the hydration shell surrounding the drug, and water molecules within the amphipathic protein pocket must be displaced. The ease with which the water is displaced from the protein pocket is described by its dissociation constant (K_d). Water that is only weakly bound to amino acid side chains within the protein pocket would have a high K_d and require fewer hydrocarbon molecules to successfully compete for access to this allosteric site. Consequently, this protein would have a lower molar water solubility cut-off. In contrast, water that is tightly bound within the pocket would have a low K_d, and therefore a high hydrocarbon concentration would be necessary to compete for access to this site. Such a protein would exhibit a high drug molar water solubility cut-off. It is possible that ion channels may have more than one amphipathic allosteric site for low-affinity interactions with inhaled anesthetics or other hydrocarbons [16–18]; however the methods employed in the present study would have identified receptor cut-off effects based only on the amphipathic allosteric site with the highest water K_d in that receptor and which would therefore exhibit the lowest hydrocarbon molar water solubility cut-off effect among all modulatory sites. Other lower water K_d sites could be important for binding and modulation by more soluble hydrocarbons and inhaled anesthetics when present at sufficient aqueous concentrations.

A second explanation for hydrocarbon molar water solubility cut-offs is possible. Desolvation of water molecules around the ligand is necessary for protein binding to occur. However, if the difference in free energy between the solvated protein-drug complex and the separated solvated protein and solvated drug is too great, then drug binding will be energetically unfavorable and no modulation of protein function will occur [19]. Larger hydrophobic drug ligands are surrounded by larger and more rigid water shells for which desolvation may be associated with greater enthalpy. The strength of water complexes around the ligand might increase to the point that drug receptor binding—and thus drug-receptor modulation can only occur if there remains sufficient entropy to overcome increased enthalpy of binding [20].

In either case, a molar water solubility hypothesis is not predicated on any particular molecular size, shape, polarity, functional groups, or atomic arrangement of the drug for low affinity interactions to take place. Indeed, the diversity of conventional anesthetics and other hydrocarbons capable of modulating a single anesthetic-sensitive ion channel, as well as the relatively minor effect differences produced by dug enantiomers [21], suggest that ligand structure itself is not crucial for binding. However, ligand structure does determine the magnitude and type of modulation for the protein it binds. Whether there is inhibition versus potentiation of K_{2P} channel currents, for example, will depend on the functional group of the hydrocarbon ligand (Table 2). Modulation magnitude also differed between functional groups; inhibition of $Na_v1.4$ channels was approximately four times greater for alcohols, alkenes, and ethers than for amines or cycloalkanes. The importance of structural elements within receptor binding pockets has also been demonstrated through mutation studies that confer resistance to conventional anesthetic or other hydrocarbon modulation [22–24], although it is unknown whether some of these changes may also have altered the water K_d or drug desolvation enthalpy that, in turn, could have affected the ability of the drug to bind the allosteric pocket.

The hydrocarbon molar water solubility cut-off value for each channel is expressed as confidence intervals, and certain error is inherent in their measurement. Butane, the smallest n-alkane studied here, is a gas at room temperature and pressure, and therefore cannot be studied at a saturated aqueous phase concentration under normobaric conditions unlike the other liquid and solid hydrocarbons. All receptors were nonetheless modulated by 90% atm of butane, but had current modulation not been observed, a true cut-off could have been inferred at this submaximal concentration. Furthermore, carbon additions to the ω-end of the hydrocarbon chain produce discrete, non-continuous changes in molar water solubility. For each series of functional groups, there is a range of solubility values that lie between the C_N modulating hydrocarbon and the C_{N+1} cut-off hydrocarbon where the receptor effect is unknown. Most important, however, is the reliance on calculated solubility values for hydrocarbons in pure water at 25 °C and pH = 7.0 rather than measured solubility values under study conditions with a 250 mOsm electrolyte solution at 22 °C and pH = 7.4. Both accurate measurement and accurate prediction of solubility values are challenging for extremely hydrophobic compounds or for large or complex molecules with multiple functional groups. To limit this problem, only simple aliphatic compounds with the functional group on the first carbon, or central and symmetrical in the case of the dialkyl ethers, were studied. Even so, increasing hydrocarbon chain length is frequently accompanied by greater divergence between calculated and measured water solubility values [25, 26].

Whole cell current cut-off responses were measured using hydrocarbons at saturated aqueous concentrations. This was done to ensure that each cut-off was independent of any particular endpoint (e.g., amnesia, unconsciousness, or immobility). Lack of receptor modulation at a saturated hydrocarbon concentration implies absent modulation at a lower pharmacologic concentration, including concentrations relevant to anesthetic endpoints. Anesthetic efficacy is in mammals is unknown for many, but not all, of the hydrocarbons tested. Primary alcohol anesthetic potency increases with increasing carbon chain length from methanol to dodecanol, after which further carbon additions do not produce anesthesia at all [27]. This anesthetic cut-off corresponds to the alcohol molar water solubility cut-off for $GABA_A$ receptors (Table 2). However, a general anesthesia cut-off effect has been reported to occur with n-alkanes and dialkyl ethers having around 11-to-15 or more carbon atoms [28] and cycloalkanes having eight or more carbons atoms [29]. These molecules are far longer and have molar water solubility values far lower than occur with the $GABA_A$ receptor cut-off. Although observed anesthetic effects might be due to glycine receptor modulation, high affinity effects on one or more other anesthetic-sensitive receptors, or even systemic toxicity, it seems very possible that anesthetic effects could be the result of potent alcohol metabolites produced by oxidation of alkanes, cycloalkanes, and ethers by cytochrome P450 enzymes [30, 31]. Since the hydroxyl group confers greater molar water solubility, primary alcohols have receptor cut-offs at longer chain lengths than either alkanes or cycloalkanes or dialkyl ethers. These long-chain alcohol metabolites are also much more potent general anesthetics than their parent compounds [32], so even tiny quantities can have narcotic effects. Identifying simple parallels between in vitro receptor cut-offs and in vivo anesthetic cut-offs thus may be complicated for certain classes of organic compounds.

Channel studies were conducted using a reductionist biological system. However, in vitro electrophysiologic responses conducted at room temperature for relevant anesthetic-sensitive ion channels in oocytes seem to correlate with anesthetic potency in animals [33–35]. Likewise, the hydrocarbons studied in Table 1 administered in vivo would be expected to similarly modulate ion channels; in the case of drugs below the solubility cut-off, no in vivo modulation would be expected at all.

Finally, the molar water solubility hypothesis could offer practical applications to the development of new and novel inhaled anesthetic agents. Conventional volatile anesthetics bind promiscuously to a variety of cell proteins, but not all of these receptor interactions are essential to their ability to produce general anesthesia. For example, NMDA receptors contribute to immobilizing actions of inhaled anesthetics able to inhibit their function, but experimental inhaled anesthetics can still be immobilizers without producing NMDA receptor inhibition [36]. Since there is nearly a 10-fold separation in the hydrocarbon molar water solubility cut-off effects between NMDA versus $GABA_A$ receptors, a volatile anesthetic might be modified to target calculated aqueous solubility values within this range to confer selectivity against higher cut-off NMDA receptors while preserving activity at lower cut-off $GABA_A$ receptors. With sufficient $GABA_A$ receptor potentiation and contributions of lower cut-off receptors, such an agent might retain immobilizing potency but lose adverse effects associated with the modulation of higher cut-off receptors. Consequently, molar water solubility could be key to identifying volatile anesthetics with new molecular mechanisms of action and improved pharmacodynamic profiles.

Conclusions

Anesthetic-sensitive ion channels and receptors all appear to exhibit allosteric cut-off effects associated with drug molar water solubility. These results support the Molar Water Solubility Hypothesis mechanism for non-specific protein interactions with drugs of varied sizes and shapes administered at relatively high aqueous phase concentrations, such as occurs with inhaled anesthetic agents. Low-affinity binding at allosteric sites may occur following successful displacement of water by a hydrocarbon molecule (or portion thereof). However, when a hydrocarbon has a molar water solubility below the allosteric cut-off for a channel, as likely determined by the dissociation constant for water at the allosteric site, that hydrocarbon cannot be delivered at a concentration sufficient to outcompete the water for binding site access. In addition to describing how anesthetics of various sizes and shapes may be able to modulate functions of different anesthetic-sensitive ion channels and receptors, the Molar Water Solubility Hypothesis and order of receptor cut-offs offers a unique tool for the development of new inhaled anesthetic agents. By changing substituents on molecules to decrease their molar water solubility, it may be possible to generate novel inhaled anesthetics that are selective against some of the ion channels or receptors normally modulated by conventional volatile anesthetics.

Abbreviations

$GABA_A$: γ-aminobutyric acid receptor type A; $Na_v1.2$: Voltage-gated sodium channels type II; $Na_v1.4$: Voltage-gated sodium channels type IV; NMDA: N-methyl-d-aspartate; TREK-1: TWIK-related potassium channel type I; TRESK: TWIK-related spinal cord potassium channel

Funding

This work was funded by the National Institutes of Health National Institutes of General Medical Sciences (Grant GM092821-02).

Authors' contributions

RJB: Conceived the idea, designed the experiments, assisted with some measurements, analyzed the data, and wrote the manuscript. TLP: Performed study measurements and reviewed the manuscript draft. Both authors read and approved the final manuscript.

Competing interests

Aspects of this work are included in intellectual property filings and issued patents regarding the identification and use of new inhalation anesthetics and analgesics. Dr. Brosnan is the inventor of record, and patents are owned by the University of California. The University of California has licensed this intellectual property to Expanesthetics, Inc. (Davis, CA), and Dr. Brosnan is Chair of the Expanesthetics Scientific Advisory Board. Neither Dr. Brosnan nor Mr. Pham has received financial compensation from Expanesthetics, Inc., and neither owns equity in Expanesthetics, Inc.

References

1. Fisher E. Einfluss der Configuration auf die Wirkung der Enzyme. Ber Dtsch Chem Ges. 1894;27(3):2985–93.
2. Brosnan RJ, Steffey EP. Inhalation anesthetics. In: Riviere JE, Papich MG, editors. Veterinary Pharmacology and Therapeutics. 10th ed. Hoboken: Wiley; 2018. p. 216–46.
3. Steffey EP, Mama KR, Brosnan RJ. Inhalation anesthetics. In: Grimm KA, Lamont LA, Tranquilli WJ, Greene SA, Robertson SA, editors. Veterinary anesthesia and analgesia. 5th ed. Ames: Wiley; 2015. p. 237–331.
4. Franks NP, Lieb WR. Selective actions of volatile general anaesthetics at molecular and cellular levels. Br J Anaesth. 1993;71(1):65–76.
5. Bhattacharya AA, Curry S, Franks NP. Binding of the general anesthetics propofol and halothane to human serum albumin. High resolution crystal structures. J Biol Chem. 2000;275(49):38731–8.

6. Brosnan RJ, Pham TL. Hydrocarbon molar water solubility predicts NMDA vs. GABAA receptor modulation. BMC Pharmacol Toxicol. 2014;15:62.
7. Brosnan RJ, Pham TL. GABAA receptor modulation by phenyl ring compounds is associated with a water solubility cut-off value. Pharmacology. 2016;98(1–2):13–9.
8. Herold KF, Hemmings HC Jr. Sodium channels as targets for volatile anesthetics. Front Pharmacol. 2012;3:50.
9. Chae YJ, Zhang J, Au P, Sabbadini M, Xie GX, Yost CS. Discrete change in volatile anesthetic sensitivity in mice with inactivated tandem pore potassium ion channel TRESK. Anesthesiology. 2010;113(6):1326–37.
10. Heurteaux C, Guy N, Laigle C, Blondeau N, Duprat F, Mazzuca M, Lang-Lazdunski L, Widmann C, Zanzouri M, Romey G, et al. TREK-1, a K+ channel involved in neuroprotection and general anesthesia. EMBO J. 2004;23(13):2684–95.
11. Mihic SJ, McQuilkin SJ, Eger EI 2nd, Ionescu P, Harris RA. Potentiation of gamma-aminobutyric acid type a receptor-mediated chloride currents by novel halogenated compounds correlates with their abilities to induce general anesthesia. Mol Pharmacol. 1994;46(5):851–7.
12. Zhang Y, Laster MJ, Hara K, Harris RA, Eger EI 2nd, Stabernack CR, Sonner JM. Glycine receptors mediate part of the immobility produced by inhaled anesthetics. Anesth Analg. 2003;96(1):97–101.
13. Horishita T, Harris RA. n-Alcohols inhibit voltage-gated Na+ channels expressed in Xenopus oocytes. J Pharmacol Exp Ther. 2008;326(1):270–7.
14. Peoples RW, Weight FF. Differential alcohol modulation of $GABA_A$ and NMDA receptors. Neuroreport. 1999;10:97–101.
15. Franks NP, Lieb WR. Temperature dependence of the potency of volatile general anesthetics: implications for in vitro experiments. Anesthesiology. 1996;84(3):716–20.
16. Brannigan G, LeBard DN, Henin J, Eckenhoff RG, Klein ML. Multiple binding sites for the general anesthetic isoflurane identified in the nicotinic acetylcholine receptor transmembrane domain. Proc Natl Acad Sci U S A. 2010;107(32):14122–7.
17. Forman SA, Miller KW. Anesthetic sites and allosteric mechanisms of action on Cys-loop ligand-gated ion channels. Can J Anaesth. 2011;58(2):191–205.
18. Bondarenko V, Mowrey DD, Tillman TS, Seyoum E, Xu Y, Tang P. NMR structures of the human alpha7 nAChR transmembrane domain and associated anesthetic binding sites. Biochim Biophys Acta. 2014;1838(5):1389–95.
19. Brooks CL, Karplus M, Pettitt BM. Proteins: a theoretical perspective of dynamics, structure, and thermodynamics. New York: Wiley; 1988.
20. Krimmer SG, Betz M, Heine A, Klebe G. Methyl, ethyl, propyl, butyl: futile but not for water, as the correlation of structure and thermodynamic signature shows in a congeneric series of thermolysin inhibitors. ChemMedChem. 2014;9(4):833–46.
21. Brosnan R, Gong D, Cotten J, Keshavaprasad B, Yost CS, Eger EI 2nd, Sonner JM. Chirality in anesthesia II: stereoselective modulation of ion channel function by secondary alcohol enantiomers. Anesth Analg. 2006;103(1):86–91.
22. Borghese CM, Werner DF, Topf N, Baron NV, Henderson LA, Boehm SL 2nd, Blednov YA, Saad A, Dai S, Pearce RA, et al. An isoflurane- and alcohol-insensitive mutant GABA(A) receptor alpha(1) subunit with near-normal apparent affinity for GABA: characterization in heterologous systems and production of knockin mice. J Pharmacol Exp Ther. 2006;319(1):208–18.
23. Borghese CM, Xiong W, Oh SI, Ho A, Mihic SJ, Zhang L, Lovinger DM, Homanics GE, Eger EI 2nd, Harris RA. Mutations M287L and Q266I in the glycine receptor alpha1 subunit change sensitivity to volatile anesthetics in oocytes and neurons, but not the minimal alveolar concentration in knockin mice. Anesthesiology. 2012;117(4):765–71.
24. Borghese CM, Blednov YA, Quan Y, Iyer SV, Xiong W, Mihic SJ, Zhang L, Lovinger DM, Trudell JR, Homanics GE, et al. Characterization of two mutations, M287L and Q266I, in the alpha1 glycine receptor subunit that modify sensitivity to alcohols. J Pharmacol Exp Ther. 2012;340(2):304–16.
25. Coates M, Connell DW, Barron DM. Aqueous solubility and octan-1-ol-water partition coefficients of aliphatic hydrocarbons. Environ Sci Technol. 1985; 19(7):628–32.
26. Amidon GL, Yalkowsky SH, Leung S. Solubility of nonelectrolytes in polar solvents II: solubility of aliphatic alcohols in water. J Pharm Sci. 1974;63(12): 1858–66.
27. Alifimoff JK, Firestone LL, Miller KW. Anaesthetic potencies of primary alkanols: implications for the molecular dimensions of the anaesthetic site. Br J Pharmacol. 1989;96(1):9–16.
28. Jeppsson R. Parabolic relationship between lipophilicity and biological activity of aliphatic hydrocarbons, ethers and ketones after intravenous injections of emulsion formulations into mice. Acta Pharmacol Toxicol (Copenh). 1975;37(1):56–64.
29. Fang Z, Sonner J, Laster MJ, Ionescu P, Kandel L, Koblin DD, Eger EI 2nd, Halsey MJ. Anesthetic and convulsant properties of aromatic compounds and cycloalkanes: implications for mechanisms of narcosis. Anesth Analg. 1996;83(5):1097–104.
30. Pennec A, Jacobs CL, Opperman DJ, Smit MS. Revisiting cytochrome P450-mediated Oxyfunctionalization of linear and cyclic alkanes. Adv Synth Catal. 2015;357(1):118–30.
31. Brady JF, Lee MJ, Li M, Ishizaki H, Yang CS. Diethyl ether as a substrate for acetone/ethanol-inducible cytochrome P-450 and as an inducer for cytochrome(s) P-450. Mol Pharmacol. 1988;33(2):148–54.
32. Eger EI 2nd, Eisenkraft JB, Weiskopf RB. The Pharmacology of Inhaled Anesthetics. 2nd ed. San Antonio: Dannemiller Memorial Education Foundation; 2003.
33. Zimmerman SA, Jones MV, Harrison NL. Potentiation of gamma-aminobutyric acidA receptor cl- current correlates with in vivo anesthetic potency. J Pharmacol Exp Ther. 1994;270(3):987–91.
34. Rehberg B, Xiao YH, Duch DS. Central nervous system sodium channels are significantly suppressed at clinical concentrations of volatile anesthetics. Anesthesiology. 1996;84(5):1223–33. discussion 1227A
35. Eger EI 2nd, Liao M, Laster MJ, Won A, Popovich J, Raines DE, Solt K, Dutton RC, Cobos FV 2nd, Sonner JM. Contrasting roles of the N-methyl-D-aspartate receptor in the production of immobilization by conventional and aromatic anesthetics. Anesth Analg. 2006;102(5):1397–406.
36. Brosnan RJ, Fukushima FB, Pham TL. Anesthetic synergy between two n-alkanes. Vet Anaesth Analg. 2017;44(3):577–88.

Permissions

All chapters in this book were first published in PT, by BioMed Central; hereby published with permission under the Creative Commons Attribution License or equivalent. Every chapter published in this book has been scrutinized by our experts. Their significance has been extensively debated. The topics covered herein carry significant findings which will fuel the growth of the discipline. They may even be implemented as practical applications or may be referred to as a beginning point for another development.

The contributors of this book come from diverse backgrounds, making this book a truly international effort. This book will bring forth new frontiers with its revolutionizing research information and detailed analysis of the nascent developments around the world.

We would like to thank all the contributing authors for lending their expertise to make the book truly unique. They have played a crucial role in the development of this book. Without their invaluable contributions this book wouldn't have been possible. They have made vital efforts to compile up to date information on the varied aspects of this subject to make this book a valuable addition to the collection of many professionals and students.

This book was conceptualized with the vision of imparting up-to-date information and advanced data in this field. To ensure the same, a matchless editorial board was set up. Every individual on the board went through rigorous rounds of assessment to prove their worth. After which they invested a large part of their time researching and compiling the most relevant data for our readers.

The editorial board has been involved in producing this book since its inception. They have spent rigorous hours researching and exploring the diverse topics which have resulted in the successful publishing of this book. They have passed on their knowledge of decades through this book. To expedite this challenging task, the publisher supported the team at every step. A small team of assistant editors was also appointed to further simplify the editing procedure and attain best results for the readers.

Apart from the editorial board, the designing team has also invested a significant amount of their time in understanding the subject and creating the most relevant covers. They scrutinized every image to scout for the most suitable representation of the subject and create an appropriate cover for the book.

The publishing team has been an ardent support to the editorial, designing and production team. Their endless efforts to recruit the best for this project, has resulted in the accomplishment of this book. They are a veteran in the field of academics and their pool of knowledge is as vast as their experience in printing. Their expertise and guidance has proved useful at every step. Their uncompromising quality standards have made this book an exceptional effort. Their encouragement from time to time has been an inspiration for everyone.

The publisher and the editorial board hope that this book will prove to be a valuable piece of knowledge for researchers, students, practitioners and scholars across the globe.

List of Contributors

I-Yun Lee, Yin-Yin Lin, Yao-Hsu Yang, Yu-Ching Cheng and Li-Hsin Shu
Department of Chinese Medicine, Chiayi Chang Gung Memorial Hospital, No.6, W. Sec., Jiapu Rd., Puzi City, Chiayi County 613, Taiwan, Republic of China

Ching-Yuan Wu
Department of Chinese Medicine, Chiayi Chang Gung Memorial Hospital, No.6, W. Sec., Jiapu Rd., Puzi City, Chiayi County 613, Taiwan, Republic of China
School of Chinese medicine, College of Medicine, Chang Gung University, Tao-Yuan, Taiwan

Yu-Shin Lin
Department of Pharmacy, Chiayi Chang Gung Memorial Hospital, Chiayi, Taiwan

Chun-Liang Lin
Departments of Nephrology, Chiayi Chang Gung Memorial Hospital, Chiayi, Taiwan
Kidney and Diabetic Complications Research Team (KDCRT), Chiayi Chang Gung Memorial Hospital, Chiayi, Taiwan

Wei-Yu Lin
Department of Urology, Chang Gung Memorial Hospital at Chiayi, Puzi City, Taiwan
Chang Gung University of Science and Technology, Chia-Yi, Taiwan

Henrique Hesse
Department of Biochemistry and Biophysics, Butantan Institute, 1500, Vital Brasil Avenue, Sao Paulo 05503-900, Brazil

Arthur Cássio de Lima Luna and Durvanei Augusto Maria
Department of Biochemistry and Biophysics, Butantan Institute, 1500, Vital Brasil Avenue, Sao Paulo 05503-900, Brazil
Department of Medical Sciences, Medical School, University of Sao Paulo, Sao Paulo, Brazil

Greice Kelle Viegas Saraiva
Department of Biochemistry, Institute of Chemistry, University of Sao Paulo, Sao Paulo, Brazil

Gilberto Orivaldo Chierice
Department of Chemistry and Molecular Physics, University of Sao Paulo, Sao Carlos, Brazil

Yingxin Zeng, Haiming Jing and Nan Zhang
Beijing Key Laboratory of Diagnostic and Traceability Technologies for Food Poisoning, Beijing Center for Disease Prevention and Control/Beijing Center of Preventive Medicine Research, Beijing 100013, China

Shan Gao and Guojun Li
Beijing Key Laboratory of Diagnostic and Traceability Technologies for Food Poisoning, Beijing Center for Disease Prevention and Control/Beijing Center of Preventive Medicine Research, Beijing 100013, China
Beijing Key Laboratory of Environmental Toxicology, School of Public Health, Capital Medical University, Beijing 100069, China

Jing-Dong J. Han and Bo Xian
Key Laboratory of Computational Biology, CAS Center for Excellence in Molecular Cell Science, Collaborative Innovation Center for Genetics and Developmental Biology, Chinese Academy of Sciences-Max Planck Partner Institute for Computational Biology, Shanghai Institutes for Biological Sciences, Chinese Academy of Sciences, 320 Yue Yang Road, Shanghai 200031, China

Weiyang Chen
College of Information, Qilu University of Technology (Shandong Academy of Sciences), Jinan 250353, China

Matthew Flavel and Markandeya Jois
School of Life Sciences, La Trobe University, Bundoora, Vic 3083, Australia

Tosapol Anukunwithaya, Pilaslak Poo, Natthaphon Hunsakunachai and Ratchanee Rodsiri
Department of Pharmacology and Physiology, Faculty of Pharmaceutical Sciences, Chulalongkorn University, Bangkok 10330, Thailand

Phisit Khemawoot
Department of Pharmacology and Physiology, Faculty of Pharmaceutical Sciences, Chulalongkorn University, Bangkok 10330, Thailand
Preclinical Pharmacokinetics and Interspecies Scaling for Drug Development Research Unit, Chulalongkorn University, Bangkok 10330, Thailand

Suchinda Malaivijitnond
Department of Biology, Faculty of Science, Chulalongkorn University, Bangkok 10330, Thailand

Preclinical Pharmacokinetics and Interspecies Scaling for Drug Development Research Unit, Chulalongkorn University, Bangkok 10330, Thailand

M Mofizul Islam and Dennis Wollersheim
Department of Public Health, La Trobe University, Melbourne, Victoria, Australia

Ian S. McRae
Research School of Population Health, ANU College of Health and Medicine, Australian National University, Canberra, Australia

Soumya Mazumdar
Healthy People and Place Unit, Population Health, Liverpool Hospital, South West Sydney Local Health District, New South Wales Health, Sydney, New South Wales, Australia

Paul Simpson and Tony Butler
The Kirby Institute, University of New South Wales, Sydney, Australia

Kaniz Fatema
Centre for Health Equity Training, Research and Evaluation (CHETRE), Sydney, New South Wales, Australia
UNSW Sydney Research Centre for Primary Health Care and Equity, Sydney, New South Wales, Australia
Population Health, South Western Sydney Local Health District, NSW Health, Sydney, New South Wales, Australia
Ingham Institute, Liverpool, New South Wales, Australia

Tinchou Li
Division of Neurosurgery, Department of Surgery, Taipei Tzu Chi Hospital, Buddhist Tzu Chi Medical Foundation, New Taipei City, Taiwan, Republic of China
Department of Surgery, School of Medicine, Tzu Chi University, Hualien City, Taiwan, Republic of China

Mingcheng Lee, Yiyin Lin and Maoliang Chen
Department of Research, Taipei Tzu Chi Hospital, Buddhist Tzu Chi Medical Foundation, New Taipei City, Taiwan, Republic of China

Fuming Tsai
Department of Research, Taipei Tzu Chi Hospital, Buddhist Tzu Chi Medical Foundation, New Taipei City, Taiwan, Republic of China
Department of Microbiology, Soochow University, Shih Lin, Taipei City, Taiwan, Republic of China

Yunhsiang Chen
Department of Life Science, Fu Jen Catholic University, New Taipei City, Taiwan, Republic of China

Filip Caisberger and Martin Valis
Department of Neurology, University Hospital Hradec Kralove, Hradec Kralove, Czech Republic

Jaroslav Pejchal, Jan Misik and Jiri Kassa
Department of Toxicology and Military Pharmacy, Faculty of Military Health Sciences, University of Defence, Hradec Kralove, Czech Republic

Kamil Kuca
Department of Chemistry, Faculty of Science, University of Hradec Kralove, Hradec Kralove, Czech Republic
Biomedical Research Center, Uiversity Hospital Hradec Kralove, Hradec Kralove, Czech Republic

Abimbola O. Opadeyi
Department of Clinical Pharmacology and Therapeutics, University of Benin, Benin-City, Edo State, Nigeria
Department of Medicine, University of Benin Teaching Hospital, Benin-City, Nigeria

Ambrose O. Isah
Department of Clinical Pharmacology and Therapeutics, University of Benin, Benin-City, Edo State, Nigeria
Department of Medicine, University of Benin Teaching Hospital, Benin-City, Nigeria
National Drug Safety Advisory Committee, National Agency for Food and Drug Administration and Control, Federal Ministry of Health, Abuja, Nigeria

Annie Fourrier-Réglat
Inserm, Bordeaux Population Health Research Center, team, Pharmacoepidemiology, University Bordeaux, UMR 1219, F-33000 Bordeaux, France
Bordeaux PharmacoEpi, INSERM CIC1401, F-33000 Bordeaux, France
CHU de Bordeaux, Pôle de santé publique, Service de Pharmacologie médicale, F-33000 Bordeaux, France

Girish Parthan, Shobhit Bhansali, Rama Walia and Anil Bhansali
Department of Endocrinology, Post Graduate Institute of Medical Education and Research, Sector- 12, Chandigarh PIN Code-160012, India

Anura V. Kurpad and Kishor Bhat
Department of Physiology, St. John's Medical College, Bangalore, India

Chia-Ling Tsai and Mu-Chan Ke
Department of Dentistry, Kaohsiung Chang Gung Memorial Hospital and Chang Gung University College of Medicine, Kaohsiung, Taiwan

Yi-Hao Chen, Hsi-Kung Kuo, Hun-Ju Yu, Chueh-Tan Chen, Ya-Chi Tseng and Pei-Chang Wu
Department of Ophthalmology, Kaohsiung Chang Gung Memorial Hospital and Chang Gung University College of Medicine, 123, Da-Pi Road, Niao-Sung District, Kaohsiung 88301, Taiwan, Republic of China

Pei-Chin Chuang
Department of Medical Research, Kaohsiung Chang Gung Memorial Hospital, and Chang Gung University College of Medicine, Kaohsiung, Taiwan
Center for Translational Research in Biomedical Sciences, Kaohsiung Chang Gung Memorial Hospital, Kaohsiung, Taiwan

Kamil Kuca, Kamil Musilek and Eugenie Nepovimova
Biomedical Research Center, University Hospital Hradec Kralove, Hradec Kralove, Czech Republic
Department of Chemistry, Faculty of Science, University of Hradec Kralove, Hradec Kralove, Czech Republic

Daniel Jun, Jana Zdarova-Karasova, Ondrej Soukup and Martina Hrabinova
Biomedical Research Center, University Hospital Hradec Kralove, Hradec Kralove, Czech Republic
Faculty of Military Health Sciences, University of Defence, Hradec Kralove, Czech Republic

John Mikler
Defence Research and Development Canada - Suffield Research Centre, Department of National Defence, Suffield, Alberta, Canada

Tanos C. C. Franca
Center for Basic and Applied Research, Faculty of Informatics and Management, University of Hradec Kralove, Hradec Kralove, Czech Republic
Department of Chemical Engineering, Military Institute of Engineering, Rio de Janeiro, RJ 22290-270, Brazil

Teodorico C. Ramalho
Center for Basic and Applied Research, Faculty of Informatics and Management, University of Hradec Kralove, Hradec Kralove, Czech Republic
Department of Chemistry, Federal University of Lavras, Lavras/MG, Brazil

Elaine F. F. Da Cunha and Alexandre A. De Castro
Department of Chemistry, Federal University of Lavras, Lavras/MG, Brazil

Martin Valis
Neurology Clinic, University Hospital Hradec Kralove, Hradec Kralove, Czech Republic

Ying Li, Qing-Shan Chen, Jing Yu and Guo-Qing Zhang
Department of Pharmacy, Eastern Hepatobiliary Surgery Hospital, Second Military Medical University, Shanghai 200438, China

Du-Xin Sun
Department of Pharmaceutical Science, College of Pharmacy, University of Michigan, Ann Arbor, MI 48109, USA

Xiu-Liang Cui
National Center for Liver Cancer, Shanghai 201805, China
The International Cooperation Laboratory on Signal Transduction, Eastern Hepatobiliary Surgery Hospital, Shanghai 200438, China

Hai Zhang
Department of Pharmacy, Shanghai First Maternity and Infant Hospital, Tongji University School of Medicine, Shanghai 201204, China

Jie Gao
Department of Pharmaceutical Sciences, Second Military Medical University, 325 Guohe Road, Shanghai 200433, China

Yufeng Zhao, Aili Yan, Di Chen, Rong Xie, Yingguang Liu, Xiangyan Liang, Yanyan Zhao, Lanlan Wei, Xi Xu and Xingli Su
The institute of Basic Medical Sciences, Xi'an Medical University, Xi'an 710021, China

Lei Zhang
Department of Gerontological Surgery, The First Affiliated Hospital, Xi'an Medical University, Xi'an 710061, China

Jun Yu
Medical Research Center, The Second Affiliated Hospital, Xi'an Medical University, Xi'an 710038, China

Aster Desalew Kassie
Boru Meda District Hospital, South Wollo Zone, Amhara Region, Southeast, Ethiopia

Berhanu Boru Bifftu and Habtamu Sewunet Mekonnen
University of Gondar, College of Medicine and Health Science, School of Nursing, Gondar, Ethiopia

Hadi Molanaei, Abdul Rashid Qureshi, Olof Heimbürger, Bengt Lindholm, Björn Anderstam and Peter Stenvinkel
Division of Renal Medicine and Baxter Novum, Department of Clinical Science, Intervention and Technology, Karolinska Institutet, Karolinska University Hospital, SE-141 86 Stockholm, Sweden

Ulf Diczfalusy
Division of Clinical Chemistry Department of Laboratory Medicine, Karolinska Institutet, Karolinska University Hospital, Stockholm, Sweden

Leif Bertilsson
Division of Clinical Pharmacology, Department of Laboratory Medicine, |Karolinska Institutet, Karolinska University Hospital, Stockholm, Sweden

Niccolò Lombardi, Giada Crescioli, Alessandra Bettiol, Ettore Marconi, Antonio Vitiello, Roberto Bonaiuti, Ersilia Lucenteforte, Alessandro Mugelli, Lisa Giovannelli and Alfredo Vannacci
Department of Neurosciences, Psychology, Drug Research and Child Health, Section of Pharmacology and Toxicology, University of Florence, viale G. Pieraccini, 6, 50139 Florence, Italy

Anna Maria Calvani
Department of Pharmacy, Anna Meyer Children's University Hospital, viale G. Pieraccini, 24, 50139 Florence, Italy

Stefano Masi
Department of Emergency Medicine, Anna Meyer Children's University Hospital, viale G. Pieraccini, 24, 50139 Florence, Italy

Tomoki Fukuyama
Department of Molecular Biomedical Sciences, College of Veterinary Medicine, North Carolina State University, Raleigh, NC, USA

Sarah Ehling, Jenny Wilzopolski and Wolfgang Bäumer
Department of Molecular Biomedical Sciences, College of Veterinary Medicine, North Carolina State University, Raleigh, NC, USA
Institute of Pharmacology and Toxicology, Faculty of Veterinary Medicine, Freie Universität Berlin, Koserstraße 20, 14195 Berlin, Germany

Aleksandra Świderska
National Health Fund Headquarters, Warsaw, Poland

Marek Wiśniewski and Jacek Sein Anand
Department of Clinical Toxicology, Medical University of Gdansk, Kartuska 4/6, 80-104, Gdansk, Poland
Pomeranian Center of Toxicology, Gdansk, Poland

Marek Wiergowski
Department of Forensic Medicine, Medical University of Gdansk, Gdansk, Poland

Anna Krakowiak
Toxicology Department, Nofer Institute of Occupational Medicine, Lodz, Poland

Lakshay Mahajan
Division of Veterinary Pharmacology and Toxicology, Faculty of Veterinary Science and Animal Husbandry, R S Pura, Jammu 181102, India

Pawan Kumar Verma
Division of Veterinary Pharmacology and Toxicology, Faculty of Veterinary Science and Animal Husbandry, R S Pura, Jammu 181102, India

Rajinder Raina
Division of Veterinary Pharmacology and Toxicology, Faculty of Veterinary Science and Animal Husbandry, R S Pura, Jammu 181102, India

Shilpa Sood
Division of Veterinary Pathology, Faculty of Veterinary Science and Animal Husbandry, R S Pura, Jammu 181102, India

Chunlan Ji, Yueming Luo, Chuan Zou, Lihua Huang, Ruimin Tian and Zhaoyu Lu
National Key Unit of Clinical Research of TCM on Chronic Kidney Diseases, Key Unit of Kidney Diseases, Guangdong Provincial Hospital of Chinese Medicine, The Second Clinical College of Guangzhou University of Chinese Medicine, 111th Dade Road, Guangzhou 510120, People's Republic of China

Rezvan Enteshari Najafabadi and Nasrin Kazemipour
Department of Basic Sciences, School of Veterinary Medicine, Shiraz University, Shiraz, Iran

Abolghasem Esmaeili and Siamak Beheshti
Cell, Molecular Biology and Biochemistry Division, Department of Biology, Faculty of Sciences, University of Isfahan, Iran

Saeed Nazifi
Department of Clinical Science, School of Veterinary Medicine, Shiraz University, Shiraz, Iran

Maria Antonietta Maselli, Antonia Ignazzi and Annunziata Scirocco
Experimental Pharmacology Laboratory, National Institute of Gastroenterology "S. de Bellis", Research Hospital - Castellana Grotte (BA), 70013 Castellana Grotte, Italy

Francesco Pezzolla and Dionigi Lorusso
Department of Surgery, National Institute of Gastroenterology "S. de Bellis", Research Hospital - Castellana Grotte (BA), 70013 Castellana Grotte, Italy

Fabrizio De Ponti
Department of Medical and Surgical Sciences, University of Bologna, 40126 Bologna, Italy

Carola Severi
Department of Internal Medicine and Medical Specialities, University Sapienza, 00161 Rome, Italy

Amir Kazemi Korayem, Shahriar Ghamami and Zahra Bahrami
Department of Chemistry, Faculty of Science, Imam Khomeini International University, Qazvin 34148-96818, Iran

Robert J. Brosnan and Trung L. Pham
Department of Surgical and Radiological Sciences, School of Veterinary Medicine, University of California, One Shields Avenue, Davis, CA 95616, USA

Index

Dr. REENA WILFRED, Sc 'E'